Professional's Handbook of

COMPLEMENTARY
&
ALTERNATIVE
MEDICINES

SECOND EDITION

C. W. Fetrow, PharmD
Juan R. Avila, PharmD

SPRINGHOUSE
Springhouse, Pennsylvania

Staff ✍

Senior Publisher
Donna O. Carpenter

Editorial Director
William J. Kelly

Clinical Director
Marguerite S. Ambrose, RN, MSN, CS

Creative Director
Jake Smith

Art Director
Elaine Kasmer Ezrow

Drug Information Editor
Tracy Roux, RPh, PharmD

Senior Associate Editor
Ann E. Houska

Clinical Project Editor
Eileen Cassin Gallen, RN, BSN

Editor
Barbara Hodgson

Clinical Editors
Heather Rischel Burcher, RN; Margaret Friant Cramer, RN, MSN; Christine M. Damico, RN, MSN, CPNP; Nancy Laplante, RN, BSN; Lori Musolf Neri, RN, MSN, CCRN, CRNP; Kimberly A. Zalewski, RN, MSN, CEN

Copy Editors
Leslie Dworkin, Dolores Connors Matthews

Designers
Arlene Putterman (associate design director), Joseph John Clark, ON-TRAK Graphics, Inc.

Illustrator
Debra Moloshok

Typographer
Diane Paluba (manager)

Manufacturing
Patricia K. Dorshaw (manager), Otto Mezei (book production manager)

Editorial Assistants
Carol A. Caputo, Arlene P. Claffee, Beth Janae Orr

Indexer
Barbara Hodgson

Visit our Web site at eDrugInfo.com

Contents ✍

Complementary and alternative medicines

Appendices and index

About the authors ✍

C. W. Fetrow, *PharmD*, is the coordinator of Pharmacokinetics and the Outpatient Anticoagulant and Drug Evaluation Services at St. Francis Medical Center in Pittsburgh. He is a member of the American Society of Health-System Pharmacists, teaches a pharmacokinetics course at Duquesne University, and is a member of the adjunct faculty at the University of Pittsburgh, School of Pharmacy. Dr. Fetrow teaches pharmacology through the medical residency program at St. Francis, is a consultant pharmacist for nursing homes, and lectures on alternative medicines throughout the United States.

Juan R. Avila, *PharmD*, is a medical therapeutic liaison for Sanofi-Synthelabo, Inc. He has served on the faculty at the schools of pharmacy at Shenandoah University in Winchester, Va., and Duquesne University in Pittsburgh. Dr. Avila also teaches psychopharmacology as a clinical instructor at St. Francis Medical Center in Pittsburgh. He is a member of the American Association of Colleges of Pharmacy and the American Society of Health-System Pharmacists.

Acknowledgments ✎

Typically, a book of this magnitude involves many dedicated and talented people. Without the involvement of such people, we might not have completed *Professional's Handbook of Complementary & Alternative Medicines,* Second Edition, in a timely manner. We thank and express our gratitude to those who have assisted us from behind the scenes.

To our immediate families and close friends, whose emotional support and continued excitement in our work made it all the more meaningful, especially Crystal Turner-Avila, whose support has never wavered.

To our contributors (both rookies and veterans), who helped us compile these informative monographs and who, we hope, are proud to be associated with this work.

To the St. Francis Health Sciences Medical Library staff, especially David Brennan, Jackie Wire, Vi Brown, and Mary Lee Fazio, for their tireless pursuit and retrieval of difficult-to-locate journal articles.

To our seemingly endless supply of pharmacy students, who often found themselves immersed in projects at a moment's notice.

To our colleagues and coworkers, who covered for us when we needed time to work on the book.

To our friend Bill Burley, whose wealth of knowledge of plants and plant taxonomy enabled us to update and correct oversights associated with the plant portion of the herbal entries. We believe that his supervision and insight have set us far apart from other herbal medicine texts.

And to the patients, personnel, and medical staff of St. Francis Medical Center in Pittsburgh, Shenandoah University, and Sanofi-Synthelabo, whose continued encouragement and interest in our work provided the stimulus that kept us hungry for more information and a second edition.

Our special thanks to our friend and colleague, Thom Bache, RPh, director of pharmacy at St. Francis Medical Center, for the many years of patience and supervision he invested in the fledgling era of our careers; for granting us the freedom to pursue the clinical issues we found most exciting and most challenging; for often shining light on the more human aspect of the story; and finally, for more than 25 years of tireless devotion to and protection of the people and patients of St. Francis Medical Center. We dedicate this edition to Thom, in hopes that it, too, will persevere for years to come.

C. W. Fetrow, PharmD
Juan R. Avila, PharmD

Contributors and consultants

Sandra Axtell, PharmD
Clinical Coordinator
    Pharmacy Services
Kaleida Health-Millard
    Fillmore Hospital
Buffalo

Cathy L. Bartels, PharmD
Associate Professor, Director
    of Drug Information
School of Pharmacy & Allied
    Health Sciences
University of Montana
Missoula

**Jamie Brobeck-Holowka,
PharmD**
Clinical Pharmacist
University of Pittsburgh
    Medical Center Health
    System
Pittsburgh

**Mary L. Brubaker, Pa-C,
PharmD, FASHP, BCPS, BCNSP,
CHES**
Clinical Assistant Professor
Northern Arizona University
Flagstaff

Patrick Bryant, PharmD, FSCIP
Director, Drug Information
    Center
Clinical Associate Professor
School of Pharmacy
University of Missouri-
    Kansas City

William Burley
Consultant for Botanical
    Nomenclature
Seattle

Paula J. Ceh, PharmD
Assistant Professor
Butler University
Clinical Pharmacist
The Center for
    Complementary Medicine
Indianapolis

Paula H. Cippel, RPh
Pharmacist
Klingensmith's Drug Stores,
    Inc.
Ford City, Pa.

Kevin A. Clauson, PharmD
Fellow, Natural Product
    Research
University of Missouri-
    Kansas City

Umberto Conte, PharmD
Clinical Pharmacist
Mount Sinai Medical Center
New York

James C. Coons, PharmD
Staff Pharmacist
University of Virginia Health
    System
Charlottesville

Colleen M. Culley, PharmD
Drug Information Specialist
University of Pittsburgh
    Medical Center
Assistant Professor
University of Pittsburgh
    College of Pharmacy

Eric J. Culley, PharmD
D.U.R. Clinical Pharmacy
    Services Specialist
Highmark Blue Cross Blue
    Shield
Pittsburgh

Brent Ednie, MD
Internist
Indiana Hospital
Indiana, Pa.

Amy L. Gruel, PharmD
Clinical Assistant Professor,
    Drug Information
    Specialist
University of Montana
Missoula

Andrea Ho-Kean, PharmD
Drug Information/HIV
    Clinical Pharmacist
Stadtlanders/Procare
Clinical Instructor
University of Pittsburgh

**Michelle L. Holbrook, RPh,
PharmD**
Clinical Pharmacy Services
    Specialist
Highmark Blue Cross Blue
    Shield
Pittsburgh

**Pamela Hucko Koerner,
PharmD**
Clinical Pharmacist
Medicine Shoppe Pharmacy
Pittsburgh

**B.J. Komoroski, PharmD candi-
date**
University of Pittsburgh
    School of Pharmacy

Robert V. Laux, PharmD
Assistant Professor
Duquesne University
Pittsburgh
Clinical Specialist
Thomas Jefferson University
    Hospital
Philadelphia

**Mandy Leonard, PharmD,
BCPS**
Manager, Drug Information
    Service
The Cleveland Clinic
    Foundation

Bradley A. Long, MSLS
Senior Information Services
    Librarian
Scott Memorial Library
Thomas Jefferson University
Philadelphia

Scott F. Long, RPh, PhD
Assistant Professor of
    Pharmacology and
    Toxicology
School of Pharmacy
Southwestern Oklahoma
    State University
Weatherford

Lee Ann McDowell, PharmD
Clinical Pharmacy Specialist
University of Pittsburgh
    Medical Center-Passavant
Clinical Instructor
Duquesne University
University of Pittsburgh

Cydney E. McQueen, PharmD
Fellow, Natural Product
    Research
University of Missouri-
    Kansas City
School of Pharmacy
University of Missouri-
    Kansas City

Linda M. Nicolaus, PharmD
Clinical Consultant
  Pharmacist
Apothecare Collaborative
  Services, Inc.
Moon Township, Pa.

Christine K. O'Neil, PharmD
Associate Professor
Duquesne University
Clinical Pharmacist
St. Francis Medical Center
Pittsburgh

Julianne S. Orlowski, DO
Chief Resident, Internal
  Medicine
St. Francis Medical Center
Pittsburgh

Dana L. Osicki, RPh
Drug Information
  Pharmacist
The Cleveland Clinic
  Foundation

Brian N. Peters, PharmD, MS
Manager of Patient Care
  Services
Department of Pharmacy
Children's Hospital
Columbus

John P. Rose, PharmD, Pa-C
Critical Care Medicine
Upper Chesapeake Medical
  Center
Bel Air, Md.

Paul L. Schiff, Jr., PhD
Professor
School of Pharmacy
University of Pittsburgh

Douglas Slain, PharmD, BCPS
Assistant Professor
West Virginia University
Morgantown

Scott K. Stolte, PharmD
Assistant Professor
Bernard J. Dunn School of
  Pharmacy
Shenandoah University
Winchester, Va.

James A. Tjon, PharmD
Director, Drug Information
  and Pharmacoepidemiol-
  ogy Center
Assistant Professor of
  Pharmacy and Thera-
  peutics
University of Pittsburgh

David A. White, BSc, RPh
Drug Information/Restricted
  Drug Placement
The Cleveland Clinic
  Foundation

Kris M. Williams, RPh
Pharmacist Manager
Klingensmith's Drug Stores,
  Inc.
Kittanning, Pa.

Marian S. Williams, RPh
Staff Pharmacist
Armstrong County
  Memorial Hospital
Kittanning, Pa.

Maria B. Yaramus, PharmD
Clinical Specialist,
  Informatics and Research
  Coordinator
Integrative Medicine Center
University of Pittsburgh
  Medical Center–
  Pittsburgh Cancer
  Institute
Assistant Professor
University of Pittsburgh
  School of Pharmacy

Chris Ann Yeschke, RPh
Sterile Products Supervisor
St. Francis Medical Center
Pittsburgh

Foreword ✍

Prior to the publication of the first edition of *Professional's Handbook of Complementary & Alternative Medicines*, there was no reliable, comprehensive, unbiased source of information on the use of alternative medicines. The proliferation of herbs available to the public has now spawned a rapidly increasing number of scientific studies that attempt to determine whether these natural products have therapeutic usefulness. Basing their observations on scientific trials worldwide, the authors of this book have analyzed more than 300 commonly used herbs. Each monograph provides information that, because of its impartiality, lets you make appropriate decisions regarding the therapeutic use of a specific herb your patient is taking.

Undeniably, alternative medicines are here to stay. Because so many patients use herbs today, all health care professionals—nurses, physicians, and pharmacists—as well as students and everyone else involved with drug therapy for patients, need to know as much as possible about these nontraditional remedies.

By using this book, you'll be able to discern fact from myth and to answer with certainty the questions your patients may have about herbal therapy. The references and analyses provided for every entry offer insight into the therapeutic usefulness of each herb.

The authors, both widely respected and highly experienced, have pored through dozens of books, hundreds of journal articles, and thousands of pages of government documents to update this most comprehensive handbook. You won't find a more detailed, up-to-date, professional resource about herbal medicines anywhere, nor one presented with such a keen eye toward presenting the facts, rather than the folklore, about herbs.

Regardless of your field of expertise, and no matter how many patients you care for or provide services to, you'll want to keep the *Professional's Handbook of Complementary & Alternative Medicines,* Second Edition, handy—for your sake and that of your patients.

Simeon Margolis, MD, PhD
Professor of Medicine and Biological Chemistry
The Johns Hopkins University School of Medicine
Baltimore

Preface ●

In the preface to the first edition of the *Professional's Handbook of Complementary & Alternative Medicines*, we described a case of a patient referred to us because she was experiencing an adverse event and her physician could not determine the cause. After reviewing all her herbal medicines, we lamented the lack of referenced clinical information regarding many herbal products and set out to develop a useful handbook for health care providers like ourselves. The book has received positive feedback, and our belief that traditional health care providers are searching for peer-reviewed, balanced information regarding complementary and alternative medicines has been reinforced.

Since the publication of the first edition, there has been an explosion of literature regarding complementary and alternative medicines, especially herbal medicines and nutraceuticals. This increased volume of information reflects the important force that herbal medicines have become. With more research being conducted, the need for a comprehensive, easy-to-read, referenced handbook has become more important than ever for busy clinicians. Some studies are published in well-respected, peer-reviewed journals, but the sources of most of the information flooding practitioners and patients alike are manufacturers and advocacy groups. Also, most of the information is derived from animal or laboratory data or comes from small, single-site human trials that may or may not be controlled.

In this edition of the *Professional's Handbook of Complementary & Alternative Medicines*, we have continued our efforts to review innumerable studies on the most commonly used herbal and nutraceutical products and present the information as a cohesive, comprehensive, and scientifically valid reference for the health care provider. We have added a number of new products and have reviewed and updated products previously included. We also enlisted the assistance of a botanical expert experienced in plant taxonomy in an effort to keep abreast of plant nomenclature and related plant species.

One of our colleagues once told us to listen to patients in a nonjudgmental way and recognize the negative forces that propel alternative ways of thinking and the positive forces that foster self-improvement. We agree wholeheartedly with this philosophy. As health care providers, we need to reinforce the positive efforts a patient exerts in achieving wellness and at the same time gently guide that patient's enthusiasm toward therapies of proven efficacy through education. We must take care not to extinguish a patient's hope but be wary of propagating false promises. *Professional's Handbook of Complementary & Alternative Medicines*, Second Edition, will help clinicians fulfill these worthwhile goals.

We encourage the continued quest to gather scientifically valid data about alternative medicines that so many patients rely on as part of their treatment. This edition of *Professional's Handbook of Complementary & Alternative Medicines* will help you learn the facts about herbal medicines. Only then will your patients receive meaningful information that will allow them to make informed decisions with respect to their health care.

C. W. Fetrow, PharmD
Juan R. Avila, PharmD

How to use this book ✎

One of the first books of its kind written specifically for health care professionals, *Professional's Handbook of Complementary & Alternative Medicines* takes a scientific and comprehensive look at complementary and alternative medicines, focusing mainly on herbs. The book's features and format are designed to accommodate the wide-ranging needs of health care professionals seeking information about alternative medicines.

FEATURES
An introductory chapter explains the history of complementary and alternative medicines and discusses the uses, risks, and regulations of alternative versus traditional medicine. This chapter is followed by monographs on more than 300 alternative medicines organized alphabetically by generic name for quick access.

References are placed at the end of each monograph so they can be found easily. Each monograph is consistent, with clearly marked headings, so you can locate specific information quickly. Special features help enhance knowledge and skills:

• An alert symbol (✦**ALERT**) calls your attention to warnings, cautions, and other critical information about the use of the product.
• Look for the "Research findings" logo in selected entries, to read about important studies, results, and conclusions.
• A "Folklore" logo leads you to interesting background information on an alternative medicine, such as the history of its use or other herb-related facts.
• Numerous appendices providing additional information make the book even more useful.

MONOGRAPHS
Each monograph provides detailed information about the alternative medicine. A guide word at the top of each page identifies the generic name of the alternative medicine covered on that page. Each monograph is complete in itself and doesn't require flipping to other sections of the book for more information. Headings within each monograph follow this sequence: generic name, synonyms, taxonomic class (when appropriate), common trade names, common forms, source, chemical components, actions, reported uses, dosage, adverse reactions, interactions, contraindications and precautions, special considerations, points of interest (when appropriate), commentary, and references.

Synonyms
In each monograph, the generic name is followed by an alphabetized list of its synonyms.

Taxonomic class
When applicable, the taxonomic classification of the herb is given. This enables you to locate herbs that are botanically related. If the alternative medicine described is not an herb (for example, melatonin), no taxonomic class is given.

Common trade names
This section is an alphabetical list of the common trade names associated with the alternative medicine. Several commercial agents are produced by different manufacturers and may occur in combination with other agents. The mention of a trade name does not imply endorsement of that product or guarantee its legality.

Common forms
This section lists known preparations available for each agent—for instance, tablets, capsules, extracts, tinctures. Available dosage forms and standardized strengths are listed, if known.

Source
This section provides information about the source plant's botanical name and other data about the occurrence of the agent in nature.

Chemical components
This section summarizes the key chemical composition of the alternative medicine and offers data relevant to the product's reported actions.

Actions
This section describes how the alternative medicine is thought to achieve its therapeutic effects, based on in vitro, animal, and human studies. Keep in mind that an alternative medicine's action depends on the chemical components of the plant or other natural substance and their concentrations within each product.

Reported uses
This section describes anecdotal uses of the agent, based on clinical studies with humans and case reports. These uses are not meant to be recommendations but rather unproven claims of use. This section also summarizes significant results from key scientific and clinical studies.

Dosage
This section lists the routes of administration and general dosage information for each form of the alternative medicine and, where available, information about its reported use. This information has been gathered from scientific literature, anecdotal reports, and available clinical data on alternative medicines. However, not all uses have specific dosage information; often, no consensus on dosage exists. Dosage notations reflect current clinical trends and should not be considered as recommendations of the authors or publisher.

Adverse reactions
Here, categorized by body system, you'll find undesirable effects that may follow use of the alternative medicine. Some of these effects have not been reported but are theoretically possible, given the chemical composition or action of the agent.

Interactions
This section lists each agent's clinically significant interactions with other drugs or foods. The interaction is followed by the effect of the interaction

and then a specific suggestion for avoiding the interaction itself. As with adverse reactions, some interactions have not been proven but are theoretically possible. The interacting drug or food is italicized for at-a-glance review.

Contraindications and precautions
This section lists any condition, especially a disease, in which the use of the agent is undesirable, and provides recommendations for cautious use as appropriate.

Special considerations
This section offers helpful information for clinicians, such as monitoring techniques and methods of preventing and treating adverse reactions. Overdose and treatment information is included, as appropriate. Particularly important reactions and overdose information are highlighted with an Alert symbol. Patient-teaching tips that focus on educating the patient about the agent's purpose, preparation, administration, and storage are included, as are suggestions for promoting patient compliance with the therapeutic regimen and steps the patient can take to prevent or minimize the risk or severity of adverse reactions.

Points of interest
Anecdotal information, historical facts, or other relevant data about selected alternative medicines can be found in this section.

Commentary
In this section, the authors evaluate anecdotal reports and scientific literature to separate facts from myths about the alternative medicine's uses. The analysis summarizes exactly where each agent stands from a scientific point of view and offers advice about use or recommendations for further study, as appropriate.

References
This section lists key clinical studies referred to in the monograph. The authors and reviewers conducted an exhaustive review of literature from around the world—including numerous foreign publications and obscure research studies.

APPENDICES
In the book's appendices, you'll find therapeutic monitoring guidelines, potentially unsafe plants, alternative medicines to avoid during pregnancy, plant families, a resource list for alternative medicine, and an alternative medicine information sheet for patients.

INDEX
The index lists generic name, synonyms, and reported uses for each alternative medicine.

Abbreviations

ACE	angiotensin-converting enzyme
AIDS	acquired immunodeficiency syndrome
ALT	alanine aminotransferase
AST	aspartate aminotransferase
b.i.d.	twice daily
BUN	blood urea nitrogen
cAMP	cyclic 3',5' adenosine monophosphate
CBC	complete blood count
CK	creatine kinase
CNS	central nervous system
COPD	chronic obstructive pulmonary disease
CSF	cerebrospinal fluid
CV	cardiovascular
DNA	deoxyribonucleic acid
FDA	Food and Drug Administration
g	gram
G	gauge
GI	gastrointestinal
G6PD	glucose-6-phosphate dehydrogenase
H_1	histamine$_1$
H_2	histamine$_2$
HIV	human immunodeficiency virus
I.M.	intramuscular
INR	international normalized ratio
IU	international unit
I.V.	intravenous
kg	kilogram
MAO	monoamine oxidase
mcg	microgram
mg	milligram
MI	myocardial infarction
ml	milliliter
NSAID	nonsteroidal anti-inflammatory drug
PABA	para-aminobenzoic acid
P.O.	by mouth
P.R.	by rectum
PT	prothrombin time
PTT	partial thromboplastin time
q.i.d.	four times daily
RBC	red blood cell
RNA	ribonucleic acid
t.i.d.	three times daily
WBC	white blood cell

COMPLEMENTARY
&
ALTERNATIVE MEDICINES

Overview of complementary and alternative medicines

The use of complementary and alternative medicines has become a phenomenon too massive to ignore. Schools are granting doctorates in naturopathy; traditional schools of medicine, pharmacy, and nursing are offering courses in alternative medicines. Among patients who see mainstream health care providers, 33% to 42% use alternative medicine remedies. Many of these patients fail to disclose this fact to their primary health care providers. Market sales of herbs in the United States were an estimated $14 billion in 2000, and the rate of growth has increased dramatically in recent years. About 80% of the world's population uses herbs for medicinal purposes; some of this use is not by choice but rather because of a lack of traditional health care.

Despite efforts by health care providers to keep pace with an ever-growing body of factual medical evidence, to share that knowledge with patients, and to offer new, FDA-approved pharmaceuticals, devices, and procedures at an almost alarming rate, the general public still feels the need to reach out for something more. In an increasing number of instances, that something is herbal medicine.

Studies indicate that many patients who use alternative medicines and also seek conventional treatment exercise more; are more careful about avoiding fatty foods, tobacco, and alcohol; are more compliant with their regular medication regimen; and make lifestyle modifications more readily than patients who seek conventional health care alone. Consequently, today's health care providers need to know which complementary and alternative medicines are helpful, which are harmful, which are ineffective, and which lack sufficient data about safety and efficacy. An understanding of phytomedicine and its components is the first step in this education.

Phytomedicine

Phytomedicine—the practice of using plants or plant parts to achieve a therapeutic cure—has been around for at least several centuries and is in common use throughout the world. The United States is one of the last nations to embrace it.

The National Institutes of Health (NIH) estimates that in the United States, about one in three persons pursues some form of complementary or alternative medical therapy, such as herbal medicine, homeopathy, acupuncture, biofeedback, color therapy, music therapy, hypnotherapy, aromatherapy, Ayurvedic medicine, or Bach flower remedies. The use of such therapies is probably greatest in certain subgroups of the population, such as the terminally or chronically ill.

Partly in response to the popularity of alternative remedies, the NIH established the Office of Alternative Medicines to study and compile data. In other countries, similar committees, such as Commission E in Germany, have reviewed the safety and efficacy of herbs and published the results to resolve product debates.

HISTORY

Early Native Americans used plants to treat various maladies, but the practice of phytomedicine fell out of favor over the years and for generations has remained largely outside the realm of contemporary American medical practice. Germany, certain Asian countries, Italy, Spain, the Netherlands, and Belgium have taken a more aggressive approach.

Herbal medicine in Germany

Germany markets about 700 therapeutic herbs. About 70% of German health care providers prescribe phytopharmaceuticals to their patients. Furthermore, Commission E, a branch of the German government similar to the FDA, has compiled monographs for more than 300 herbs that discuss their safety and efficacy.

Herbal medicine in the United States

Despite a slow start, the commercial herbal industry in the United States is booming. More than 750 herbs are now marketed here. Mass marketing and media blitzes aimed at health food stores, supermarkets, and retail pharmacies have prompted rapid growth in the sales of herbal supplements.

Public access to these products, along with limited regulation, has led to tremendous growth. Herbs and dietary supplements can be purchased in malls, pharmacies, grocery stores, and convenience stores, as well as through mail-order catalogs, wholesalers, and the Internet. This unlimited and unrestricted access to herbal products will most likely continue; herbal manufacturers will flourish; and attempts at regulation or standardization of the industry will prove only marginally effective.

PHARMACOGNOSY

The study of chemicals from natural sources for their medicinal application is *pharmacognosy.* Although it usually refers to the study of chemical entities in higher plants such as bushes, shrubs, and trees and in components of lower plants such as fungi, molds, and yeasts, land and marine animals, fish, and insects can also serve as potential medicinal agents.

About 250,000 species of flowering plants exist in the world today. Only a small percentage of these have been adequately studied for pharmacologic activity. Many more valuable agents may lie waiting to be discovered in plants yet to be screened for therapeutic applications.

Determining the species of plant to pursue for pharmacologic activity is often difficult, especially with so many plants to explore. Anecdotal reports of therapeutic efficacy and local medical folklore are usually seen as effective ways to identify potentially therapeutic plant components.

Manufacturing an herb

In most industrialized nations, crude drugs—defined as natural substances collected and dried before manufacturing—are seldom used as chief therapeutic agents. More commonly, certain components of the plant are identified, removed, modified, and applied therapeutically in a consistent manner.

Many plants can be grown in climates that resemble the plant's native land. Compatibility of the plant to a particular region and the cost of harvesting the plant in that same area determine the availability of crude drugs. National and international restrictions on the collection of wild plants limit availability of plant resources and drive up the cost of production. These factors force countries to specialize in producing only certain types of phytomedicinal resources.

Despite the tendency for a country to produce only certain resources, the quality of crude drugs is often questionable. By the time a crude drug arrives at a manufacturing center, it has been subjected to adulteration, deterioration, or contamination. Deliberate adulteration most commonly occurs with expensive natural substances or natural substances that are in short supply.

Cultivating specific plants ensures a reliable source of the plant with less risk of adulteration. The age of the plant can dramatically affect the quality and concentration of active plant constituents, as can environmental conditions such as temperature, rainfall, length of daylight, altitude, atmosphere, and soil.

Before drying the plant, insect- or disease-infested plant parts and unwanted materials (dirt, debris, unnecessary components) are removed. The process should be repeated before packaging and storage.

Drying can last anywhere from a few hours to a few weeks, depending on the relative humidity of the local climate and the physical nature of the plant components. Drying by artificial heat (hot water pipes, stoves, belt dryers) carries the advantage of shorter drying times. Veterans of the process have learned when to halt the drying phase to prevent plant parts from becoming too brittle and dried out.

Deterioration of the dried product can occur when it is exposed to moisture in the surrounding air (usually about 10% to 15%) and sunlight. Some processes introduce sterilization as a way to minimize microbial contamination. Proper storage and preservation must take place to ensure quality of the product until delivery to the manufacturing facility, where the crude drug undergoes various grinding, crushing, extraction, or distillation processes before being transformed into an herbal pharmaceutical.

Standards of quality for herbal medicines

Official standards are critical for ensuring the quality of herbal products. Such standards are not well established or well recognized in the United States, much less anywhere else in the world. On the forefront of strengthening official standards, outside the United States, lies the European Scientific Cooperative for Phytotherapy, a committee composed of manufacturers of herbal medicines and herbal associations working with European research groups.

As far as standards within the United States are concerned, in 1995 the United States Pharmacopeia (USP) commissioned an advisory panel on natural products whose mission was to establish standards and develop information concerning herbal and dietary supplements. Supplemental monographs created by this endeavor address various issues associated with the standardization of individual herbs. The following list of section headings outlines the information found in each monograph:

1. Title: identifies the most commonly accepted name of the entity.
2. Definition: describes plant parts used, genus, species, authority, and family of botanical.
3. Packaging and storage: cites appropriate packaging and storage conditions designed to promote integrity of the product.
4. Labeling: states requirements for label nomenclature.
5. Reference standards: identifies appropriate reference standards.
6. Botanic characteristics: describes visible and microscopic shape and structure characteristics of whole plant or plant parts.
7. Identification: describes pharmacognostic tests used to identify the entity.
8. Total ash: sets limits for amount of inorganic residue remaining after incineration of plant.
9. Acid-insoluble ash: sets limits for amount of foreign inorganic residue remaining after boiling the total ash with $3N$ hydrochloric acid (an indication of how much dirt and soil remain in the sample).
10. Water-soluble ash: sets limits for the residue remaining after boiling the total ash with water.
11. Foreign organic matter: limits amount of non–drug-containing matter.
12. Loss on drying: sets criteria for loss limits of water, volatile oils, and other volatile chemical compounds.
13. Water content: limits variation in water content of dried botanicals.
14. Alcohol-soluble or water-soluble extractives: sets thresholds for minimum acceptable amount of aqueous-, alcohol-, or aqueous alcohol-soluble extractives.
15. Volatile oil: describes the quantity of volatile oil present in botanical.
16. Heavy metals: limits quantity of heavy metals present in botanical.
17. Pesticide residue: sets strict limits on pesticide content.
18. Microbial limits: sets limits on total bacteria and mold count.
19. Marker substances and content tests: establishes standards for quantitative chemical analysis of botanical for the presence of certain marker substances that aid in proper identification.

Other agencies and organizations have begun to develop standards within this industry. In 1997, an ad-hoc advisory board for the FDA proposed the development of a special working group to develop industry standards for good manufacturing practices (GMPs) of dietary supplements. Work began in 1998 and continues as a voluntary program followed by a few manufacturers.

The National Nutritional Foods Association (NNFA) is a U.S.-based organization of representatives from several thousand manufacturers, retailers, suppliers, and distributors of natural products, health foods, and dietary supplements. The NNFA offers a type of accreditation program to its members that includes inspections of member manufacturing facilities to determine whether they meet NNFA-specified standards of GMPs. Once accredited by the NNFA, a manufacturer is entitled to display the seal of the NNFA on its products. The NNFA seal began to appear on some dietary supplement products as early as 1999. In 1990, the NNFA initiated the TruLabel program, which randomly evaluates some portion of more than 25,000 dietary supplement products registered with the organization to assure that the product contents are the same as those indicated on the label. Aside from their role as a key lobbying force for passage of the Dietary Supplement Health and Education Act and having representation within the FDA's special working group, the NNFA has submitted guidelines for GMPs to the FDA.

Despite these attempts to provide consistency in a rapidly growing marketplace, few laws exist that govern manufacturer adherence or deviation from policies and guidelines developed by these agencies.

Regulating the herbal industry

A major contention of herbal medicine advocates is the notion that because herbal medicines are natural products, they are somehow safer or more effective. The majority of alternative medicine products are essentially unregulated and are not yet required to demonstrate safety, efficacy, or quality in the same manner as prescription medicines before becoming commercially available.

EARLY ATTEMPTS AT REGULATION

The first attempt by the U.S. government to regulate any medicine—herbal or traditional—was the Food and Drugs Act of 1906, which prohibited the adulteration and misbranding of drugs. The act focused on the quality of products being marketed and did not address the safety and efficacy of the medicines themselves. The Food and Drugs Act arose from public pressure imposed on the government after a series of fraudulent incidents involving patent medicine manufacturers and meat-packing firms.

It was not until the late 1930s that the issue of product safety was finally addressed. The FDA had been established by Congress in 1928 but had been given little authority and even less guidance about how to proceed. In 1937, a newly marketed product, elixir of sulfanilamide, was found to be toxic and contributed to the deaths of more than 100 persons. This tragedy became the impetus for the passage of the Federal Food, Drug, and Cosmetic Act the next year, which mandated that all drugs sold in the United States be proved safe before being marketed.

Only the issue of product efficacy remained unregulated. That changed in 1962, when senators Kefauver and Harris amended the Federal Food, Drug, and Cosmetic Act to require that any drug originating after 1962 be proved both safe and effective before reaching the marketplace.

CURRENT REGULATIONS

In the United States, debate continues about what role the FDA should play in regulating and approving alternative medicines. The FDA regulates the pharmaceutical industry by requiring manufacturers of new products to file a New Drug Application, which must detail scientifically sound laboratory and clinical trials that demonstrate a drug product's safety and efficacy. Because these trials can be expensive, the pharmaceutical industry tends to focus on entities that it can patent, which excludes naturally occurring products, such as plants and other alternative medicines.

Products approved before 1962 that showed evidence of safety but lacked evidence of efficacy were "grandfathered in" and allowed to stay on the shelf as long as their manufacturers made no claims of the agents' efficacy. In the late 1980s, the FDA decided to examine these grandfathered drugs and commissioned a study of OTC drugs, including many herbal products. Evidence of a few herbal products supported claims of safety and efficacy, but most were deemed unsafe or ineffective. In some cases, insufficient data were available to evaluate the agents' efficacy. Although the FDA lists many herbs as safe, herbal manufacturers cannot legally claim therapeutic efficacy of their products without evidence to support the claim.

As the popularity of alternative medicines continued to grow, it became clear that some manufacturers in the herbal industry were trying to circumvent the intent of the Federal Food, Drug, and Cosmetic Act. Despite the fact that the manufacturers of herbal medicines could not put therapeutic claims directly on the container or label, many pamphlets, books, and advertisements for the product were available on request or within arm's reach from where the product sat on the shelf. As this practice became more prevalent, the FDA began to intervene, which led to political confrontations between the two sides. The climax of this huge debate yielded the Dietary Supplement, Health, and Education Act of October 1994. The act defined herbal products as neither food nor drugs but something called dietary supplements and protected them from regulation as food additives or as drugs unless the product's labeling contained therapeutic claims of efficacy. The term *dietary supplement* refers not only to herbal medicines derived from plants but also to chemical entities commonly known as nutraceuticals. *Nutraceuticals* are typically endogenous compounds found within cells or tissues of humans or mammals or structurally related to chemicals found within the body. Usually, the specific purpose, function, or metabolic pathway of these entities in the body is incompletely understood.

For all dietary supplements introduced before October 1994, the burden of proof to demonstrate safety was now in the hands of the FDA, not the manufacturer. The act stipulates that all products introduced after that date must be proved safe by the manufacturer. Also, information regarding therapeutic claims for herbal products can be disseminated into the marketplace as long as the information is neither misleading nor product-specific and is physically separated from the product and without product stickers affixed to it.

Since 1994, a few changes have occurred. In 1997, the FDA published additional clarifications for claims herbal manufacturers were permitted to make. As before, no dietary supplement manufacturer could claim efficacy for any disease on the label, but structure or function claims were allowed. For example, the manufacturer of a cranberry dietary supplement could not claim on the package label that "ingestion of cranberry treats urinary tract infections." But the manufacturer could claim that "ingestion of cranberry supports normal, healthy function of the urinary tract," a typical structure or function claim.

In 1999, the FDA mandated that manufacturers include a "Supplement Facts" panel on the dietary supplement's package label. Warnings to manufacturers designed to regulate any claims made with respect to pregnant women have also emerged from the office of the FDA.

Herbal use and traditional medicine

Health care providers should look closely at the risks and benefits of herbal medicines, just as they do at the risks and benefits of traditional therapies.

SUPPORTING HERBAL USE

Proponents of herbal medicine cite three main reasons for supporting the use of herbal rather than traditional medicines.

An estimated 25% of today's relied-on, contemporary pharmaceuticals have originated in part or entirely from naturally occurring chemicals from plants. Advocates of herbal therapy rely heavily on this fact as support for herbal pharmaceuticals. Herbal constituents or their derivatives have provided therapeutic agents for cancer, constipation, edema, heart failure, hypercoagulable states, inflammation, pain, tissue congestion, and many other conditions. Well-known therapeutic agents derived from herbal sources include capsaicin (red pepper plant), pilocarpine (jaborandi tree), taxol (Pacific yew tree), and warfarin (sweet clover). Examination of these constituents provides a compelling argument for the clinical application of future herbal agents.

Herbal medicine has been around for centuries and is said to be valuable because the philosophies and practices of herbal medicine have not perished. No one knows for certain when or where the first attempt at using a plant to effect a therapeutic cure was made. Some references suggest that Neanderthal man might have been one of the first phytomedicine practitioners. Ancient Middle Easterners appear to have been the first to rigorously document the use of plants for various diseases, compiling the first known pharmacopoeia, titled *Materia Medica.* The Greek historian Herodotus recounted how Egyptians worshiped certain plants, believing that some herbs held the secret to a healthy life and longevity. Not to be outdone by the Egyptians, the Greeks also incorporated various plants and flowers into several aspects of Greek mythology.

Plant use and herb worship have become as diverse and intertwined as the branches of a tree. The overwhelming majority of lay literature directed toward the consumer freely endorses the use of herbal medicines. Various advocacy texts cite anecdotal accounts of so-called cures to promote uses for the plants. There is no lack of legends, folklore, or anecdotal stories to support any herbalist's suggestions. Occasionally, these stories of success with herbs have taken on almost mythical or supernatural proportions.

RISKS

As with modern, tested pharmaceuticals, herbal medicines have some risk associated with their use. The fact that a plant is completely natural does not necessarily make the use of agents derived from that plant risk-free. Several plants, when consumed in their most natural form, can cause grave illness or even death in humans and animals. Many of these plants are routinely avoided by herbalists, scientists, and the general public because of their risks. Hundreds of herbs and alternative medicines exist, most of which have not been studied adequately, particularly in relation to their toxicology.

Adverse reactions to herbal medicines can be directly related to exposure to one or more chemical components of the plant or to an inappropriate or incorrect manufacturing process during the preparation of a dietary or herbal supplement. Laws do not require that adverse effects of dietary supplements be reported to the FDA, but many have been documented. A review of adverse effects reported in the medical literature between 1992 and 1996 highlights cases of hypersensitivity reactions, hepatotoxic reactions, and renal damage associated with various herbal products. One of the more infamous adverse events was associated with the amino acid L-tryptophan, touted for its ability to reduce pain and promote sleep. During the late 1980s, it was discovered that tablet fillers contained in a few L-tryptophan products caused the rare but reportedly fatal eosinophilia-myalgia syndrome.

Dietary supplements and weight-loss products containing ephedra alkaloids raised public concern because of a number of adverse effects, such as increased blood pressure, tremors, arrhythmias, seizures, strokes, heart attacks, and death. These effects were documented in several hundred incident reports sent to the FDA between 1993 and 1997.

A study designed to assess the prevalence of herbal product use and its associated morbidity in an adult asthmatic population found an increase in the number of hospitalizations for patients who used herbs and black coffee or tea. A large retrospective study of admissions to a Taiwanese hospital found that 4% of admissions were related to herbal drug use, ranking herbal medicines third among drug categories most responsible for adverse effects.

Inadequate or inappropriate dissemination of information to the public, combined with weak regulation, can lead unwary consumers to use herbal medicines that can cause dangerous adverse reactions. Manufacturers of dietary supplements and herbal drugs spend millions of dollars each year on advertising their products. Existing regulations for product labeling of herbal supplements fail to provide ample warning of risks to consumers. Many advertisements could be considered misleading or at least of questionable accuracy, despite FDA restrictions to limit manufacturers' claims to those that relate only to proper health maintenance.

The Internet has a huge potential for increasing the use of herbal products. If the marketing information of alternative medicines is left unreviewed by government agencies, dangerous consequences may result. Herbal products otherwise unobtainable in the United States have been purchased over the Internet and have been associated with substantial morbidity.

HERBAL REGULATIONS

Dietary supplement and herbal medicine manufacturers are generally not required to comply with the same standards and regulations that apply to major pharmaceutical companies. As a result, the public can face significant dangers related to herbal medicine use.

In the spring of 1998, for instance, the FDA issued a warning regarding an herbal medicine named Sleeping Buddha. Apparently, the product contained an unlabeled sedative, the benzodiazepine estazolam. Fortunately, no adverse effects from this product were reported. At this same time, the FDA issued another warning regarding an herb called plantain, a plant that contains digitalis-like glycosides. Consumption of the herb by geriatric patients or patients with heart disease could cause subsequent cardiac problems. Potential dangers of this sort fall into the category of "extrinsic misadventures." These are usually related to a lack of standardization or to contamination, adulteration, or substitution of the products. They may also be related to a misidentification or misbranding.

The quantity of pharmacologically active chemical components of many plants can vary considerably, depending on the time of year during harvest, age of the plant, or method of pollination. Other variables include the amount of water given to the plants, wind, inclement weather, and soil condition.

Consumers may be exposed to various compounds when herbal supplements are ingested. Manufacturers do not always separate active chemical ingredients of the plant. As a result, patients may ingest many chemicals that occur naturally in the plant, along with the reportedly active constituents.

Several published reports of chemical analysis of products taken off the health food store shelf and then evaluated demonstrate the need for standardization in the industry. These reports have routinely shown that product reliability is in question. Some reports demonstrate that products are contaminated with heavy metals, such as lead, mercury, or even arsenic. Other studies reveal the persistence of herbicides and pesticides in some products. Case reports after injuries find that herbal manufacturers have adulterated products with other known anxiolytic drugs such as diazepam or added analgesics such as mefenamic acid, phenylbutazone, or aspirin. Other contaminants, including caffeine, theophylline, diuretics, corticosteroids, and atropine, have been discovered in reportedly pure herbal products. Interestingly, one study evaluating the ingredients of 44 feverfew products, an herbal product touted to treat migraine headaches, found that 22% of the products tested had no active feverfew in the dosage form. Another study found that one-third of the 24 ginseng products were devoid of any active ginseng component.

Additional concerns arise from the notable lack of product stability and bioavailability testing. These data are usually not available on the label or anywhere else.

LACK OF CONSENSUS

An overwhelming lack of consensus exists about the therapeutic use of herbal medicine. Recommended dosages vary considerably among sources, even among noted advocates in the field. No standards exist for monitoring adverse effects or efficacy.

The time a person spends evaluating his response to an herbal supplement could be spent seeking professional medical advice and using proven pharmacotherapy. In cases of severe depression or other severe mental illnesses or in a patient with a life-threatening disease, a delay in seeking professional help could prove the difference between life and death.

ABUSES

Unlike their prescription-only counterparts, herbal medicines can be purchased and consumed freely by virtually anyone. Purchases and use can take place without forethought or advice, without restriction or limitation, without even something as seemingly insignificant as confirming a person's age. In stark contrast, a person is required to be a certain age before purchasing cigarettes or alcohol. People who want to purchase these chemicals must demonstrate proof of the minimum age requirement by displaying a valid driver's license. In general, such identification is required of minors because society believes they are not mature enough and perhaps lack sufficient education to handle the potential dangers and responsibilities that accompany the use of chemicals that can intoxicate, addict, and cause physiologic damage.

Herbal medicines are not without the potential for abuse, the potential to harm, and, in some cases, the potential to addict or intoxicate. Perhaps similar legislation should be passed to require consumers who want to purchase certain herbal agents to provide some kind of identification before such a purchase can be made.

Among many cultures, traditional healers and religious leaders have used psychoactive plants as part of their rituals, yet the perception remains that plants are safe and pose no danger of abuse or dependence. Many plants may have been safely used for hundreds of years in controlled settings, such as religious rituals, but when used indiscriminately by the general public, the use of these plants can lead to problems.

The leaves of the coca shrub, for instance, have been chewed by the Incas and their descendants for countless generations to help them work in the high altitudes of the Andes. The anxiolytic kava has been used in Polynesia for hundreds of years without reported adverse consequences; it is now known that the drug increases the effects of alcohol. By itself, kava can lead to intoxicating effects. Kava users continue to consume the agent even after they develop adverse effects, such as the skin reactions that can occur from chronic use.

The abuse potential of a drug may not be identified immediately; most often, it is identified after one or more controlled clinical trials. Herbal products do not have to undergo rigorous trials before being marketed, so problems can be identified only after many people experience a particular adverse effect, such as dependence.

Cost

Although herbal medicines are less expensive than their FDA-labeled counterparts, the hidden cost of herbs can be substantial. The cost of delayed effective therapy, treatment of adverse effects and drug interactions, and subsequent hospital admissions adds significantly to the cost of using ineffective herbal remedies in place of more effective traditional therapy. As herbal medicine becomes more popular and as herbal medicine manufacturers spend increasing amounts of their profit on advertising, the cost of herbs, in many cases, has begun to exceed the cost of traditional allopathic medicines by a significant margin.

Educating patients about herbal use

A stepwise approach to patient counseling allows health care providers to carefully broach the subject of alternative therapies with their patients. Patients who are prescribed traditional medications deserve and are routinely given specific advice about the drugs they are receiving. Patients who use herbal or alternative medicines should receive comparable advice.

All patients should be reminded to disclose all medications they take, alternative or otherwise. Health care providers should routinely include herbal medicines when asking about the patient's drug use and explain that full information about current medications is needed to help prevent or solve problems related to adverse effects or drug interactions. If it does not pose a great inconvenience for the patient, he should be asked to bring his medications with him to the health care provider's office. In the event of an adverse reaction, having the containers at hand could provide valuable data about chemical content, brand names, manufacturer names, frequency of dosage, and other important information.

The patient should be told that alternative medicines may be beneficial as well as harmful and that herbal medicines may interact adversely with the patient's existing medications or adversely affect the patient's disease. Using herbs may also lead to significant delays in the time it takes for the patient to enter the mainstream health care system and receive more appropriate and effective therapy for his condition.

Every patient should be aware of the quality of alternative products and the frequent lack of scientific evidence about herbs as compared with more traditional agents. It may be especially relevant to discuss the quality of products produced in the alternative industry versus that of the modern pharmaceutical industry or to offer comparisons between products for both industries with respect to cost, frequency of dosage, and potential adverse effects.

Patients should be instructed to watch for unusual signs or symptoms while taking any medicine but particularly alternative medicines. These symptoms may represent significant adverse reactions to the herbal medicines or drug interactions between an herbal and a traditional medicine.

Realistic and appropriate therapeutic goals should be discussed with each patient. If patients are unwilling to consider traditional pharmaceuticals, they should at least agree to monitor their goals of therapy along with the health care provider. If, after a sufficient trial of alternative medicine, these goals have not been achieved, the health care provider may be able to persuade the patient to return to more appropriate conventional pharmacotherapy.

Future of herbal medicine

Herbal medicine has evolved distinctly, isolated from the mainstream of modern medicine. The lack of available medical literature and clinical documentation makes it seem as though the growth of herbal medicine has occurred in some parallel universe. Precedent suggests that it may be foolish to ignore promising chemical constituents in the herbal compendium.

Experts in pharmacognosy suggest that only a small percentage of Earth's plants have been thoroughly investigated for their pharmacologic activity. An estimated 25% of traditional medicines are derived from plants. Many dominant pharmaceutical companies appear to have forgotten this fertile reservoir of unique chemical entities and instead concentrate on revisions or spin-offs of existing successful agents and new compounds in biotechnology. Profitable sales success stories in the dietary supplement marketplace have encouraged a few pharmaceutical companies to take on manufacturing their own line of popular dietary supplements, despite the lack of patent protection. Simultaneously, a veritable explosion of new information and clinical research regarding dietary supplement products has hit the medical literature because of the public's increasing and undaunting interest in these therapies. The potential for new and uniquely valuable entities derived from this group of agents is exciting, but the time-tested and labor-intensive process of investigation and development of any new pharmaceutical entity should not fall short of determining its risk-versus-benefit profile. Enthusiasm for these products should be tempered with the fact that adequate information regarding safety and efficacy is needed before health care providers—or patients, for that matter—can make intelligent, informed decisions about their own health care.

ACIDOPHILUS

ACIDOPHILUS MILK, *LACTOBACILLUS ACIDOPHILUS*,
PROBIOTICS, YOGURT

Common trade names
Bacid, DDS-Acidophilus, Florajen Acidophilus Extra Strength, Kyo-Dophilus, Lactinex (mixed culture of *Lactobacillus acidophilus* and *Lactobacillus bulgaricus*), MoreDophilus, Probiata, Pro-Bionate, Superdophilus

Common forms
Available in various dosages, in cultures ranging from 500 million to 4 billion viable organisms of *L. acidophilus,* in capsules, granules, powders, softgels, suppositories, and tablets as well as in milk and yogurt.

Source
L. acidophilus is usually commercially prepared as concentrated, dried, viable cultures. The cultures can be found in varying quantities in many dairy products, especially milk and yogurt.

Chemical components
L. acidophilus and other *Lactobacillus* species (*L. bulgaricus, L. catenaforme, L. fermentum, L. jensenii,* and *L. minutus*) are anaerobic, gram-positive, nonsporulating bacilli that typically inhabit the vagina and GI tract of mammals. There is some evidence that *L. acidophilus* may produce a compound that improves its ability to survive in environments that contain competing bacteria. Although usually nonpathogenic, lactobacilli have been implicated as possible causes of some infections.

Actions
L. acidophilus may aid digestion and absorption of food nutrients and produce B complex vitamins and vitamin K. The bacterium normally resides in the GI tract with about 400 other species of bacteria and yeasts. It helps to maintain a balance of bacterial diversity and prevent the overgrowth of any single species. As part of the normal GI flora, *L. acidophilus* inhibits the growth of other organisms by competing for nutrients, altering the pH of the environment, or producing bacteriocins, such as hydrogen peroxide, lactic acid, and acetic acid.

Some exogenous antibacterial compounds produced by *L. acidophilus* affect interferon production. Others may exert antibacterial activity against *Helicobacter pylori* and other intestinal bacteria.

Human studies have shown that the ingestion of *L. acidophilus* reduces the concentration of certain fecal enzymes that promote the formation of carcinogens in the colon. It is not known whether or not this reduction influences the prevalence of colon cancer.

Reported uses

Acidophilus cultures are commonly used to prevent or treat uncomplicated diarrhea caused by antimicrobials that disrupt normal intestinal flora. These cultures are also claimed to be useful in patients with diverticulitis, *H. pylori*–induced gastric ulcers, infectious diarrhea, irritable bowel syndrome, or ulcerative colitis, but evidence to support these claims is lacking.

Acidophilus may be useful in the prevention and treatment of bacterial vaginosis and vaginal yeast infections caused by *Candida albicans*. Clinical trials have been inconclusive (Fredricsson et al., 1989).

Limited evidence suggests that acidophilus may offer relief to patients with fever blisters, hives, canker sores, and acne, but these skin conditions are largely self-limiting and study results are inconclusive.

Attempts to document a cholesterol-lowering effect for acidophilus products in humans have proved unsuccessful.

Dosage

Dosage is based on the number of live organisms in a commercial acidophilus culture.

For most reported uses, 1 to 10 billion viable organisms/day in divided doses t.i.d. or q.i.d. is cited as a reasonable regimen.

Adverse reactions

GI: flatulence.

Interactions

Warfarin: May enhance intestinal production and absorption of vitamin K, decreasing warfarin's efficacy. Monitor appropriately.

Contraindications and precautions

Lactose-sensitive patients may find it difficult to tolerate dairy products that contain acidophilus cultures.

Special considerations

• To be effective, acidophilus products must provide viable *L. acidophilus* organisms that can survive the hostile environment of the GI tract. Proper manufacturing techniques, packaging, and storage are needed to ensure viability. Some manufacturers require refrigeration of their products, depending on which subspecies is used for the parent cultures.

• Inform the patient that some dairy sources of acidophilus, particularly yogurt and milk, may not contain viable cultures because of dramatic temperature fluctuations during transport.

• Advise the patient that the FDA does not consider acidophilus products safe and effective for use as antidiarrheals.

• Tell the patient to expect some flatus, at least initially. This reaction subsides with continued use.

Bold italic type indicates that reaction may be life-threatening.

Points of interest
● Many acidophilus products contain questionable levels of *L. acidophilus* as well as other bacterial species of uncertain benefit.
● Significant variations in potency and stability have been observed.
● Products made by the same company but having different lot numbers have produced conflicting results in clinical trials.

Commentary
Data supporting the use of *L. acidophilus*–containing products for their antidiarrheal benefits and for maintaining normal levels of intestinal and vaginal bacteria and yeasts stem mainly from in vitro studies and theoretical evidence. Clinical trials in humans have not yielded many positive results. To further complicate the issue, variability of the quality of acidophilus cultures ingested might have influenced these results. Standardization of these products must be accomplished before conducting studies that evaluate their efficacy for therapeutic use.

References
Fredricsson, B., et al. "Bacterial Vaginosis Is Not a Simple Ecological Disorder," *Gynecol Obstet Invest* 28:156, 1989.

ACONITE

FRIAR'S CAP, HELMET FLOWER, MONKSHOOD, SOLDIER'S CAP, WOLFSBANE

Taxonomic class
Ranunculaceae

Common trade names
No commercially prepared products are available in the United States.

Common forms
Available as a liniment, tea, or tincture.

Source
Active components are obtained from leaves, flowers, and roots of *Aconitum napellus*. An erect perennial herb with tuberous roots, aconite is native to mountainous regions in Europe, Japan, China, India, and North America.

Chemical components
Aconite contains the alkaloids aconine, aconitine, napelline, picraconitine, and others responsible for the plant's primary toxicities. Potency depends on the plant's alkaloid content, which varies with the season and the altitude at which the plant is cultivated. The leaves and roots usually have the highest alkaloid content.

Other components found in the plant include malonic acid, succinic acid, itaconic acid, aconitic acid, sugars, starches, fats, and resin.

Actions
Aconite's action is primarily cardiotoxic because of its effect on the inward sodium channels. It prolongs cardiac repolarization, and as a result, various arrhythmias—primarily ventricular—can occur.

In one study, aconite (0.6 mg/kg) administered intraperitoneally to a rabbit damaged the myelin sheath of the visceral pathway, spinal cord, and peripheral nerves (Kim et al., 1991). Because the drug can be absorbed through the skin, picking the flowers or other parts of the *A. napellus* plant can cause toxicity.

Reported uses
The first reported therapeutic use of aconite in the United States was in tincture preparations in the 1800s. It was believed to be useful for treating fever, headache, inflammation, and neuralgia. Few sources now promote this plant for therapeutic use because of its potential for serious toxicity. In some countries, aconite is incorporated into topical liniments that are claimed to create congestion in local blood vessels and subsequent redness of the skin.

Some literature suggests using aconite in the treatment of hypertension.

Animal models suggest that aconite possesses antibacterial, antifungal, and antitumor activity, but these effects have not been demonstrated in humans.

Dosage
No forms of this plant are recommended for human consumption.

Adverse reactions
CNS: paresthesia, weakness.
CV: *arrhythmias (ventricular tachycardia), bradycardia.*
EENT: blurred vision, mydriasis, numbness of the oral mucosa, increased salivation, *throat tightness.*
GI: diarrhea, nausea, vomiting.
Metabolic: *acidosis,* hypokalemia.
Other: *death.*

Interactions
Antiarrhythmics, antihypertensives, beta blockers, calcium channel blockers, diuretics: May increase toxicity. Avoid administration with aconite.

Contraindications and precautions
Aconite is contraindicated for all conditions, especially in patients with arrhythmias, CV disease, or hemodynamic instability; in those with known hypersensitivity to the plants; and in those who are pregnant or breast-feeding.

Special considerations
▲ **ALERT** Ventricular tachycardia may occur. Aconite-induced arrhythmias are usually unresponsive to traditional antiarrhythmics, cardioversion, and pacing. In most cases, bypass machines were used until the ar-

rhythmia resolved on its own or death occurred (Fitzpatrick et al., 1994; Tai et al., 1992).

ALERT Death has resulted from as little as 5 ml of aconite tincture, 2 mg of pure aconite, 1 g of crude plant parts, or 6 g of cured aconite; no known antidote exists.

• Instruct the patient to avoid consuming any part of the plant.

• Inform the patient that aconite should remain in the garden. The plant should be handled only with gloves that retard absorption of plant oils through the skin.

Points of interest

• Aconite extract has been implicated in numerous suicides and was once used as a poison for arrows (Fatovich, 1992).

• The results of feline studies indicate that atropine may antagonize cardiac depressive and hypersalivation effects related to aconite. Human data are inconclusive.

Commentary

Case reports and available clinical information about aconite toxicity and fatalities clearly illustrate the danger of this herb (But et al., 1994). Aconite has no therapeutic value and poses a grave danger to patients who use it even in small quantities.

References

But, P., et al. "Three Fatal Cases of Herbal Aconite Poisoning," *Vet Hum Toxicol* 36:212-15, 1994.

Fatovich, D. "Aconite: A Lethal Chinese Herb," *Ann Emerg Med* 21:309-11, 1992.

Fitzpatrick, A.J., et al. "Aconite Poisoning Management with a Ventricular Assist Device," *Anesth Intens Care* 22:714-17, 1994.

Kim, S.H., et al. "Myelo-Optic Neuropathy Caused by Aconite in Rabbit Model," *Jpn J Ophthalmol* 35:417, 1991.

Tai, Y., et al. "Cardiotoxicity After Accidental Herb-Induced Aconite Poisoning," *Lancet* 340:1254-56, 1992.

AGAR

AGAR-AGAR, CHINESE GELATIN, COLLE DU JAPON, E406, GELOSE, JAPANESE GELATIN, JAPANESE ISINGLASS, LAYOR CARANG, VEGETABLE GELATIN

Common trade names

Multi-ingredient preparations: Agarbil, Agoral, Agoral Plain, Demosvelte-N, Falqui, Lexat, Paragar, Pseudophage

Common forms

Available as a dry powder and in flakes and strips.

Source

Agar is an aqueous extract from the cell walls of various species of red algae, including *Gelidium cartilagineum* and *Gracilaria confervoides*.

Chemical components

Agar is composed primarily of the calcium salt of a sulfuric acid ester of the complex polysaccharide agarose-agropectin. The powdered form is soluble in boiling water. The resultant solution gels when cool, even at concentrations as low as 5%.

Actions

The pharmacokinetics of agar have not been well studied in humans. Poorly absorbed from the GI tract, agar promotes fecal bulk and may influence absorption of dietary minerals, proteins, and fat.

In one study, five patients were placed on a high-fiber diet (agar-agar) for 5 days. During that time, protein and fat digestibility was markedly decreased and fecal excretion of cholesterol increased (Kaneko et al., 1986).

In animal studies, rats fed 10% agar-agar experienced reduced absorption of calcium, iron, zinc, copper, chromium, and cobalt. A notable increase in fecal dry matter indicated that agar was not absorbed (Harmuth-Hoene et al., 1980; Kondo et al., 1996). The results of other animal studies show that agar decreases protein digestibility and reduces nitrogen retention (Harmuth-Hoene, 1976; Harmuth-Hoene et al., 1979). These effects may result from partial breakdown of agar by intestinal flora and a resultant inhibition of proteolytic enzymes.

Reported uses

Agar has long been used as a culture medium in bacteriology. It is also used as an emulsifying and suspending agent in many pharmaceutical and food products. Agar was formerly used frequently as a bulk-forming laxative. It has been found to be less effective than phototherapy and phenobarbital in the treatment of neonatal hyperbilirubinemia (Vales et al., 1990).

Dosage

As a bulk-forming laxative, 4 to 16 g P.O. once daily or b.i.d.

Adverse reactions

GI: bowel obstruction, esophageal obstruction.
Metabolic: decreased absorption of vitamins, minerals, and nutrients (especially calcium, iron, zinc, copper, chromium, and cobalt).
Respiratory: *aspiration* (when administered with insufficient liquids).

Interactions

Alcohol: Dehydration and precipitation of agar from solutions. Avoid use with agar.
Electrolyte solutions: Partial dehydration and decreased viscosity of agar solutions. Avoid use with agar.
Tannic acid: Precipitation of agar from solutions. Avoid use with agar.

Bold italic type indicates that reaction may be life-threatening.

Contraindications and precautions
Agar is contraindicated in patients with impaired consciousness (because of aspiration risk) and in pregnant or breast-feeding patients. Use cautiously in patients with a history of esophageal or bowel obstruction, throat problems, or difficulty swallowing.

Special considerations
• Bowel and esophageal obstruction are potential risks. Instruct the patient to take this herb with plenty of water (at least 8 oz) to minimize the risk of obstructions and aspiration.

• Advise the patient to report abdominal pain; chest pain, tightness, or pressure; difficulty swallowing or breathing; or vomiting to his health care provider.

• Inform the patient that products containing agar should be taken on an empty stomach to minimize the risk of decreased absorption of vitamins and minerals.

• Advise the patient to anticipate a change in the bulk and appearance of stools. If appropriate, offer a stool softener to patients who might have difficulty tolerating increased fecal bulk.

Commentary
Because no long-term human studies have assessed agar's effects on mineral and nutrient absorption and because more effective agents, such as psyllium, are available, products that contain agar should not be routinely used to treat constipation.

References
Harmuth-Hoene, A.E. "The Effect of Non-protein Food Constituents on the Nutritive Value of Radiation-Sterilized Casein," *Int J Vitam Nutr Res* 46:348-55, 1976.

Harmuth-Hoene, A.E., et al. "Effect of Dietary Fiber on Mineral Absorption in Growing Rats," *J Nutr* 110:1774-84, 1980.

Harmuth-Hoene, A.E., et al. "Effect of Indigestible Polysaccharides on Protein Digestibility and Nitrogen Retention in Growing Rats," *Nutr Metab* 23:399-407, 1979.

Kaneko, K., et al. "Effect of Fiber on Protein, Fat and Calcium Digestibility and Fecal Cholesterol Excretion," *J Nutr Sci Vitaminol* 32:317-25, 1986.

Kondo, H., et al. "Influence of Dietary Fiber on the Bioavailability of Zinc in Rats," *Biomed Environ Sci* 9:204-08, 1996.

Vales, T.N., et al. "Pharmacologic Approaches to the Prevention and Treatment of Neonatal Hyperbilirubinemia," *Clin Perinatol* 17:245-73, 1990.

AGRIMONY

CHURCH STEEPLES, COCKLEBURR, LIVERWORT,
PHILANTHROPOS, STICKLEWORT, STICKWORT

Taxonomic class
Rosaceae

Common trade names
Potter's Piletabs (England)

Common forms
Available as tablets and teas.

Source
The leaves, stems, and flowers of the dried herb
Agrimonia eupatoria are used to make compresses,
gargles, and teas. Agrimony commonly grows in the
Western United States, Europe, and Asia.

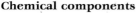

Chemical components
Active elements in agrimony include agrimonolide, ascorbic acid, an essential oil, flavonoids (luteolin and apigenin), polysaccharides, silicic
acid, tannins (ellagitannins and trace gallotannins), urosolic acid, and
vitamins B_1 and K. The seeds contain linoleic, linolenic, and oleic acids.

Actions
Anecdotal reference to stringent and mild antiseptic properties are
reported. In one animal study, agrimony extracts decreased the
blood glucose level and slowed the rate of weight loss in mice with
streptozocin-induced diabetes (Swanston-Flatt et al., 1990).

Reported uses
Agrimony is claimed to be useful for many purposes, such as diarrhea,
mucositis, pharyngitis, and other inflammatory conditions, but human
clinical trials involving agrimony are lacking. (See *Agrimony: Fact and
fiction.*)

Dosage
Little is known about doses of agrimony for any reported use. One
source suggests adding 2 to 4 tsp of dried leaves per cup of water to
make a tea that can be taken once daily. Other sources suggest using agrimony in a poultice applied topically to treat sores.

Adverse reactions
Skin: photosensitivity.
Other: *hypersensitivity reactions.*

Interactions
None reported.

Bold italic type indicates that reaction may be life-threatening.

FOLKLORE
Agrimony: Fact and fiction

Numerous claims for agrimony have been made over the centuries. The Greeks supposedly used agrimony to treat eye problems. Anglo-Saxons referred to the herb as *garclive* and apparently used it for wounds. In combination with mugwort and vinegar, agrimony was reportedly used for back pain.

Agrimony is regarded by some herbalists as a popular pre-event gargle for speakers and singers to soothe their throats and make them supple. Other claims include the herb's use as an antiasthmatic, antitumorigenic, cardiotonic, coagulant, decongestant, diuretic, and sedative, as well as a remedy for gallbladder problems and a topical agent for corns and warts.

One early herbal remedy for internal bleeding involved swallowing a mixture of agrimony, human blood, and pulverized frog parts.

Contraindications and precautions
Agrimony is contraindicated in patients with a history of hypersensitivity to plants in the rose family and in pregnant or breast-feeding patients.

Special considerations
• Monitor the patient for dermatologic reactions, especially if agrimony is being applied topically.
• Inform the patient that little scientific data about this herb exist. Although no known chemical interactions have been reported, consideration must be given to the pharmacologic properties of the herbal product and the potential for interference with the intended therapeutic effect of conventional drugs.
• Caution the patient to avoid strong sunlight; agrimony may predispose patients to sunburn.

Points of interest
• Agrimony has been used as a dye. It is pale yellow in September and deep yellow later in the year.

Commentary
This plant is not recommended for medicinal use because little is known about its safety and efficacy.

References
Swanston-Flatt, S.K., et al. "Traditional Plant Treatments for Diabetes: Studies in Normal and Streptozotocin Diabetic Mice," *Diabetologia* 33:462-64, 1990.

ALFALFA

BUFFALO HERB, LUCERNE, MEDICAGO, *MEDICAGO SATIVA*,
PURPLE MEDICK

Taxonomic class
Fabaceae

Common trade names
None available.

Common forms
Available in capsules (374 mg, 380 mg, 550 mg), dried herb, liquid extract,
powder (350 mg), and tablets (44 mg, 50 mg, 60 mg, 100 mg, 500 mg).

Source
This legume grows throughout the world under widely varying conditions. The whole plant is used medicinally.

Chemical components
Various acids (lauric acid, malic acid, maleic acid, oxalic acid, myristic
acid, palmitic acid, and quinic acid), alkaloids (pyrrolidine-type [stachydrine, homostachydrine] and pyridine-type [trigonelline]), and
amino acids (arginine, asparagine, canavanine, cysteine, histadine, isoleucine, leucine, lysine, methionine, phenylalanine, threonine, tryptophan, and valine) exist in alfalfa. A coumarin (medicagol), isoflavonoids
(coumestrol, biochanin A, daidzein, formononetin, and genistein), saponins (arabinose, galactose, glucuronic acid, glucose, rhamnose, and
xylose), steroids (campesterol, cycloartenol, beta-sitosterol, alphaspinasterol, and stigmasterol), carbohydrates, vitamins (A, B_1, B_6, B_{12},
C, E, K), calcium, carotene, magnesium, potassium, protein, minerals,
and trace elements are also found in the plant.

Actions
Alfalfa leaves and stems contain saponins that have been reported to
decrease the plasma cholesterol level without changing the HDL level.
Other, unidentified components in alfalfa decrease intestinal absorption
of cholesterol and increase the excretion of neuronal steroids and bile
acids. In one study, the plasma cholesterol level declined by 20% and
HDL-LDL ratio improved by 40% (Malinow et al., 1979).

The manganese content of alfalfa produces a hypoglycemic effect. The
results of a study using mice in whom diabetes had been induced that
were fed alfalfa demonstrated a proportional increase in insulin secretion from pancreatic beta cells of the mice (Gray and Flatt, 1997). These
results support the insulin-releasing and insulin-like activities of alfalfa.

Alfalfa root saponins exhibit toxicity toward *Candida* species, *Geotrichum candidum, Rhodotorula gluinis* yeasts, and *Torulopsis* species.
The medicago component has also been effective against yeasts.

The isoflavonoids biochanin A, coumestrol, daidzein, and genistein
possess estrogenic properties.

Bold italic type indicates that reaction may be life-threatening.

L-Canavanine is similar structurally to arginine. This component, found mainly in alfalfa sprouts, binds to arginine-dependent enzymes, which alters the intercellular calcium level as well as the ability of some T- and B-cell lines to regulate antibody synthesis. In two patients, this reaction has reactivated systemic lupus erythematosus (SLE). In animal studies, the reaction provoked pancytopenia and reduced serum complement levels.

An investigation into alfalfa's effect on hepatic drug-metabolizing enzymes in rats showed that alfalfa potentiated the activity of aminopyrine N-demethylase. This enzyme is responsible for some methylation reactions associated with phase II liver detoxification.

Reported uses

Alfalfa is a great source of vitamins A, C, E, and K as well as calcium, iron, phosphorus, and potassium. Patients with hypercholesterolemia have reportedly used alfalfa in conjunction with other treatments. Anecdotally, postmenopausal women have used this herb to alleviate hot flashes.

Dosage

Dried herb: 5 to 10 g P.O. or as an infusion t.i.d.
Liquid extract (1:1 in 25% alcohol): 5 to 10 ml P.O. t.i.d.

Adverse reactions

Hematologic: blood dyscrasias.
Metabolic: hypoglycemia.
Skin: photosensitivity.
Other: *lupuslike reactions.*

Interactions

Anticoagulants: May potentiate activity and increase risk of bleeding because of coumarin content in plant. Avoid use with alfalfa.
Chlorpromazine: Drug-induced photosensitivity. Advise patient to take precautions.
Hormonal therapies (oral contraceptives and replacement therapies): Estrogenic effects may alter pharmacologic activity. Avoid use with alfalfa.
Hypoglycemic drugs: May potentiate hypoglycemic events. Monitor blood glucose level.
Insulin: Increases risk of hypoglycemic events. Monitor blood glucose level.
Vitamin E: Potentiates alfalfa. Avoid use with alfalfa.
Vitamin K: Reverses effects of warfarin. It is not known whether the plant's coumarin content or vitamin K will predominate on warfarin.

Contraindications and precautions

Alfalfa is contraindicated in patients with SLE and in those receiving anticoagulation or hormone therapy. Avoid its use in women who are pregnant or breast-feeding.

Special considerations
• Advise the patient to consult his health care provider before using herbal preparations because a treatment that has been clinically researched and proved effective may be available.
• Inform the patient receiving hormonal therapy that alfalfa's potential interactions with other drugs are unknown. More frequent monitoring of blood glucose levels and coagulation may be needed.
🖢 ALERT Caution the patient about the potential for lupuslike reactions.
• Instruct the patient to report unusual symptoms, such as bleeding, breast tenderness, dizziness, and hot flashes, promptly to his health care provider.

Commentary
Alfalfa might emerge as an adjunctive therapy for hypercholesterolemia and diabetes. Considerably more study is needed before it is possible to visualize a role in the treatment of either of these or other disorders. Notably, this herb might effect significant therapeutic consequences when used with other drugs because of its ability to enhance hepatic metabolism and potentiate the effects of anticoagulants and hypoglycemics.

References
Gray, A.M., and Flatt, P.R. "Pancreatic and Extra-pancreatic Effects of the Traditional Anti-diabetic Plant, *Medicago sativa (lucerne)*," *Br J Nutr* 78(2):325-34, 1997.
Malinow, M.R., et al. "Comparative Effect of Alfalfa Saponins and Alfalfa Fiber on Cholesterol Absorption in Rats," *Am J Clin Nutr* 32(9):1810-12, 1979.

ALLSPICE

CLOVE PEPPER, JAMAICA PEPPER, PIMENTA, PIMENTO

Taxonomic class
Myrtaceae

Common trade names
None known.

Common forms
Fluidextract: essential oil
Pimento water (aqua pimentae): contains oil of pimento, 1 fl oz
Powdered fruit: 10 to 30 grains
    Available as a condiment in various commercial preparations.

Source
Active chemicals are derived from the dried, unripened berries of a tree (*Pimenta dioica* or *Eugenia pimenta*) native to Central America, Mexico, and the West Indies.

Chemical components
The active components of allspice include eugenol, caryophyllene, and methyleugenol in a volatile oil. Other components include glycosides,

---

gum, minerals, quercetin, resin, sesquiterpenes, sugar, tannin, and vitamins (A, C, niacin, riboflavin, thiamine). The volatile oil can be obtained through distillation of the fruit. The rind of the berries is thought to lead to the greatest medicinal activity.

Actions

Several in vitro studies of allspice provide evidence of antibacterial and antifungal activity (Hitokoto et al., 1980; Moleyar and Narasimham, 1992; Nadal et al., 1973). It is also claimed to act as a GI stimulant and an antiflatulent.

Limited data are available on the pharmacokinetic actions of the active ingredients. Two metabolites have been identified: homomandelic acid and homovanillic acid.

In animal models, about 1% of the active ingredient eugenol is demethylated. It causes CNS depression, inhibits prostaglandin activity in human colonic tissue, and increases the activity of certain digestive enzymes, including trypsin, a protein-digesting enzyme. Eugenol's antioxidant properties have been reproduced in a few in vitro studies. Despite this effect, some data suggest that eugenol may promote cancer growth (Oya et al., 1997).

Pimentol, derived from methanol extract of allspice, acts as a hydroxyl radical scavenger in in vitro models.

In animal studies, ethanolic and aqueous extracts administered I.V. to rats caused analgesia, CNS depression, dose-related hypotension, and hypothermia (Suarez et al., 1997).

Reported uses

The essential oil derived from the allspice berry has been claimed to be therapeutically useful in treating flatulence and indigestion in traditional medicine, but there is little or no data to support these claims.

Other unsupported claims of therapeutic usefulness include treatment of colds, diabetes, diarrhea, fatigue, hysterical paroxysms, and menstrual cramps. No human clinical trials are reported in the literature.

Crushed allspice berries have been applied topically to treat bruises and soothe sore joints and muscles. The anesthetic properties of eugenol may be the rationale for this application. Indeed, eugenol is used by dentists as a local anesthetic and antiseptic for teeth and gums.

Dosage

As a vehicle for purgative medicines, 1 to 2 fl oz (5 parts bruised pimento to 200 parts water, distilled down to 100 parts).

For flatulence, 2 or 3 gtt of allspice oil on sugar.

For indigestion, 1 to 2 tsp of allspice powder per cup of water, up to 3 cups daily.

For muscle pain, allspice powder may be mixed with enough water to make a paste to be applied topically.

For toothache pain, 1 or 2 gtt of allspice oil may be applied to painful area. Do not administer more often than q.i.d.

Adverse reactions
CNS: seizures (with excessive use).
GI: gastroenteritis, nausea, vomiting.
Skin: contact dermatitis.

Interactions
Iron and other minerals: Interference with absorption of minerals. Avoid using together.

Contraindications and precautions
Allspice is contraindicated in patients with chronic GI disorders, such as diverticulitis, diverticulosis, duodenal ulcers, reflux disease, spastic colitis, and ulcerative colitis. It is also contraindicated in patients with cancer or those who are at high risk for cancer. Avoid its use in pregnant or breast-feeding patients.

Special considerations
• Monitor the patient using allspice topically for hypersensitivity reactions.
• Inform the patient that eugenol may pose an undetermined potential risk of cancer.
• Advise the patient that some sources recommend that allspice consumption should be limited to an amount normally contained in foods as a condiment.
⬌ **ALERT** Caution the patient that seizures may result with excessive use.

Points of interest
• Allspice is commonly used as an aromatic spice in foods and to provide flavor in toothpaste and other products. The FDA considers it safe for external use.

Commentary
Except for a few in vitro and animal studies and human toxicology case reports, data supporting the use of allspice for any of its alleged therapeutic uses are limited. Most of the information available is found in the lay literature, not peer-reviewed journals. Allspice and eugenol have been widely used in foods, dental products, and other pharmaceuticals and can be considered safe for consumption in small quantities. Controlled clinical trials are needed to explore historical therapeutic claims.

References
Hitokoto, H., et al. "Inhibitory Effects of Spices on Growth and Toxin Production of Toxigenic Fungi," *Appl Environ Microbiol* 39:818-22, 1980.

Kanerva, L., et al. "Occupational Allergic Contact Dermatitis from Spices," *Contact Dermatitis* 35:157-62, 1996.

Moleyar, V., and Narasimham, P. "Antibacterial Activity of Essential Oil Components," *Int J Food Microbiol* 16:337-42, 1992.

Nadal, N., et al. "Antimicrobial Properties of Bay and Other Phenolic Essential Oils," *Cosmet Perum* 88:37-38, 1973.

Oya, T., et al. "Spice Constituents Scavenging Free Radical and Inhibiting Pentosidine Formation in a Model System," *Biosci Biotechnol Biochem* 61:263-66, 1997.

Bold italic type indicates that reaction may be life-threatening.

Suarez, U.A., et al. "Cardiovascular Effects of Thanolica and Aqueous Extracts of *Pimenta dioica* in Sprague-Dawley Rats," *J Ethnopharmacol* 5:107-11, 1997.

ALOE

ALOE BARBADENSIS, ALOE VERA, BARBADOS ALOE, BURN PLANT, CAPE ALOE, CURACAO ALOE, ELEPHANT'S GALL, FIRST-AID PLANT, HSIANG-DAN, LILY OF THE DESERT, LU-HUI, MEDICINE PLANT, MIRACLE PLANT, PLANT OF IMMORTALITY, SOCOTRINE ALOE, VENEZUELA ALOE, ZANZIBAR ALOE

Taxonomic class
Asphodelaceae or Liliaceae

Common trade names
Multi-ingredient preparations: All Natural Aloe Vera Gel, AloeCeuticals Snow and Sun Sunburn Spray (Lip Balm, Gel), Aloe Flex Orthopedic Cream, Aloe Grande, Aloe Life, Aloe Shield (Soft Gel Capsules), Aloe Vera Gel, Aloe Vera Inner Leaf Capsules, Aloe Vera Jelly, Aloe Vera Juice, Aloe Vera Ointment, Aloe Vesta Perineal, Benzoin Compound Tincture, Carrasyn Gel Wound Dressing, Dermaide Aloe, Whole Leaf Aloe Vera Juice

Common forms
Capsules: 75 mg, 100 mg, 200 mg aloe vera extract or aloe vera powder
Gel: 98%, 99.5%, 99.6% aloe vera gel
Juice: 99.6%, 99.7% aloe vera juice
   Also available as cream, hair conditioner, jelly, juice, liniment, lotion, ointment, shampoo, skin cream, soap, and sunscreen as well as in facial tissues.

Source
Aloe gel is obtained from the center parenchymatous tissues of the large bladelike leaves of *Aloe vera* (also referred to as *Aloe barbadensis, Aloe vulgaris* hybrids, *Aloe africana, Aloe ferox, Aloe perryi,* and *Aloe spicata*). Orally ingested preparations are composed of either the colorless juice from secretory cells located just below the leaf epidermis or a solid yellow latex obtained by evaporating the juice.
   Commercial products are available as topical and oral preparations. Topical preparations contain a colorless mucilaginous gel called aloe gel or aloe vera gel. Sometimes this gel is erroneously called aloe juice. Aloe gel is prepared by various methods, with variable consistencies and stability, although fresh gel from the plant may be preferred.

Chemical components
The chemical composition of aloe varies, depending on the species and the environmental growing conditions. The juice and latex contain hydroanthraquinone derivatives (10-C-D-glucosyl diastereoisomers of aloe-emodin anthrone), including anthraquinone glycosides aloin A

and B (formerly known as barbaloin and isobarbaloin, respectively). A reddish black glistening residue known as aloin (a mixture of aloin A and aloin B) is produced when the latex is filtered and dried.

Aloe gel, in contrast, is mostly water. Other gel compounds include bradykininase, a serine carboxypeptidase, magnesium lactate, organic acids, steroids, sugars, vitamins, and the polysaccharides acemannan and glucomannan. Because mechanical separation of gel from latex is not always complete, aloe gel may accidentally contain anthraquinone glycosides from the latex.

Actions

When taken internally, aloin is cleaved by intestinal bacteria and produces a metabolite that irritates the large intestines and stimulates colonic motility, propulsion, and transit time. In addition, aloin causes active secretion of fluids and electrolytes in the lumen and inhibits reabsorption of fluids from the colon. These actions produce a feeling of distention and increase peristalsis. The cathartic effect occurs 8 to 12 hours after ingestion.

When used externally, besides acting as a moisturizer on burns and other wounds, aloe reduces inflammation, possibly by blocking production of thromboxane A_2, inactivating bradykinin, inhibiting prostaglandin A_2, and inhibiting oxidation of arachidonic acid.

Aloe's antipruritic effect may result from blockage of the conversion of histidine to histamine as a result of the inhibition of histidine decarboxylase. Wound healing is believed to result from increased blood flow to the wounded area.

Some in vitro studies have demonstrated that aloe juice and aloe gel preparations inhibit the growth of bacteria and fungi commonly isolated from wounds and burns (Grindlay and Reynolds, 1986). Other studies have found inconsistent activity in this regard. Conflicting results may be due to variable content of the aloe preparations and deterioration of some of the active compounds. Because the identification and stability of the active components are unknown, the clinical relevance of claims of antibacterial and antifungal effects remains unknown.

In vitro and murine studies suggest that aloe-emodin may hold some promise as a useful entity for treating neuroectodermal tumors because of its unique cytotoxicity profile (Pecere et al., 2000).

Reported uses

Therapeutic claims center on aloe's use externally as a topical gel for cuts, frostbite, minor burns, skin irritation, sunburn, and other dermal wounds and abrasions. Numerous studies have validated these claims by demonstrating that topical application of aloe gel decreases acute inflammation, promotes wound healing, reduces pain, and exerts an antipruritic effect (Heggers et al., 1987).

Internally, the dried latex has been claimed to be useful as a stimulant laxative. Other claims for use of aloe include amenorrhea, asthma, bleeding, colds, seizures, and ulcers. No medical evidence supports the clinical application of aloe for these conditions.

Bold italic type indicates that reaction may be life-threatening.

Aloe preparations have also been considered for use in the treatment of acne, AIDS, arthritis, asthma, blindness, bursitis, cancer, colitis, depression, diabetes, glaucoma, hemorrhoids, multiple sclerosis, peptic ulcers, and varicose veins. Few, if any, well-controlled clinical trials substantiate the use of aloe for any of these disorders.

One controlled trial comparing a gel formulation of aloe, allantoin, and silicon dioxide failed to show a significant clinical benefit for the therapy of recurrent oral aphthous ulcers (Garnick et al., 1998). Another trial failed to find benefit of an acemannan hydrogel dressing derived from aloe vera over that of moist saline gauze for the treatment of pressure ulcers (Thomas et al., 1998).

Although several significant criticisms of the study can be made, one preliminary trial suggests a potential benefit for the combination of aloe tincture (1 ml P.O. b.i.d.) and melatonin (20 mg/day) in the therapy of patients with advanced solid tumors (Lissoni et al., 1998).

Dosage
For burns, pruritus, skin irritation, and other wounds (external forms), aloe may be applied liberally as needed. Although internal use is not recommended, some sources suggest 100 to 200 mg of aloe or 50 to 100 mg of aloe extract P.O., taken in the evening. Information about dosages for aloe juice is lacking.

Adverse reactions
GI: *damage to intestinal mucosa (may be irreversible),* harmless brown discoloration of intestinal mucosa (with frequent use), painful intestinal spasms, severe hemorrhagic diarrhea.
GU: kidney damage, red discoloration of urine (with frequent use).
Hematologic: *accumulation of blood in pelvic region* (with large doses).
Metabolic: fluid and electrolyte loss from frequent use, hypokalemia.
Skin: contact dermatitis, delayed wound healing because of reduced oxygen permeability (topical forms).
Other: *spontaneous abortion* or premature birth (during the third trimester of pregnancy).

Interactions
Antiarrhythmics, cardiac glycosides, loop diuretics, other potassium-wasting drugs, corticosteroids, thiazides: Increased effects of these drugs when aloe is used internally. Avoid internal use of aloe.

Contraindications and precautions
External aloe preparations are contraindicated in patients known to be hypersensitive to aloe or in those with a history of allergic reactions to plants in the Liliaceae family (garlic, onions, and tulips). Internal use is contraindicated in pregnant or breast-feeding patients, during menstruation, in children, and in patients with renal or cardiac disease (because of the potential for hypokalemia and, possibly, disturbance of cardiac rhythm).

Special considerations

ALERT Inform the patient that oral use can cause severe abdominal discomfort and serious hypokalemia and other electrolyte imbalance.

ALERT Unapproved use of aloe vera injections for cancer has been associated with the death of four patients (Anon., 1998). Use of injectable aloe vera preparations or chemical constituents of aloe vera is not recommended.

ALERT Reflex stimulation of uterine musculature may cause spontaneous abortion or premature birth during the third trimester of pregnancy.

ALERT Overdose may result in severe hemorrhagic diarrhea, kidney damage and, possibly, death.

• Caution the patient against the internal use of aloe vera gel and aloe vera juice.

Commentary

Aloe has a long history of popular use, and topical application is generally considered safe. The FDA does not recommend aloe for any specific condition. Fresh aloe may be useful for the treatment of burns and minor tissue injury, but studies are not well documented. Because aloe laxatives that contain anthraquinone produce dramatic cathartic effects, less toxic laxatives should be used. Few studies support the use of aloe juice for internal consumption. Although a recent in vitro study found that aloe-emodin exerts genotoxic activity (Muller et al., 1996), further research is needed regarding its use as an anticancer agent.

References

Anon. "License Revoked for Aloe Vera Use," *Nat Med Law* 1:1-2, 1998.

Garnick, J.J., et al. "Effectiveness of a Medicament Containing Silicon Dioxide, Aloe and Allantoin," *Oral Surg Oral Med Oral Pathol Oral Radiol Endod* 86(5):550-56, 1998.

Grindlay, D., and Reynolds, T. "The Aloe Vera Phenomenon: A Review of the Properties and Modern Uses of the Leaf Parenchyma Gel," *J Ethnopharmacol* 16:117-51, 1986.

Heggers, J.P., et al. "Beneficial Effects of Aloe in Wound Healing," *Phytotherapy Res* 7:S48-S52, 1987.

Lissoni, P., et al. "Biotherapy with the Pineal Immunomodulating Hormone Melatonin Versus Melatonin Plus Aloe Vera in Untreatable Advanced Solid Neoplasms," *Nat Immun* 16(1):27-33, 1998.

Muller, S.O., et al. "Genotoxicity of the Laxative Drug Components Emodin, Aloe-Emodin, and Danthron in Mammalian Cells: Topoisomerase II-Mediated," *Mutat Res* 371:165-73, 1996.

Pecere, T., et al. "Aloe-emodin Is a New Type of Anticancer Agent with Selective Activity Against Neuroectodermal Tumors," *Cancer Res* 60(11):2800-4, 2000.

Thomas, D.R., et al. "Acemannan Hydrogel Dressing Versus Saline Dressing for Pressure Ulcers. A Randomized Controlled Trial," *Adv Wound Care* 11(6):273-76,1998.

Bold italic type indicates that reaction may be life-threatening.

AMERICAN CRANESBILL

ALUM BLOOM, ALUM ROOT, AMERICAN KINO, CHOCOLATE FLOWER, CROWFOOT, DOVE'S-FOOT, *GERANIUM ROBERTIANUM*, HERB ROBERT, OLD MAID'S NIGHTCAP, SHAMEFACE, SPOTTED CRANESBILL, STINKING CRANESBILL, STORKSBILL, WILD CRANESBILL, WILD GERANIUM

Taxonomic class
Geraniaceae

Common trade names
None known.

Common forms
Available as decoctions, extracts, poultices, teas, and tinctures.

Source
Forms for internal use are prepared using the dried rhizome and leaves of *Geranium maculatum,* a perennial herb found commonly in the Eastern United States and Canada. Topical preparations are usually created using flowers of the plant.

Chemical components
Tannin, which is hydrolyzed to gallic acid, is the principal active ingredient of American cranesbill. It occurs in high concentrations in the dried rhizomes of *G. maculatum.*

Actions
Precise mechanisms of action have not been adequately described in primary medical literature.

Reported uses
Internal use of the extract has been claimed to be useful for cancer, cholera, diarrhea, dysentery, inflammation of the bladder or lip, leukorrhea, menorrhagia, metrorrhagia, plague, and renal bleeding and as a contraceptive.

Claims for external use include burns, hemorrhoids, sores, sore throat, and stomatitis. Modern medical literature has not justified these claims. One in vitro study found no antibacterial activity of American cranesbill against organisms that cause cholera (Guevara et al., 1994).

Dosage
Decoction: 1 or 2 tsp of rhizome in 1 cup of water P.O. t.i.d.
Infusion: 1 oz of plant material in 1 pt of water P.O.
Tincture: 2 to 4 ml P.O. t.i.d.

Adverse reactions
Hepatic: *hepatotoxicity* (with high tannin concentrations).

Interactions
None reported.

Contraindications and precautions

American cranesbill is contraindicated in pregnant or breast-feeding patients.

Special considerations

• Although no known chemical interactions have been reported, consideration must be given to the pharmacologic properties of the herbal product and the potential for interference with the intended therapeutic effect of conventional drugs.

• Caution the patient not to self-treat symptoms before appropriate medical evaluation because this may delay diagnosis of a potentially serious medical condition.

• Advise the patient to avoid consuming American cranesbill because not enough is known about its effects.

• Advise the patient who wants to use this herb to report unusual symptoms to his health care provider.

• Monitor the patient's liver function test results.

Commentary

Because safety and efficacy data of American cranesbill are unavailable, its use should be avoided.

References

Guevara, J.M., et al., "The In Vitro Action of Plants on *Vibrio cholerae*," *Rev Gastroenterol Peru* 14:27-31, 1994. Abstract.

ANDROSTENEDIONE

4-ANDROSTENE-3,17-DIONE

Common trade names

Androstenedione, Androsurge, Andro 100, Andro 250.

Multi-ingredient preparations: Andro-Max (with 300 mg of *Tribulus terrestris*), AndroPlex 700, Androstat, AndroStat Poppers, AndrosteDERM (Percutaneous Gel Matrix), 19-NorAndro 250, 19-Nor 3-Andro, NorAndro Blend, and TriAndroBlend

Common forms

Available in various dosages ranging from 50 to 300 mg as capsules or tablets, percutaneous gel, and sublingual spray.

Source

Androstenedione is produced in small quantities by mammalian adrenal glands and gonads. Subsequently, it is found in small quantities in dietary animal meats.

Chemical components

Androstenedione, an anabolic steroid, is an important precursor for androgens and estrogens. It is endogenously synthesized from DHEA in the adrenal cortex. Although men and women appear to handle androstenedione differently, 5% to 6% of circulating androstenedione is

---

Bold italic type indicates that reaction may be life-threatening.

metabolized by the liver into testosterone, a potent androgenic steroid (MacDonald et al., 1979). Androstenedione release is probably mediated by way of beta-adrenergic stimulation. A significant percentage of an androstenedione dose is aromatized into estradiol and estrone (King et al., 1999). As with testosterone, androstenedione production reaches a plateau by ages 25 to 30 and steadily declines after age 40.

Actions

Androstenedione is a potent anabolic steroid with weak androgenic properties that are about equivalent to 10% to 20% that of testosterone (Nelson, 1980). Anabolic effects typical of this class of steroid include anticatabolism and increased skeletal muscle mass and aggressiveness.

Androstenedione has been shown to significantly reduce (12%) serum HDL levels (King et al., 1999). Systemic bioavailability of orally administered androstenedione is considered poor because of a possible hepatic first-pass effect. This possibility has been suggested because of low rates (1.8%) of conversion to testosterone after oral doses compared with I.V. doses (5.9%; Horton and Tait, 1966). Single oral doses of androstenedione have increased serum androstenedione levels by 175% to 350%.

Reported uses

Because of its close association with testosterone, androstenedione is touted as an ergogenic agent. Androstenedione supplementation is promoted as a "legal steroid" to increase strength and muscle mass, speed recovery of muscles, increase energy and sexual arousal, and enhance well-being. Studies have produced varying results with respect to androstenedione's ability to increase serum testosterone levels. With regard to androstenedione supplementation, no clinical trial has proved an anabolic effect for androstenedione. Studies have attempted to demonstrate one or more of the following: an increase in lean body mass, a reduction in fat body mass, an anabolic effect on muscle or muscle metabolism, or an increase in strength. None of the effects was considered superior to those seen in the placebo group.

Dosage

Dosages vary considerably. Most studies have used 100 to 300 mg P.O. administered once daily or in divided doses b.i.d.

Adverse reactions

CNS: aggressive behavior (with supplementation of some anabolic steroids).
GU: gynecomastia.
Hepatic: elevated liver function test results (with supplementation of some anabolic steroids).
Musculoskeletal: muscle catabolism (Rasmussen et al., 2000).
Other: hirsutism (females), suppression of endogenous testosterone secretion (controversial).

Interactions

None reported. However, anastrozole and other aromatase inhibitors could potentiate the effects of androstenedione by preventing its conversion to endogenous estrogens.

Contraindications and precautions

Androstenedione is contraindicated in patients with a history of or at risk for developing certain cancers (such as cancer of breast, pancreas, or prostate). Pregnant women especially and women in general should probably avoid using androstenedione.

Special considerations

• Significant reduction in HDL levels (reported with androstenedione consumption) increases the relative risk of coronary disease and myocardial infarction.
• Advise the patient that although controversial, androstenedione supplementation may increase the risk of certain hormone-sensitive cancers (such as prostate and breast cancer).
• Inform the patient that it is difficult to predict the effects of commercially available products that combine mixtures of androstenedione with other related steroids (such as DHEA and 4-androstene-3β,17β-diol).

Points of interest

• Androstenedione is a popular supplement with both amateur and professional weight lifters and bodybuilders.
• The U.S. Olympic Committee and the National Collegiate Athletic Association consider androstenedione a banned substance for athletic competition.
• 4-Androstenedione-3β,17β-diol is a primary metabolite of androstenedione. In vitro evidence suggests that it might yield a higher percentage of testosterone than androstenedione. Clinical trial data have failed to support this premise.

Commentary

Data surrounding supplementation of androstenedione appear to refute its value as an anabolic or ergogenic aid. Clinical trials offer conflicting data regarding the androstenedione's ability to raise the serum testosterone level. No data support a clinically relevant anabolic effect for healthy eugonadal males. Also, theoretical concerns exist regarding its undesirable effects on HDL levels and the supplement's ability to significantly elevate the serum estrogen level. Another unknown is whether this agent has any detrimental effect on hormone-sensitive cancers. Androstenedione supplementation cannot be recommended.

References

Earnest, C.P., et al. "In Vivo 4-Androstene-3,17-dione and 4-Androstene-3β,17β-diol Supplementation in Young Men," *Eur J Appl Physiol* 81:229-32, 2000.

Horton, R., and Tait, J.F. "Androstenedione Production and Interconversion Rates Measured in Blood and Studies on the Possible Sites of Its Conversion to Testosterone," *J Clin Invest* 45:301-13, 1966.

Bold italic type indicates that reaction may be life-threatening.

King, D.S., et al. "Effect of Oral Androstenedione on Serum Testosterone and Adaptions to Resistance Training in Young Men. A Randomized Controlled Trial," *JAMA* 281(21):2020-28, 1999.

Leder, B.Z., et al. "Oral Androstenedione Administration and Serum Testosterone Concentrations in Young Men," *JAMA* 283(6):779-82, 2000.

MacDonald , P.C., et al. "Origin of Estrogen in Normal Men and Women with Testicular Feminization," *J Clin Endocrinol Metab* 49:905-16, 1979.

Nelson, D.H. "Adrenal Androgens," in *The Adrenal Cortex.* Edited by Smith, L.H., Jr. Philadelphia: W.B. Saunders, 102-12, 1980.

Rasmussen, B.B., et al. "Androstenedione Does Not Stimulate Muscle Protein Anabolism in Young Healthy Men," *J Clin Endocrinol Metab* 85:55-59, 2000.

Wallace, M.B., et al. "Effects of Dehydroepiandrosterone vs Androstenedione Supplementation in Men," *Med Sci Sports Exerc* 31(12):1788-92, 1999.

ANGELICA

ANGELICA ROOT, ANGELIQUE, DONG QUAI, ENGELWURZEL, GARDEN ANGELICA, HEILIGENWURZEL, ROOT OF THE HOLY GHOST, TANG-KUEI, WILD ANGELICA

Taxonomic class
Apiaceae

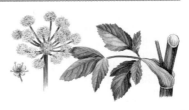

Common trade names
The species *Angelica sinensis,* from which this agent gets its name, is known as dong quai or tang-kuei.

Common forms
Available as cut, dried, or powdered root; essential oil; liquid extract; or tincture.

Source
Active compounds are derived from the fruits, leaves, rhizomes, and roots of many species of *Angelica,* a perennial in the parsley family that includes *A. acutiloba, A. archangelica, A. astragalus, A. atropurpurea, A. dahurica, A. edulis, A. gigas, A. japonica, A. keiskei, A. koreana, A. polymorpha, A. pubescens, A. radix,* and *A. sinensis.*

Chemical components
Various coumarins (angelicin, bergapten, imperatorin, oreoselone, osthol, oxypeucedanin, umbelliferone, xanthotoxol, and xanthotoxin) have been isolated from different *Angelica* species. The phenolic compound ferulic acid has been obtained from *A. sinensis.* Decursinol angelate is purified from the root of *A. gigas.* Two chalcones (xanthoangelol and 4-hydroxyderricin) have been isolated from *A. keiskei.*

Other compounds have been isolated from the roots and fruits of *A. archangelica,* such as terpene hydrocarbons, alcohols, esters, lactones, aliphatic carbonyls, and other aromatic compounds. Polysaccharides, palmitic acid, and the flavonoid archangelenone have also been isolated. Other compounds found in the volatile oils include alpha- and beta-phellandrene, alpha-pinene, alpha-thujene, limonene, beta-carophyllene, linalool, borneol, acetaldehyde, and some macrocyclic lactones.

Actions

Antitumorigenic properties have been noted in several animals. Decursinol angelate has cytotoxic and protein kinase C–activating activities (Ahn et al., 1996). In mice with skin cancer, chalcones from the root extract of *A. keiskei* exhibited potent antitumorigenic properties. Extracts from *A. archangelica* reduced the mutagenic effects of thiotepa in mouse bone marrow cells, and *A. radix* increased the production of tumor necrosis factor in mice. Several furanocoumarin compounds extracted from the root of *A. japonica* showed inhibitory activity against human adenogastric carcinoma (MK-1) cell growth (Fujioka et al., 1999).

Immunostimulatory properties were observed in vitro with angelan, a polysaccharide isolated from *A. gigas*. Angelan increased expression of interleukin (IL)-2, IL-4, IL-6, and interferon-gamma, resulting in activation of macrophages and natural killer cells involved in nonspecific immunity (Han et al., 1998).

Anti-inflammatory and analgesic properties have also been noted. Compounds isolated from the roots of *A. pubescens* inhibited centrally and peripherally mediated inflammatory substances. In vitro data show prominent inhibitory effects on both 5-lipoxygenase and cyclooxygenase (Liu et al., 1998).

Coumarin osthole inhibits platelet aggregation in vivo and in vitro (Hoult and Paya, 1996). *A. sinensis* significantly inhibited thromboxane A_2 formation and mildly affected prostaglandin I_2 production in animals compared with aspirin.

Angelica polysaccharide has been shown to promote the proliferation and differentiation of hematopoietic progenitor cells in healthy and anemic mice (Wang and Zhu, 1996).

Coumarins and ferulic acid from *A. dahurica* root have antimicrobial actions (Kwon et al., 1997). Two chalcones isolated from *A. keiskei* also showed antibacterial activity against gram-positive bacteria.

The aqueous extract of *A. sinensis* given I.V. decreased myocardial injury and the incidence of premature ventricular contractions and arrhythmias induced by myocardial reperfusion. Furanocoumarins inhibited the in vitro binding of diazepam to CNS benzodiazepine receptors in rat cells (Bergendorff et al., 1997).

A. sinensis and nifedipine improved pulmonary function and decreased mean arterial pulmonary pressures in chronic obstructive pulmonary disease patients with pulmonary hypertension. *A. polymorpha* has been found to selectively inhibit the production of allergic antibodies in asthmatics.

Uterine stimulant effects in the mouse and relaxation of the trachea in animals have been documented.

Bold italic type indicates that reaction may be life-threatening.

Polysaccharides isolated from the root of *A. sinensis* demonstrated dose-dependent protective effects on GI mucosa in rats administered the gastric irritants ethanol and indomethacin (Cho et al., 2000).

Antihypertensive effects were observed in rats administered an ACE inhibitor compound extracted from *A. keiskei* (Shimizu et al., 1999).

A. astragalus reduced serum levels of total cholesterol and triglycerides to the same extent as pravastatin and further lowered levels of LDL cholesterol and apolipoprotein B in rats with puromycin aminonucleoside-induced nephrotic syndrome. Attenuation of renal injury also was observed, as evidenced by a reduction of the glomerular sclerosing index value in treated rats (Lu et al., 1997).

Reported uses
This Chinese herb has been claimed to be of therapeutic usefulness for many disorders. It has been called a "cure-all" for gynecologic disorders and been promoted for such conditions as anemia, menstrual discomfort, and postmenopausal symptoms as a result of its purported estrogen-like effects and erythropoietic potential. No controlled studies have corroborated these benefits.

In a study of young women with leukorrhagia and insufficient luteal function, angelica root extract, in combination with several other Chinese herbs, regulated the menstrual cycle and reduced the severity of leukorrhagia.

Other claims include angelica's ability to improve circulation in the extremities; to treat anemia, backaches, and headaches; and to relieve asthma, eczema, hay fever, and osteoporosis.

Most studies of angelica have been conducted on animals, making it difficult to determine therapeutic benefits in humans.

Dosage
No consensus exists. Studies conducted with angelica used various concentrations of extracts, aqueous solutions, and powders, making identification of standardized dosage difficult.

Adverse reactions
CV: hypotension (from coumarins derived from *A. pubescens*; Hoult and Paya, 1996).
Hematologic: increased risk of bleeding (when used with such drugs as heparin and warfarin).
Skin: *phototoxicity* (effect of furanocoumarins).

Interactions
Warfarin: Significantly prolonged PT when *A. sinensis* is administered with warfarin. Avoid use with angelica.

Contraindications and precautions
Avoid using angelica in pregnant or breast-feeding patients because of potential stimulant effects on the uterus.

Special considerations
• Monitor the patient taking angelica for signs of bleeding, especially if he is also taking an anticoagulant.
• Inform the patient that using angelica may increase the risk of cancer.
• Urge the patient to promptly report signs of allergic reactions.
• Advise the patient to take precautions against direct sun exposure while taking angelica preparations.

Points of interest
• *A. atropurpurea* last appeared in the USP around 1860.
• Concerns have been raised regarding the potential carcinogenic risk of angelica, which led the International Fragrance Commission to recommend a limit of 0.78% angelica root in commercial preparations of suntan lotions.

Commentary
Although angelica is widely used in traditional Chinese medicine, its efficacy appears to be supported only by anecdotal evidence. The herb has been studied extensively in animal models, but scientifically valid human studies are lacking. Until more conclusive data are available, it is difficult to justify the therapeutic use of angelica for specific disorders.

References
Ahn, K.S., et al. "Decursinol Angelate: A Cytotoxic and Protein Kinase-C Activating Agent from the Root of *Angelica gigas*," *Planta Med* 62:7-9, 1996.

Bergendorff, O., et al. "Furanocoumarins with Affinity to Brain Benzodiazepine Receptors In Vitro," *Phytochemistry* 44:1121-24, 1997.

Cho, C.H., et al. "Study of the Gastrointestinal Protective Effects of Polysaccharides from *Angelica sinensis* in Rats," *Planta Med* 66(4):348-51, 2000.

Fujioka, T., et al. "Antiproliferative Constituents from Umbelliferae Plants. Furanocoumarin and Falcarindiol Furanocoumarin Ethers from the Root of *Angelica japonica*," *Chem Pharm Bull* 47(1):96-100, 1999.

Han, S.B., et al. "Characteristic Immunostimulation by Angelan Isolated from *Angelica gigas* Nakai," *Immunopharmacology* 40(1):39-48, 1998.

Hoult, J.R., and Paya, M. "Pharmacological and Biochemical Actions of Simple Coumarins: Natural Products with Therapeutic Potential," *Gen Pharmacol* 27:713-22, 1996.

Kwon, Y.S., et al. "Antimicrobial Constituents of *Angelica dahurica* Roots," *Phytochemistry* 44:887-89, 1997.

Liu, J.H., et al. "Inhibitory Effects of Angelica pubescens f. biserrata on 5-Lipoxygenase and Cyclooxygenase," *Planta Med* 64(6):525-29, 1998.

Lu, Y., et al. "Effect of Astragalus Angelica Mixture on Serum Lipids and Glomerulosclerosis in Rats with Nephrotic Syndrome," *Chung Kuo Chung His I Chieh Ho Tsa Chih* 17(8):478-80, 1997.

Shimizu, E., et al. "Effects of Angiotensin I-Converting Enzyme Inhibitor from Ashitaba (*Angelica keiskei*) on Blood Pressure of Spontaneously Hypertensive Rats," *J Nutr Sci Vitaminol* 45(3):375-83, 1999.

Wang, Y., and Zhu, B. "The Effect of Angelica Polysaccharide on Proliferation and Differentiation of Hematopoietic Progenitor Cells," *Chung Hua I Hsueh Tsa Chih* 76:363-66, 1996.

Wei, L., et al. "Treatment of Complications Due to Peritoneal Dialysis for Chronic Renal Failure with Traditional Chinese Medicine," *J Tradit Chin Med* 19(1):3-9, 1999.

ANISE

ANISEED, ANISE OIL, SWEET CUMIN

Taxonomic class
Apiaceae

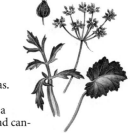

Common trade names
Beech Cough Drops, Bronhillor Natural Source Cough Candies & Throat Discs

Common forms
Available as an extract and in lozenges and teas. Also available in trace quantities as flavoring agents in liqueurs, lozenges, and teas as well as a fragrance in soaps, creams, perfumes, foods, and candies.

Source
Pimpinella anisum, the anise plant, is native to the Mediterranean area. The dried ripe fruit of the plant is referred to as aniseed. Anise oil is extracted from aniseed by steam distillation. Anise oil can also be obtained from the Chinese star anise plant (*Illicium verum*).

Chemical components
Anise extract typically contains 1% to 3% volatile anise oil. The primary constituent of anise oil is anethole (80% to 90%). Other components include alpha-pinene, linalool, anisaldehyde, and methyl chavicol. The composition of anise oil from *I. verum* resembles that of anise oil obtained from *P. anisum* but also contains trace quantities of safrole and myristicin. Naturally occurring coumarins and sitosterols have been found in tissue cultures of the *P. anisum* root.

Actions
Despite weak anticonvulsant effects, animal models have failed to justify claims of anise in this therapeutic application. One report suggests that aniseed extract exhibits mild sympathomimetic activity. Mucociliary transport velocity increased when patches of ciliated epithelium of frog esophagus were exposed to anise oil extract. However, another study showed that other volatile oils have more pronounced sympathomimetic effects than does anise oil.

Anise oil has been shown to exert varying effects on tracheal and ileal smooth muscle of the guinea pig (Reiter and Brandt, 1985). Anise oil extract exerts estrogenic, antifungal, and antibacterial properties. Anethole, a component of anise, gives licorice its characteristic flavor and odor (Caldwell and Sutton, 1988).

Reported uses

Therapeutic claims surround the use of this agent as an antasthmatic, an antiflatulent, an antispasmodic, a cough suppressant, and an expectorant. Modern medical literature describing well-designed trials do not confirm these therapeutic benefits in humans. The primary use of anise oil remains as a flavoring agent in foods and beverages. It has also been used as an insect repellent and insecticide.

In a Russian study, a combination of volatile oils was given to decrease mental fatigue in a group of aviation flight controllers. Combinations of anise, brandy mint, and lavender were shown to prevent occupation-induced changes in mental capacity, blood content, and oxygen tension of the cerebrovascular circulation (Leshchinskaia et al., 1983).

Anecdotal reports suggest that anethole ointment has been used to treat lice and scabies (Chandler and Hawkes, 1984).

Dosage

For intestinal gas, 0.1 ml anise oil P.O. t.i.d.

Small quantities of anise are commonly found in baked goods, beverages, and cough drops.

Adverse reactions

CNS: seizures.
EENT: inflammation of the lip and stomatitis (when used in toothpaste).
GI: nausea and vomiting.
Metabolic: pseudo-Conn's syndrome (hypermineralocorticism).
Respiratory: *pulmonary edema.*
Skin: contact dermatitis.
Other: *hypersensitivity reactions.*

Interactions

Iron: May enhance iron absorption across the intestinal mucosa. Avoid use with anise.

Contraindications and precautions

Anise is contraindicated during pregnancy (potential for estrogenic activity). Use cautiously in patients who are prone to atopy or contact dermatitis.

Special considerations

• Pure anise oil should not be taken internally except under the supervision of a health care provider.

🔺 **ALERT** Nausea, pulmonary edema, seizures, and vomiting have occurred with ingestion of 1 to 5 ml of anise oil.

🔺 **ALERT** Pseudo-Conn's syndrome may develop after intoxication of anise-based beverage (Trono et al., 1983).

• A study with rats suggests that anise extract may promote the absorption of iron across the intestinal mucosa (el-Shobaki et al., 1990). This effect has not been studied in humans.

Bold italic type indicates that reaction may be life-threatening.

• Instruct the patient to store anise in a tightly sealed, light-resistant container at room temperature.

• Monitor the patient for weight gain as a result of sodium and water retention.

• Advise the patient against ingesting pure anise oil because of its potential toxicity.

Points of interest

• Anise oil is generally considered safe by the FDA.

• Japanese star anise *(Illicium anisatum)* is poisonous.

Commentary

Although ancient medical folklore suggests many applications for anise oil, actual therapeutic benefits appear limited. Until more data become available, anise should be used only as a flavoring agent and fragrance. Ingestion of large quantities (at least several milliliters) of anise oil should probably be avoided because of potential gastrotoxicity.

References

Caldwell, J., and Sutton, J.D. "Influence of Dose Size on the Disposition of Trans-methoxy-14C Anethole in Human Volunteers," *Food Chem Toxicol* 26:87-91, 1988.

Chandler, R.F., and Hawkes, D. "Aniseed: Spice, Flavor, Drug," *Can Pharm J* 117:28-29, 1984.

Leshchinskaia, I.S., et al. "Effect of Phytonocides on the Dynamics of the Cerebral Circulation in Flight Controllers During Their Occupational Activity," *Kosm Biol Aviakosm Med* 17:80-83, 1983.

Reiter, M., and Brandt, W. "Relaxant Effects on Tracheal and Ileal Smooth Muscles of the Guinea Pig," *Arzneimittelforschung* 35:408-14, 1985.

el-Shobaki, F.A., et al. "The Effect of Some Beverage Extracts on Intestinal Iron Absorption," *Z Ernahrungswiss* 29:264-69, 1990.

Trono, D., et al. "Pseudo-Conn's Syndrome Due to Intoxication with Non-alcoholic Pastis," *Schweiz Med Wochenschr* 113:1092-95, 1983.

ARNICA

ARNICA FLOWERS, ARNICA ROOT, COMMON ARNICA, LEOPARD'S BANE, MEXICAN ARNICA, MOUNTAIN ARNICA, MOUNTAIN DAISY, MOUNTAIN TOBACCO, SNEEZEWORT, WOLF'S BANE

Taxonomic class

Asteraceae

Common trade names

Arnicaid, Arnica Spray, Arniflora (Gel), Traumeel-S (homeopathic formulation of arnica and other plant extracts manufactured in Italy)

Common forms

Available as a spray for topical application and in creams (preferred in Europe), gels, ointments, sublingual preparations, tablets, teas, and tinctures. Creams typically contain 15% arnica oil; salves should contain 20% to 25% arnica oil.

Source
Active components are usually extracted from the flowers and rootstocks of *Arnica montana, A. fulgens, A. sororia,* and *A. cordofolia.* Mexican arnica is derived from *Heterotheca inuloides.* Certain species of *Arnica* are native from Alaska to the Western United States and Mexico. Others are native to Europe and Siberia.

Chemical components
Arnica's active ingredients are thought to be flavonoid glycosides and sesquiterpenoid lactones, including anthoxanthine, arnisterol (arnidiol), choline, dihydrohelenalin, faradiol, and helenalin. Arnica also contains a group of polysaccharides with a content of 65% to 100% galacturonic acid and 0.5% to 1% resins, tannins, and volatile oils.

Actions
Four sesquiterpenoids isolated from *H. inuloides* in one study demonstrated antibacterial activity in vitro. One compound exhibited grampositive antibacterial activity and minimal bactericidal concentrations of 12.5 mcg/ml against methicillin-resistant *Staphylococcus aureus* (Kubo et al., 1994). Another in vitro study supported arnica's inhibitory effect against a few gram-positive organisms, but the effect was considered minor.

An *A. montana* extract has been shown to increase phagocytosis in mice (Wagner and Jurcic, 1991).

In a Dutch study, most arnica flavonoids demonstrated moderate to low cytotoxicity in vitro when compared with cisplatin. Helenalin, a sesquiterpene lactone, displayed the strongest cytotoxicity (Willuhn et al., 1994). Another study apparently found a quicker recovery from carbon tetrachloride–induced hepatic injury in rats when the rats were given a preparation of phenolic compounds of *A. montana.* Other studies in rats have also supported a role of arnica extracts in reducing lipid peroxidation and restoration of glutathione activity in the carbon tetrachloride–induced hepatic injury.

An in vitro study found that helenalin and dihydrohelenalin inhibited platelet function in humans. Another study in healthy human volunteers failed to find significant effects on blood-clotting parameters immediately after use of an arnica extract (Baillargeon et al., 1993).

In vitro studies have documented an anti-inflammatory effect for some components of arnica (Schaffner, 1997). Traumeel-S, a homeopathic mixture containing arnica, was found to reduce rat paw edema. This was associated with a decrease in interleukin-6 production in the animals (Lussignoli et al., 1999).

Reported uses
Arnica is claimed to be useful for relieving muscle and joint aches and is frequently cited in herbal literature as being able to promote wound

---

Bold italic type indicates that reaction may be life-threatening.

RESEARCH FINDINGS
Analgesic effects of arnica

A study involving 118 patients with impacted wisdom teeth examined a tincture of *Arnica montana* for its analgesic and wound-healing abilities (Kaziro, 1984). Random assignment of metronidazole 400 mg, arnica 200 centisemal dilutions in neutral tablets, or placebo was given twice daily to patients who had had teeth extracted. The subjects were also given a regularly scheduled narcotic analgesic.

Double-blind assessment of pain as measured by edema, trismus (mouth-opening), visual analogue scale, and wound healing was conducted in all patients in each group at postoperative days 4 and 8. On day 4, pain-relief scores were not significantly different. On day 8, results indicated a statistically significant difference in analgesia in favor of metronidazole when compared with either arnica or placebo.

Metronidazole was also more effective than either arnica or placebo in its ability to prevent swelling and promote healing. Arnica was not favored in any of the outcome measurements. In fact, the investigators found that arnica seemed to increase pain and edema. Although this study found differences favoring metronidazole, the statistical test used is questionable for the data evaluated. Results should be assessed with that caution in mind.

healing. In veterinary medicine, the agent is classified as a counterirritant, an effect probably related to the isomeric alcohol component of arnica.

Analgesic effects failed to be verified in a double-blind study of arnica, metronidazole, and a placebo among postoperative dental patients (Kaziro, 1984). (See *Analgesic effects of arnica* .)

Similarly, a homeopathic dose of arnica was tested against a placebo in a population of post abdominal hysterectomy patients. No significant difference was found between the two groups (Hart et al., 1997). In a small study of marathon runners, another formulation of arnica failed to produce statistically significant benefits in muscle stiffness, laboratory measurements of muscle injury, or healing time of muscle injuries. Notably, a systematic review of placebo-controlled trials published before 1998 failed to find any support of efficacy for arnica as a homeopathic medicinal (Ernst and Pittler, 1998).

Dosage
No consensus exists. Homeopathic doses (trace quantities) appear to be most popular.

Adverse reactions
CNS: *coma,* nervous disorders.
CV: *arrhythmias, cardiotoxicity,* hypertension.
EENT: mouth ulcers (with undiluted commercial mouthwash preparation of oil of peppermint and arnica).
GI: gastroenteritis, nausea, vomiting.
Hematologic: increased risk of bleeding (conflicting data).
Hepatic: *hepatic failure.*
Musculoskeletal: muscle weakness.
Skin: arnica-induced *Sweet's syndrome* (acute febrile neutrophilic dermatosis clinically resembling *erythema multiforme*), contact dermatitis (with topical use).
Other: *death, organ damage.*

Interactions
Antihypertensives: May reduce effectiveness of these drugs. Avoid use with arnica.

Contraindications and precautions
Avoid using arnica in pregnant patients because of the risk of uterine oxytocic activity and lack of knowledge about arnica's teratogenic potential.

Special considerations
• Instruct the patient not to apply arnica to abraded skin or open wounds.
◗ **ALERT** Keep arnica preparations out of the reach of children. Coma, nausea, organ damage, vomiting, and even death have occurred in children from ingestion of arnica flowers or roots. Induce emesis and perform gastric lavage to remove undigested contents. Supportive care may be needed.
• Explain to the patient that when taken orally, arnica may cause allergic reactions, cardiotoxicity, hypertension, renal dysfunction, and vertigo because of the activity of sesquiterpene lactones and components of the essential oil.
• Advise the patient to avoid prolonged topical use because of the potential for allergic reactions.

Points of interest
• Arnica has been approved by the German Commission E as a topical agent with effective analgesic, antibacterial, and anti-inflammatory properties. The FDA, however, has classified arnica as an unsafe herb.

Commentary
Despite interesting in vitro studies and exciting possibilities for use of this agent, clinical trials have failed to document therapeutic benefits of arnica. A systematic analysis also failed to find significant proof of efficacy for homeopathic application of arnica. External use is discouraged because of the risk of allergic reactions. The results of well-conducted clinical trials that verify a favorable risk-benefit ratio are needed before therapeutic applications of arnica can be considered.

Bold italic type indicates that reaction may be life-threatening.

References

Baillargeon, L., et al. "The Effects of *Arnica montana* on Blood Coagulation: A Randomized, Controlled Trial," *Can Fam Physician* 39:2362-67, 1993.

Ernst, E., and Pittler, M.H. "Efficacy of Homeopathic Arnica. A Systematic Review of Placebo-controlled Trials," *Arch Surg* 133:1187-90, 1998.

Hart, O., et al. "Double-Blind, Placebo-controlled, Randomized Clinical Trial of Homeopathic Arnica C30 for Pain and Infection After Total Abdominal Hysterectomy," *J R Soc Med* 90:73-78, 1997.

Kaziro, G.S. "Metronidazole and *Arnica montana* in the Prevention of Post-surgical Complications: A Comparative Placebo-controlled Trial," *Br J Oral Maxillofac Surg* 22:42-49, 1984.

Kubo, I., et al. "Antimicrobial Agents from *Heterotheca inuloides*," *Planta Med* 60:218-21, 1994.

Lussignoli, S., et al. "Effect of Traumeel S, a Homeopathic Formulation, on Blood-induced Inflammation in Rats," *Complement Ther Med* 7(4):225-30, 1999.

Schaffner, W. "Granny's Remedy Explained at the Molecular Level: Helenalin Inhibits NF-kappa B," *Biol Chem* 378:935, 1997. Editorial.

Wagner, H., and Jurcic , K. "Immunologic Studies of Plant Combination Preparations: In Vitro and In Vivo Studies on the Stimulation of Phagocytosis," *Arzneimittelforschung* 10:1072-76, 1991.

Willuhn, G., et al. "Cytotoxicity of Flavonoids and Sesquiterpene Lactones from *Arnica* Species Against GLC4 and the COLO 320 Cell Lines," *Planta Med* 60:434-37, 1994.

ASH

BIRD'S TONGUE, COMMON ASH, EUROPEAN ASH, *FRAXINUS AMERICANA*, *FRAXINUS ATROVIRENS*, *FRAXINUS HETEROPHYLLA*, *FRAXINUS JASPIDA*, *FRAXINUS POLEMONIIPOLIA*, *FRAXINUS SIMPLIFOLIA*, *FRAXINUS VERTICILLATA*, WEEPING ASH, WHITE ASH

Taxonomic class
Oleaceae

Common trade name
Multi-ingredient preparation: Phytodolar

Common forms
Liquid extract: combination product containing common ash *(Fraxinus excelsior)* bark, aspen *(Populus tremula)* leaves and bark, and goldenrod *(Solidago virgaurea)* aerial, alcohol 45.6%

Source
The crude drug is prepared from the leaves and bark of the *F. excelsior* tree.

Chemical components
Ash leaf extracts contain varying amounts of flavonoids (including rutin 0.1% to 0.9%), iridoide monoterpenes, mannitol (16% to 28%), mucilages (10% to 20%), phenolic acids, phytosterols, tannins, and triterpenes, depending on the time of year the plants are harvested.

Extracts of ash bark contain hydroxycoumarins, including aesculin, fraxin, and isofraxidin.

Actions
Limited studies have been conducted on the actions of ash alone. Available information pertains to the activity of ash as an anti-inflammatory. Ash has been shown to inhibit the enzyme myeloperoxidase, which is released by activated granulocytes and produces the destructive agent hypochloric acid (von Kruedener et al., 1996). Ash also inhibits the enzyme dihydrofolate reductase. Alone and in combination, ash significantly reduced rat paw edema to varying degrees and decreased arthritic paw volume. This anti-inflammatory activity was comparable to the tested doses of diclofenac (el-Ghazaly et al., 1992).

Reported uses
Historically, the dried powders of ash leaf extracts were used as a mild diuretic and tonic.

Studies have been conducted for the use of ash, alone and in combination with aspen and goldenrod, as an anti-inflammatory in patients with rheumatoid arthritis. Clinical studies with combination products have noted similar efficacy in arthritic conditions with NSAIDs (Klein-Galczinsky, 1999).

Dosage
Reported dosage for the combination product ranges from 20 to 40 gtt P.O. t.i.d. or q.i.d. mixed with water or a fluid of choice. A standard dosage has not been established.

Adverse reactions
None reported.

Interactions
None reported.

Contraindications and precautions
The combination product should be used with caution in patients who are hypersensitive to salicylates. Effects in pregnancy are unknown.

Special considerations
• Find out why the patient has been taking ash.
• Although no chemical interactions have been reported in clinical studies, consideration must be given to the herbal product's pharmacologic properties and the potential for interference with the intended therapeutic effect of conventional drugs.
• Caution the patient not to self-treat symptoms of arthritis before receiving appropriate medical evaluation because this may delay diagnosis of a serious medical condition.

Bold italic type indicates that reaction may be life-threatening.

• Advise the patient to consult a health care provider before using herbal preparations because a treatment that has been clinically researched and proved effective may be available.
• Keep ash extracts away from children and pets.

Points of interest
• *F. excelsior* is listed in the FDA Poisonous Plant Database.
• The German Commission E, which oversees drug use in Germany, considers ash an unapproved product.

Commentary
Although there is information about the use of ash in a fixed combination product for treating arthritic conditions, information about ash alone is limited. Additional safety and efficacy data are needed to assess the risks and benefits of ash.

References
el-Ghazaly, M., et al. "Study of the Anti-inflammatory Activity of *Populus tremula, Solidago virgaurea* and *Fraxinus excelsior*," *Arzneimittelforschung* 42(3):333-36, 1992.

Klein-Galczinsky, C. "Pharmacological and Clinical Effectiveness of a Fixed Phytogenic Combination Trembling Poplar *(Populus tremula)*, True Goldenrod *(Solidago virgaurea)* and Ash *(Fraxinus excelsior)* in Mild to Moderate Rheumatic Complaints," *Wien Med Wochenschr* 149(8-10):248-53, 1999.

Strehl, E., et al. "Inhibition of Dihydrofolate Reductase Activity by Alcoholic Extracts from *Fraxinus excelsior, Populus tremula* and *Solidago virgaurea*," *Arzneimittelforschung* 45(2):172-73, 1995.

von Kruedener, S., et al. "Effects of Extracts from *Populus tremula L., Solidago virgaurea L.* and *Fraxinus excelsior L.* on Various Myeloperoxidase Systems," *Arzneimittelforschung* 46(8):809-14, 1996.

ASTRAGALUS

HUANG CHI, HUANG QI, MILK VETCH, MONGOLIAN MILK VETCH, YELLOW LEADER

Taxonomic class
Fabaceae

Common trade names
Astragalus Power, Astragalus Supreme, Biomune OSF Plus, Nature's Way Astragalus Root, Neo-Cardio, Phytisone, Phyto Complete, Phytogen, Super Immuno-Tone, Thymucin

Common forms
Available in capsules (100 mg, 150 mg, 200 mg, 250 mg, 400 mg, 470 mg, 500 mg), extract, tea, and tincture.

Source
The herb is derived from the root of the astragalus or *Astragalus membranaceous* plant, which is native to China, Korea, and Japan. The root

may be fried with honey or chewed untreated; it has a sweet, licorice flavor.

Chemical components

Astragalus contains betaine, beta-sitosterol, choline, glycosides (astragalosides I through VII), plant acids (AMon-S, hexuroic acid), polysaccharides (astroglucans A through C), rumatakenin, sugar, saponins (more than 40 identified), and vitamin A.

Actions

Animal studies suggest effects that include stimulation of the immune system, possibly by the saponin and multiple polysaccharide constituents found in the astragalus root. Mice subjected to testing for stamina and stress resistance (swimming long distances and exposure to extreme temperatures) performed better when fed astragalus root.

Several test tube and rodent studies suggest that the herb successfully combats the scarring, inflammation, and other heart damage caused by the Coxsackie B virus.

Astragalus root saponins have been found to have diuretic activity. These saponins have also been identified as having anti-inflammatory and antihypertensive activity.

Reported uses

Astragalus is mainly used in traditional Chinese medicine to support and enhance the immune system. One study examined immune system stimulation for AIDS patients, and the preliminary results appeared favorable. A series of Chinese reports claim that a mixture of herbs including astragalus could induce seronegative conversion in a small number of HIV patients. Some people use the herb to speed healing because it may provide antibacterial activities or enhance one's own immune system. Others use astragalus as a protectant for the liver and kidneys.

Ten patients suffering from Coxsackie B viral myocarditis with depressed natural killer (NK) activity were given astragalus I.M. for 3 to 4 months. After treatment, the NK activity increased from 11.5% to 44.9%, whereas the control group NK activity remained unchanged (Yang et al., 1990). In another study, researchers observed an improved cellular immunity in blood samples of patients suffering from viral myocarditis.

According to various studies, astragalus may be beneficial for repair of the heart muscle. One study suggests that patients using astragalus experienced less anginal pain and improved electrocardiography readings compared with subjects using nifedipine (Peirce, 1999). Another study demonstrated significant improvement of left ventricular function in post–myocardial infarction patients treated with astragalus compared with patients who did not receive the herb over a 4-week period. This study hypothesized that astragalus's antioxidant effects contributed to the benefits observed.

Dosage
Dried root: 1 to 4 g P.O. t.i.d.
Tincture: 1 dropperful P.O. b.i.d. or t.i.d.

Adverse reactions
None reported.

Interactions
Antihypertensives: Interference with or increased hypotensive effects. Avoid using together.

Contraindications and precautions
Use astragalus cautiously in patients taking immunosuppressants or those with autoimmune diseases.

Special considerations
• Find out why the patient has been taking astragalus.
• Although no known chemical interactions have been reported in clinical studies, consideration must be given to the herbal product's pharmacologic properties and the potential for interference with the intended therapeutic effect of conventional drugs.
• Caution the patient not to self-treat symptoms of cardiac or immune dysfunction before receiving appropriate medical evaluation because this may delay diagnosis of a potentially serious medical condition.
• Advise the patient to consult a health care provider before using herbal preparations because a treatment that has been clinically researched and proved effective may be available.

Commentary
Astragalus has demonstrated some intriguing behaviors on the immune system. Although this herb is thought to have minor toxicities, research is in its infancy. Caution should be used when considering it for the treatment of serious insults to the immune system, such as AIDS, cancer, hepatitis, HIV infection, and myocarditis.

References
Peirce, A. *The American Pharmaceutical Association Practical Guide to Natural Medicines.* New York: William Morrow & Co., Stonesong Press, 1999.
Yang, Y.Z., et al. "Effect of *Astragalus membraneous* on Natural Killer Cell Activity and Induction with Coxsackie B Viral Myocarditis," *Chin Med J* 103(4):304-7, 1990.

AVENS

BENEDICT'S HERB, CITY AVENS, CLOVE ROOT, COLEWORT, GEUM, GOLDY STAR, HERB BENNET, WAY BENNET, WILD RYE, WOOD AVENS

Taxonomic class
Rosaceae

Common trade names
Few or no commercially prepared products are available in the United States.

Common forms
Available as a tea and tincture.

Source
The drug is a volatile oil extracted from the dried herb, rhizome, or root of *Geum urbanum,* a member of the rose family.

Chemical components
The volatile oil primarily contains eugenol, along with gum, resin, and tannins. The roots contain caffeic, chlorogenic, and gallic acids.

Actions
The mechanism for eugenol's anti-inflammatory activity is thought to involve the potent inhibition of cyclooxygenase. Other factors may be involved as well, including inhibition of prostaglandin production (Tunon et al., 1995).

Reported uses
Avens is claimed to have anti-inflammatory, antiseptic, aromatic, astringent, and tonic properties. In earlier times, avens was used as a treatment for insect bites, plague, and stomach ills. More recently, folk medicine has claimed that the extract is effective in the treatment of chills, chronic hemorrhage, diarrhea, dysentery, gastric irritation, headache, intermittent fever, leukorrhea, sore throat, and wounds. Medical literature does not justify these claims.

Dosage
Various dosages have been used: 1 dram (liquid extract of the herb), ½ to 1 dram (liquid extract of the root), or 15 to 30 grains as a tonic (powdered herb or root) P.O. t.i.d.

Adverse reactions
GI: GI bleeding, indigestion.
GU: decreased renal function.

Interactions
Antihypertensives: May antagonize the effects of these drugs. Avoid concomitant use.

Contraindications and precautions
Avoid using avens in pregnant or breast-feeding patients.

Special considerations
• Although no known chemical interactions have been reported in clinical studies, consideration must be given to the herbal product's pharmacologic properties and the potential for interference with the intended therapeutic effect of conventional drugs.

Bold italic type indicates that reaction may be life-threatening.

• Advise the patient that little scientific information exists concerning the pharmacologic actions of avens and that other pharmaceutical remedies, such as NSAIDs, have known risks and benefits.
• Advise the patient who wants to consume avens to report unusual symptoms to his health care provider.
• Keep avens away from children and pets.

Points of interest
• Avens has been revered in Europe since the 12th century. Some people believe that it can ward off evil spirits and deter poisonous creatures.

Commentary
In vitro data suggest only potential efficacy as an anti-inflammatory compared with available NSAIDs. Data on safety and randomized, controlled trials evaluating efficacy are needed before use of this drug can be considered.

References
Tunon, H., et al. "Evaluation of Anti-inflammatory Activity of Some Swedish Medicinal Plants: Inhibition of Prostaglandin Biosynthesis and PAF-Induced Exocytosis," *J Ethnopharmacol* 48:61-76, 1995.

BALSAM OF PERU

BLACK BALSAM, INDIAN BALSAM, MYROSPERUM PEREIRA, MYROXYLON, TOLUIFERA PEREIRA

Taxonomic class
Fabaceae

Common trade names
None known.

Common forms
Many commercial products, such as conditioners, lotions, salves, and shampoos, contain small quantities of balsam of Peru.

Source
Balsam of Peru is obtained from a boiled extract of battered and scorched tree bark of *Myroxylon pereirae* (*M. balsamum*). The balsam of Peru tree, a legume, grows in Florida, Central America, and Peru.

Chemical components
Balsam of Peru is 50% to 65% cinnamein, a volatile oil, and 20% to 28% resin. Cinnamein is composed of benzoic acid esters, benzyl alcohol, benzyl cinnamate, cinnamic acid esters (such as styracin), and the ester form of the alcohol peruviol, often considered equivalent to nerolidol (a sesquiterpene alcohol). Coumarin, styrene, and vanillin occur in trace amounts. The resin contains benzoic and cinnamic acids.

Actions
Balsam of Peru is reported to possess mild antiseptic and antibacterial properties and is claimed to promote skin growth.

Reported uses
This agent is claimed to be useful as an anthelmintic, an antineoplastic, an antihemorrhoidal drug, a diuretic, an expectorant, a pediculocide, and a stimulant. Balsam of Peru is also used in topical preparations to treat anal pruritus, dandruff, diaper rash, hemorrhoids, indolent ulcers, pressure ulcers, rheumatoid conditions, scabies, wounds, and other skin problems. Dentists have used balsam of Peru in dental impression media and to treat postextraction alveolitis, commonly called dry socket.

Dosage
For hemorrhoids: 1.8- to 3-mg suppositories P.R.

Adverse reactions

Skin: contact dermatitis (may relate to cinnamein, with frequent use).
Other: *systemic toxicity* in infants after application on nipples of breast-feeding mother.

Interactions

Sulfur-containing compounds: Separation of resin component from the balsam. Avoid administration with balsam of Peru.

Contraindications and precautions

Avoid using balsam of Peru in pregnant or breast-feeding patients. Use cautiously in patients who are prone to contact dermatitis.

Special considerations

• Advise the patient to watch for allergic reactions to topical forms of balsam of Peru.
• Inform the patient that little information exists to support therapeutic claims for internal use.
• Advise the female patient to avoid using balsam of Peru during pregnancy or when breast-feeding.

Points of interest

• Balsam of Peru has a pleasing odor and vanilla-like flavor, which make it useful in pharmaceutical preparations as well as shampoos and conditioners. It can also be found in small quantities (0.0015%) in baked goods, chocolate candies, frozen dairy desserts, gelatins, puddings, and other food products.
• Germany allows use of this agent for many dermatologic conditions.
• Balsam of Peru is nearly insoluble in water but soluble in alcohol, chloroform, and glacial acetic acid.

Commentary

Contact dermatitis limits use of balsam of Peru. Few scientific data exists to support the agent for medicinal purposes. Balsam of Peru will probably remain in use only as a fragrance in the pharmaceutical and cosmetic industries.

References

"Peruvian Balsam," in *Remington's Pharmaceutical Sciences.* Easton, Pa.: Mack Publishing Co., 1990.
"Peruvian Balsam," in *The United States Dispensatory.* Philadelphia: Lippincott-Raven Pubs., 1993.

BARBERRY

BERBERRY, COMMON BARBERRY, EUROPEAN BARBERRY, JAUNDICE BERRY, OREGON GRAPE, PEPPERRIDGE BUSH, SOUR-SPINE, SOWBERRY, TRAILING MAHONIA, WOOD SOUR

Taxonomic class
Berberidaceae

Common trade names
Oregon Grape Root

Common forms
Available as an extract, liquid, tablets (400 mg), and tea.

Source
Barberry comes from the roots, wood, and bark of *Mahonia vulgaris* and *M. aquifolium* (also known as *Berberis aquifolium* and *B. vulgaris*), plants that have edible, red-orange fruitlike berries. *Mahonia* species are native to Europe and some parts of North America and have long been used as landscape shrubs.

Chemical components
Barberry species contain tannins and many isoquinoline alkaloids, including berbamine, berberine, bervulcine, columbamine, jatrorrhizine, magnoflorine, and oxycanthine.

Actions
Berberine, the most extensively studied component of barberry, may possess anthelmintic, anticonvulsant, and sedative properties and exerts local anesthetic effects when injected subcutaneously. It has also demonstrated in vitro antibacterial activity against several species that exceeds that of chloramphenicol.

An ethanolic extract of *B. vulgaris* has shown anti-inflammatory activity in in vitro and animal studies. Other alkaloid isolates of the plant are less potent in their anti-inflammatory effects than the total ethanol extract (Ivanovska and Philipov, 1996).

A few of the isoquinoline alkaloids exert uterine-stimulating effects in animals (Farnsworth et al., 1975). Other studies have shown antiarrhythmic and hypotensive effects with berbamine and antiarrhythmic activity with berberine.

Reported uses
Barberry is claimed to be of therapeutic usefulness as an antidiarrheal, an antipyretic, and a cough suppressant as well as in ameliorating jaundice.

In the past, berberine was used as an astringent in various ophthalmic preparations but is seldom used in these forms today. It has been shown to be more effective than a placebo in resolving *Vibrio cholerae*–induced diarrhea but had no benefit over placebo in patients with diarrhea due to other causes (Maung et al., 1985).

Bold italic type indicates that reaction may be life-threatening.

Dosage
In one study, a dosage of 400 mg P.O. daily was used to ameliorate acute diarrhea (Maung et al., 1985).

Adverse reactions
CNS: confusion, stupor.
GI: diarrhea.
GU: nephritis.
Other: spontaneous abortion.

Interactions
Antiarrhythmics: May increase antiarrhythmic effects. Monitor closely.
Antihypertensives: May increase hypotensive effects. Discourage use.

Contraindications and precautions
Barberry is contraindicated in pregnant patients because of the risk of spontaneous abortion. Use cautiously in women of childbearing age.

Special considerations
⚫ ALERT Some references suggest that symptoms of poisoning from this plant may appear as confusion, diarrhea, nephritis, and stupor. Toxic dosage is unknown.
• Monitor for signs and symptoms of poisoning and alert the patient's primary health care provider if they occur.
• Caution the patient against consuming large quantities of barberry because it contains potentially toxic chemicals.
• Inform the patient that little evidence exists to support medicinal uses of barberry.
• Caution the female patient to avoid using barberry during pregnancy.

Points of interest
• Berberine gives the rootwood of the barberry plant its characteristic bright golden yellow color.
• Berberine salts derived from barberry have been used as an astringent in eyedrops and eye washes.

Commentary
More evidence needs to be collected before barberry or its components can be considered useful for therapeutic application. This compound needs further evaluation as an antidiarrheal before it can be recommended for acute diarrhea.

References
Farnsworth, N.R., et al. "Potential Value of Plants as Sources of New Antifertility Agents," *J Pharm Sci* 64:535-98, 1975.

Ivanovska, N., and Philipov, S. "Study on the Anti-inflammatory Action of *Berberis vulgaris* Root Extract, Alkaloid Fractions, and Pure Alkaloids," *Int J Immunopharmacol* 10:553-61, 1996.

Maung, K.U., et al. "Clinical Trial of Berberine in Acute Watery Diarrhea," *BMJ* 291:1601, 1985.

BARLEY

FOXTAIL GRASS, HARE BARLEY, *HORDEUM* SPP.
(*DISTICHON, IRREGULARE, JUBATUM, LEPORINUM,
VULGARE*), MILLED BARLEY, PEARL BARLEY, PERLATUM,
POT BARLEY, SCOTCH BARLEY, WILD BARLEY

Taxonomic class
Gramineae

Common trade names
None known.

Common forms
As an additive in malt beverages, breakfast cereals, and animal feed, barley is prepared as barley flakes, barley grits, distilled barley water, malt extracts, and whole-grain barley (made into flour).

Source
Barley is an annual cereal grass with flowers, fruit, leaves, stems, and roots. The medicinal chemicals are extracted from the grain itself. Malted barley is prepared from germination of barley seeds. The grass is native to Asia and Ethiopia but cultivated worldwide.

Chemical components
Barley contains fatty oil (linoleic and oleic acids), hydroxycoumarins (aesculetin, gramine, herniarin, hordenine, scopoletin, tyramine, and umbelliferone), monosaccharides and oligosaccharides (fructose, glucodifructose, glucose, raffinose, and saccharose), polysaccharides (fructans and starch), proteins (albumins, globulins, glutelins, and prolamines), and vitamins (B_2, B_6, E, and nicotinic, pantothenic, and folic acids).

Actions
Because of its demulcent properties, barley is claimed to have a soothing effect on the alimentary tract (Gruenwald et al., 1998; Spoerke, 1980). In animals, germinated barley foodstuff was shown to improve intestinal damage by increasing luminal short-chain fatty acid production (Mitsuyama et al., 1998). Hordenine, or *N,N*-dimethyltyramine, which is present in the rootlets of barley, may exert sympathomimetic effects on the intestine.

Reported uses
Barley is most commonly used as stock feed or a minor source of flour and for malting. It has been reported to treat diarrhea, gastritis, and inflammatory bowel conditions (Gruenwald et al., 1998). Human studies suggest that the consumption of barley may have cholesterol-lowering effects (Bourdon et al., 1999; Ikegami et al., 1996; Lupton et al., 1994; McIntosh et al., 1991). Hypoglycemic effects in healthy patients who consumed barley have been reported (Liljeberg et al., 1996; Thorburn et

---

Bold italic type indicates that reaction may be life-threatening.

al., 1993). These studies also suggest that barley is an important component of diets in patients with diabetes (Liljeberg et al., 1996; Thorburn et al., 1993). Barley has been claimed to prevent cancer as well.

Dosage
Various amounts of barley are contained in foods.

Adverse reactions
None known.

Interactions
None reported.

Contraindications and precautions
Barley is contraindicated in pregnant patients.

Special considerations
• Barley is not known to cause adverse effects in humans, but it has caused fatal muscle dystrophy in calves (Hidiroglou et al., 1977).
• Feeding barley has little or no effect on milk supply (Casper et al., 1990), but it may decrease milk proteins (Weiss et al., 1989).
• Animal poisonings have occurred with the consumption of barley that was contaminated with fungus (Spoerke, 1980).
• Although no known chemical interactions have been reported in clinical studies, consideration must be given to the herbal product's pharmacologic properties and the potential for interference with the intended therapeutic effect of conventional drugs.
• Caution the patient not to self-treat symptoms of GI problems before receiving appropriate medical evaluation because this may delay diagnosis of a potentially serious medical condition.
• Advise the patient to consult a health care provider before using herbl preparations because a treatment that has been clinically researched and proved effective may be available.

Points of interest
• Ancient folklore cites barley as a food for potency and vigor. Roman gladiators, known as *hordearii* (barley eaters), ate barley for strength.
• Barley is referred to as "medicine for the heart" in Pakistan. Examples of supposed cholesterol-lowering recipes include banana-barley bread, barley-bran muffins, barley tabouli, and rieska (flatbread).
• Less processed barley probably produces more beneficial therapeutic effects.

Commentary
Barley is used extensively in foods and malted drinks. Although there are reports of barley's use in diabetes, GI conditions, and hypercholesterolemia, safety and efficacy data are still lacking. Until well-controlled human studies confirm the use of barley for these conditions, it is not recommended outside normal dietary consumption.

References

Bourdon, I., et al. "Postprandial Lipid, Glucose, Insulin, and Cholecystokinin Responses in Men Fed Barley Pasta Enriched with Beta-glucan," *Am J Clin Nutr* 69(1):55-63, 1999.

Bruneton, J. *Pharmacognosy, Phytochemistry, Medicinal Plants.* New York: Lavoisier Publishing, 1995.

Casper, D.P., et al. "Response of Early Lactation Dairy Cows Fed Diets Varying in Source of Nonstructural Carbohydrate and Crude Protein," *J Dairy Sci* 68:2027-32, 1990.

Gruenwald, J., et al., eds. *PDR for Herbal Medicines.* Montvale, N.J.: Medical Economics Co., 1998.

Hidiroglou, H., et al. "Influences of Barley and Oat Silages for Beef Cows on Occurrence of Myopathy in Their Calves," *J Dairy Sci* 60:1905-9, 1977.

Ikegami S., et al. "Effect of Boiled Barley-Rice-Feeding in Hypercholesterolemic and Normolipemic Subjects," *Plant Foods Hum Nutr* 49(4):317-28, 1996.

Liljeberg, H.G., et al. "Products Based on a High Fiber Barley Genotype, but Not on Common Barley or Oats, Lower Postprandial Glucose and Insulin Responses in Healthy Humans," *J Nutr* 126(2):458-66, 1996.

Lupton, J.R., et al. "Cholesterol-lowering Effect of Barley Bran Flour and Oil," *J Am Diet Assoc* 94(1):65-70, 1994.

McIntosh, G.H., et al. "Barley and Wheat Foods: Influence on Plasma Cholesterol Concentrations in Hypercholesterolemic Men," *Am J Clin Nutr* 53(5):1205-9, 1991.

Mitsuyama, K., et al. "Treatment of Ulcerative Colitis with Germinated Barley Foodstuff Feeding: A Pilot Study," *Ailment Pharmacol Ther* 12(12):1225-30, 1998.

Spoerke, D.G. *Herbal Medications.* Santa Barbara, Calif.: Woodbridge Press Publishing Co., 1980.

Thorburn, A., et al. "Carbohydrate Fermentation Decreases Hepatic Glucose Output in Healthy Subjects," *Metabolism* 42(6):780-5, 1993.

Weiss, W.P., et al. "Barley Distillers Grains as a Protein Supplement for Dairy Cows," *J Dairy Sci* 72:980-7, 1989.

BASIL

COMMON BASIL, GARDEN BASIL, HOLY BASIL, SWEET BASIL

Taxonomic class
Lamiaceae

Common trade names
None known.

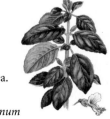

Common forms
Available as chopped or powdered leaves and a tea.

Source
The crude drug is derived from the leaves of *Ocimum basilicum* (sweet or common basil) or *Ocimum sanctum* (holy basil), members of the mint family (Labiatae).

Bold italic type indicates that reaction may be life-threatening.

Chemical components
The active components of basil include eugenol, linalool, and methyl chavicol (estragole). Other components include monoterpenes (such as camphor, cineol, geraniol, and ocimene), phenylpropanes (such as methyl cinnamate), and sesquiterpenes.

Actions
In human trials, *O. sanctum* and *Ocimum album* significantly lowered urine glucose as well as fasting and postprandial blood glucose levels in 40 patients with type 2 diabetes. Total cholesterol levels were also slightly decreased (Agrawal et al., 1996).

Animal studies have revealed some peripherally mediated analgesic effects of the fixed oil of *O. sanctum* (Singh and Majumdar, 1995). Another trial in guinea pigs found antasthmatic and anti-inflammatory properties in extracts from fresh leaves and the essential oils of *O. sanctum* leaves (Singh and Agrawal, 1991). In studies with rats, *O. basilicum* components (aqueous extracts, flavonoid glycosides, and methanol extracts) were found to have antiulcerative effects (Akhtar et al., 1992).

Reported uses
Basil is claimed to possess analgesic, anti-inflammatory, antioxidant, antiseptic, antiulcerative, and hypoglycemic properties.

Dosage
The dosage reported in one trial was 2.5 g of fresh, dried leaf powder once daily (Agrawal et al., 1996). A tea can be made by placing 2.5 g of fresh, dried leaf powder in ½ cup of water, straining, and drinking once or twice daily, as needed.

Adverse reactions
Hepatic: *hepatocellular carcinoma.*
Metabolic: hypoglycemia.

Interactions
Insulin, sulfonylureas, other antidiabetics: May increase hypoglycemic effects. Avoid administration with basil.

Contraindications and precautions
Avoid using basil in pregnant or breast-feeding patients because of the potential for increased menstrual flow and the mutagenic effects of estragole. Use cautiously in diabetic patients.

Special considerations
● Monitor the diabetic patient for hypoglycemia if he consumes basil in quantities that exceed amounts typically used for foods.
● Instruct the patient to avoid long-term use of basil because of its potential mutagenic effect. Estragole is a known hepatocarcinogen in animals.
● Advise the female patient not to use basil during pregnancy or when breast-feeding.

Points of interest
• Cultivation practices and soil variations can significantly change the chemical composition of basil.

Commentary
Few human studies examine the effects of basil for medicinal purposes. One study showed significant reductions in blood glucose levels, which led the investigators to comment on basil's usefulness in the treatment of type 2 diabetes (Agrawal et al., 1996). Although the results of this small study are suggestive, they have not yet been duplicated in a large, controlled trial. Claims of efficacy in other diseases have not been substantiated in human trials.

References
Agrawal, P., et al. "Randomized Placebo Controlled, Single-blind Trial of Holy Basil Leaves in Patients with Non-Insulin-Dependent Diabetes Mellitus," *Int J Clin Pharmacol Ther* 34:406-9, 1996.

Akhtar, M.S., et al. "Antiulcerogenic Effects of *Ocimum basilicum* Extracts, Volatile Oils and Flavonoid Glycosides in Albino Rats," *Int J Pharmacognosy* 30:97-104, 1992.

Brinker, F. *The Toxicology of Botanical Medicines,* rev. 2nd ed. Sandy, Ore.: Eclectic Medicinal Publications, 1996.

Dey, B.B., and Chaundhuri, M.A. "Essential Oil of *Ocimum sanctum* and Its Antimicrobial Activity," *Indian Perfum* 28:82-86, 1984.

Singh, S., and Agrawal, S.S. "Antasthmatic and Anti-inflammatory Activity of *Ocimum sanctum,*" *Int J Pharmacognosy* 29:306-10, 1991.

Singh, S., and Majumdar, D.K. "Analgesic Activity of *Ocimum sanctum* and Its Possible Mechanism of Action," *Int J Pharmacognosy* 33:188-92, 1995.

BAY

BAY LAUREL, BAY LEAF, BAY TREE, SWEET BAY

Taxonomic class
Lauraceae

Common trade names
Various manufacturers provide the entire leaf or crushed leaves as a condiment. No medicinal products are known.

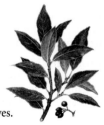

Common forms
Available as berries, essential oils, extracts, and leaves.

Source
Leaves and berries of *Laurus nobilis,* a small tree native to the Mediterranean, are commonly used to obtain bay. Another species of bay tree grows in California; its product is more bitter and used primarily for extracts.

Chemical components

The volatile oil contains alpha-pinene, camphene, cineole, eugenol, geraniol, limonene, linalool, phenylhydrazine, piperidine, and sabinene. Other constituents include boldine, catechins, costunolide, isodomesticine, launobine, laurenobiolide, nandergine, neolitsine, proanthocyanidins, and reticuline.

Actions

Eugenol acts as a sedative in rodents. Cineole has shown antibacterial activity against *Vibrio parahaemolyticus*. In mice, costunolide has had a hepatic microsomal enzyme inductive effect on liver glutathione s-transferase enzyme (Wada et al., 1997). Other studies with mice suggest chemotherapeutic effects (Rao and Hashim, 1995). Aqueous extracts of *L. nobilis* seeds reportedly demonstrated antiulcerative properties in experiments of ethanol-induced gastric injury of rat models (Afifi et al., 1997). Other rat studies suggest that methanolic extracts of bay may slow gastric emptying (Matsuda et al., 1999).

Reported uses

Because of the plant's strong aromatic qualities, herbalists claim that bay leaves are useful for common colds. Additional claims include the use of bay as an antirheumatic, a diuretic, and a stimulant. Bay is a common ingredient in natural toothpastes because of its purported antiseptic properties. Extracted oil has been used to treat muscle sprains and strains.

Dosage

The leaves are most commonly used to season foods and, if whole, are typically removed before consumption. Bay leaves should be thoroughly dried and crushed before ingestion. Bay extracts have been applied topically or used in baths and soaks.

Adverse reactions

GI: GI impaction, *perforation.*
Respiratory: *asthma.*
Skin: contact dermatitis.

Interactions

Insulin: Increased hypoglycemic actions (bay leaf extract). Monitor concomitant use carefully.

Contraindications and precautions

Avoid use in pregnant or breast-feeding patients.

Special considerations

• Caution the patient that the essential oil from bay leaves should not be consumed because of the risk of allergic reaction and asthma attack.
🔊 **ALERT** Bay leaves are largely indigestible, have sharp serrated edges, and should not be consumed intact. The leaves can become lodged in the esophagus or intestines and often require surgical removal (Panzer, 1983).

- Urge the diabetic patient to closely monitor blood glucose levels.
- Caution the patient not to ingest whole, intact bay leaves.
- Advise the female patient to avoid using bay during pregnancy or breast-feeding.

Points of interest
- Bay increases insulin's effects more than threefold and, therefore, nutritionists recommend it to diabetic patients.

Commentary
Bay leaf is a popular seasoning, but no therapeutic claim for treating diabetes or other diseases can be clinically verified.

References
Afifi, F.U., et al. "Evaluation of Gastroprotective Effect of *Laurus nobilis* Seeds on Ethanol Induced Gastric Ulcer in Rats," *J Ethnopharmacol* 58(1):9-14, 1997.

Hausen, B.M., and Hjorth, N. "Skin Reactions to Topical Food Exposure," *Dermatol Clin* 2:567-78, 1984.

Matsuda, H., et al. "Preventive Effects of Sesquiterpenes from Bay Leaf on Blood Ethanol Elevation in Ethanol-loaded Rat: Structure Requirement and Suppression of Gastric Emptying," *Bioorg Med Chem Lett* 20:9(18):2647-52, 1999.

Panzer, P.E. "The Dangers of Cooking with Bay Leaves," *JAMA* 250:164-65, 1983. Letter.

Rao, A.R., and Hashim, S. "Chemopreventive Action of Oriental Food-Seasoning Spices Mixture Garam Masala on DMBA-Induced Transplacental and Translactational Carcinogenesis in Mice," *Nutr Cancer* 23:91-101, 1995.

Wada, K., et al. "Inductive Effects of Bay Leaf and Its Component Costunolide on the Mouse Liver Glutathione S-Transferase," *Fac Natural Medicines* 51:283-85, 1997.

BAYBERRY

CANDLEBERRY, MYRICA, SOUTHERN WAX MYRTLE, SPICEBUSH, SWEET OAK, TALLOW SHRUB, VEGETABLE TALLOW, WAXBERRY, WAX MYRTLE PLANT

Taxonomic class
Myricaceae

Common trade names
Bayberry Bark

Common forms
Available as capsules (450 mg, 475 mg), extract, liquid, and tea.

Source
Bayberry is native to Texas and the eastern United States. Medicinal extracts are usually obtained from the dried root bark of *Myrica cerifera*.

Chemical components
Various portions of the bayberry plant are rich in tannins. Other compounds include the triterpenes myricadiol, taraxerol, and taraxerone

---

Bold italic type indicates that reaction may be life-threatening.

and the flavonoid glycoside myricitrin. Gum, starch, and an acrid astringent resin also occur. Bayberry wax contains lauric, myristic, and palmitic acid esters.

Actions
The pharmacokinetics of bayberry are incompletely known. Some data suggest that myricadiol exerts mineralocorticoid activity. Myricitrin may stimulate the secretion of bile. Dried bayberry root is reported to possess antibiotic, antipyretic, and emetic effects (Paul et al., 1974). The high tannin content of bayberry bark gives the herb its astringent properties.

Reported uses
Bayberry in tea preparations is claimed to be useful as an antidiarrheal, an agent for jaundice, an emetic, a gargle for sore throats, a stimulant, and a topical agent to promote wound healing.

Dosage
No consensus exists. Many references suggest consumption as a tea.
Liquid extract (1:1 in 45% alcohol): 0.6 to 2 ml P.O. t.i.d.

Adverse reactions
EENT: allergic rhinitis.
GI: gastric irritation, vomiting.
Hepatic: hepatic damage (may relate to tannin content).
Other: *hypersensitivity reactions* (Jacinto et al., 1992).

Interactions
Antihypertensives: Large doses may cause mineralocorticoid effects (sodium and water retention); hypotensive effects are antagonized. Avoid using together.

Contraindications and precautions
Avoid ingestion of bayberry plant parts because of the high tannin content; tannins are known to cause GI irritation and hepatic damage. Bayberry is contraindicated in pregnant or breast-feeding patients; effects are unknown.

Special considerations
• Monitor the patient for weight gain and hypertension related to sodium and water retention.
• Monitor the patient for hypersensitivity reactions.
• Bayberry may be carcinogenic; data from studies using rodents are conflicting.
• Advise the female patient to avoid using bayberry during pregnancy or when breast-feeding.

Points of interest
• Bayberry is best known for its small, bluish white berries, from which the wax is extracted to make fragrances and candles.

Commentary

Little medical evidence exists to support therapeutic claims for bayberry. Hypersensitivity reactions from the pollen extract may limit its use. Bayberry's high tannin content precludes oral use because of the potential for gastric distress and hepatic damage.

References

Jacinto, C.M., et al. "Nasal and Bronchial Provocation Challenges with Bayberry (*Myrica cerifera*) Pollen Extract," *J Allergy Clin Immunol* 90:312-18, 1992.

Paul, B.D., et al. "Isolation of Myricadiol, Myriciatrin, Taraxerol, and Taxerone from *Myrica cerifera* Root Bark," *J Pharm Sci* 63:958-59, 1974.

BEARBERRY

ARCTOSTAPHYLOS, BEARSGRAPE, CROWBERRY, FOXBERRY, HOGBERRY, KINNIKINNICK, MANZANITA, MOUNTAIN BOX, ROCKBERRY, UVA-URSI

Taxonomic class

Ericaceae

Common trade names

Multi-ingredient preparations: Arctuvan, Solvefort, Uroflux, Uvalyst

Common forms

Available as drops, tablets, and tea.

Source

The crude drug is obtained from the dry leaves (not berries) of the low, trailing evergreen shrub *Arctostaphylos uva-ursi* (also *Arctostaphylos coactylis* and *Arctostaphylos adenotricha*).

Chemical components

Leaves contain hydroquinone derivatives (mainly arbutin), hydroquinone monoglucoside, and small amounts of methylarbutin. Other compounds include arbutin gallic acid ester, gallotannin, iridoid glycoside monotropein, paracoumaric flavonoids, piceoside, phenol carboxylic acids (mainly gallic), syringic acids, and triterpenes.

Actions

Bearberry contains 5% to 15% arbutin, which hydrolyzes when ingested and releases hydroquinone (Jahodar et al., 1978). Hydroquinone is the principal antiseptic and astringent constituent of the plant (Turi et al., 1997). Isoquercetin (a flavonoid pigment) and ursolic acid (a triterpene derivative) contribute to the diuretic action of the extract. Evidence in rats suggests that this effect is minimal.

One study in mice indicated that bearberry may counter the symptoms of diabetes, particularly weight loss, without affecting glycemic control (Swanston-Flatt et al., 1989). A Japanese study reports that bearberry increases the inhibitory effect of dexamethasone, indomethacin, and prednisolone in inflammatory and allergic responses (Matsuda et

---

Bold italic type indicates that reaction may be life-threatening.

al., 1992). Antityrosinase activity has been described with some constituents of bearberry (Matsuo et al., 1997).

Reported uses

Bearberry is claimed to be modestly effective as a diuretic and urinary tract antiseptic. It has also been used as a diuretic in veterinary medicine.

Dosage

Doses of 1 to 10 g P.O. daily have been suggested. Doses as high as 20 g have been reported with no adverse effects, but CNS toxicity may appear in some patients from as little as 1 g.

Adverse reactions

GI: nausea, vomiting.
GU: green-colored urine.
Skin: cyanosis.

Interactions

Diuretics: Increased electrolyle loss. Avoid administration with bearberry.
Urinary acidifiers (ascorbic acid, methenamine): Inactivation of bearberry in urine. Avoid administration with bearberry.

Contraindications and precautions

Avoid using bearberry in pregnant or breast-feeding patients; effects are unknown. Use cautiously in patients taking diuretics; bearberry may promote electrolyte disturbances.

Special considerations

● Alert laboratory technicians conducting urinalyses that the patient's urine may be green because of the effects of bearberry.
● Advise the patient that traditional diuretics should be considered over the use of bearberry.
● Taken in large doses (more than 20 g as a single dose), bearberry may cause CV collapse, seizures, tinnitus, and vomiting.
● Caution the patient taking diuretics that concomitant use of bearberry could lead to excessive electrolyte loss and may increase the likelihood of CV collapse, dizziness, muscle cramps, palpitations, and weakness.
● Advise the patient that his urine may turn green.
● Advise women to avoid using bearberry during pregnancy or when breast-feeding.

Points of interest

● Urine must have an alkaline pH before bearberry can act as a urinary tract antiseptic.

Commentary

Inadequate data prevent the recommendation of bearberry for any disease state. Further study of this agent and its constituents is needed; bearberry may have potential as an anti-inflammatory or a weak diuretic.

References

Jahodar, L., et al. "Investigation of Iridoid Substances in *Arctostaphylos uva-ursi*," *Pharmazie* 33:536-37, 1978.

Matsuda, H., et al. "Effects of Water Extract From *Arctostaphyllos uva-ursi* on the Antiallergic and Anti-inflammatory Activities of Dexamethasone Ointment," *Yakugaku Zasshi* 112:73-77, 1992. Abstract.

Matsuo, K, et al. "Anti-tyrosinase Activity Constituents of *Arctostaphylos uva-ursi*," *Yakugaku Zasshi* 117(2):1028-32, 1997.

Swanston-Flatt, S.K., et al. "Evaluation of Traditional Plant Treatments for Diabetes: Studies in Streptozocin Diabetic Mice," *Acta Diabetol Lat* 26:51-55, 1989.

Turi, M., et al. "Influence of Aqueous Extracts of Medicinal Plants on Surface Hydrophobicity of *E. coli* Strains of Different Origin," *APMIS* 105:956-62, 1997. Abstract.

BEE POLLEN

BUCKWHEAT POLLEN, MAIZE POLLEN, PINE POLLEN, POLLEN PINI, PUHUANG, RAPE POLLEN, SONGHUAFEN, TYPHA POLLEN

Common trade names
Multi-ingredient preparations: Aller G Formula 25

Common forms
Capsules: 500 mg, 1,000 mg
Granules: 300 mg
Tablets: 500 mg, 1,000 mg
    Also available as candy bars, liquid, and wafers.

Source
Bee pollen consists of flower pollen and nectar, mixed with digestive enzymes (saliva) from worker honeybees (*Apis mellifera*). It is harvested at a beehive entrance as bees travel through a wire mesh, which forces them to brush their legs against a collection vessel. Commercial quantities of pollen can be obtained directly from flowers.

Chemical components
Bee pollen consists of carbohydrates; essential fatty acids, comprising largely alpha-linolenic and linoleic acids; minerals; and protein. It also contains small amounts of B complex vitamins, vitamin C, and various amino acids, coenzymes, enzymes, and hormones.

Actions
Many nutrients occur in concentrated amounts in bee pollen. Bioflavonoids, for example, function as strong antioxidants within the body and can reduce cholesterol, strengthen and stabilize capillaries, reduce inflammation, and act as antiallergens, antihistamines, and antivirals.

    The effects of bee pollen extract on acetaminophen toxicity in rats were studied. Researchers concluded that early intervention with bee pollen (within 1 hour) could potentially increase survival. All untreated

---

Bold italic type indicates that reaction may be life-threatening.

rats died within 24 hours; many of the rats that received bee pollen survived 72 hours or longer.

The results of other in vitro tests suggest that bee pollen bioflavonoids may exert antioxidant activity and promote the detoxification of metabolically stressed cells.

Reported uses
Bee pollen is claimed to be useful for treating allergies, asthma, and impotence. Because of its antioxidant properties, bee pollen is also claimed to be useful for lowering the risk of cancer and heart disease. Cholesterol- and triglyceride-lowering effects of bee pollen have prompted its use for atherosclerosis, hemorrhoids, hypertension, varicose veins, and various circulatory problems.

Bee pollen has been suggested as a treatment for prostatitis and other inflammatory conditions as well. No clinical studies exist to support these claims.

Dosage
Most sources suggest 500 to 1,000 mg P.O. t.i.d. 30 minutes before meals.

Adverse reactions
Other: *allergic reactions*, ranging from self-limiting nausea and vomiting to ***anaphylaxis*** (Broadhurst, 1997).

Interactions
Insulin, other antidiabetics: May promote hyperglycemia in diabetics. Avoid administration with bee pollen.

Contraindications and precautions
Bee pollen is contraindicated in patients with a history of atopy or an allergy to pollen or plant products because of the risk of hypersensitivity reactions. It is also contraindicated in diabetic patients.

Special considerations
- Refrigerate fresh pollen to maintain its quality.
- Imported pollens are often subject to sterilization techniques during customs inspections and, therefore, lack many enzymes and nutrients.
- Find out why the patient has been taking bee pollen.
- Advise the patient to consult a health care provider before using herbal preparations because a treatment that has been clinically researched and proven effective may be available.

Points of interest
- Bee pollen achieved renewed notoriety during the late 1970s after several famous athletes provided testimony on its behalf.
- Germany allows use of bee pollen as an appetite stimulant.

Commentary
The concept behind manipulating the immune response with bee pollen does not differ appreciably from the allopathic concept of an allergy shot. Both techniques introduce an allergen into the body, which stimu-

lates an immune response. The difference lies in the fact that because bee pollen must be taken orally (it is largely destroyed during digestion), a patient requires 10,000 times the amount of a typical injected-allergen challenge to elicit an immune response.

Bee pollen products are not standardized. The agent typically contains pollen from many kinds of plants. Pollen composition varies from week to week and hive to hive. This lack of standardization means that product efficacy varies from one dose to another.

The overall lack of scientific data for bee pollen mandates that therapeutic applications be avoided until appropriate studies are performed.

References

Broadhurst, L. *Information About Bee Pollen.* Botanical Medicine Conference. Philadelphia, 1997.

Griffith, H.W. "Bee Pollen," in *The Complete Guide to Vitamins, Minerals, and Supplements.* Tucson, Ariz.: Fisher Books, 1988.

BENZOIN

BENJAMIN TREE, BENZOE, BENZOIN TREE, GUM BENJAMIN, SIAM BENZOIN, SUMATRA BENZOIN

Taxonomic class
Styracaceae

Common trade names
Multi-ingredient preparations: Balsam of the Holy Victorious Knight, Friar's Balsam, Jerusalem Balsam, Pfeiffer's Cold Sore Preparation, Turlington's Balsam Of Life, Ward's Balsam

Common forms
Available as compound benzoin tincture USP, which contains 10% benzoin, 2% aloe, 8% storax, 4% tolu balsam, and 75% to 83% alcohol. Benzoin is also an ingredient in cold sore creams, lotions, and ointments.

Source
Benzoin is a balsamic resin usually obtained by wounding the bark of *Styrax benzoin* trees that are at least 7 years old. It can also be obtained from the bark of *Styrax paralleloneurus* and *Styrax tonkinensis*.

Chemical components
Sumatra benzoin (*S. benzoin*) is composed primarily of benzoic and cinnamic acids and their esters. It also contains small quantities of benzaldehyde, phenylpropyl cinnamate and benzyl cinnamate, styracin, styrene, and vanillin. Sumatra benzoin yields at least 75% of alcohol-soluble extract; Siam benzoin (*S. tonkinensis*) yields at least 90%. In the United States, either extract can be used in compound benzoin tincture.

Actions
Benzoin tinctures possess mild bactericidal properties, but the efficacy and spectrum of these properties are poorly described. Benzoin, which has a characteristic balsamic aroma, also has adhesive properties and mucosal protectant activity.

Reported uses
Benzoin has been used for more than 100 years, but most uses are anecdotal and have not been systematically studied. The agent has been applied topically as an antiseptic and a wound adhesive. A comparative trial of compound benzoin tincture and gum mastic found mastic to be a superior wound adhesive that was better tolerated than benzoin tincture (Lesesne, 1992). Benzoin tincture has been painted on the skin before applying adhesive tape for supportive dressings.

The American Dental Association accepts benzoin tincture as a topical mucosal protectant and for symptomatic relief of pain from canker sores, gingivitis, and oral herpetic lesions (Council on Dental Therapeutics, 1984).

Benzoin has been used in cough and cold products for its claimed expectorant properties. Compound benzoin tincture has been added to hot water to create a volatile steam inhalation, but this may be no more effective than unmedicated water vapor (Covington, 1993).

Dosage
For mucosal protection, in adults and children older than age 6 months, a few drops applied topically no more than once every 2 hours. The tincture should be used in infants only under medical supervision.
For steam inhalation, about 5 ml of compound benzoin tincture added to 1 pt of hot water. Alternatively, place the tincture on a handkerchief for inhalation.

Adverse reactions
GI: gastritis, *GI hemorrhage* if ingested (Arys and Awasthi, 1987).
Respiratory: *asthma* (inhalation).
Skin: contact dermatitis, urticaria.
Other: *allergic reactions.*

Interactions
None reported.

Contraindications and precautions
Inhalation of benzoin products is contraindicated in patients with reactive airway diseases, such as asthma. Benzoin is toxic if taken internally. (See *Gastritis from benzoin ingestion,* page 72.) Use products that contain benzoin cautiously in atopic patients or in those who are prone to contact dermatitis.

Special considerations
● Monitor closely for gastritis and GI hemorrhage in patients taking benzoin internally. Advise against oral consumption.

RESEARCH FINDINGS
Gastritis from benzoin ingestion

This case illustrates the need for patients to follow instructions.

A young man was prescribed compound benzoin tincture as inhalation therapy for symptomatic relief of acute bronchitis. The man mistakenly took the tincture—2 tsp b.i.d.—internally instead of by inhalation for 10 days.

He went to the hospital, complaining of gastric symptoms of increasing severity. His symptoms, including a low hemoglobin level and the presence of blood in his stools, were consistent with those that occur with significant blood loss. He was diagnosed with and treated for severe erosive gastritis (Arys and Awasthi, 1987) and recovered uneventfully.

• Monitor use of benzoin in infants closely.

🔴 **ALERT** Observe for signs and symptoms of allergic reaction, particularly in atopic patients.

• Inform the patient that topical use can discolor the skin and cause contact dermatitis.

• Advise the patient with asthma, atopy, or contact dermatitis to avoid using benzoin.

• Inform the patient that volatile steam inhalation of benzoin is not effective; unmedicated water vapor may be used instead.

Commentary

Most clinical data regarding the use of benzoin products come from case reports and a long history of use in numerous specialities. As a wound adhesive, alternative products are superior to benzoin (Lesesne, 1992). As a skin and mucosal protectant, other agents are at least as effective as benzoin and cause fewer allergic reactions (James, 1984). The inhalation of compound benzoin tincture has been used for many years but has never been systematically studied. Inhaled steam is probably at least as effective (Covington, 1993). Antiseptics with extensively studied effectiveness are preferred over benzoin tinctures. Health care providers should be aware of the potential risk of allergic reactions, especially in atopic patients.

References

Arys, T.V.S., and Awasthi, R. "Severe GI Haemorrhage Following Accidental Ingestion of Tincture Benzoin Compound," *J Assoc Physicians India* 35:805, 1987.

Council on Dental Therapeutics. *Accepted Dental Therapeutics,* 40th ed. Chicago: American Dental Association, 1984.

Covington, T.R., ed. *Handbook of Nonprescription Drugs,* 11th ed. Washington, D.C.: American Society of Hospital Pharmacists, 1993.

Bold italic type indicates that reaction may be life-threatening.

James, W.D. "Allergic Contact Dermatitis to Compound Tincture of Benzoin," *J Am Acad Dermatol* 11:847-50, 1984.

Lesesne, C.B. "The Postoperative Use of Wound Adhesives: Gum Mastic versus Benzoin USP," *J Dermatol Surg Oncol* 18:990, 1992.

BETEL PALM

ARECA NUT, BETAL, BETEL NUT, CHAVICA BETAL, HMARG, MAAG, MARG, PAAN, PAN MASALA, PAN PARAG, PINANG, SUPAI

Taxonomic class
Arecaceae

Common trade names
No known U.S. manufacturers. Betel nuts are sold under various names in ethnic grocery stores in the United States.

Common forms
Available as betel nuts, oil, and raw leaves.

Source
Betel palm is derived from the raw and sweetened leaves and nuts of *Areca catechu*, a member of the Arecaceae (Palmae) family. The plant is native to India, China, Indonesia, Sri Lanka, the Philippines, and various parts of Southeast Asia and Africa.

Chemical components
Several compounds have been identified in leaf and nut extract: arecaidine, arecaine, arecolidine, arecoline (an alkaloid related to tobacco alkaloids such as nicotine), betel-phenol, guvacine, and phenolic compounds. A volatile oil from the leaves contains allylpyrocatechol, cadinene, chaibetol, and chavicol.

Actions
Arecoline, a parasympathomimetic (cholinergic) and sympathomimetic agent, produces CNS and respiratory stimulation, elevated temperatures, and facial flushing. It also exerts mild psychoactive properties. Betel-phenol and chavicol are counterirritants and salivary stimulants. The dichloromethane fraction from *A. catechu* was found to inhibit MAO-A in the CNS of rats (Dar and Khatoon, 2000).

Reported uses
Only three drugs (caffeine, ethanol, and nicotine) are consumed more widely than betel. About 200 million people throughout the western Pacific basin, Southeast Asia, India, and Indonesia chew betel nuts and leaves. Betel is used as a mild stimulant and digestive aid. An oily extract of leaves that contain phenolic compounds is claimed to be useful for respiratory symptoms and as a gargle for sore throats and cough. Arecoline is a veterinary anthelmintic and cathartic.

Dosage
The betel nut is generally sweetened with lime (calcium hydroxide), wrapped in the leaf of the betel vine, and chewed, similar to the American habit of chewing tobacco. Chewing the "quid," as the chewing of betel nuts is called, can take as long as 15 minutes. Users may chew as many as 15 quids daily. Chewing betel leaves and betel nuts releases a highly variable quantity of arecoline.

Adverse reactions
CNS: CNS stimulation.
CV: facial flushing.
EENT: gingivitis, periodontitis (with prolonged use), red staining of teeth and oral cavity (with prolonged use).
Musculoskeletal: resorption of oral calcium and osteomyelitis (dentition; with prolonged use; related to lime).
Respiratory: *exacerbation of asthma.*
Other: fever.

Interactions
Alcoholic beverages, tobacco chewing: Increased risk of oral cancer. Avoid use with betel palm.
Antiglaucoma drugs: May increase or decrease effects. Monitor use of betel palm products in patients taking antiglaucoma drugs. Avoid administration with betel palm.
Atropine, propranolol: Abolishes temperature-elevating effects and increases CNS effects of arecoline. Avoid administration with betel palm (Chu, 1995).
Beta blockers, calcium channel blockers, digoxin: May increase heart rate–reducing effects. Avoid administration with betel palm.
MAO inhibitors, foods that contain tyramine (such as aged wine and cheese): Increased risk of hypertensive crisis. Discourage using together.

Contraindications and precautions
Arecaidine use, arecoline use, and betel chewing are contraindicated in patients who are prone to developing oral leukoplakia, fibrosis, or cancer, particularly cancer of the esophagus and squamous cell carcinoma. Avoid using betel palm products in pregnant or breast-feeding patients (Babu et al., 1996).

Special considerations
• Ask the patient of Asian or Indian descent regarding his use of this product; betel chewing may be a habit considered innocuous to him.
• When betel is chewed, there is copious production of blood-red saliva that can stain teeth and the oral mucosa. After years of chewing, the teeth can become stained reddish brown to black.
◤ **ALERT** Betel chewing may increase one's risk of developing type 2 diabetes. This was determined from examining anthropometric testing and glycemic control of 993 Bangladeshis (Mannan et al., 2000).

Bold italic type indicates that reaction may be life-threatening.

⬤ **Alert** Diarrhea, dizziness, nausea, seizures, and vomiting (with excessive chewing) similar to toxicity experienced from excessive nicotine use may occur (Ko et al., 1995; Merlidhar and Upmanyu, 1996).

• Monitor the patient for signs and symptoms of excessive autonomic stimulation, including blurred vision, bradycardia, cold sweats, constipation, cramps, diarrhea, fasciculations, GI stimulation, hallucinations, hypersalivation, hypertension, hyperthermia (sympathomimetic), miosis, mydriasis, pallor, tachycardia, voluntary muscle paralysis, and vomiting. The patient may present with a wide variety of these symptoms.

⬤ **Alert** Caution the patient about the risk of oral and esophageal cancers with prolonged oral use. In a large retrospective study, Pan masala (commercial preparation of areca nuts, lime, catechu, and other undisclosed ingredients) chewing has been directly linked to the development of oral submucous fibrosis, a premalignant state of the oral mucous membrane (Shah and Sherma, 1998).

• Caution the patient at risk for developing diabetes that betel ingestion may increase the risk.

• Advise women to avoid using betel products during pregnancy or when breast-feeding.

Commentary

Betel nut chewing in Asia and Indonesia has been compared with tobacco and alcohol use in the West; the substances are legal but potentially harmful. Chronic betel chewing may increase a person's risk of certain oral cancers and type 2 diabetes. An effort has been made in Canada to outlaw the importation of betel products but has been met with resistance (Huston, 1991). As with tobacco, there appears to be no appropriate medicinal use for betel.

References

Babu, S., et al. "Oral Fibrosis Among Teenagers Chewing Tobacco, Areca Nut, and Pan Masala," *Lancet* 348:692, 1996. Letter: Comment.

Chu, N.S. "Betel Chewing Increases the Skin Temperature: Effects of Atropine and Propranolol," *Neurosci Lett* 194:130-32, 1995.

Dar, A., and Khatoon, S. "Behavioral and Biochemical Studies of Dichloromethane Fraction from the *Areca catechu* Nut," *Pharmacol Biochem Behav* 65(1):1-6, 2000.

Huston, B. "Betel Nuts." Bureau of Food Regulatory, International and Intraagency Affairs, Health Canada. Field Compliance Guide. Citation 1991-01. Ottawa, Canada.

Ko, Y.C., et al. "Betel Quid Chewing, Cigarette Smoking and Alcohol Consumption Related to Oral Cancer in Taiwan," *J Oral Pathol Med* 24:450-53, 1995.

Mannan, N., et al. "Increased Waist Size and Weight in Relation to Consumption of *Areca catechu*; a Risk Factor for Increased Glycaemia in Asians in East London," *Br J Nutr* 83(3):267-75, 2000.

Merlidhar, V., and Upmanyu, G. "Tobacco Chewing, Oral Submucous Fibrosis and Anaesthetic Risk," *Lancet* 347:1840, 1996. Letter.

Shah, N., and Sharma, P.P. "Role of Chewing and Smoking Habits in the Etiology of Oral Submucous Fibrosis: A Case-control Study," *J Oral Pathol Med* 27(10):475-79, 1998.

BETH ROOT

BIRTHROOT, COUGHROOT, GROUND LILY, INDIAN BALM, INDIAN SHAMROCK, JEW'S-HARP PLANT, PURPLE TRILLIUM, SNAKEBITE, SQUAW ROOT, STINKING BENJAMIN, TRILLIUM, TRILLIUM PENDULUM, WAKE-ROBIN

Taxonomic class
Liliaceae

Common trade names
Multi-ingredient preparations: Trillium Complex

Common forms
Available as liquid extract, powder, and powdered root.

Source
The active agents of beth root are derived from the dried rhizomes, roots, and leaves of *Trillium erectum,* a low-lying perennial member of the lily family, which grows in Canada and eastern and central United States.

Chemical components
The chemical composition of *T. erectum* is not well documented. The plant is reported to contain tannic acids, oxalates, a cardiotonic glycoside similar to convallamarin, and a saponin called trillarin (a diglycoside of diosgenin). Diosgenin may be chemically converted to pregnenolone and progesterone.

Actions
Beth root is reported to have antiseptic, astringent, expectorant, local irritant, and tonic properties, probably because of its tannic acid content. The plant is also reported to act as a uterine stimulant, which may be attributed to the diosgenin component. (See *Origins of beth root names.*) Some components of other *Trillium* species have antifungal properties (Hufford et al., 1988).

Reported uses
Trillium Complex is used in Australia to treat menorrhagia. The dried rhizome is used by some herbalists as a uterine stimulant. Beth root is a popular cure for bleeding, skin irritations, and snakebite. It has been used as an antidiarrheal, an astringent to reduce topical irritation, and a tonic expectorant.

Dosage
Various dosages have been used, including 1 tbsp of powder in 1 pt of boiling water taken "freely in wineglassful doses," 1 dram of powdered root P.O. t.i.d., or 30 minims of liquid extract as an astringent or a tonic expectorant.

Bold italic type indicates that reaction may be life-threatening.

Adverse reactions
CV: potential *cardiotoxicity* (convallamarin-like glycoside).
GI: GI irritation, vomiting (oxalates and saponins).

Interactions
Antiarrhythmics (such as digitalis): May increase or antagonize effects of some antiarrhythmics. Avoid administration with beth root.

Contraindications and precautions
Avoid using beth root in pregnant patients because of reported uterine stimulant properties.

Special considerations
● Monitor for GI irritation and nausea. Treat symptomatically if these effects occur and consider discontinuation of beth root.
● Caution the patient taking drugs for a cardiac condition to avoid use of beth root because of its potential to influence cardiac function.
● Advise women to avoid using beth root during pregnancy.

Commentary
Beth root has been used as a folk remedy to promote parturition and control postpartum bleeding as well as to treat skin irritation, snakebites, and many other problems, but there is little clinical or scientific evidence to support these claims. The chemistry and dosage range of beth root have been poorly documented. Controlled animal and human studies are needed before beth root or its constituents can be considered medically useful.

References
Hufford, C.D., et al. "Antifungal Activity of *Trillium grandiflorum* Constituents," *J Nat Prod* 51:94-96, 1988.

BETONY

BISHOPSWORT, WOOD BETONY

Taxonomic class
Lamiaceae

Common trade names
Herb-a-Calm Formula, Herbagessic Formula, HerbVal Formula, Wood Betony

Common forms
Available as capsules and tea.

Source
Betony is derived from the flowers and leaves of *Stachys officinalis*. The plant grows in Europe, northern Africa, and Siberia.

Chemical components
Besides tannins (which constitute 15% of betony), betony contains betaine, betonicine, flavonoid glycosides, phenylethanoid glycosides, and stachydrine.

Actions
Studies in Russia suggest that some flavonoid glycosides in the plant can lower blood pressure. Tannins give the plant antidiarrheal and astringent properties. Some components of betony are toxic to some animals (Lipkan et al., 1974).

Reported uses
Folklore suggests many therapeutic applications for betony. Modern claims are made for its use in asthma, bronchitis, diarrhea, heartburn, palpitations, renal disease, roundworm infestation, seizures, stomachaches, toothaches, wounds, and more. Modern scientific studies have failed to verify these claims.

Dosage
Betony is mostly taken as an infusion or a tea.

Adverse reactions
GI: GI irritation.
Hepatic: hepatic dysfunction.

Interactions
Antihypertensives: Increased hypotensive effects. Avoid administration with betony.

Contraindications and precautions
Betony is contraindicated in pregnant patients because of the risk of uterine stimulation.

Bold italic type indicates that reaction may be life-threatening.

Special considerations
● Advise the patient to use betony cautiously because its high tannin content may cause hepatic dysfunction and GI discomfort.
● Caution the patient not to self-treat symptoms of illness before receiving appropriate medical evaluation because this may delay diagnosis of a serious medical condition.
● Advise the patient to consult a health care provider before using herbal preparations because a treatment that has been clinically researched and proved effective may be available.
● Advise women to avoid using betony during pregnancy.

Commentary
Despite various claims, available evidence does not support the use of betony for any therapeutic application.

References
Lipkan, G.N., et al. "Primary Evaluation of the Overall Toxicity and Anti-inflammatory Activity of Some Plant Preparations," *Farm Zh* 1:78-81, 1974.

BILBERRY

BILBERRIES, BOG BILBERRIES, EUROPEAN BLUEBERRIES, HUCKLEBERRY, WHORTLEBERRY

Taxonomic class
Ericaceae

Common trade names
Bilberry Extract, Bilberry Vegicap

Common forms
Available as capsules (60 mg, 80 mg, 120 mg, 450 mg), liquid extract, tincture, and dried roots, leaves, and berries.

Source
The active components of bilberry are extracted from *Vaccinium myrtillus* by a drying process. On occasion, a hydroalcoholic extraction of the leaf is prepared.

Chemical components
Bilberry extracts are composed of about 25% anthocyanosides, 1.5% to 10% tannins, and small percentages of flavonoids, plant acids, and pectins. There are more than 15 naturally occurring anthrocyanosides in bilberry.

Actions
The pharmacokinetics of *V. myrtillus* anthocyanosides (VMA) or *V. myrtillus* extract (VME) has been studied in male rats. VMA is thought to undergo both renal and biliary elimination (Morazzoni et al., 1991). The anthocyanosides are thought to be the active components, producing reductions in vascular permeability and tissue edema in some ani-

mals. Studies with animals suggest that VME decreases vascular permeability by interacting with collagen in vascular epithelium.

VMA also is thought to aid microvascular blood flow by intensifying arteriolar rhythmic diameter changes. Leaf extracts reduced serum triglyceride levels in diabetic rats immediately after feeding, possibly through increased triglyceride lipoprotein catabolism.

The results of an in vitro study indicate that VME exerts potent antioxidant effects and a protective effect on LDLs (Laplaud et al., 1997).

Studies with animals have shown that anthocyanosides speed up regeneration of visual purple in the retina, allowing better adaptation to darkness and light (Alfieri and Sole, 1964). Anthocyanosides decrease excessive platelet aggregation in rat models (Morazzoni and Magistretti, 1986). The anthocyanoside myrtillin in bilberry causes hypoglycemia, although the mechanism is unclear. In rats, bilberry anthocyanosides exert preventive and curative antiulcerative actions (Criston and Magistretti, 1986).

Reported uses
Bilberry is claimed to be useful in treating visual and circulatory problems. A human study conducted in the 1960s concluded that it had a positive effect on night vision in normal subjects (Jayle et al., 1965). Anecdotally, bilberry has also been used to treat cataracts, diabetic retinopathy, glaucoma, hemorrhoids, macular degeneration, and varicose veins. One study failed to prove a role for bilberry in improving night visual acuity. (See *Bilberry extract and night blindness*.)

Dosage
The dosage of bilberry varies considerably; standardized products consisting of 25% anthocyanoside content should be used.
For circulatory and visual problems, 240 to 480 mg P.O. in divided doses b.i.d. or t.i.d.
To improve night vision, 60 to 120 mg of bilberry extract P.O. daily.

Adverse reactions
Hepatic: hepatic dysfunction (caused by tannin content).

Interactions
Anticoagulants, other antiplatelet drugs: Inhibition of platelet aggregation, increasing the risk of bleeding if used concurrently. Monitor the patient.
Disulfiram: Disulfiram-like reaction may occur if herbal product contains alcohol. Discourage using together.

Contraindications and precautions
Bilberry is contraindicated in pregnant or breast-feeding patients. Use cautiously in patients taking anticoagulants and in those with diabetes.

Special considerations
• Caution the patient not to self-treat symptoms of circulatory or visual disturbances before receiving appropriate medical evaluation because this may delay diagnosis of a serious medical condition.

Bold italic type indicates that reaction may be life-threatening.

RESEARCH FINDINGS
Bilberry extract and night blindness

A double-blind, placebo-controlled crossover study was conducted to assess the effects of bilberry extract (25% anthocyanosides) on night visual acuity and night contrast sensitivity. The trial involved 15 men with good vision, who received bilberry extract, 160 mg three times a day, or placebo for 21 days followed by a 1-month wash-out period. Night visual acuity and night contrast sensitivity were measured throughout the study. The results indicated no difference between the group given the bilberry extract and the group given the placebo (Muth et al., 2000).

• Advise the patient to consult a health care provider before using herbal preparations because a treatment that has been clinically researched and proved effective may be available.

⚫ ALERT Monitor for toxic reactions. Long-term consumption of large doses of bilberry leaves can be poisonous. Dosages of 1.5 g/kg/day or higher may be fatal.

• Monitor the patient for signs and symptoms of bleeding if he is also taking an anticoagulant.

• Caution the patient taking disulfiram not to take liquid extracts or tinctures that contain alcohol.

Points of interest
• During World War II, British pilots ingested bilberry preserves to enhance their night vision. Native Americans used bilberry teas and tinctures to treat symptoms of diabetes.

Commentary
The use of bilberry extracts for treating vascular leakage and edema appears intriguing, but inadequate human clinical trial data exist to substantiate efficacy in this area. Studies seem to indicate that the anecdotal reports that bilberry can improve night vision are unfounded. Little is known regarding the toxicity profile of bilberry, except that dosages that exceed 480 mg daily may be dangerous.

References
Alfieri, R., and Sole, P. "Influence des anthocyanosides adminstres par voie parenteraler sur l'adaptoelectroretinogramme du lapin," *CR Soc Biol* 158:2338, 1964.

Criston, A., and Magistretti, M.J. "Antiulcer and Healing Activity of *V. myrtillus* Anthocyanosides," *Il Farmacio* 42:29-43, 1986.

Jayle, G.E., et al. "Study Concerning the Action of Anthocyanoside Extracts of *Vaccinium myrtillus* on Night Vision," *Ann Ocul* (Paris) 198:56-62, 1965.

Laplaud, P.M., et al. "Antioxidant Action of *Vaccinium myrtillus* Extract on Human Low Density Lipoproteins In Vitro: Initial Observations," *Fundam Clin Pharmacol* 11:35-40, 1997. Abstract.

Morazzoni, P., and Magistretti, M.J. "Effects of *V. myrtillus* Anthocyanosides on Prostacyclin-like Activity in Rat Arterial Tissue," *Fitoterapia* 57:11-14, 1986.

Morazzoni, P., et al. "*Vaccinium myrtillus* Anthocyanosides Pharmacokinetics in Rats," *Arzneimittelforschung* 41:128-31, 1991.

Muth, E.R., et al. "The Effect of Bilberry Nutritional Supplementation on Night Visual Acuity and Contrast Sensitivity," *Altern Med Rev* 5(2):164-73, 2000.

BIRCH

BIRCH TAR OIL, BIRCH WOOD OIL, BLACK BIRCH, CHERRY BIRCH, SWEET BIRCH OIL, WHITE BIRCH

Taxonomic class
Betulaceae

Common trade names
None known.

Common forms
Available as dried bark, essential oil (bark, wood), and tea.

Source
Active compounds of birch are derived from the dried bark and twigs of the birch species *Betula alba (Betula pendula), Betula verrucosa, Betula pubescens,* and *Betula lenta.* Several birch species are native to eastern North America, Europe, and parts of Russia.

Chemical components
Distillation of the bark of *B. alba* yields betulin, birch tar oil, creosol, cresol, guaiacol, isomeric hydrocarbons, phenol, pyrocatechol, turpentine oil, and xylenol. Avicularin, flavonoids, galactosyl-3 myricetol, glucuronyl-3 quercetol, hyperoside, and quercetin occur in the dried leaves. Sweet birch oil is produced by steam distillation of the water-softened bark of *B. lenta.* Methyl salicylate is liberated in the process. Sweet birch oil is composed almost entirely of methyl salicylate.

Actions
Methyl salicylate has analgesic, anti-inflammatory, and antipyretic properties. Hemostatic function in animals is affected by the thromboplastic agents presumably found in *B. pendula.* The mechanism of action resembles that of human tissue thromboplastin (Kudriashov et al., 1986). In other animal studies, birch has been shown to exert diuretic properties (Bisset, 1994).

Reported uses
Claims for birch include relief of headaches and other analgesic effects as well as treatment of various acute and chronic skin disorders, GI disorders, and kidney stones. Essential oils are claimed to act against bladder infections, gout, neuralgias, rheumatism, and tuberculous cervical lymphadenitis. In veterinary medicine, essential oil of birch wood has been used to treat various skin diseases (Budavari et al., 1996).

Bold italic type indicates that reaction may be life-threatening.

Dosage
Extracts or teas can be made by steeping 2 to 3 g of the bark in boiling water for 10 to 15 minutes; the infusion may be ingested several times daily.

Adverse reactions
Skin: acute contact dermatitis.
EENT: allergic rhinitis.
Other: cross-sensitization with other plant allergens, such as celery and mugwort pollen (Vallier et al., 1988).

Interactions
None reported.

Contraindications and precautions
Birch is contraindicated in pregnant or breast-feeding patients. Use cautiously in patients with seasonal allergic rhinitis or hypersensitivity to plant allergens.

Special considerations
• Monitor for signs and symptoms of allergic reaction, particularly in patients with allergies to celery, mugwort, or other plants.
🔺 **ALERT** Caution the patient to keep birch preparations out of the reach of children. Sweet birch oil is composed of 98% methyl salicylate, which can be fatal to children when applied topically to the skin. Poisonings have been reported with as little as 4.7 g of methyl salicylate applied topically.
• Advise the patient that topical preparations may irritate the skin and mucous membranes. Encourage him to report new or unusual dermatologic manifestations.
• Advise women to avoid using birch products during pregnancy or when breast-feeding.

Points of interest
• Betulin is being evaluated for its antitumorigenic properties.
• In Germany, leaves of *B. pendula* are used as a diuretic during irrigation therapy for urinary tract infections.

Commentary
Chemical compositions from birch possess some interesting properties. However, until more clinical research becomes available, these agents have no role in modern medicine. The risk of hypersensitivity reactions makes OTC use a cause for concern.

References
Bisset, N.G., ed. *Herbal Drugs and Phytopharmaceuticals.* Boca Raton, Fla.: CRC Press, 1994.
Budavari, S., et al., eds. *The Merck Index*, 12th ed. Whitehouse Station, N.J.: Merck and Co., Inc., 1996.
Kudriashov, B.A., et al. "Hemostatic System Function as Affected by Thromboplastic Agents from Higher Plants," *Nauchnye Doki Vyss Shkoly Biol Nauki* 4:58-61, 1986.

Lahti, A., and Hannuksela, M. "Immediate Contact Allergy to Birch Leaves and Sap," *Contact Dermatitis* 6:464-65, 1980.

Vallier, P., et al. "A Study of Allergens in Celery with Cross-Sensitivity to Mugwort and Birch Pollens," *Clin Allergy* 18:491-500, 1988.

BISTORT

ADDERWORT, COMMON BISTORT, EASTER LEDGES, EASTER MANGIANT, KNOTWEED, ODERWORT, OSTERICK, PATIENCE DOCK, SNAKEROOT, SNAKEWEED, TWICE WRITHEN

Taxonomic class
Polygonaceae

Common trade names
None known.

Common forms
Available as a dried or cut root, powder, or tea.

Source
Different folk cultures use different parts of *Polygonum bistorta,* a member of the buckwheat family. Rhizomes and roots are most prized and gathered in the fall. Leaves are gathered in the spring. Bistort is native to Europe and naturalized in North America.

Chemical components
There have been reports that *P. bistorta* contains phenolic compounds. Aqueous extracts are rich in tannins (Duwiejua et al., 1994). Rhizomes and roots contain flavonoids, gallic acid, phlobaphene, starch, and a trace of emodin, an anthraquinone.

Actions
The pharmacokinetics of bistort have not been studied. Bistort is one of the strongest botanical astringents known. In a study with rats, bistort significantly inhibited acute and chronic phases of adjuvant and carrageenan-induced inflammation (Duwiejua et al., 1994). This effect has not been confirmed in human trials.

Reported uses
Extracts of underground plant parts have long been used to stop external and internal bleeding. Bistort has been used externally for hemorrhoids, insect bites, measles, snakebites, and small burns or wounds; as a mouthwash or gargle for canker sores, gum problems, laryngitis, and sore throat; and to reduce pulmonary secretions.

Internally, bistort has been used to treat dysentery, gastric and pulmonary hemorrhage, irritable bowel syndrome, jaundice, peptic ulcers, and ulcerative colitis. It has also been used as an anthelmintic, an antidote for certain poisons, and a douche for excessive vaginal discharge or bleeding.

The 1983 British Herbal Pharmacopoeia reports that bistort exerts an

---

Bold italic type indicates that reaction may be life-threatening.

anti-inflammatory activity and lists it as useful in treating diarrhea in children.

Dosage
Some sources recommend that 1 tsp of the powdered root can be combined with 1 to 1½ cups of boiling water and taken P.O. for diarrhea. More than 3 cups daily is not recommended.

Adverse reactions
GI: GI irritation.
Hepatic: hepatic dysfunction.

Interactions
None reported.

Contraindications and precautions
Avoid using bistort in pregnant or breast-feeding patients; effects are unknown.

Special considerations
- Monitor the patient for signs and symptoms of GI irritation.
- Monitor liver function test results for signs of hepatic dysfunction.
- Caution the patient not to take bistort internally for longer than a few weeks at a time.
- Advise women to avoid using bistort during pregnancy or when breast-feeding.

Points of interest
- The rhizome of bistort is rich in starch and has been roasted and eaten as a vegetable.

Commentary
Bistort may have practical value as an astringent for poultices. Its antarthritic and anti-inflammatory properties appear promising. Overall, bistort has significant anecdotal data but few scientific studies supporting its use. The lack of scientific trials for any of the therapeutic claims should limit bistort use until such clinical trials can define more precisely bistort's role in modern medicine.

References
British Herbal Pharmacopoeia, consolidated ed. London: British Herbal Medicine Association, 1983.

Duwiejua, M., et al. "Anti-inflammatory Activity of *Polygonum bistorta, Guaiacum officinale,* and *Hamamelis virginiana* in Rats," *J Pharm Pharmacol* 46:286-90, 1994.

BITTER MELON

BITTER GOURD

Taxonomic class
Cucurbitaceae

Common trade names
None known.

Common forms
Available in a decoction or tincture and as juice or a whole fruit.

Source
Bitter melon is derived from the tropical tree *Momordica charantia*, which is native to Asia, East Africa, South America, and parts of the Caribbean. Seeds, vines, and leaves are used medicinally, but the fruit of the tree is most commonly used and generally thought to be the safest.

Chemical components
Bitter melon contains the proteins alpha- and beta-momorcharin, along with serine protease inhibitors BGIA (bitter gourd inhibitor against amino acid–specific proteins) and BGTI (bitter gourd trypsin inhibitor). Also present is the plant protein MAP30; charantin, which is a mixture of steroidal saponins; and insulin-like peptides and alkaloids.

Actions
Recombinant MAP30 has been shown to inhibit HIV-1 and to have antitumorigenic effects with no untoward effects on normal human cells (Lee-Huang et al., 1995). MAP30 also may enhance the activity of dexamethasone and indomethacin as weak HIV antagonists by causing inactivation of viral DNA and specific cleavage of 28 S ribosomal RNA (Bourinbaiar and Lee-Huang, 1995).

A crude extract of bitter melon was reported to be both cytostatic and cytotoxic to human leukemic lymphocytes and yet had no harmful effect on normal human lymphocytes in vitro (Takemoto et al., 1982). These effects were observed within 2 hours, and the researchers theorize that the effect may result from quick entrance of the factor into the cells.

A later study in mice led to the conclusion that the antileukemic properties exhibited by bitter melon may be caused, at least in part, by the activation of natural killer cells in the host (Cunnick et al., 1990).

Reported uses
Bitter melon has been used as a food substance and to treat cancer, diabetes, and some types of infections. Beer, soups, and teas have been made from both the leaves and the fruit. Wax produced by the berries has been used in candlemaking.

A 1981 study (Leatherdale et al.) measured the effect of a fruit extract of bitter melon on nine patients with type 2 diabetes. The extract was given and followed by a glucose tolerance test, which revealed an improvement in glucose tolerance that was small but possibly clinically significant. No increase in serum insulin levels was noted in these patients.

Dosage
The typical dose is one small unripe melon, the equivalent of about 50 ml of juice in divided doses b.i.d. or t.i.d. Up to 100 ml of the decoction or 5 ml of the tincture may be consumed daily, also in divided dos-

---

Bold italic type indicates that reaction may be life-threatening.

es. No dosing information for patients with renal or hepatic impairment is available.

Adverse reactions
GI: diarrhea, stomach pain (overdose).

Interactions
Antidiabetics: May cause additive effects, resulting in excessive hypoglycemia. Monitor blood glucose levels and patient closely.

Contraindications and precautions
Bitter melon is contraindicated in patients with hypoglycemia because it may exacerbate this condition, causing dangerously low blood glucose levels. It is also contraindicated in young children, who may be overly sensitive to the hypoglycemic effect. Avoid using bitter melon in women who are pregnant because alpha- and beta-momorcharin have abortifacient properties (Leung et al., 1987). Data regarding the use of bitter melon in women who are breast-feeding are lacking.

Special considerations
- No dosage form can effectively mask the extremely bitter taste of bitter melon and its preparations.
- Monitor the patient for adverse GI reactions because they may be signs of overdose.
- Monitor the patient's blood glucose levels if he is taking bitter melon for its hypoglycemic effect.

Commentary
The best-substantiated use for bitter melon is as an antidiabetic agent. Without clinical data on effective dosing and predictability of response, bitter melon should be used with care and probably not with other antidiabetic drugs until more is known about its potency. Bitter melon may show some value as adjunctive therapy for HIV-infected or leukemic patients in the future, but additional studies are needed to fully evaluate its efficacy and clinical relevance. Use of bitter melon as an anti-infective remains unsubstantiated.

References
Bourinbaiar, A.S., and Lee-Huang, S. "Potentiation of Anti-HIV Activity of Anti-inflammatory Drugs, Dexamethasone and Indomethacin, by MAP30, the Antiviral Agent from Bitter Melon," *Biochem Biophys Res Commun* 208(2):779-85, 1995.

Cunnick, J.E., et al. "Induction of Tumor Cytotoxic Immune Cells Using a Protein from the Bitter Melon *(Momordica charantia)*," *Cell Immunol* 126(2):278-89, 1990.

Leatherdale, B., et al. "Improvement in Glucose Tolerance Due to *Momordica charantia (karela)*," *Br Med J (Clin Res Ed)* 282(6279):1823-24, 1981.

Lee-Huang, S., et al. "Anti-HIV and Anti-tumor Activities of Recombinant MAP30 from Bitter Melon," *Gene* 161(2):151-56, 1995.

Leung, S., et al. "The Immunosuppressive Activities of Two Abortifacient Proteins Isolated from the Seeds of Bitter Melon," *Immunopharmacology* 13(3):159-71, 1987.

Takemoto, D.J., et al. "The Cytotoxic and Cytostatic Effects of the Bitter Melon *(Momordica charantia)* on Human Lymphocytes," *Toxicon* 20(3):593-99, 1982.

BITTER ORANGE

BIGARADE ORANGE, NEROLI

Taxonomic class
Rutaceae

Common trade names
Aurantii Amarai Cortex (USP)

Common forms
Available in liquid extracts, teas, and tinctures.

Source
Bitter orange is the fruit of the flowering evergreen *Citrus aurantium.* The tree is native to parts of Asia and cultivated to some extent in the Mediterranean region.

Chemical components
Bitter orange contains large amounts of the furanocoumarin oxypeuce-danin as well as hesperidin and neohesperidin.

Actions
One study (Kim et al., 2000) tested the fruit of bitter orange for an inhibitory effect against rotavirus and found that the component hesperidin had a 50% inhibitory concentration of 25 micromol/ml and that neohesperidin had a 50% inhibitory concentration of 10 micromol/ml.

Susceptibility testing has indicated that the peel oil extract of bitter orange may be effective as a mosquito larvae insecticide (Mwaiko, 1992).

Reported uses
Bitter orange has been used in Puerto Rico and other parts of the world as a sedative and to treat GI disorders.

One study (Ramadan et al., 1996) evaluated the efficacy of oil of bitter orange in treating superficial dermatophyte infections. Sixty patients with tinea corporis, tinea cruris, or tinea pedis were randomly divided into three equivalent groups. One group was treated with a 25% emulsion of oil of bitter orange three times daily, another group was treated with 20% oil in alcohol three times daily, and the third group received pure oil of bitter orange once daily. The 25% emulsion group showed cure rates of 80% in 1 to 2 weeks and 20% in 2 to 3 weeks. The 20% oil group showed cure rates of 50% in 1 to 2 weeks, 30% in 2 to 3 weeks, and 20% in 3 to 4 weeks. Twenty-five percent of patients in the pure oil group did not finish the study, and cure rates for the remaining patients

---

Bold italic type indicates that reaction may be life-threatening.

were 33.3% in 1 week, 60% in 1 to 2 weeks, and 6.7% in 2 to 3 weeks. Mild skin irritation was the only adverse reaction noted and was observed only with the pure oil treatment.

Dosage
No consensus exists.

Adverse reactions
CNS: headache, insomnia, nervousness.
EENT: sore throat.
GI: appetite loss, indigestion.
Musculoskeletal: gout.
Skin: photosensitivity, skin irritation with redness and swelling.

Interactions
None reported.

Contraindications and precautions
Avoid using bitter orange in pregnant or breast-feeding patients; effects are unknown.

Special considerations
● Oxypeucedanin can cause phototoxicity (Naganuma et al., 1985). Caution the patient to minimize exposure to the sun.
● Although no known chemical interactions have been reported in clinical studies, consideration must be given to the herbal product's pharmacologic properties and the potential for interference with the intended therapeutic effect of conventional drugs.
● Caution the patient not to self-treat symptoms of skin infections before receiving appropriate medical evaluation because this may delay diagnosis of a serious medical condition.
● Advise the patient to consult a health care provider before using herbal preparations because a treatment that has been clinically researched and proved effective may be available.

Points of interest
● Bitter orange is used as the flavoring for the liqueur curaçao.
● Bitter orange is less expensive than other treatments for superficial dermatophyte infection.

Commentary
The results of one study indicate that there is some promise for bitter orange as a topical antifungal (Ramadan et al., 1996). Additional trials are needed to determine the most appropriate dose and to properly evaluate adverse effects associated with this use. Further study is also needed to determine the efficacy and proper clinical role of bitter orange as a treatment for or protection against rotavirus infection. Other claims of clinical applications for bitter orange are unproven.

References

Kim, D., et al. "Inhibitory Effect of Herbal Medicines on Rotavirus Infectivity," *Biol Pharm Bull* 23(3):356-58, 2000.

Mwaiko, G. "Citrus Peel Oils as Mosquito Larvae Insecticides," *East Afr Med J* 69(4):223-26, 1992.

Naganuma, M., et al. "A Study of the Phototoxicity of Lemon Oil," *Arch Dermatol Res* 278(1):31-36, 1985.

Ramadan, W., et al. "Oil of Bitter Orange: New Topical Antifungal Agent," *Int J Dermatol* 35(6):448-49, 1996.

BLACK CATECHU

ACACIA CATECHU, ACACIA DI CACHOU, ACACIE AU CACHOU, AMARAJA, CAKE CATECHU, CATECHU, CUTCH, ERH-CH'A, HAI-ERH-CH'A, KADARAM, KATECHU AKAZIE, KATESU, KHAIR, PEGU KATECHU, WU-TIEH-NI

Taxonomic class
Fabaceae

Common trade names
Multi-ingredient preparations: Diarcalm, Élixir Bonjean, Enterodyne, Hemo Cleen, Katha, Shanti Bori (used in rural Bangladesh as a component of oral contraceptives), Spanish Tummy Mixture (may contain pale catechu or black catechu as replacement product)

Common forms
Available as a dry powder, in a dried extract or liquid for oral use (0.3 to 2 g), as a local injection for hemorrhoids, and as a tincture.

Source
The crude drug is prepared as a dried extract from the heartwood of *Acacia catechu*, a leguminous tree that is native to Burma and eastern India and naturalized in Jamaica. The extract is prepared by boiling heartwood pieces in water, evaporating this mixture to a syrup, and then cooling to molds. The dried molds are then broken into pieces.

Chemical components
A. catechu contains 20% to 35% catechutannic acid, 2% to 10% acacatechin, catechu-red (a flavonoid), quercetin, and gum.

Actions
No pharmacokinetic studies are known. Most animal studies, both in vivo and in vitro, suggest possible physiologic activities, but these activities are poorly described. Studies have suggested that the herb exerts hypoglycemic effects (Singh et al., 1976) and hypotensive effects (Sham et al., 1984) and may have antileukemic (Agrawal and Agrawal, 1990) and contraceptive activity (Azad Chowdhury et al., 1984).

Reported uses
A. catechu is claimed to be useful as a topical agent for sore gums and mouth ulcers. It is a powerful astringent and indicated in numerous countries (not including the United States) for treating diarrhea and other GI problems. This agent has been commonly used in India as an ointment for indolent ulcers and has been used in rural Bangladesh as a component of an antifertility pill (Azad Chowdhury et al., 1984). Other claims include arresting nosebleeds, assisting healing in nipple fissures, and acting as a contraceptive. In the late 1800s, chronic gonorrhea was treated with an infusion of catechu.

Dosage
Dried extract can be given in doses of 0.3 to 2 g P.O. or by infusion (tea). The tincture is given in doses of 2.5 to 5 ml of a 1:5 dilution in 45% alcohol.

Adverse reactions
CV: hypotension.
GI: constipation.

Interactions
Anticholinergics, opioid analgesics: Increases risk of constipation. Avoid administration with black catechu.
Antihypertensives: Increases risk of hypotension. Avoid administration with black catechu.
Captopril: Additive hypotensive effect of catechu (Sham et al., 1984). Avoid administration with black catechu.
Immunosuppressants: Increases risk of fungal infection. Avoid administration with black catechu.
Iron-containing products: May bind iron products and gelatin, creating an insoluble complex. Do not administer together.

Contraindications and precautions
Avoid using black catechu in pregnant or breast-feeding patients. Products of the catechu family are contraindicated in patients undergoing immunosuppressive therapy. This herb is also known as a dietary carcinogen (Morton, 1992).

Special considerations
• Long-term effects of chronic use of black catechu are unknown.
🔺 **ALERT** Inform the patient that unstandardized products may contain high amounts of inactive ash and fungal contaminants such as aflatoxin, a toxic metabolite of *Aspergillus* that is associated with certain cancers.
• Monitor blood pressure.
• Black catechu is incompatible with iron or zinc sulfate preparations (Pharmaceutical Society of Great Britain, 1979).
• Caution the patient taking anticholinergics, opioid analgesics, or other drugs known to cause significant constipation about the additive effects with catechu.

• Caution the patient about the risk of hypoglycemia, especially if he has diabetes.
• Inform the patient that catechu is not a clinically proven antifertility drug and thus should not replace conventional oral contraceptive therapy.
• Advise women to avoid using black catechu during pregnancy or when breast-feeding.

Points of interest
• Although *A. catechu* and pale catechu have the name catechu in common, pale catechu is a different plant—*Uncaria gambir,* a member of the Rubiaceae family—and used primarily in the dye industry and as a veterinary astringent.

Commentary
Black catechu products were popular both in the United States and abroad during the mid-1800s and early 1900s. The drug is used as an antidiarrheal and antifertility drug in some parts of the world. Human clinical trials are lacking, and few animal studies have been conducted. Clinical efficacy in chronic diarrhea has not been proved. Acute and chronic toxic effects are also unknown. Although this agent has been used in women with cracked nipples, it is unknown whether these patients were breast-feeding at the time. Although pharmacologically interesting, black catechu cannot be recommended for any ailment until more is known about its risks and benefits.

References
Agrawal, S., and Agrawal, S.S. "Preliminary Observations on Leukaemia-Specific Agglutinins from Seeds," *Indian J Med Res* 92:38-42, 1990.

Azad Chowdhury, A.K., et al. "Antifertility Activity of a Traditional Contraceptive Pill Comprising *Acacia catechu, A. arabica,* and *Tragia involuceria,*" *Indian J Med Res* 80:372-74, 1984.

Morton, J.F. "Widespread Tannin Intake via Stimulants and Masticatories, Especially Guarana, Kola Nut, Betel Vine, and Accessories," *Basic Life Sci* 59:739-65, 1992. Abstract.

Pharmaceutical Society of Great Britain, Department of Pharmaceutical Sciences, ed. *The Pharmaceutical Codex,* 11th ed. London: The Pharmaceutical Press, 1979.

Roy, A.K., et al. "Aflatoxin Contamination of Some Common Drug Plants," *Appl Environ Microbiol* 54:842-43, 1988.

Sham, J.S.K., et al. "Hypotensive Action of *Acacia catechu,*" *Planta Med* 50:177-80, 1984.

Singh, K.N., et al. "Hypoglycaemic Activity of *Acacia catechu, Acacia suma,* and *Albizzia odaratissima* Seed Diets in Normal Albino Rats," *Indian J Med Res* 64:754-57, 1976.

BLACK COHOSH

BLACK SNAKE ROOT, BANEBERRY, BUGBANE, BUGWORT, CIMICIFUGA, RATTLE ROOT, RATTLEWEED, SQUAW ROOT

Taxonomic class
Ranunculaceae

Bold italic type indicates that reaction may be life-threatening.

Common trade names
Agnukliman, Black Cohosh, Cefakliman mono, Cimisan, Cirkufemal, Femilla N, Feminon C, Klimadynon, Menofem, Remifemin

Multi-ingredient preparations: Biophylin, Bronchicough, Bronchicum, Bronchicum SB (FM), CX, Dong Quai Complex, Esten (FM), Estrocare, Estroven, Female Balance, Femisana N, Femtrol, GNC Menopause Formula, Harpagophytum Complex, Helonias Compound, Herbal PMS Formula, Husten-Tee Bronchiflux (FM), Iodocafedrina (FM), Lifesystem Herbal Formula 4 Womens's Formula, Ligvites, Medinat Esten, NewPhase, One-A-Day Menopause Health, Perpain (FM), PMT Complex, Proesten, Remifemin Plus, Salagesic, Super Mega B+C, Vegetable Cough Remover, Vegetex, Viburnum Complex, Women's Formula Herbal Formula 3

Common forms
Caplets: 40 mg, 400 mg, 420 mg
Capsules: 25 mg, 525 mg

Source
The crude drug is extracted primarily from the dried rhizomes and roots of *Cimicifuga racemosa (Actaea racemosa)*. Other sources include other *Cimicifuga* species and *Macrotys actaeoides*. These plants are native to eastern North America.

Chemical components
Several chemical compounds have been extracted from the black cohosh plant, including acteina, cimigoside, steroidal terpenes, and 27-deoxyactein (Berger et al., 1988). Other constituents include tannins, salicylic acid, and an isoflavone, formononetine.

Actions
Physiologic effects of black cohosh include vascular and estrogenic activity. The vascular action is attributed to acteina, which in animals produces a hypotensive effect through vagal nerve activity (Genazzani and Sorrentino, 1962).

Most research has focused on the plant's estrogenic activity. In studies with rats, active constituents of the plant were found to bind directly to estrogen receptors and suppress luteinizing hormone (LH) release (Jarry and Harnischfeger, 1985; Jarry et al., 1985; Duker et al., 1991). A commercial extract reduced LH secretion without affecting follicle-stimulating hormone in a group of menopausal women. (See *Effect of black cohosh on luteinizing hormone,* page 94.) A study of hysterectomy patients failed to show any advantage of using black cohosh over conventional hormone replacement therapy (HRT; Lehmann-Willenbrock and Riedel, 1988). Black cohosh improved bone mineral density in rats that were administered a low-calcium diet (Kadota et al., 1996), but this effect has not been demonstrated in human studies.

RESEARCH FINDINGS
Effect of black cohosh on luteinizing hormone

An ethanolic extract of the rhizome of *Cimicifuga racemosa* (Remifemin) was evaluated for estrogenic activity in 55 menopausal women. One group of women received 8 mg of extract daily for 8 weeks; a control group of another 55 women received a placebo. At the end of the period, serum levels of luteinizing hormone (LH) and follicle-stimulating hormone (FSH) were decreased in the group receiving the herb compared with those who received a placebo. Only LH suppression was statistically significant. This selective effect was interpreted as an example of the extract's estrogenic activity.

The investigators reproduced these effects in rats that had their ovaries removed. Results indicate that the difference in hormonal suppression between *C. racemosa* and placebo is caused by FSH secretion, which is less sensitive than LH to estrogenic feedback inhibition (Duker et al., 1991).

Reported uses
Black cohosh has been used primarily for gynecologic-related conditions, such as dysmenorrhea, menopausal symptoms, osteoporosis, and uterine spasms. It has also reportedly been used to treat arthritis, diarrhea, diuresis, dyspepsia, kidney problems, malaise, malaria, snakebite, and sore throat and as an insect repellent.

Dosage
Dosages vary and are not standardized. In studies, dosages ranged from 8 to 2,400 mg P.O. daily.

Adverse reactions
CV: ***bradycardia,*** hypotension.
GI: nausea, vomiting.
Other: increased perspiration, miscarriage or premature birth.

Interactions
Anesthetics, antihypertensives, sedatives: May increase hypotensive effect. Avoid administration with black cohosh.
Estrogen supplements, oral contraceptives: May increase effects. Avoid administration with black cohosh.

Contraindications and precautions
Black cohosh is contraindicated in patients with a history of estrogen-dependent tumors (such as estrogen receptor–positive breast cancer), uterine cancer, or thromboembolic disorders and in pregnant or breast-feeding patients. Hypotensive effects of acteina may be additive when taken with anesthetics, antihypertensives, or sedatives.

Bold italic type indicates that reaction may be life-threatening.

Special considerations
- Inform the patient taking an antihypertensive or a sedative of the potential additive effects of black cohosh. Monitor blood pressure closely in hypertensive patients to avoid hypotension.
- Discontinue black cohosh 2 weeks before surgery to avoid hypotensive reactions with anesthetics.
- Caution the pregnant patient that black cohosh, if taken in large doses, may cause spontaneous abortion.
- Overdose may cause CNS and visual disturbances, dizziness, headache, and tremor.
- Use of black cohosh should be limited to 6 months' duration because long-term studies on toxicity are lacking.

Points of interest
- Historically, black cohosh was one of several natural ingredients in Lydia Pinkham's Vegetable Compound in the early 1900s.

Commentary
Animal and human studies on the use of black cohosh are limited. Data from these studies suggest that the herb's hormonal effects may be beneficial primarily in controlling hot flashes associated with menopause. Most clinical data regarding this plant are derived from German studies that evaluated only a small number of women. The full estrogenic activity of black cohosh has not been conclusively demonstrated in humans, and therefore, it should not be recommended as a substitute for conventional forms of hormone replacement therapy. Additional, well-controlled trials are needed to clearly define the role of black cohosh as a natural form of hormone replacement therapy.

References
Berger, S., et al. "27-Deoxyactein: A New Polycyclic Triterpenoid Glycoside from *Actaea racemosa*," *Planta Med* 54:579-80, 1988.

Duker, E., et al. "Effects of Extracts of *Cimicifuga racemosa* on Gonadotropin Release in Menopausal Women and Ovariectomized Rats," *Planta Med* 57:420-24, 1991.

Genazzani, E., and Sorrentino, L. "Vascular Action of Acteina, Active Constituent of *Actaea racemosa* L," *Nature* 194:544-45, 1962.

Jarry, H., and Harnischfeger, G. "Studies on the Endocrine Effects of the Contents of *Cimicifuga racemosa*: 1. Influence on the Serum Concentration of Pituitary Hormones on Ovariectomized Rats," *Planta Med* 1:46-49, 1985.

Jarry, H., et al. "Studies on the Endocrine Effects of the Contents of *Cimicifuga racemosa*: 2. In Vitro Binding of Compounds to Estrogen Receptors," *Planta Med* 4:316-19, 1985.

Kadota, S., et al. "Effects of Cimicifugae Rhizome on Serum Calcium and Phosphate Levels in Low Calcium Dietary Rats and on Bone Mineral Density in Ovariectomized Rats," *Phytomed* 3(4):379-85, 1996/97.

Lehmann-Willenbrock, E., and Riedel, H.H. "Clinical and Endocrinologic Studies of the Treatment of Ovarian Insufficiency: Manifestations Following Hysterectomy with Intact Adnexa," *Zentralbl Gynakol* 110:611-18, 1988.

BLACK HAW

CRAMP BARK, NANNYBERRY, SHEEPBERRY, SHONNY, SLOE,
STAGBUSH, SWEET HAW

Taxonomic class
Caprifoliaceae

Common trade names
Black Haw, PMS Serene, Utero-Tone

Common forms
Available as a liquid extract and the root bark and in capsules and tablets in combination with other herbs and extracts.

Source
The root bark of *Viburnum prunifolium*, a deciduous shrub found in the eastern United States, has traditionally been used for medicinal purposes.

Chemical components
Scopoletin (6-methoxy-7-hydroxy-coumarin) and other coumarins are thought to contribute to black haw's antispasmodic action. Other constituents of the root bark include isovaleric acid, resin, salicin, tannin, and volatile oil. A hemimellitate acid derivative, 1-methyl 2,3-dibutyl hemimellitate, has also been identified in aqueous extracts of stem bark; this compound has not been shown to exert antispasmodic properties (Jarobe et al., 1969).

Actions
The uterine relaxant properties of black haw and other *Viburnum* species have been studied in animals. In one investigation, extracts prepared from black haw, *Viburnum opulus*, and two other *Viburnum* species caused complete relaxation of uterine tissue in rats. Further chemical analyses of extracts from black haw and *V. opulus* identified at least four constituents that have uterine relaxant properties (Jarobe et al., 1966).

Reported uses
Black haw has been used most commonly as a uterine relaxant and general antispasmodic. Specific indications include prevention of spontaneous abortion and the treatment of chronic diarrhea, dysmenorrhea, general musculoskeletal spasms, and uterine pain. Human clinical trials are looking to verify these claims.

Dosage
Black haw tincture or bark can be used in a tea and taken t.i.d.

Adverse reactions
GI: GI irritation.

Bold italic type indicates that reaction may be life-threatening.

Interactions
Anticoagulants: Increased anticoagulant effects. Avoid administration with black haw.

Contraindications and precautions
Black haw is contraindicated in patients who are hypersensitive to this plant or related species. It is also contraindicated in pregnant or breast-feeding patients.

Special considerations
● Monitor the patient for signs of bleeding and hypersensitivity reactions.
● Advise the patient to consider traditional uterine relaxants before using black haw; controlled studies on this agent have not been conducted in humans.
● Advise women to avoid using black haw during pregnancy or breast-feeding.

Commentary
Available data on the pharmacologic effects of black haw are based on animal studies. Although black haw has been used for many years and was formerly included in the United States Dispensatory, human clinical data are lacking. Most important, information on the safety and adverse effects of black haw is not available. This agent should be avoided until more is known about its risks and benefits.

References
Jarobe, C.H., et al. "Uterine Relaxant Properties of *Viburnum*," *Nature* 5064:837, 1966.
Jarobe, C.H., et al. "1-Methyl 2,3-Dibutyl Hemimellitate: A Novel Component of *Viburnum prunifolium*," *J Org Chem* 34:4202-3, 1969.

BLACK ROOT
BOWMAN'S ROOT, BRINTON ROOT, CULVER'S PHYSIC, CULVERIS ROOT, HIGH VERONICA, HINI, *LEPTANDRA*, *LEPTANDRA VIRGINICA*, PHYSIC ROOT, QUITEL, TALL SPEEDWELL, *VERONICA*, *VERONICA VIRGINICA*

Taxonomic class
Scrophulariaceae

Common trade names
None known.

Common forms
Available as dried root or tincture.

Source
Black root is made from the dried rhizome and roots of *Veronicastrum virginicum*, which grows in Canada and the United States.

Chemical components
Tannic acid, verosterol (a volatile oil), cinnamic and paramethoxycin-namic acids, gum, resin, mannite, and d-mannitol have been isolated from black root. Early studies yielded a substance called leptandrin, which was thought to be the active component (Wood and Bache, 1907). No recent data support this.

Actions
Black root has a bitter, nauseating taste and irritates GI mucosa, pri-marily because of the herb's tannin content (Millspaugh, 1974). Tannic acid has astringent properties that act locally on GI mucosa. Tannic acid also forms insoluble complexes with alkaloids, glycosides, and certain heavy metal ions.

Black root also has antisecretory and antiulcerative effects in the GI tract as a result of an inhibitory action on the gastric enzyme system.

Mannite and d-mannitol are considered osmotic diuretics and work by increasing the transport of sodium and water out of the loop of Henle. Some data also suggest that cinnamic acid exerts some choleretic effect. In animal studies, cinnamic acid injections increased bile acid flow by 50% (Galecka, 1969). Other animal studies confirmed this ef-fect (Das et al., 1976).

Reported uses
Black root is claimed to be useful as a cathartic and an emetic. Because of its purported biliary action within the GI tract, it has been claimed to be beneficial in relieving jaundice and other symptoms related to he-patic or biliary congestion. Human trials are lacking.

Dosage
Black root possesses cathartic and emetic properties at 15 to 40 grains (1 to 2.6 g); the usual reported dose is 1 g. Tea may be made by mixing 1 to 2 tsp of dried black root in cold water, boiling this solution, and then simmering it for 10 minutes. The dosage of this solution is typical-ly 1 cup t.i.d. The tincture has been administered in doses of 1 to 2 ml t.i.d.

Adverse reactions
CNS: drowsiness, headache.
GI: abdominal pain or cramps, changes in stool color or odor, nausea, vomiting.
Hepatic: *hepatotoxicity.*

Interactions
None reported.

Contraindications and precautions
Black root is contraindicated in pregnant or breast-feeding patients; effects are unknown. Avoid large amounts of black root, especially in patients with existing hepatic disease, because of the potential toxic ef-fects of tannic acid on the liver.

Bold italic type indicates that reaction may be life-threatening.

Special considerations
● Alkaloids such as atropine and scopolamine, glycosides such as digoxin, and products that contain iron may form insoluble complexes with tannins. Advise the patient to avoid taking black root along with these drugs.

■ **ALERT** Hepatotoxicity after ingestion of large amounts of dried tea leaves (in the range of 1½ lb of tea every 3 to 4 days) has been reported (Haddad and Winchester, 1990).

■ **ALERT** Caution the patient to discontinue using this herb if abnormal increases in hepatic transaminase levels occur.

● Inform the patient that few scientific data exist to support therapeutic uses for this plant in humans.
● Monitor liver function test results.
● Instruct the patient to immediately report symptoms of hepatic dysfunction, such as fever, jaundice, and right upper quadrant pain. The patient should have periodic assessment of serum liver enzyme levels.
● Advise women to avoid using black root during pregnancy or when breast-feeding.

Points of interest
● Settlers gathered knowledge of black root from Native Americans. The Delaware referred to the plant as *quitel;* the Missouri and Osage called it *hini* (Lloyd, 1921).
● Early American doctors used black root as a cure for bilious fevers (Wood and Bache, 1907).

Commentary
Little information is available about black root's therapeutic uses or efficacy. No human trials have supported therapeutic claims for this herb. The lack of clinical trials limits the usefulness of anecdotal or historical data.

References
Das, P.K., et al. "Pharmacology of Kutkin and Its Two Organic Constituents, Cinnamic Acid and Vanillic Acid," *Indian J Exp Biol* 14:456-58, 1976.

Galecka, H. "Choleretic and Cholagogic Effects of Certain Hydroxy Acids and Their Derivatives in Guinea Pigs," *Acta Pol Pharm* 26:479-84, 1969.

Haddad, L.M., and Winchester, J.F. *Clinical Management of Poisoning and Drug Overdose,* 2nd ed. Philadelphia: W.B. Saunders Co., 1990.

Lloyd, J.B. *Origin and History of All the Pharmacopeial Vegetable Drugs, Chemicals, and Preparations.* 8th and 9th decennial revisions, vol. 1. Cincinnati: The Caxton Press, 1921.

Millspaugh, C.F. *American Medicinal Plants.* New York: Dover Publications, Inc., 1974. Reprint of 1892 edition.

Wood, G.B., and Bache, F. *Dispensatory of the United States of America,* 19th ed. Philadelphia: Lippincott-Raven, 1907.

BLESSED THISTLE

CARDO SANTO, CHARDON BENIT, HOLY THISTLE, KARDOBENEDIKTENKRAUT, ST. BENEDICT THISTLE, SPOTTED THISTLE

Taxonomic class
Asteraceae

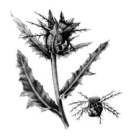

Common trade names
Blessed Thistle Combo, Blessed Thistle Herb

Common forms
Available as 325- and 340-mg capsules, 1-oz packets of dried herb, 1-oz containers of tincture, and tea.

Source
The crude drug is obtained from the leaves and, especially, the flowers of the blessed thistle, an annual plant found primarily in Asia and Europe. Blessed thistle, *Cnicus benedictus (Carbenia benedicta, Carduus benedictus),* is related to daisies, asters, and other flowering plants.

Chemical components
The aerial parts of blessed thistle contain the sesquiterpene lactones cnicin and salonitenolide. Concentration of sesquiterpene lactones is quite variable in the Asteraceae family and depends on climate, season, geographic location, and soil quality at harvest.

Actions
Blessed thistle purportedly exerts effects on the stomach, liver, heart, blood, mammary glands, and uterus. The pharmacokinetics of blessed thistle compounds have not been well documented. In vitro cytotoxicity has been demonstrated for cnicin (Barrero et al., 1997).

The antibiotic activity of cnicin and other components of blessed thistle has also been investigated.

Reported uses
Blessed thistle is claimed to be useful for several GI and hepatic disorders and for memory improvement, stimulation of lactation, and relief from menstrual symptoms.

Dosage
Various dosages have been suggested, depending on the intended use and method of administration. Lack of human trials makes it difficult to arrive at specific dosage recommendations. Besides capsules and tinctures, some sources recommend blessed thistle as a tea.

Adverse reactions
GI: nausea, vomiting.
Skin: contact dermatitis.

Bold italic type indicates that reaction may be life-threatening.

Interactions
Other herbal drugs based on Asteraceae family: Possible cross-sensitivity. Avoid administration with blessed thistle.

Contraindications and precautions
Blessed thistle is contraindicated in pregnant or breast-feeding patients; effects are unknown. Use cautiously in patients with a history of contact dermatitis, especially in relation to other members of the Asteraceae family.

Special considerations
● Monitor for contact dermatitis in susceptible patients. Airborne contact dermatitis is possible because of cross-sensitivity with other members of the Asteraceae family. (Sesquiterpene lactones are sensitizers.)
● Inform the patient who wants to take blessed thistle that few scientific data on therapeutic benefits are available.
● Advise women to avoid using blessed thistle during pregnancy or when breast-feeding.

Points of interest
● According to legend, blessed thistle was a popular folk remedy and tonic used by monks during the Middle Ages. It was also used to treat bubonic plague.
● Germany allows use of this herb in the treatment of dyspepsia and loss of appetite.

Commentary
Many anecdotal claims are made for this agent, but there are no animal or human clinical data to support them.

References
Barrero, A.F., et al. "Biomimetic Cyclization of Cnicin to Malacitanolide, a Cytotoxic Eudesmanolide from *Centaurea malacitana*," *J Nat Prod* 60:1034-35, 1997.

Crellin, J.K., and Philpott, J. *Herbal Medicine Past and Present. A Reference Guide to Medicinal Plants*, vol. 2. Durham, N.C.: Duke University Press, 1990.

Reynolds, J.E.F., et al., eds. *Martindale, The Extra Pharmacopeia*, 31st ed. London: Royal Pharmaceutical Society of Great Britain, 1996.

Zeller, W., et al. "The Sensitizing Capacity of Compositae plants. VI. Guinea Pig Sensitization Experiments with Ornamental Plants and Weeds Using Different Methods," *Arch Dermatol Res* 277:28-35, 1985.

BLOODROOT
INDIAN PAINT, RED PUCCOON, REDROOT, TETTERWORT

Taxonomic class
Papaveraceae

Common trade names
Multi-ingredient preparations: Lexat, Viadent

Common forms
Available as an ingredient (sanguinarine) in some toothpastes and oral rinses.

Source
The alkaloid sanguinarine is extracted from the rhizome of *Sanguinaria canadensis*, a herbaceous perennial that is native to North America.

Chemical components
Bloodroot contains several pharmacologically active alkaloids, including the isoquinolone derivatives chelerythrine, homochelidonine, protopine, sanguidimerine, and sanguinarine. Other compounds extracted from bloodroot include berberine, coptisine, and sanguirubine.

Actions
Sanguinarine, the most extensively studied agent in bloodroot, is poorly absorbed from the GI tract. It has broad antimicrobial activity and anti-inflammatory properties. Minimum inhibitory concentrations of sanguinarine range from 1 to 32 mcg/ml for most species of bacteria that promote dental plaque (Godowski, 1989).

Sanguinarine converts to a negatively charged iminiun ion that permits the compound to bind to plaque (Godowski, 1989). Sanguinarine also can induce mild CNS depression and has a papaverine-like action on smooth muscle and cardiac muscle.

Reported uses
Bloodroot was formerly used as an expectorant, but because of its toxicity, it fell into disuse. Other claims include use as a digestive stimulant, an emetic, and a laxative.

The efficacy of sanguinarine as an antiplaque agent has been well documented in numerous clinical trials (Godowski, 1989; Kopczyk et al., 1991). In contrast, a study of periodontal disease treatments showed no significant advantage to using a sanguinarine dentrifice and oral rinse in conjunction with initial periodontal therapy, such as oral hygiene instruction, scaling, and root planing (Cullinan et al., 1997).

Because of its ability to chemically corrode and destroy tissue, bloodroot has been prescribed as a cure for surface cancers, fungal growths, nasal polyps, and ringworm. In humans, it has been tested topically for the treatment of ear and nose carcinomas. Mouthwashes generally contain dilute concentrations of sanguinarine.

Dosage
Extract (1:1 in 60% alcohol): 0.06 to 0.3 ml P.O. t.i.d.
Tincture: 0.3 to 2 ml P.O. t.i.d.

Adverse reactions
CNS: CNS depression (with large doses), ***coma*** (with excessive doses in animals), headache.
CV: hypotension, ***shock.***

Bold italic type indicates that reaction may be life-threatening.

EENT: eye and mucous membrane irritation and degradation (from contact with root dust or components).

GI: nausea, vomiting.

Interactions
Sanguinarine extract and zinc: Synergistic enhancement of antimicrobial efficacy of sanguinarine (Eisenberg et al., 1991). Discuss concomitant use with knowledgeable practitioner.

Contraindications and precautions
Avoid using bloodroot during pregnancy. Use cautiously under medical supervision on abraded or healing tissue.

Special considerations
• Caution the patient against using bloodroot or its components unless under strict supervision and guidance of his dentist or other primary health care provider.

• Advise the patient to consult a health care provider before using herbal preparations because a treatment that has been clinically researched and proved effective may be available.

🕭 **ALERT** The powdered rhizome and juice of bloodroot are potentially destructive to mammalian tissues. Advise the patient to avoid oral ingestion.

• Advise women to avoid using bloodroot during pregnancy.

Points of interest
• The FDA has classified bloodroot as an herb that is unsafe for use in foods, beverages, or drugs. However, the herb is used in homeopathic medicine.

Commentary
Most clinical data support using sanguinarine as an ingredient in toothpaste and oral rinses to control dental plaque. However, a study by Cullinan and coworkers (1997) showed no benefit of sanguinarine when used with routine periodontal care. The study also questioned the use of sanguinarine because it offers no advantage over routine periodontal care and is potentially dangerous if ingested orally.

Sanguinarine's efficacy in treating topical cancers, fungal infections, and nasal polyps has not been demonstrated in controlled clinical trials, and oral ingestion is associated with tissue destruction. Its use cannot be recommended without additional studies.

References
Cullinan, M.P., et al. "Efficacy of a Dentrifice and Oral Rinse Containing *Sanguinaria* Extract in Conjunction with Initial Periodontal Therapy," *Aust Dent J* 42:47-51, 1997.

Eisenberg, A.D., et al. "Interactions of Sanguinarine and Zinc on Oral Streptococci and *Actinomyces* Species," *Caries Res* 25:185-90, 1991.

Godowski, K.C. "Antimicrobial Action of Sanguinarine," *J Clin Dent* 1:96-101, 1989.

Kopczyk, R.A., et al. "Clinical and Microbiological Effects of a *Sanguinaria-* Containing Mouth Rinse and Dentrifice with and without Fluoride During Six Months of Use," *J Periodontol* 62:617-22, 1991.

BLUE COHOSH

BLUE GINSENG, *CAULOPHYLLUM*, PAPOOSE ROOT, SQUAWROOT, YELLOW GINSENG

Taxonomic class
Berberidaceae

Common trade names
Blue Cohosh Low Alcohol, Blue Cohosh Root, Blue Cohosh Root Alcohol Free, Blue Cohosh Root Low Alcohol

Common forms
Available as capsules (500 mg), a dried powder, tablets, tea, and tinctures (1 oz, 2 oz).

Source
The aerial parts, roots, and rhizomes of *Caulophyllum thalictroides* have been used to extract active ingredients. This herb is found in parts of eastern United States and in Canada. The seeds are bright blue.

Chemical components
Rhizome and root extracts contain the alkaloids anagyrine, baptofoline, magnoflorine, and methylcytisine (caulophylline); the saponins caulosaponin and cauloside D; and citrollol, gum, phosphoric acid, phytosterol, resin, and starch. Hydrolysis of cauloside D yields hederagenin.

Actions
A glycoside component of blue cohosh stimulates smooth muscle in the coronary vessels, small intestine, and uterus in various animals (Ferguson and Edwards, 1954).

Antifertility actions have been documented in animal studies (Chaudrasekhar and Sarma, 1974; Chaudrasekhar and Raa Vishwanath, 1974). Some anti-inflammatory and antimicrobial actions have been reported as well (Benoit et al., 1976, and Anisimov et al., 1972, respectively). Methylcytisine has pharmacologic activity similar to that of nicotine, causing elevations in blood pressure and blood glucose levels and increased peristalsis (Scott and Chen, 1943).

Reported uses
Early claims for this herb include its use as an anticonvulsant, an agent to increase menstrual flow, an agent to induce labor, an antirheumatic, and an antispasmodic. In a national survey of certified nurse-midwives, blue cohosh was reported (by questionnaire) to be used 65% of the time by those nurse-midwives who endorsed herbal medicine use. Blue cohosh was often used with other herbal preparations to induce labor (McFarlin et al., 1999).

Bold italic type indicates that reaction may be life-threatening.

Dosage
Dried rhizome or root: 0.3 to 1 g P.O. t.i.d.
Liquid extract (1:1 in 70% alcohol): 0.5 to 1 ml P.O. t.i.d.

Adverse reactions
CV: chest pain, hypertension.
GI: abdominal cramps, GI irritation, severe diarrhea.
Metabolic: hyperglycemia.
Skin: mucous membrane irritation after contact with powdered extract.
Other: *poisoning in children* after ingestion of seeds.

Interactions
Antianginals: May interfere with therapy, leading to increased chest pain and discomfort. Avoid administration with blue cohosh.
Antidiabetics: May antagonize hypoglycemic effects of these drugs. Avoid administration with blue cohosh.
Antihypertensives: May interfere with therapy, leading to increased blood pressure. Avoid administration with blue cohosh.
Nicotine replacements: Increased effects of nicotine. Avoid administration with blue cohosh.

Contraindications and precautions
Blue cohosh is contraindicated in pregnant patients because of its potential uterine-stimulating and teratogenic effects. At least two cases of severe neonatal heart failure have been linked to consumption of blue cohosh during pregnancy (Gunn and Wright, 1996; Jones and Lawson, 1998). Also, N-methylcytisine, an alkaloid of blue cohosh, has demonstrated teratogenic effects in a rat embryo culture (in vitro method; Kennelly et al., 1999).
    Blue cohosh is also contraindicated in patients with heart disease.

Special considerations
- The active agent in blue cohosh, methylcytisine, is pharmacologically similar to but much less potent than nicotine.
- Monitor the patient for signs and symptoms of overdose, which could resemble nicotine poisoning. Initiate gastric lavage or induce emesis and provide appropriate supportive measures.
- Monitor blood pressure and blood glucose levels in patients taking this drug.
- Advise women to avoid using blue cohosh during childbearing years and pregnancy.

⚑ ALERT Advise the patient to keep blue cohosh products out of the reach of children. The bright blue seeds are attractive but poisonous.

Commentary
Blue cohosh offers encouraging opportunities for investigation as a therapeutic agent for inflammatory disease or as a contraceptive. The potential for toxicity and worsening of the disease requires considerable investigation to assess the herb's risks and benefits before it can be recommended for use. Pregnant women should be reminded to reconsider

using this herbal preparation during pregnancy because of significant risks to the fetus.

References

Anisimov, M.M., et al. "The Antimicrobial Activity of the Triterpene Glycosides of *Caulophyllum robustum* Maxim," *Antibiot Khimioter* 17:834, 1972.

Benoit, P.S., et al. "Biochemical and Pharmacological Evaluation of Plants. XIV: Anti-inflammatory Evaluation of 163 Species of Plants," *Lloydia* 393:160-71, 1976.

Chaudrasekhar, K., and Raa Vishwanath, C. "Studies on the Effect of Implantation on Rats," *J Reprod Fertil* 38:245-46, 1974.

Chaudrasekhar, K., and Sarma, G.H.R. "Observations on the Effect of the Low and High Doses of Caulophyllum on the Ovaries and the Consequential Changes in the Uterus and Thyroid in Rats," *J Reprod Fertil* 38:236-37, 1974.

Ferguson, H.C., and Edwards, L.D. "A Pharmacological Study of a Crystalline Glycoside of *Caulophyllum thalictroides*," *J Am Pharm Assoc* 43:16-21, 1954.

Gunn, T.R., and Wright, I.M.R. "The Use of Blue and Black Cohosh in Labour," *NZ Med J* 109:410-11, 1996.

Jones, T.K., and Lawson, B.M. "Profound Neonatal Congestive Heart Failure Caused by Maternal Consumption of Blue Cohosh Herbal Medication," *J Pediatr* 132:550-52, 1998.

Kennelly, E.J., et al. "Detecting Potential Teratogenic Alkaloids from Blue Cohosh Rhizomes Using an In Vitro Rat Embryo Culture," *J Nat Prod* 62(10):1385-89, 1999.

McFarlin, B.L., et al. "A National Survey of Herbal Preparation Use by Nurse-midwives for Labor Stimulation. Review of the Literature and Recommendations for Practice," *J Nurse Midwifery* 44(3):205-16, 1999.

Scott, C.C., and Chen, K.K. "The Pharmacologic Action of *N*-Methylcytisine," *Therapeutics* 79:334, 1943.

BLUE FLAG

DAGGER FLOWER, DRAGON FLOWER, FLAG LILY, FLEUR-DE-LIS, FLOWER-DE-LUCE, LIVER LILY, POISON FLAG, SNAKE LILY, WATER FLAG, WILD IRIS

Taxonomic class
Iridaceae

Common trade names
Iridin, Irisin

Common forms
Liquid extract: 0.5 to 1 fluid dram (2.5 to 5 ml)
Powdered root: 20 grains (1,300 mg)
Solid extract: 10 to 15 grains (650 to 975 mg)
Tincture: 1 to 3 fluid drams (5 to 15 ml)

Source
The rhizome of *Iris versicolor* yields iridin and an oleoresin. *I. versicolor* is a perennial herb found abundantly in swamps and low-lying areas throughout eastern and central North America.

Bold italic type indicates that reaction may be life-threatening.

Chemical components
The rhizome contains starch, gum, tannin, 25% acrid resinous matter, 0.025% furfural (a volatile oil), 0.002% isophthalic acid, traces of salicylic acid, lauric acid, stearic acid, palmitic acid, and I-triacontanol. Other constituents include beta-sitosterol, iridin, and iriversical. A number of substances contained in the rhizome are unidentified.

Actions
Little is known about the phytochemical, therapeutic, or toxicologic properties of blue flag and its components. The acute oral toxicity for furfural is 127 mg/kg (Newall et al., 1996). The root is claimed to possess anti-inflammatory, dermatologic, diuretic, and laxative properties. The commercial products Iridin and Irisin are powdered root extracts with diuretic and intestinal stimulant properties.

Reported uses
Blue flag was used by Native Americans as a cathartic and an emetic. It has been called the liver lily because of its purported ability to cure hepatic diseases. Externally, the poulticed root was used as an anti-inflammatory on sores and bruises. Powdered root preparations have been used as diuretics and intestinal stimulants.

Dosage
Available data on dosages relate to use of blue flag as a cathartic.
Liquid extract, tinctures: 0.5 to 3 fluid drams P.O.
Solid extract, powdered root: 10 to 20 grains P.O.

Adverse reactions
CNS: headache.
GI: nausea, vomiting.
Hepatic: *hepatotoxicity* (caused by tannin content).
Skin: mucous membrane irritation (caused by furfural component).

Interactions
None reported.

Contraindications and precautions
Blue flag is contraindicated in pregnant or breast-feeding patients; effects are unknown.

Special considerations
• Advise the patient to avoid taking blue flag internally.
• Inform the patient that contact of this herb with eyes, nose, or mouth causes severe irritation.
ALERT Severe nausea and vomiting can occur after ingestion of fresh root preparations.
ALERT Iridin has caused poisoning in humans and livestock.
• Caution parents to keep all parts of this plant out of the reach of children.
• Advise women to avoid using blue flag during pregnancy or when breast-feeding.

Points of interest
● The fresh rhizome emits a slight, peculiar odor and has a pungent, acrid taste.
● The rhizome of *I. versicolor* is an official pharmaceutical ingredient in the USP.
● When not in bloom, blue flag can easily be mistaken for sweet flag (*Acorus calamus*).

Commentary
Blue flag is a known intestinal irritant and may be dangerous in some conditions; therefore, its use cannot be recommended. The fact that little is known about the phytochemical and toxicologic properties of blue flag and its constituents indicates that this herb is best avoided until further information is available.

References
Newall, C.A., et al. *Herbal Medicines: A Guide for Health-Care Professionals*. London: Pharmaceutical Press, 1996.

BOGBEAN

BUCK BEAN, MARSH TREFOIL, WATER SHAMROCK

Taxonomic class
Gentianaceae

Common trade names
Bogbean and Figwart Capsules

Common forms
Available as dried leaf, liquid extract, and tincture.

Source
Bogbean extract is made from the leaves of *Menyanthes trifoliata*. This plant is native to swamps and marshes in Europe and North America.

Chemical components
Several acids (caffeic, chlorogenic, ferulic, folic, palmitic, salicylic, vanillic), alkaloids (choline, gentianin, gentianidine), and flavonoids (hyperin, kaempferol, quercetin, rutin, trifolioside) are present in bogbean. Other components include a coumarin, scopoletin, iridoids, carotene, and ceryl alcohol.

Actions
Bogbean is claimed to have diuretic properties. An in vitro study suggests that compounds isolated from bogbean may be valuable analgesics. The isolation of eight compounds from the dried rhizomes of *M. trifoliata* and their inhibition on prostaglandin synthesis was reported. Two of the eight compounds showed significant inhibition of prostaglandin synthesis, with compounds 2 to 14 times more potent than as

---

pirin. The other isolated compounds did not affect prostaglandin synthesis (Huang et al., 1995).

Tertiary references suggest that bile-stimulating properties have been described for both caffeic and ferulic acid. Bogbean extracts have also demonstrated antibactericidal properties (Bishop and MacDonald, 1951).

Reported uses
Bogbean has been reported to be an antirheumatic, an appetite stimulant, a cathartic laxative, and an agent for fevers, scurvy, and dropsy (edematous state). Human trials evaluating bogbean for safety and efficacy are lacking.

Dosage
Dried leaf: 1 to 2 g in a tea P.O. t.i.d.
Extract (1:1 in 25% alcohol): 1 to 2 ml P.O. t.i.d. with plenty of juice or water at mealtimes.

Adverse reactions
GI: nausea, vomiting.
Hematologic: *bleeding*, hemolysis (Giaceri, 1972).

Interactions
Anticoagulants (heparin, warfarin): May potentiate action of anticoagulants because of coumarin derivative in bogbean. Avoid administration with bogbean.
Antiplatelet drugs (aspirin, clopidrogrel, ticlopidine): May increase risk of bleeding. Avoid administration with bogbean.

Contraindications and precautions
Bogbean is contraindicated in pregnant or breast-feeding patients.

Special considerations
• Monitor for signs of bleeding, especially in patients receiving concomitant anticoagulation or antiplatelet therapy.
🖐 **ALERT** Inform the patient that ingestion may result in severe, protracted nausea and vomiting.
• Advise the patient to keep liquid extracts away from children because of poisoning risk.
• Advise the patient to report abdominal pain, dizziness, or vomiting. Urge him to stop taking bogbean if symptoms persist.

Points of interest
• The fruit of *M. trifoliata*, a plant found predominantly in swamps and bogs, resembles a small bean; hence the name bogbean.
• Small quantities of bogbean are used as a natural food flavoring in Europe.

Commentary
Although animal studies have documented a few therapeutic pharmacologic uses for bogbean, definitive validation from human clinical tri

als is not available to justify its use for any therapeutic claims. Questions about safety remain unanswered.

References
Bishop, C.J., and MacDonald, R.E. "A Survey of Higher Plants for Antibacterial Substances," *Botany* 15:231-59, 1951.
Giaceri, G. "Chromatographic Identification of Coumarin Derivatives in *Menyanthes trifoliata*," *Fitoterapia* 43:134-38, 1972.
Huang, C., et al. "Anti-inflammatory Compounds Isolated from *Menyanthes trifoliata* L.," *Acta Pharm Sinica* 30:621-26, 1995.

BOLDO
BOLDINE, BOLDO-DO-CHILE

Taxonomic class
Monimiaceae

Common trade names
Boldo is a minor ingredient in more than 60 preparations used principally in South America and Europe (for example, Boldaloin and Hepatica).

Common forms
Available as an extract, a tea, and a tincture.

Source
Boldine, an alkaloid, is the principal constituent of the leaves and bark of the Chilean boldo tree, *Peumus boldus* (*Boldea boldus*). This small evergreen is native to Chile and Peru and naturalized in the Mediterranean region. Boldine has also been found in more than a dozen other trees and shrubs in the laurel, magnolia, and monimia families.

Chemical components
At least 17 alkaloids occur in the leaves and bark of the boldo tree. Dried boldo leaves have a total alkaloid content of 0.25% to 0.5%. Boldine is the principal alkaloid, constituting about 0.1% of the dried leaf. The bark is much richer in alkaloids, with boldine accounting for about 75% of the total alkaloid content. Other compounds include a coumarin, flavonoids, resin, tannins, and volatile oils.

Actions
Although boldo is a widely used medicinal plant, its physiologic effects and mechanisms of action are not well known. Pharmacokinetic, pharmacodynamic, and physiologic data in humans are lacking. In studies with dogs, boldo was found to exert a diuretic effect, increasing urinary excretion by 50% (Speisky and Cassels, 1994). In other animal studies, boldo relaxed smooth muscle and prolonged intestinal transit time, a process mediated at least in part through anticholinergic actions (Gotteland et al., 1995).

Boldine acted as an alpha blocker and calcium antagonist in rats. When administered parenterally, boldine exerts some inhibitory CNS action, possibly mediated by dopamine receptor blockade (Speisky and Cassels, 1994).

Laboratory tests have shown boldine to be a more potent antioxidant than vitamin E. Other laboratory studies indicate that boldine offers in vitro protection of cytochrome P-450 enzyme systems from damage caused by exposure to peroxidative attack (Kringstein and Cederbaum, 1995). These findings have led to speculation that boldine may have value as a hepatoprotective agent or as a treatment in free radical–mediated disease states.

Studies have demonstrated that boldine is not mutagenic or genotoxic (Speisky and Cassels, 1994; Tavares and Takahashi, 1994). However, data show that a hydroalcoholic extract of boldine has abortive and teratogenic effects in rats. Also, the boldo extract was associated with changes in blood glucose and serum ALT, AST, bilirubin, cholesterol, and urea levels in rats (Almedia et al., 2000).

Reported uses
Boldo is one of the most widely used medicinal plants in Chile. Its principal therapeutic claims are for treating digestive and hepatobiliary disorders. Some human clinical trials appear to validate its use in digestive disorders. (See *GI effects of boldo,* page 112.)

Boldo-based preparations are also used for colds, dyspepsia, earache, flatulence, generalized edema, gonorrhea, gout, headache, menstrual pain, nervousness, rheumatism, syphilis, and weakness. Other therapeutic claims include use as an anthelmintic, a diuretic, a laxative, a mild hypnotic, and a sedative.

Dosage
Human clinical trials have used 2.5 g of dried boldo extract P.O. daily.

Adverse reactions
CNS: exaggerated reflexes, lack of coordination, *seizures.*

Interactions
None reported.

Contraindications and precautions
Boldo is contraindicated in patients with existing CNS or respiratory system disorders and in pregnant or breast-feeding patients.

Special considerations
🔺 ALERT Although reports are conflicting, boldo volatile oil may be toxic. In large doses, boldo may cause paralysis of motor and sensory nerves and, eventually, the muscle fibers, causing death due to respiratory arrest. Toxicologic studies in animals seem to reflect favorably on the claimed low toxicity of boldo. In mice and guinea pigs, 500 to 1,000 mg/kg of boldine P.O. was needed to produce death; 15 g of boldine P.O. was needed to cause death in a 26-lb (12-kg) dog. Death in these cases was caused by respiratory depression. In another study, rats

RESEARCH FINDINGS
GI effects of boldo

A study was conducted to assess the effects of boldo on mouth-to-cecum transit time in healthy humans. Twelve volunteers received either 2.5 g of a dry boldo extract or a glucose placebo during two successive 4-day periods. On day 4 of each period, the subjects received 20 g of lactulose. The level of exhaled hydrogen was then measured every 15 minutes to detect changes that would reflect mouth-to-cecum transit time. These results suggested that transit time was significantly greater after the administration of boldo than after the placebo. Some investigators believe that this study helps to explain the mechanism and efficacy of boldo in the treatment of digestive disorders (Gotteland et al., 1995). Another study examined boldo given with rhubarb, gentian, and cascara in treating GI complaints. Although useful in treating appetite loss, flatulence, and itching, boldo and cascara were more effective than other herbal combinations in treating constipation (Borgia et al., 1981).

showed no signs of toxicity after ingesting up to 3,000 mg/kg of boldine extract P.O. (Speisky and Cassels, 1994).

• Instruct the patient to keep boldo preparations and plant parts out of the reach of children.

• Advise the patient with existing CNS or respiratory problems to avoid using boldo products.

• Inform the patient that additional studies are needed before boldo or its components can be recognized for the treatment of any disorder.

• Instruct the patient to avoid ingestion of boldo volatile oil because its toxicity index is unknown.

• Urge the patient to periodically undergo assessment of his liver function and blood glucose levels.

• Advise women to avoid using boldo during pregnancy or when breast-feeding.

Points of interest

• Fossilized boldo leaves more than 13,000 years old imprinted with human teeth have been found in Chile. It is not known whether ancient Chileans used these leaves for medicinal purposes or chewed them simply for their pleasant and refreshing taste (Speisky and Cassels, 1994).

• More than 60 preparations registered in various countries include boldo as an active ingredient, usually as a minor constituent. Most of these products are indicated for digestive or hepatobiliary disorders. Chile exports about 800 tons of dried boldo leaves annually, mainly to Argentina, Brazil, Italy, France, and Germany (Speisky and Cassels, 1994).

Bold italic type indicates that reaction may be life-threatening.

Commentary
Further studies are needed to clarify the pharmacology, pharmacokinetics, and toxicology of boldo. Findings about boldo's antioxidant and hepatoprotective properties warrant additional investigation. Until the safety and efficacy of boldo preparations are established, this herb cannot be recommended for human use.

References
Almedia, E.R., et al. "Toxicological Evaluation of the Hydro-alcohol Extract of the Dry Leaves of *Peumus boldus* and Boldine in Rats," *Phytother Res* 14(2):99-102, 2000.

Borgia, M., et al. "Pharmacological Activity of an Herbs Extract. A Controlled Clinical Study," *Curr Ther Res* 29:525-36, 1981.

Gotteland, M., et al. "Effect of a Dry Boldo Extract on Oro-cecal Transit in Healthy Volunteers," *Rev Med Chil* 123:955-60, 1995.

Kringstein, P., and Cederbaum, A.I. "Boldine Prevents Human Liver Microsomal Lipid Peroxidation and Inactivation of Cytochrome P4502E1," *Free Radic Biol Med* 18:559-63, 1995. Abstract.

Speisky, H., and Cassels, B.K. "Boldo and Boldine: An Emerging Case of Natural Drug Development," *Pharmacol Res* 29:1-12, 1994.

Tavares, D.C., and Takahashi, C.S. "Evaluation of the Genotoxic Potential of the Alkaloid Boldine in Mammalian Cell Systems In Vitro and In Vivo," *Mutat Res* 321:139-45, 1994. Abstract.

BONESET

AGUEWEED, CROSSWORT, EUPATORIUM, FEVERWORT, INDIAN SAGE, SWEATING PLANT, THOROUGHWORT, VEGETABLE ANTIMONY

Taxonomic class
Asteraceae

Common trade names
Multi-ingredient preparations: Catarrh Mixture, Nature's Answer Boneset Low Alcohol

Common forms
Available as an extract, a tea, and a topical cream.

Source
The crude drug is obtained from the dried leaves and flowering tops of the perennial herb *Eupatorium perfoliatum,* which grows throughout much of the United States and parts of Canada.

Chemical components
Boneset contains crystalline wax; flavonoids, such as astragalin, kaempferol, quercetin, and rutin; eupatorin, a bitter, crystalline glycoside; gallic acid; inulin; polysaccharides; resin; sterols; sugars; tannin; terpenoids; triterpenes; and volatile oil.

Actions

Although boneset is an old herbal standby, especially as an antipyretic, comparatively little is known about its pharmacologically active constituents. Animal studies suggest that boneset exhibits immunostimulatory actions on granulocytes and macrophages of sesquiterpene lactones and polysaccharide fractions of *E. perfoliatum* (Wagner et al., 1985).

Several studies attribute diaphoretic and emetic properties to boneset. Also, weak to moderate anti-inflammatory activity has been documented for some of the flavonoids and for an alcoholic extract of boneset. Although most members of the genus *Eupatorium* contain hepatotoxic pyrrolizidine alkaloids, they have not been found in boneset (Smith and Culvenor, 1981).

Reported uses

Despite more than 200 years of anecdotal use as an antipyretic, no human clinical trial has been reported that establishes boneset's efficacy for this use. A study in Germany failed to find any difference between a homeopathic boneset remedy and aspirin for discomfort of the common cold (Gassinger et al., 1981). Other traditional uses are as a treatment for acute bronchitis, congestion of the respiratory mucosa, and influenza and as an expectorant and a sedative.

Dosage

Extract: 10 to 40 gtt (2 to 4 g of plant material) mixed in a liquid P.O. daily.
Tea: 2 to 6 tsp of crushed dried leaves and flowering tops steeped in 1 cup to 1 pt of boiling water.

Adverse reactions

GI: diarrhea, vomiting.
Hepatic: *hepatotoxicity.*
Other: *allergic reactions.*

Interactions

None reported.

Contraindications and precautions

Boneset is contraindicated in pregnant or breast-feeding patients; effects are unknown.

Special considerations

• Monitor liver function test results periodically.
• Inform the patient that insufficient data exist to recommend boneset as a treatment for any disease state and that many proven anti-inflammatory compounds with known risks and benefits exist.
• Advise women to avoid using boneset during pregnancy or when breast-feeding.

Bold italic type indicates that reaction may be life-threatening.

Points of interest
• It has been suggested that boneset derived its name from an alleged ability to alleviate dengue fever, also known as breakbone fever.
• Despite its inclusion in the USP for almost a century (1820-1916) and the National Formulary for almost 25 years (1926-1950), boneset's use was never advocated by the traditional medical community. More recently, boneset has been included in homeopathic formulations and herbal mixtures marketed in Europe and to practicing herbalists.
• Boneset was used by Native Americans to treat malaria. (See *Native Americans fought fever with boneset*.)

Commentary
Medicinal use of boneset should be discouraged until more is known about its safety and efficacy. Because many substantiated allopathic

therapies already exist for the range of boneset's claimed therapeutic applications, it is unlikely that additional research will be pursued.

References
Gassinger, C.A., et al. "A Controlled Clinical Trial for Treating the Efficacy of the Homeopathic Drug *Eupatorium perfoliatum* D2 in the Treatment of the Common Cold," *Arzneimittelforschung* 31:732-36, 1981.

Smith, L.W., and Culvenor, C.C. "Plant Sources of Hepatotoxic Pyrrolizidine Alkaloids," *J Nat Prod* 44:129-52, 1981.

Wagner, H., et al. "Immunostimulating Polysaccharides (Heteroglycans) of Higher Plants," *Arzneimittelforschung* 35:1069, 1985.

BORAGE
BEEBREAD, *BORAGINIS FLOS*, *BORAGINIS HERBA*, BORETSCH, COMMON BORAGE, COMMON BUGLOSS, COOL TANKARD, OX'S TONGUE, STARFLOWER

Taxonomic class
Boraginaceae

Common trade names
Borage Oil, Borage Oil Capsules, Borage Power

Common forms
Capsules (softgels): 240 mg, 500 mg, 1,300 mg borage seed oil (oil contains 20% to 26% gamma linolenic acid [GLA]).

Source
Active components of the drug are obtained from the leaves, stems, flowers, and especially the seeds of borage (*Borago officinalis*), a hardy annual that grows in Europe and eastern United States.

Chemical components
Borage seed contains a mucilage, tannin, an essential oil, malic acid, and potassium nitrate. The fatty acid component of the seed oil consists of linoleic acid, GLA, oleic acid, and saturated fatty acids. The oil also contains small amounts of pyrrolizidine alkaloids, notably amabiline, a known hepatotoxin.

Actions
The mucilage component of borage produces an expectorant-like action. The malic acid and potassium nitrate components produce a mild diuretic effect.

GLA from borage seeds may suppress inflammation and joint tissue injury. It is rapidly converted to dihomogammalinoleic acid, an immediate precursor of monoenoic prostaglandin E_1, which has potent anti-inflammatory activity (Levanthal et al., 1993).

Topical borage oil may be effective for dermatitis because of uptake of GLA into the stratum corneum, thereby increasing the water-binding capacity of the stratum corneum, resulting in a smooth surface (Nissen et al., 1995).

Borage may increase dihomogammalinolenic acid, possibly resulting in increased prostaglandin E_1, which has vasodilator and bronchodilator effects in pulmonary vasculature (Christophe et al., 1994).

Borage teas are claimed to have soothing effects. Studies in rats and humans have suggested that borage can calm the CV response to stress. In one study, borage oil reduced systolic blood pressure and heart rate and reportedly improved the ability to perform tasks. This clinical trial used daily doses of 1.3 g for 28 days but involved only 10 persons. The mechanism of action is unknown (Mills, 1989).

Reported uses
Borage leaves have been part of European herbal medicine for centuries. During medieval times, the leaves and flowers were steeped in wine and taken to dispel melancholy. Borage has been used to treat bronchitis and colds and is claimed to possess anti-inflammatory, diaphoretic, expectorant, and tonic properties. (See *Treating joint inflammation with borage.*) More recently, it has been used to treat rheumatoid arthritis (Leventhal et al., 1993; Karlstad et al., 1993; Zurier et al., 1996), and study results show moderate improvement in symptoms (Zurier et al.,

---

Bold italic type indicates that reaction may be life-threatening.

RESEARCH FINDINGS
Treating joint inflammation with borage

Three clinical trials show promising results using gamma-linolenic acid (GLA) in borage seed oil in the treatment of joint disorders.

A randomized, double-blind, placebo-controlled 12-month trial was conducted in 56 patients who have rheumatoid arthritis. The patients were randomized to receive either 2.8 g of GLA or placebo for 6 months. The GLA groups showed a statistically significant moderate improvement in duration of morning stiffness, degree of disability, improvement in swollen joint count, and score compared with baseline ($P<.05$). Patients in the placebo group didn't show significant improvement in any measure. All patients then received GLA for the next 6 months. An evaluation of patients 15 months after study entry showed that most had experienced an exacerbation of their disease (Zurier et al., 1996).

A randomized, double-blind, placebo-controlled 24-week trial was conducted using 37 patients who had rheumatoid arthritis and active synovitis. The treatment group receiving GLA (1.4 g) as borage seed oil daily showed significant reduction of signs and symptoms of disease activity ($P<.05$). Thirty-six percent of the subjects experienced fewer tender joints and 28% had fewer swollen joints. The placebo group showed no such improvement. Of note, many of the patients in both groups also received NSAIDs and some received up to 10 mg of prednisone daily. No patients withdrew from GLA treatment (Leventhal et al., 1993).

In an uncontrolled trial, seven healthy patients and seven patients with rheumatoid arthritis received nine capsules of GLA (1.1 g) daily for 12 weeks. All the patients also received NSAIDs alone, prednisone and NSAIDs, or just acetaminophen. Eighty-five percent of the arthritic patients exhibited apparent clinical improvement, as a result of the administration of GLA (Pullman-Mooar et al., 1990).

1996). Borage oil has been used to treat atopic dermatitis, eczema, and infantile seborrheic dermatitis (Henz et al., 1999). It has been studied in cystic fibrosis patients as well, demonstrating statistically nonsignificant increases in vital capacity and forced expiratory volume (Christophe et al., 1994).

Dosage
For atopic dermatitis and eczema: 2 to 3 g of borage oil P.O. in divided doses, or 3% to 10% borage oil applied topically b.i.d. (Nissen et al., 1995).

For infantile seborrheic dermatitis: 0.5 ml applied topically to the scalp b.i.d. until lesions clear and then 2 to 3 times/week until age 6 to 7 months.

For rheumatoid arthritis: 1.4 g GLA (6 to 7 g of borage) P.O. in divided doses t.i.d. after meals.

Adverse reactions
CNS: temporal lobe epilepsy.
GI: belching, constipation, flatulence, loose stools.
Hepatic: hepatic dysfunction.

Interactions
Anticonvulsants: May decrease efficacy of these drugs. Avoid administration with borage.
Antihypertensives: May increase hypotensive effect of these drugs. Avoid administration with borage.
CNS stimulants, epileptogenics: May increase reduction in seizure threshold. Avoid administration with borage.

Contraindications and precautions
Borage is contraindicated in patients who are hypersensitive to this herb or any of its components and in pregnant or breast-feeding patients; effects are unknown. Schizophrenics and patients receiving epileptogenic drugs are at increased risk for temporal lobe epilepsy (Newall et al., 1996). Borage may be carcinogenic and hepatotoxic (Blumenthal et al., 1998).

Special considerations
• Monitor liver function test results periodically in patients who take borage.
• Urge the patient with liver impairment to avoid using borage because it may cause further hepatic dysfunction.
• Caution the patient with a seizure disorder to avoid using borage.
• Advise women to avoid using borage during pregnancy or when breast-feeding.

Points of interest
• Borage oil (starflower oil) is used as an alternative to evening primrose oil as a source of GLA.

Commentary
A few studies in rats and humans suggest that borage has value as an anti-inflammatory for rheumatoid arthritis. Two controlled clinical trials have demonstrated improvements in signs and symptoms of rheumatoid arthritis and active synovitis. Its exact role in therapy and questions about its efficacy and safety remain unresolved. Borage may also be effective for atopic dermatitis, eczema, and infantile seborrheic dermatitis. Other claims for this product are largely unsubstantiated.

References

Blumenthal, M., et al. *Herb Guide by Pharmacological Action (Unapproved Herbs). The Complete German Commission E Monographs: Therapeutic Guide to Herbal Medicines.* Austin, Tex.: The American Botanical Council, 1998:473-74.

Christophe, A., et al. "Effect of Administration of Gamma-Linolenic Acid on the Fatty Acid Composition of Serum Phospholipids and Cholesteryl Esters in Patients with Cystic Fibrosis," *Ann Nutr Metab* 38(1):40-47, 1994.

Henz, B.M., et al. "Double-blind, Multicentre Analysis of the Efficacy of Borage Oil in Patients with Atopic Eczema," *Br J Dermatol* 140(4):685-88, 1999.

Karlstad, M.D., et al. "Effect of Intravenous Lipid Emulsions Enriched with Gamma-linolenic Acid on Plasma n-6 Fatty Acids and Prostaglandin Biosynthesis After Burn and Endotoxin Injury in Rats," *Crit Care Med* 21:1740-49, 1993.

Leventhal, L.J., et al. "Treatment of Rheumatoid Arthritis with Gamma-linolenic Acid," *Ann Intern Med* 119:867-73, 1993.

Mancuso, P., et al. "Dietary Fish Oil and Fish and Borage Oil Suppress Intrapulmonary Proinflammatory Eicosanoid Biosynthesis and Attenuate Pulmonary Neutrophil Accumulation in Endotoxic Rats," *Crit Care Med* 25:1198-1206, 1997.

Mills, D.E. "Dietary Fatty Acid Supplementation Alters Stress Reactivity and Performance in Man," *J Hum Hypertens* 3:111-16, 1989.

Newall, C.A., et al. *Herbal Medicines, A Guide for Health-Care Professionals.* London: The Pharmaceutical Press, 1996.

Nissen, H.P., et al. "Borage Oil: Gamma-Linolenic Acid in the Oil Decreases Skin Roughness and TEWL and Increases Skin Moisture in Normal and Irritated Human Skin," *Cosmetics Toiletries Mag* 110:71-73, 76, 1995.

Pullman-Mooar, S., et al. "Alteration of the Cellular Fatty Acid Profile and the Production of Eicosanoids in Human Monocytes by Gamma-linolenic Acid," *Arthritis Rheum* 33:1526-33, 1990.

Zurier, R.B., et al. "Gamma-Linolenic Acid Treatment of Rheumatoid Arthritis: A Randomized, Placebo-Controlled Trial," *Arthritis Rheum* 39(11):1808-17, 1996.

BOSWELLIA

FRANKINCENSE, OLIBANUM, SALAI GUGGAL

Taxonomic class
Burseraceae

Common trade names
Multi-ingredient preparations: Boswellia Extract Standardized, Boswellia Resin (various manufacturers), Boswellin, Boswellin Cream, Frankincense Oil, Joint Assist (462 mg of glucosamine and boswellin), Maxi-Boz

Common forms
Capsules and tablets: 150 mg, 250 mg, 300 mg, 325 mg, 350 mg, 500 mg

Source
Most preparations use the resin of *Boswellia serrata*, which is collected by stripping away the bark of the tree. The resin is allowed to dry and forms a gummy exudate. Some preparations use an alcoholic or ethanolic extract of this gum resin.

Chemical components

The gum resin contains triterpene acids that are generally referred to as boswellic acids. The four major acids are beta-boswellic acid, 3-*O*-acetyl-beta-boswellic acid, 11-keto-beta boswellic acid, and 3-*O*-acetyl-11-keto-beta boswellic acid.

Actions

Boswellic acids appear to have some anti-inflammatory properties. Several animal and in vitro studies show that boswellic acids inhibit lipoxygenase, an enzyme responsible for leukotriene synthesis (Wildfeuer et al., 1998; Safayhi et al., 1997). Other animal studies demonstrated anti-inflammatory effects of *Boswellia* extract in mice and rats (Singh and Atal, 1986).

Other in vitro studies demonstrate an inhibitory effect of boswellic acid on the synthesis of DNA, RNA, and protein in human leukemia HL-60 cells. Although cellular growth rate slowed, cell viability was not affected (Shao et al., 1998).

Reported uses

Boswellia extract has a history of being used to treat a wide variety of disorders, including arthritis, asthma, diarrhea, syphilis, and tumors. A double-blind study examined the effect of *Boswellia* resin extract in 37 patients with active rheumatoid arthritis. Despite daily doses of 3,600 mg, no beneficial effect was noted between the *Boswellia* extract and placebo on swelling, pain, or number of doses of NSAIDs taken (Sander et al., 1998).

Another study evaluated the effect of boswellic acids on patients with asthma. In a double-blind, placebo-controlled study, 40 patients were given 300 mg three times a day for 6 weeks. Seventy percent of the treatment group showed improvement by a decrease in dyspnea and in the number of attacks or an increase in forced expiratory volume, or both. Twenty-seven percent of the control group also showed improvement in these areas (Gupta et al., 1998).

Boswellia gum resin was also tested in patients with ulcerative colitis. The Boswellia resin preparation (350 mg three times a day) was compared with sulfasalazine (1 g three times a day) for 6 weeks of treatment. Both groups showed similar results and improvement in stool properties; histopathology of rectal biopsies; serum levels of iron, calcium, phosphorus, and proteins; and total leukocyte and eosinophil counts (Gupta et al., 1997).

Dosage

The range used in studies was from 300 mg P.O. t.i.d. up to 3,600 mg daily.

The LD50 (lethal dose at which 50% of rats die) was greater than 2 g/kg in mice and rats.

Adverse reactions

None reported.

Bold italic type indicates that reaction may be life-threatening.

Interactions
None reported.

Contraindications and precautions
Avoid using boswellia in pregnant or breast-feeding women; effects are unknown.

Special considerations
- Find out why the patient has been taking boswellia.
- Although no known chemical interactions have been reported in clinical studies, consideration must be given to the herbal product's pharmacologic properties and the potential for interference with the intended therapeutic effect of conventional drugs.
- Advise the patient to consult a health care provider before using herbal preparations because a treatment that has been clinically researched and proved effective may be available.
- Urge the patient to report symptoms of arthritis, asthma, or ulcerative colitis to his health care provider.
- Advise women to avoid using boswellia during pregnancy.

Points of interest
- B. serrata should not be confused with B. carteri, also known as frankincense or "incense." Unlike the serrata species, B. carteri is used for its aromatic properties and considered obsolete as a medicinal herb.

Commentary
Although some data support the use of Boswellia resin for inflammatory conditions, the results are inconclusive. The human trials have few participants, have vague results, and show no statistical differences between the Boswellia resin and placebo. The in vitro studies that claim a potential benefit in leukemia are interesting, but no clinical studies support this claim.

References
Gupta, I., et al. "Effects of Boswellia serrata Gum Resin in Patients with Bronchial Asthma: Results of a Double-blind, Placebo-controlled, 6-Week Clinical Study," Eur J Med Res 3(11):511-14, 1998.

Gupta, I., et al. "Effects of Boswellia serrata Gum Resin in Patients with Ulcerative Colitis," Eur J Med Res 2(1):37-43, 1997.

Safayhi, H., et al. "Inhibition by Boswellic Acids of Human Leukocyte Elastase," J Pharmacol Exp Ther 281(1):460-63, 1997.

Sander, O., et al. "Is H15 (Resin Extract of Boswellia serrata, "Incense") a Useful Supplement to Established Drug Therapy of Chronic Polyarthritis? Results of a Double-blind Pilot Study," Z Rheumatol 57(1):11-16, 1998.

Shao, Y., et al. "Inhibitory Activity of Boswellic Acids from Boswellia serrata Against Human Leukemia HL-60 in Culture," Planta Med 64(4):328-31, 1998.

Singh, G.B., and Atal, C.K. "Pharmacology of an Extract of Salai Guggal Ex-Boswellia serrata, a New Non-steroidal Anti-inflammatory Agent," Agents Actions 18(3-4):407-12, 1986.

Wildfeuer, A., et al. "Effects of Boswellic Acids Extracted from an Herbal Medicine on the Biosynthesis of Leukotrienes and the Course of Experimental Autoimmune Encephalomyelitis," *Arzneimittelforschung* 48(6):668-74, 1998.

BREWER'S YEAST

FAEX MEDICINALIS, MEDICINAL YEAST, *SACCHAROMYCES CEREVISIAE*

Common trade names
None known.

Common forms
Available in liquid, powder, and tablets (650 mg).

Source
Brewer's yeast is recovered after being used in the beer-brewing process.

Chemical components
Brewer's yeast is a rich source of vitamins (especially B complex), protein, minerals (particularly chromium), glucans, and mannans.

Actions
Brewer's yeast has been used to improve glucose tolerance in diabetic patients because of its high chromium content. Chromium is thought to increase insulin release, but this is controversial.

Medicinal yeast has also shown benefit to those suffering from such GI maladies as flatulence and diarrhea. In one study, brewer's yeast helped to facilitate the treatment of persistent *Clostridium difficile,* and in another study, it was used to treat enterotoxigenic *Escherichia coli* (Izadnia et al., 1998). Brewer's yeast also reduced water and electrolyte influx into the intestines stimulated by the *Vibrio cholerae* toxin. The success of brewer's yeast in the treatment of infectious diarrhea appears to be due to its ability to reestablish normal balances of the intestinal flora by increasing the activity of disaccharidases, saccharidases, maltase, and lactase.

There have been some reports of brewer's yeast's ability to modulate the immune system by stimulating phagocytosis, but evidence to support these claims is insufficient.

Reported uses
Brewer's yeast has been used in the treatment of GI maladies, including dysbiosis, infectious diarrhea, and loss of appetite. Some people use this supplement for its vitamin and mineral content to treat acne and contact dermatitis.

Dosages
For the chromium content, some sources recommend 1 or 2 tbsp of the powder P.O. t.i.d. This dosage provides about 360 mcg of chromium per day (RDA is 50 to 200 mcg/day). The average daily dose of brewer's yeast is 6 g.

Bold italic type indicates that reaction may be life-threatening.

Adverse reactions
CNS: migrainelike headaches in sensitive people (allergy related).
GI: flatulence, intestinal discomfort.
Skin: *allergic reactions.*

Interactions
MAO inhibitors: May increase blood pressure. Avoid administration with brewer's yeast.

Contraindications and precautions
Brewer's yeast is contraindicated in immunosuppressed patients.

Special considerations
ALERT Caution the patient not to confuse brewer's yeast with baker's yeast.
• Caution the patient not to self-treat symptoms of GI illnesses or dermatitis before receiving appropriate medical evaluation because this may delay diagnosis of a serious medical condition.
• Advise the patient to consult a health care provider before using any alternative medication because a treatment that has been clinically researched and proved effective may be available.
• Monitor the patient for severe headaches.
• Urge the diabetic patient to closely monitor blood glucose levels while taking brewer's yeast.

Commentary
Brewer's yeast appears to be a reasonable source of vitamins and minerals. It may be an alternative product for people who have difficulty swallowing drugs because it is typically sprinkled on foods. The use of brewer's yeast for its ability to stimulate the immune system warrants further research before any recommendations can be made.

References
Izadnia, F., et al. "Brewer's Yeast and *Saccharomyces boulardii* Both Attenuate *Clostridium difficile*–induced Colonic Secretion in the Rat," *Dig Dis Sci*, 43(9):2055-60, 1998.

BROOM

BANNAL, BROOMTOPS, GENISTA, GINSTERKRAUT, HOGWEED, IRISH TOPS, SAROTHAMNI HERB, SCOTCH BROOM, SCOTCH BROOM TOP

Taxonomic class
Fabaceae

Common trade names
None known.

Common forms
Available as cigarettes, extracts, root, and teas.

Source

The crude drug is prepared from the twigs and flowers of *Cytisus scoparius* (*Sarothamnus scoparius*). Broom has been naturalized from Europe to the United States and Canada. This plant should not be confused with Spanish broom (*Spartium junceum*), used in trace amounts in foods and cosmetics.

Chemical components

Broom tops (flowers) contain the alkaloid sparteine. The concentration of this alkaloid ranges from 0.01% to 0.22% in floral parts and up to 1.5% in twigs. Broom also contains the flavone glycosides genitoside, isoquercetin, lupanine, oxysparteine, scoparoside, and spiraeoside. Caffeic acid derivatives, essential oils (containing phenylethyl alcohol, phenols, and acids), isoflavones (sarothamnoside), kaempferol, and quercetin derivatives have also been reported. Broom seeds contain phytohemagglutinins, or lectins.

Actions

The metabolism of sparteine has been repeatedly documented in humans. Studies with rodents show that sparteine inhibits sodium and potassium transport across the cell membrane. This action in cardiac cells mimics the actions of type IA antiarrhythmics, such as quinidine and procainamide. Sparteine produces a negative chronotropic effect and, possibly, a negative inotropic effect (Pugsley et al., 1995; Raschack, 1974).

Sparteine undergoes oxidative metabolism by way of the cytochrome P-450 system in the liver. Cardiac drugs that share the same CYP2D6 pathway have demonstrated the ability to inhibit sparteine metabolism (Belpaire and Bogaert, 1996). All drugs known to share this metabolic pathway have the potential to interfere with the metabolism of sparteine. Sparteine is also a known oxytocic.

Another component of broom, scoparoside, possesses diuretic properties.

Reported uses

Medical folklore and homeopathy have endowed broom with antiarrhythmic, cathartic, diuretic, and emetic properties at high doses. Smoking broom cigarettes is reported to produce euphoria and relaxation. Some researchers argue that these effects are unlikely to occur because of the small quantity of alkaloids taken into the body through smoking of the plant.

Lectins isolated from broom seeds have been used as pharmacologic markers (Young et al., 1984). They have also been used to classify red cell polyagglutinability (Bird and Wingham, 1980). Sparteine, like debrisoquin, is used to characterize metabolizers of the oxidative metabolic pathway CYP2D6 in the liver (Belpaire and Bogaert, 1996).

Dosage

No consensus exists.

Bold italic type indicates that reaction may be life-threatening.

Adverse reactions

CNS: headache, mind-altering sensations (from smoking plant parts).

CV: *arrhythmias,* worsening of heart failure.

Respiratory: fungal pneumonia (increased risk when contaminated broom tops are smoked as cigarettes).

Other: spontaneous abortion (from effects of sparteine), uterine contractions.

Interactions

Antihypertensives: May alter effectiveness of some antihypertensives. Avoid administration with broom.

Beta blockers, other cardiac drugs, tricyclic antidepressants, and other drugs that undergo metabolism by way of CYP2DG: May enhance the effects of these drugs; increases risk of serious arrhythmias, such as ventricular fibrillation, ventricular tachycardia, bradycardia, and heart block. Avoid administration with broom.

Cardiac pacemakers: May interfere with proper function of pacemaker. Avoid use of broom in patients with pacemakers.

Contraindications and precautions

Broom is contraindicated in pregnant patients because it is known to cause spontaneous abortion. It is also contraindicated in patients with hypertension or significantly impaired cardiac function because of the potential for arrhythmias and the agent's ability to increase the tone of the vascular system.

Special considerations

⚫ ALERT Poisoning from overdose is possible. At toxic concentrations, broom may cause a clinical picture similar to that of nicotine poisoning: diarrhea, mental status changes, nausea, shock, tachycardia, and vertigo.

- Caution the patient to avoid ingesting or smoking broom preparations because of potentially dangerous effects on the vascular system.
- Inform the patient that broom is a dangerous herb and lacks approval for any therapeutic use.
- Advise the patient not to confuse this plant with Spanish broom (S. junceum).
- Caution women to avoid using broom during pregnancy.

Points of interest

- Before the use of hops, broom was used to enhance the taste and intoxicating power of beer.
- The FDA considers this plant unsafe for human consumption. The German Commission E, which oversees drug use in Germany, considers broom effective for certain cardiac disorders.

Commentary

Although broom contains interesting and potentially useful therapeutic agents, the risks appear to outweigh any purported benefits. Besides, safer and more effective drugs are available for all the potential therapeutic applications for broom. Additional data are needed to determine more completely the risks and benefits of the pharmacologic alkaloids contained in this plant.

References

Belpaire, F.M., and Bogaert, M.G. "Cytochrome P450: Genetic Polymorphism and Drug Interactions," *Acta Clin Belg* 51:254-60, 1996.

Bird, G.W., and Wingham, J. "Lectins for Polyagglutinable Red Cells: *Cytisus scoparius, Spartium junceum* and *Vicia villosa*," *Clin Lab Haematol* 2:21-23, 1980.

Leung, A.Y. *Encyclopedia of Common Natural Ingredients Used in Food, Drugs, and Cosmetics.* New York: Wiley-Interscience, 1980.

Pugsley, M.K., et al. "The Cardiac Electrophysiological Effects of Sparteine and Its Analogue BRB-I-28 in the Rat," *Eur J Pharmacol* 27:319-27, 1995.

Raschack, V.M. "Wirkungen von Spartein und Spartein-derivaten auf Herz and Kreislauf," *Arzneimittelforschung* 24:753, 1974.

Young, N.M., et al. "Structural Differences Between Two Lectins from *Cytisus scoparius*, Both Specific for D-galactose and N-acetyl-D-galactosamine," *Biochem J* 222:41, 1984.

BUCHU

AGATHOSMA, *BAROSMA BETULINA*, BETULINE, BOCCO, *DIOSMA BETULINA*

Taxonomic class
Rutaceae

Common trade names
Multi-ingredient preparations: Alvita Teas Buchu, Buchu Essential Oil, Cranberry/Buchu Concentrate, Gaia Herbs Buchu Leaves, Gaia Herbs Plantain/Buchu

Common forms
Available as dried leaves (for infusion) and a tincture.

Source
Active components of buchu are derived from a volatile oil in the leaves of *Barosma betulina* (*Agathosma betulina*) and the related species *Barosma serratifolia* and *Barosma crenulata*, low-lying shrubs that grow in South Africa. The leaves are harvested while the plants are flowering or bearing fruit.

Chemical components
The volatile oil of *B. betulina* leaves contains more than 100 chemicals. Those that may be responsible for the pharmacologic properties attributed to the herb include diosphenol (buchu camphor), pulegone, terpene-4-ol, and a number of flavonoids. Mucilage, resin, and coumarins have been reported in other *Barosma* species.

Actions
Little information is available on the action of buchu. In studies with rats, diosmin, a buchu flavonoid, acted as an anti-inflammatory (Farnsworth and Cordell, 1976).

Bold italic type indicates that reaction may be life-threatening.

Reported uses
Buchu is claimed to be useful as an antirheumatic and a diuretic and in the treatment of colds, coughs, stomachaches, and urogenital tract infections. The use of buchu leaves and the volatile oil has been popular among the inhabitants of South Africa for hundreds of years.

Dosage
Infusion: 1 small glass of the infusion (1 oz of dried leaves added to 1 pt of boiling water).
Tincture: 1 to 2 ml P.O. t.i.d. or q.i.d.

Adverse reactions
GI: diarrhea, nausea, vomiting (volatile oil).
GU: increased menstrual flow (pulegone), nephritis (volatile oil).
Hepatic: *hepatotoxicity* from volatile oil constituent (pulegone).
Other: *spontaneous abortion* (pulegone).

Interactions
Anticoagulants: May potentiate effects of anticoagulants. Avoid administration with buchu.

Contraindications and precautions
Buchu is contraindicated in pregnant or breast-feeding patients; pulegone has abortifacient activity and increases menstrual flow. It is also contraindicated in patients who are prone to kidney infections or those with urinary tract infections, mild to moderate renal disease, or hepatic dysfunction because the herb may exacerbate these conditions.

Special considerations
● Monitor liver function test results in patients using buchu because of its potential for causing hepatic dysfunction.
● Instruct the patient to avoid ingesting this plant; little is known about buchu, and some components could be toxic.
● Advise women to avoid using buchu during pregnancy or when breast-feeding.

Points of interest
● Buchu was once included in the U.S. National Formulary as an antiseptic and a diuretic. In 1821, it was listed in the British Pharmacopoeia as a medicine for catarrh of the bladder, cystitis, nephritis, and urethritis.
● In Germany, buchu is used as a treatment for kidney and urinary tract infections and as a diuretic. German health authorities, however, do not endorse its use because its purported actions for those conditions have not been substantiated.
● Buchu is used as a "cooling diuretic" in Ayurvedic medicine (Frawley and Lad, 1986).

Commentary

Buchu's efficacy has not been demonstrated in clinical trials or animal studies. Because of its potential for causing hepatic dysfunction, this herb cannot be recommended.

References

Farnsworth, N.R., and Cordell, G.A. "A Review of Some Biologically Active Compounds Isolated from Plants as Reported in the 1974-1975 Literature," *Lloydia* 39:420-55, 1976.

Frawley, D., and Lad, V. *The Yoga of Herbs.* Twin Lakes, Wisc.: Lotus Press, 1986.

Simpson, D. "Buchu—South Africa's Amazing Herbal Remedy," *Scott Med J* 43(6):189-91, 1998.

BUCKTHORN

COMMON BUCKTHORN, EUROPEAN BUCKTHORN, HARTSHORN, PURGING BUCKTHORN, WAYTHORN

Taxonomic class

Rhamnaceae

Common trade names

Multi-ingredient preparations: Herbal Laxative, Herbalene, Laxysat Mono Abführ-Tee Nr.2, Neo-Cleanse, Neo-Lax

Common forms

Available as a syrup.

Source

The drug is extracted from the berries of the thorny shrub or tree *Rhamnus cathartica.* Buckthorn is native to Europe and naturalized in parts of the United States and Canada.

Chemical components

Buckthorn berries are believed to contain acetic acid, albumen, sugar, tannin, and an azotized substance composed primarily of glucosides. Rhamnocathartin, a bitter, yellow amorphous substance, is soluble in water and alcohol. Rhamnin, found in the berries of the shrub, is barely soluble in cold water but soluble in hot alcohol. Rhamnegine breaks down into crystallizable sugar when heated with a dilute mineral acid. Rhamnotannic acid, formed during the separation of rhamnin, is an amorphous, friable, bitter mass that is soluble in alcohol and insoluble in water.

Actions

Buckthorn is reported to exert powerful cathartic effects. One study with animals found that the herb may be hepatotoxic in mice, possibly resulting from deposits of monoparticulate glycogen in the cytoplasm. Compounds in *R. cathartica* are thought to interfere with glycogen metabolism (Lichtensteiger et al., 1997).

Bold italic type indicates that reaction may be life-threatening.

Reported uses
Buckthorn's main use, as a cathartic, has declined drastically because of its violent mechanism of action and severe adverse effects. A powder or decoction of the bark has been used as a gentle astringent or tonic for skin ailments.

Dosage
No consensus exists.

Adverse reactions
CNS: anxiety, trembling.
GI: abdominal pain, diarrhea, nausea, vomiting.
Hepatic: *hepatotoxicity* (caused by tannin content).
Metabolic: dehydration.
Respiratory: *decreased respirations.*

Interactions
None reported.

Contraindications and precautions
Buckthorn is contraindicated in pregnant or breast-feeding patients; effects are unknown. Use cautiously in patients with GI disorders such as Crohn's disease, irritable bowel syndrome, peptic ulcer disease, and ulcerative colitis because of worsened symptoms.

Special considerations
- Although no known chemical interactions have been reported in clinical studies, consideration must be given to the herbal products' pharmacologic properties and the potential for interference with the intended therapeutic effect of conventional drugs.
- Caution the patient about potential GI problems associated with using buckthorn. Gentler, more predictable laxatives should be recommended, especially for older patients and young children.
- Instruct the patient to keep berries and all buckthorn preparations out of the reach of children.
- Advise women to avoid using buckthorn during pregnancy or when breast-feeding.

Points of interest
- Buckthorn is primarily used as a dye. The juice of the berries produces a saffron-colored dye and the bark, a brilliant yellow. The ripened berries of the plant are typically mixed with alum, which results in a sap-green color commonly used for watercoloring.
- Until the 19th century, syrup of buckthorn was the common form. The syrup was prepared by boiling the juice of a buckthorn with pimento, ginger, and sugar. Because of the severity of the resulting drug's actions, use of the herb was discontinued in humans. The herb was occasionally given to animals as a laxative and was mixed with equal parts of castor oil. The discovery of a more gently acting relative, *Rhamnus purshiana*, has led to a more limited use of *R. cathartica*.

Commentary

No clinical trials support the medicinal use of *R. cathartica*. Its violent actions and severe adverse effects suggest that the risks of administration outweigh the benefits. Medications with a lower incidence of adverse effects and more predictable efficacy should be considered.

References

Lichtensteiger, C.A., et al. "*Rhamnus cathartica* (Buckthorn) Hepatocellular Toxicity in Mice," *Toxicol Pathol* 25:449-52, 1997.

Millspaugh, C.F. *American Medicinal Plants*. New York: Dover Publications, Inc., 1974. Originally published in 1892.

BUGLEWEED

CARPENTER'S HERB, COMMON BUGLE, EGYPTIAN'S HERB, FARASYON MAIY, GYPSY-WEED, GYPSYWORT, MENTA DE LOBO, MIDDLE COMFREY, PAUL'S BETONY, SICKLEWORT, SU FERASYUNU, WATER BUGLE, WATER HOREHOUND

Taxonomic class

Lamiaceae

Common trade names

Bugleweed Extract, Bugleweed Motherwort Compound

Common forms

Available as a dried herb, liquid extract, and tincture.

Source

Pharmacologically active compounds are extracted from the roots, stems, leaves, and flowers of *Lycopus virginicus* and *Lycopus europaeus*. These members of the mint family are native to Europe and North America.

Chemical components

Active constituents of *L. europaeus* include lithospermic, chlorogenic, caffeic, ellagic, and rosmarinic acids as well as the flavone glycoside luteolin-7-glucoside. Other compounds include amino acids, minerals, sugars, tannin, ursolic acid, and sinapinic acid. *L. virginicus* was found to contain rosmarinic and caffeic acids (Horhammer et al., 1962). *L. europaeus* was found to contain catechol oxidase from diterpene metabolites.

Actions

Certain active compounds in *Lycopus* species have demonstrated complex endocrine effects in animal models, including a dose-related decrease in immunoglobulin G (IgG) antibody activity. The plant also inhibits IgG stimulation of adenylate cyclase in human thyroid membranes and thyroid iodine release in mice in vivo. It is unclear why bugleweed extracts interact with thyroid-stimulating hormone (TSH) and IgG antibody activity (Auf'Mkolk et al., 1985).

Bold italic type indicates that reaction may be life-threatening.

A study in horses found that oxidized *Lycopus* plant constituents inhibited serum gonadotropin levels in pregnant mares. These constituents also inhibited human chorionic gonadotropin (HCG) and prolactin in vitro (Brinker, 1990).

Reported uses
Bugleweed is claimed to have astringent and mild narcotic qualities and has been used for years in the symptomatic treatment of Graves' disease. *Lycopus* was compared with digitalis during the 19th century and was found to lower the pulse rate without accumulating in the system (Millspaugh, 1974). *L. europaeus* has also been used as a remedy for intermittent fever.

Dosage
For antithyroidal and antigonadal effects, 25 to 50 mg/kg parenterally or 200 to 1,000 mg/kg P.O. in animals (Brinker, 1990; Winterhoff et al., 1994).

Adverse reactions
Metabolic: hyperthyroidism (controversial).

Interactions
Beta blockers: May mask symptoms of hyperthyroidism. Avoid administration with bugleweed.
Thyroid hormone replacement: May interfere with thyroid replacement therapy. Avoid administration with bugleweed.

Contraindications and precautions
Bugleweed is contraindicated in pregnant or breast-feeding patients; effects are unknown. Use with extreme caution in patients with primary or secondary hypopituitarism, pituitary adenoma, primary or secondary hypogonadism, TSH-stimulating tumors, or related disorders. Use cautiously in patients with systolic dysfunction or heart failure.

Special considerations
- Bugleweed suppresses follicle-stimulating hormone (FSH), luteinizing hormone (LH), HCG, and TSH levels. Depending on the patient's hormone levels, concurrent *Lycopus* administration could enhance or antagonize the effects of these hormones.
- Bugleweed has not been evaluated in other thyroid conditions, such as multinodular goiters and subacute thyroiditis.
- *Lycopus* and related species should not be substituted for antithyroid drugs, such as propylthiouracil and methimazole.
- No adverse effects have been reported in animal studies with *L. europaeus; L. virginicus* inhibits testicular growth in rats (Sourgens et al., 1980).
- Instruct the patient with a history of thyroid or cardiac disease or osteoporosis to consult a health care provider before taking bugleweed because of its unclear effect on thyroid function.

• Advise the patient taking oral contraceptives or fertility drugs to consult a health care provider before taking bugleweed.
• Advise women to avoid using bugleweed during pregnancy or when breast-feeding.

Points of interest
• *L. europaeus* is frequently sold as *L. virginicus*.

Commentary
Knowledge of bugleweed's physiologic effects is derived from in vivo and in vitro animal studies using freeze-dried extracts. Although the results of animal studies do not necessarily apply to humans, they should inspire caution. This agent inhibits various hormones, such as FSH, TSH, LH, and HCG, but the level of inhibition has not been evaluated. It is difficult to determine the place, if any, of bugleweed in the treatment of Graves' disease, but research suggests that this plant should be investigated more thoroughly.

References
Auf'Mkolk, M., et al. "Extracts and Auto-oxidized Constituents of Certain Plants Inhibit the Receptor-Binding and the Biological Activity of Graves' Immunoglobulins," *Endocrinology* 116:1687-93, 1985.

Brinker, F. "Inhibition of Endocrine Function by Botanical Agents," *J Naturopath Med* 1:1-14, 1990.

Horhammer, L., et al. "Studies on the Ingredients of *Lycopus europaeus*," *Arzneimittelforschung* 12:1-7, 1962.

Kohrle, J., et al. "Iodothyronine Deiodinases: Inhibition by Plant Extracts," *Acta Endocrin* Suppl 16:188-92, 1981.

Millspaugh, C.F. *American Medicinal Plants.* New York: Dover Publications, 1974. Reprint of 1892 edition.

Sourgens, H., et al. "Antihormonal Effects of Plant Extracts on Hypophyseal Hormone in the Rat," *Acta Endocrin* 234:49, 1980.

Winterhoff, H., et al. "Endocrine Effects of *Lycopus europaeus* L. Following Oral Application," *Arzneimittelforschung* 44:41-45, 1994.

BURDOCK

BARDANA, BARDANCE RADIX, BEGGAR'S BUTTONS, BURR SEED, CLOT-BUR, COCKLEBURR, COCKLE BUTTONS, CUCKOLD, EDIBLE BURDOCK, FOX'S CLOTE, GOBO, GREAT BURR, GREAT BURDOCK, HAPPY MAJOR, HARDOCK, HAREBURR, LAPPA, LOVE LEAVES, PERSONATA, PHILANTHROPIUM, THORNY BURR, WILD GOBO

Taxonomic class
Asteraceae

Common trade names
Multi-ingredient preparations: Anthraxiviore, Burdock Blend Extract, Burdock Root, Burdock Sarsaparilla Compound

---

Bold italic type indicates that reaction may be life-threatening.

Common forms
Available as capsules (425 mg, 475 mg, cream for topical administration, dried root, liquid extract, tea, and tincture (made from crushed seeds).

Source
The crude drug is extracted from the dried root of the great burdock, *Arctium lappa*, or common burdock, *Arctium minus*. The seeds and leaves of burdock plants have also been used in folk medicine. Burdock is a large biennial herb grown in China, Europe, and the United States. The plant can be identified in the spring by the round heads of its purple flowers.

Chemical components
The principal component of burdock root is a carbohydrate, inulin, which can account for up to 50% of the total plant mass. Additional components include anthroquinone glycosides; nonhydroxy acids; a plant hormone, gamma-guanidino-*n*-butyric acid; polyacetylenes; polyphenolic acids; tannins; and volatile acids. Seeds contain chlorogenic acid, fixed oils, a germacranolide, a glycoside (arctiin), lignans, and other compounds. Some commercial teas that contain burdock have been prone to contamination with atropine.

Actions
Burdock is claimed to exert antimicrobial, antipyretic, diaphoretic, and diuretic activities. Uterine stimulation has been reported in in vivo studies. In animal studies, burdock extracts have reportedly demonstrated strong hypoglycemic activity (Lappinina and Sisoeva, 1964) and antagonism of platelet activating factor (Iwakami et al., 1992).

Various in vitro and animal studies have found that burdock possesses antimutagenic effects (Dombradi and Foldeak, 1966; Tsujita et al., 1979).

Reported uses
Burdock is claimed to be useful for a wide range of ailments, including arthritis; cystitis; gout; hemorrhoids; lumbar pain; rheumatism; sciatica; skin disorders, such as acne, canker sores, dry skin, eczema, and psoriasis; and ulcers. It has also been used as a blood purifier. In the Far East, burdock is used to treat cancer, impotence, and sterility. Some studies have reported the use of burdock in the treatment of kidney stones and HIV infection.

Dosage
Burdock is taken internally as a tea or used externally as a compress.
Dried root: 2 to 6 g P.O. t.i.d.
Liquid extract (1:1 in 25% alcohol): 2 to 8 ml P.O. t.i.d.
Tea: 1 cup P.O. t.i.d. or q.i.d.
Tincture (1:10 in 45% alcohol): 8 to 12 ml P.O. t.i.d.

Adverse reactions
Skin: allergic dermatitis (Rodriguez et al., 1995).
Other: *allergic reactions.*

Interactions
Insulin, oral antidiabetics: May increase hypoglycemic effects. Avoid administration with burdock.

Contraindications and precautions
Burdock is contraindicated during pregnancy—especially in the first trimester—because of the effects of anthraquinone glycosides found in the roots of burdock plants. It is also contraindicated in patients who are hypersensitive to the herb or related plant species.

Special considerations
• Allergic reactions have been demonstrated in people who are sensitive to the Asteraceae/Compositae family. Other members of this family include chrysanthemum, daisy, mangold, and ragweed.

🍂 **ALERT** Poisoning caused by atropine contamination of some commercial burdock teas can occur. Signs and symptoms of toxicity include blurred vision, dilated pupils, and rapid pulse rate. Treatment, if needed, includes physostigmine reversal (Bryson, 1978; Bryson and Rumack, 1978; Rhoads and Anderson, 1985).

• Inform the patient that burdock products may be significantly contaminated with atropine and that toxicity has resulted from this contamination.

• Inform the diabetic patient that burdock may increase the risk of hypoglycemia and that insulin or oral antidiabetic drug doses may need to be reduced.

• Inform the patient that few scientific data evaluate burdock's effects in humans.

• Caution women to avoid using burdock during pregnancy or when breast-feeding.

Points of interest
• Burdock root is commonly eaten in Asia, less often in the United States.

Commentary
Animal and in vitro studies suggest that burdock use might offer therapeutic benefits. Clinical trials are needed to support these claims. Also, data regarding the safety and efficacy of burdock are lacking.

References
Bryson, P.D. "Burdock Root Tea Poisoning," *JAMA* 240:1586, 1978.

Bryson, P.D., and Rumack, B.H. "Burdock Root Tea Poisoning," *JAMA* 239:2157, 1978.

Dombradi, C.A., and Foldeak, S. "Antitumor Activity of *A. lappa* Extracts," *Tumori* 52:173-75, 1966.

Gruenwald, J., et al. *PDR for Herbal Medicines.* Montvale, N.J.: Medical Economics Company, Inc., 1998.

Iwakami, S., et al. "Platelet Activating Factor (PAF) Antagonists Contained in Medicinal Plants: Ligans and Sesquiterpenes," *Chem Pharm Bull* 40:1196, 1992.

Jellin, J.M., et al. *Natural Medicines Comprehensive Database.* Stockton, Calif.: Therapeutic Research Faculty, 1999.

Bold italic type indicates that reaction may be life-threatening.

Lappinina, L.O., and Sisoeva, T.F. "Investigation of Some Plants to Determine Their Sugar Lowering Action," *Farmatsevt Zh* 19:52-58, 1964.

Rhoads, P.M., and Anderson, R. "Anticholinergic Poisonings Associated with Commercial Burdock Root Tea," *Clin Toxicol* 22:581-84, 1985.

Rodriguez, P., et al. "Allergic Contact Dermatitis Due to Burdock (*Arctium lappa*)," *Contact Dermatitis* 33:134-35, 1995.

Tsujita, J., et al. "Comparison of Protective Activity of Dietary Fiber Against the Toxicities of Various Food Colors in Rats," *Nutr Rep Int* 20:635-42, 1979.

BUTCHER'S BROOM

BOX HOLLY, KNEE HOLLY, PETTIGREE, SWEET BROOM

Taxonomic class
Liliaceae

Common trade names
Multi-ingredient preparations: Butcher's Broom Extract 4:1, Butcher's Broom Root, Hemodren Simple, Ruscorectal

Common forms
Capsules: 75 mg, 110 mg, 150 mg, 400 mg, 470 mg, 475 mg
    Also available as liquid extract and tea.

Source
Butcher's broom is extracted from the leaves, rhizomes, and roots of *Ruscus aculeatus*, a low-lying evergreen of the lily family. It is native to the Mediterranean region but also grows in southern United States.

Chemical components
The major active components of butcher's broom are the steroidal saponins ruscogenin and neoruscogenin. Coumarins, flavonoids, glycolic acid, sparteine, and tyramine have also been isolated.

Actions
In a study of dog veins, the saponins in butcher's broom produced vasoconstriction by directly activating postjunctional alpha$_1$ and alpha$_2$ receptors (Marcelon et al., 1983).
    Studies with animals have evaluated the effect of *R. aculeatus* on the diameter of arterioles and venules (Bouskela et al., 1993) and the effect of local changes in temperature on venous responsiveness to *R. aculeatus* (Rubanyi et al., 1984). Clinical trials suggest that a *Ruscus* preparation relieved symptoms of chronic phlebopathy of the legs (Cappelli et al., 1988). The extract of this plant possesses anti-inflammatory properties as well.

Reported uses
Butcher's broom is claimed to be helpful in treating arthritis, hemorrhoids, leg edema, peripheral vascular disease, and varicose veins. It has also been used as a diuretic and a laxative. Human clinical data to support these claims are limited.

Dosage

For venous phlebopathy in the lower limbs, the dosage of butcher's broom tested in humans was 99 mg P.O. daily (in combination with ascorbic acid and hesperidin).

Adverse reactions

None reported.

Interactions

Anticoagulants: May increase effects of these drugs. Monitor closely.
Antihypertensives: May reduce effects of alpha blockers, such as prazosin, doxazosin, terazosin; reduces effectiveness of therapy for benign prostatic hyperplasia (BPH). Avoid administration with butcher's broom.
MAO inhibitors: May cause hypertensive crisis from tyramine in butcher's broom. Avoid administration with butcher's broom.

Contraindications and precautions

Butcher's broom is contraindicated in pregnant or breast-feeding patients; effects are unknown. Use cautiously in patients with hypertension or BPH or those who are receiving alpha antagonist therapy.

Special considerations

• Inform the patient that more effective agents exist to treat his disease and that long-term effects of butcher's broom are unknown.
• Caution the patient with circulatory disorders that butcher's broom may interfere with other drugs he is taking.
• Advise women to avoid using butcher's broom during pregnancy or when breast-feeding.

Points of interest

• Butchers in Europe and the Mediterranean at one time used the leaves and twigs of this plant to scrub chopping blocks clean, hence the name butcher's broom.

Commentary

Butcher's broom possesses vasoconstrictive properties, but clinical data about these effects are limited. One study suggests that butcher's broom is beneficial in patients with chronic venous insufficiency and varicose veins. The study involved only 40 patients and *R. aculeatus* was used in combination with hesperidin and ascorbic acid.

Butcher's broom may be well tolerated, but additional studies are needed to evaluate its efficacy in treating venous disease and other vascular conditions. No clinical data support the use of butcher's broom for treating arthritis or hemorrhoids.

References

Bouskela, E., et al. "Effects of *Ruscus* Extract on the Internal Diameter of Arterioles and Venules of the Hamster Cheek Pouch Microcirculation," *J Cardiovasc Pharmacol* 22:221-24, 1993.
Cappelli, R., et al. "Use of Extract of *Ruscus aculeatus* in Venous Disease in the Lower Limb," *Drugs Exp Clin Res* 14:277-83, 1988.

Bold italic type indicates that reaction may be life-threatening.

Marcelon, G., et al. "Effect of *Ruscus aculeatus* on Isolated Canine Cutaneous Veins," *Gen Pharmacol* 14:103, 1983.

Rubanyi, G., et al. "Effect of Temperature on the Responsiveness of Cutaneous Veins to the Extract of *Ruscus aculeatus*," *Gen Pharmacol* 15:431-34, 1984.

BUTTERBUR

EUROPEAN PESTROOT, SWEET COLTSFOOT, WESTERN COLTSFOOT

Taxonomic class
Asteraceae

Common trade names
Multi-ingredient preparations: Alzoon, Butterbur Root Extract, Feverfew/Dogwood Supreme, Neurochol, Petaforce, Wild Cherry Supreme

Common forms
Available as 25-mg standardized capsules, *Petasites* extract, and liquid *Petasites* extract (concentration may vary).

Source
Active compounds of butterbur are extracted from the leaves, flowers, stems, and root stock of *Petasites hybridus*, *P. officinalis*, or *Tussilago petasites*. Some formulas use extract from the leaves and roots of *P. frigidus*, also known as *P. palmatus*, *T. palmatum*, or western coltsfoot. These plants are low-lying perennial herbs of the Compositae family.

Chemical components
The active components of *P. hybridus* are believed to be isopetasin, oxopetasin esters, and petasin. Several studies have found petasin, a sesquiterpene ester of petasol and angelic acid, to be the most active component (Weiss, 1988). Isopetasin and oxopetasin esters have been isolated. Other alkaloids isolated from *P. hybridus* include the pyrrolizidine alkaloids integerrimine, senecionine, and senkirkine (Luthy et al., 1983) as well as petasol and isopetasol (Predescu et al., 1980). *P. frigidus* contains petasin and related esters, saponins, resins, and volatile oils as well as small amounts of pyrrolizidine alkaloids. The latter occur in young leaves but not in the roots, which are more often used in commercial extracts (Moore, 1995).

Actions
Studies with animals have found that *P. hybridus* extracts possess anti-inflammatory and spasmolytic properties. The extracts reduced intestinal ulcerations and blocked gastric damage in rats. The effects were dose-dependent.

Extracts also inhibited peptido-leukotriene biosynthesis in mouse peritoneal macrophages and did not affect prostaglandin synthesis. Pro posed mechanisms include inhibition of 5-lipoxygenase or interference with the use of calcium ions in leukotriene production (Brune et al., 1993).

In 1953, studies found a cytostatic effect of *Petasites* extract on fertilized sea urchin eggs, leading to the agent being used later as an analgesic for cancer patients (Weiss, 1988). This effect is not substantiated in other available literature.

Some work is being done examining *P. hybridus'* effects on dopamine$_2$ and histamine$_1$ receptors (Berger, 1998).

Reported uses

Butterbur has been used for thousands of years for GI disorders and GI-related pain as well as for asthma, cough, skin diseases, and spasms of the urogenital tract (Brune et al., 1993). Other therapeutic claims include its use as an antarthritic, an astringent for cosmetic purposes, a diuretic, and a sedative. Butterbur was prescribed in ancient times as an ointment for ulcers and sores (Bianchini and Corbetta, 1977). References have also been made to an analgesic effect of *Petasites* extracts, but this effect may be secondary to the herb's spasmolytic properties.

P. frigidus may be taken as a tea or smoked. It may also be used as a poultice by patients who reside in areas where the plant is endemic, including the United States (Moore, 1995).

Dosage

No consensus exists.

Adverse reactions

EENT: eye discoloration.
GI: abdominal pain or pressure, sustained constipation, discoloration of stool, dysphagia, severe nausea, vomiting.
GU: difficulty urinating.
Hepatic: *hepatotoxicity.*
Respiratory: *difficulty breathing.*
Skin: skin discoloration.

Interactions

None reported, but administration of butterbur with anticholinergics may not be advisable.

Contraindications and precautions

Avoid using *Petasites* extracts in pregnant or breast-feeding patients; effects are unknown. Also avoid using butterbur in patients with decreased GI or bladder motility because symptoms of these disorders may worsen.

Special considerations

• Discourage the use of butterbur in patients with disorders that might be worsened by any effect on leukotriene synthesis or calcium-modulated smooth-muscle contractility, especially in the GI tract. Also discourage its use in patients with underlying disorders that may become dangerous if inadequately treated, such as asthma.

Bold italic type indicates that reaction may be life-threatening.

◖ ALERT Carcinogenic and hepatotoxic effects may result from the presence of pyrrolizidine alkaloids in the plant (Luthy et al., 1983).

• Monitor for adverse reactions, and notify the health care provider if any occur.

• Advise women to avoid using butterbur during pregnancy or when breast-feeding.

Commentary

Despite the use of butterbur extracts for centuries, little information is available to establish safety and efficacy in the prevention or treatment of any diseases in humans. Although studies with animals suggest a possible mechanism of action for reducing smooth-muscle spasms and inflammation, studies in humans are lacking.

Further research may reveal a beneficial effect of the more active components of *Petasites* extracts, but purification and standardization of these extracts are needed before reliable claims can be made. The active components of *Petasites* extract can vary from one batch to another, and potentially hazardous alkaloids have been identified in these plants.

References

Berger, D., et al. "Influence of *Petasites hybridus* on Dopamine-D2 and Histamine-H1 Receptors," *Pharm Acta Helv* 72(6):373-75, 1998.

Bianchini, F., and Corbetta, F. *Health Plants of the World: Atlas of Medicinal Plants.* New York: Newsweek Books, 1977.

Brune, K., et al. "Gastroprotective Effects by Extracts of *Petasites hybridus*: The Role of Inhibition of Peptido-leukotriene Synthesis," *Planta Med* 59:494-96, 1993.

Luthy, J., et al. "Pyrrolizidine Alkaloids in *Petasites hybridus* and *P. albus*," *Pharm Acta Helv* 58:98-100, 1983. Abstract.

Moore, M. *Medicinal Plants of the Pacific West.* Santa Fe, N.M.: Red Crane Books, 1995.

Predescu, I., et al. "Contributions to the Chromatographic and Spectral Study of *Petasites hybridus* Extract," *Farmacia Bucharest* 28:241-48, 1980.

Weiss, R.F. *Herbal Medicine.* Beaconsfield, England: Beaconsfield Publishers Ltd., 1988.

C

CABBAGE
BRASSICA, COLEWORT

Taxonomic class
Fabaceae

Common trade names
None known.

Common forms
Available in preparations from chopped or pressed cabbage and juices.

Source
Active components are extracted from the leaves of *Brassica oleracea*. Cabbage is originally from the Mediterranean, but cultivated varieties are found in damp and temperate climates worldwide.

Chemical components
Compounds isolated from *B. oleracea* include various mustard oils, allyl mustard oil, methyl sulfonyl alkyl isothiocyanates, and methyl sulfonyl alkyl isothiocyanates; 3-hydroxy-methyl indole; 5-vinyl-oxazolidine-2-thion (goitrin); rhodanides; alkyl nitriles; and amino acids.

Actions
Cruciferous vegetables such as cabbage have a high glucosinate content. These substances are precursors that are converted to isothiocyanates. Many isothiocyanates inhibit the neoplastic effects of various carcinogens (Verhoeven et al., 1997).

Brassinin, a phytoalexin first identified as a constituent of cabbage, was synthesized and demonstrated a dose-dependent inhibition in mouse mammary and skin tumors (Mehta et al., 1995). Similar studies have reinforced the efficacy of cabbage as a suppressor of cancer in animal models (Bresnick et al., 1990; Beecher, 1994).

Hypoglycemic effects of *Brassica* vegetables have been noted in a limited number of studies (Platel and Srinivasan, 1997).

Reported uses
Cabbage has been promoted for its cancer-preventive effects, hypoglycemic activity, and use in relieving breast engorgement.

Numerous case-control and cohort studies have examined the association between the consumption of *Brassica* or cruciferous vegetables and cancer. Six cohort studies have demonstrated an inverse relation between the consumption of *Brassica* vegetables and the risk of lung cancer, stomach cancer, and all cancers taken together. Sixty-four percent of the case-control studies showed this inverse association. The association was most consistent for colorectal, lung, and stomach cancers and least consistent for endometrial, ovarian, and prostate cancers (van Poppel et al., 1999).

A prospective cohort study reported a weak association between total vegetable and fruit intake and bladder cancer risk. In this study, only the associations for broccoli and cabbage were statistically significant (Michaud et al., 1999).

The effect of cabbage on breast engorgement has been studied using various forms, such as a cream containing cabbage extract and application of the actual leaf. In one small placebo-controlled study involving 21 lactating women, there was no difference between the cabbage extract cream and placebo. Breast-feeding had a greater effect on relieving breast engorgement than either cream (Roberts et al., 1998). Other studies have compared the efficacy of applying cabbage leaves, chilled or at room temperature, with using standard care with chilled gel packs. Although mothers who used the cabbage leaves preferred this method and generally breast-fed longer, there was no statistically significant difference between the groups with regard to relieving breast engorgement (Roberts et al., 1995; Nikoderm et al., 1993).

Dosage
Traditional uses suggest the following doses:
Oral: 1 tsp of cabbage juice t.i.d. for gastritis; 1 L of juice daily to supplement the diet.
Topical: Apply leaves to inflamed tissue or use as an extract in a cream.

Adverse reactions
None reported.

Interactions
Acetaminophen, oxazepam, warfarin: May decrease efficacy of these drugs because of induced hepatic metabolism. Monitor the patient's PT and INR.

Contraindications and precautions
Cabbage may exacerbate goiters and hypothyroidism by reducing iodine uptake by the thyroid gland. Ingesting large quantities of cabbage may elevate thyroid-stimulating hormone levels. In pregnant and breast-feeding patients, avoid using in amounts greater than those typically found in foods.

Special considerations
● Educate the patient regarding the use of cabbage as a cancer preventive.
● Caution the patient that cabbage may decrease the effectiveness of other drugs he is taking.
● Caution the patient not to self-treat symptoms of illness before seeking appropriate medical evaluation because this may delay diagnosis of a serious medical condition.

Bold italic type indicates that reaction may be life-threatening.

• Advise the patient to consult a health care provider before using herbal preparations because a treatment that has been clinically researched and proved effective may be available.

Points of interest
• Besides cabbage, *Brassica* vegetables include broccoli, Brussels sprouts, cauliflower, and kale.

Commentary
Most of the evidence concerning the cancer-preventive effects of *Brassica* vegetables and their proposed active ingredients comes from animal studies. Human epidemiological evidence supports the association between high consumption of cruciferous vegetables such as cabbage and a decreased risk of certain cancers. Critics caution that this effect may be due to consumption of vegetables in general, not just *Brassica* vegetables. Further epidemiological research and controlled trials in humans are needed to define the role of *Brassica* vegetables in cancer prevention. Cabbage leaves do not appear to relieve breast engorgement but may provide a cooling effect. Cabbage is a savory vegetable and when consumed in a realistic quantity does not appear to produce adverse effects.

References
Beecher, C.W. "Cancer Preventive Properties of Varieties of *Brassica oleracea*: A Review," *Am J Clin Nutr* 59(5 Suppl):1166S-70S, 1994.

Bresnick, E., et al. "Reduction in Mammary Tumorigenesis in the Rat by Cabbage and Cabbage Residue," *Carcinogenesis* 11(7):1159-63, 1990.

Mehta, R.G., et al. "Cancer Chemopreventive Activity of Brassinin, a Phytoalexin From Cabbage," *Carcinogenesis* 16(2):399-404, 1995.

Michaud, D.S., et al. "Fruit and Vegetable Intake and Incidence of Bladder Cancer in a Male Prospective Cohort," *J Natl Cancer Inst* 91(7):605-13, 1999.

Nikoderm, V.C., et al. "Do Cabbage Leaves Prevent Breast Engorgement? A Randomized, Controlled Study," *Birth* 20(2):61-64, 1993.

Platel, K., and Srinivasan, K. "Plant Foods in the Management of Diabetes Mellitus: Vegetables as Potential Hypoglycemic Agents," *Nahrung* 41(2):68-74, 1997.

Roberts, K.L., et al. "A Comparison of Chilled and Room Temperature Cabbage Leaves in Treating Breast Engorgement," *J Hum Lact* 11(3):191-94, 1995.

Roberts, K.L., et al. "Effects of Cabbage Leaf Extract on Breast Engorgement," *J Hum Lact* 14(3):231-36, 1998.

van Poppel, G., et al. "*Brassica* Vegetables and Cancer Prevention. Epidemiology and Mechanisms," *Adv Exp Med Biol* 472:159-69, 1999.

Verhoeven, D.T., et al. "A Review of Mechanisms Underlying Anticarcinogenicity by *Brassica* Vegetables," *Chem Biol Interact* 103(2):79-129, 1997.

CALUMBA
COCCULUS PALMATUS, COLOMBO, COLUMBO ROOT

Taxonomic class
Menispermaceae

Common trade names
Multi-ingredient preparations: Amaro Maffioli, Appetiser Mixture, Bitteridina, Ducase, Elixir Spark, Padma-Lax, Richelet, Travel-Caps

Common forms
Available as capsules and an elixir that is often prepared without heating as a cold infusion.

Source
The root of the *Jatorhiza palmata* plant is dried and powdered. The powder changes color from green to brownish black as it rapidly absorbs moisture from the air and decomposes. The plant is native to Mozambique and Madagascar.

Chemical components
The plant yields columbamine, jateorhizine, palmatine, three yellow crystalline alkaloids, and columbin, a colorless crystalline principle.

Actions
In studies with anesthetized mice, columbin decreased the time of urethane- and alpha-chloralose–induced sleep and prolonged the sleep time of hexobarbital-treated mice (Wada et al., 1995).

Reported uses
No human studies have been reported, but anecdotal evidence suggests calumba's use as an antidiarrheal and antiflatulent and for treating chronic enterocolitis, gastritis, and indigestion. It is seldom used as a cathartic or digestive aid because of its morphinelike effects.

Dosage
In an animal study using mice, 20 to 40 mg/kg/day P.O. was given for 5 days.
Traditional uses suggest the following doses:
Oral: 2 tsp of boiled root as tea every hour.
Single drops: 20 gtt of extract or 2.5 g of tincture can be used.

Adverse reactions
GI: constipation, epigastric pain and vomiting (with large doses).

Interactions
Antacids, histamine$_2$ antagonists: May produce an additive effect in the GI tract. Reevaluate the need for both acid-modifying entities.

Contraindications and precautions
Avoid using calumba in pregnant or breast-feeding patients; effects are unknown.

Special considerations
• Recommend other drugs to the patient who needs an antidiarrheal.
• Advise the patient to consult a health care provider before using herbal

preparations because a treatment that has been clinically researched and proved effective may be available.
- Calumba overdose can lead to paralysis and unconsciousness.
- Advise women to avoid using calumba during pregnancy or when breast-feeding.

Points of interest
- Calumba is cultivated for use as a flavoring agent and a dye.

Commentary
Because human clinical trials are lacking, calumba cannot be recommended for use. More studies are needed in animals and humans to establish safety and efficacy. Given the safety and efficacy of approved antidiarrheals, further investigation and development of calumba for this application are of questionable value.

References
Colombo. *Natural Medicines Comprehensive Database.* Therapeutic Research Faculty. 1999, p. 280.
Wada, K., et al. "Columbin Isolated from *Calumbae radix* Affects the Sleep Time of Anesthetized Mice," *Biol Pharm Bull* 18:634-36, 1995.

CAPSICUM

BELL PEPPER, CAPSAICIN, CAYENNE, CHILI PEPPER, HOT PEPPER, PAPRIKA, PIMIENTO, RED PEPPER, TABASCO PEPPER

Taxonomic class
Solanaceae

Common trade names
Capsin, Cap-Stun, Capzasin, Dolorac, No Pain HP, Pepper Defense, R-Gel, Zostrix (HP)

Common forms
Cream: 0.025%, 0.075%, 0.25%
Gel: 0.025%
Lotion: 0.025%, 0.075%
Self-defense spray: 5%, 10%

Source
Capsaicinoids are derived from the dried fruit of the plants of the Solanaceae family. The species most commonly used are *Capsicum frutescens* and *Capsicum annum.* Before the actual capsaicin can be isolated, a concentrate called oleoresin capsicum is formed from the peppers. Extraction of capsaicin forms water-insoluble needles (highly alcohol- and fat-soluble). Other species of *Capsicum* used include *C. baccatum, C. chinensis,* and *C. pubescens.* These peppers should not be

confused with the plants that give us common black pepper and white pepper (*Piper* species, family Piperaceae).

Chemical components

Capsicum species can contain up to 1.5% of a capsaicinoid oleoresin. The major components of the oleoresin responsible for the plant's pungent appeal are capsaicin, 6,7-dihydrocapsaicin, homocapsaicin, homodihydrocapsaicin, and nordihydrocapsaicin. Many volatile oils, carotenoids (capsanthin, capsorubin, carotene, lutein), proteins, fats, and high amounts of vitamins A and C are present. The amount of vitamin C present may be four to six times that found in an orange. Provitamins E, P, B_1, B_2, and B_3 have also been identified as components.

Other plant material contains steroidal alkaloidal glycosides (solanine and solasadine) and scopoletin (coumarin). Each chili pepper contains about 0.14% of capsaicin, with the highest concentrations in the yellowish red placenta of the fruit and its attachments.

Actions

Although topical capsaicin produces an intense irritation at the contact point, vesicles usually do not form. The initial dose of capsaicin causes profound pain, but repeated applications produce desensitization, with analgesic and even anti-inflammatory effects. Heat sensation is caused by the stimulation of specific local afferent nerve fibers. Analgesic effects may be explained by capsaicin-induced neuronal depletion of substance P, believed to be a mediator in the transmission of painful stimuli from the periphery to the spinal cord. The analgesic effect can also result from the methoxyphenol portion of the capsaicin molecule that may interfere with the lipoxygenase and cyclooxygenase pathways.

Capsaicin does not cause blistering or redness because it does not act on the capillaries or other blood vessels. An externally applied 0.1% capsaicin solution inhibits flare formation after intradermal injection of histamine. Areas of skin (control) without pretreatment of capsaicin developed a wheal, flare, and itching. Flare response is believed to be substance P–mediated.

Juices from the fruits have shown antibacterial properties in vitro. I.V. infusion of capsaicin has been reported to stimulate secretion of epinephrine and norepinephrine from the adrenal medulla of rodents.

Reported uses

Traditional claims surrounding the use of capsicum include treatment of bowel disorders, chronic laryngitis, and peripheral vascular disease. Various preparations of capsicum have been applied topically as counterirritants and external analgesics. Topical capsaicin preparations are useful for treating pain associated with diabetic neuropathy, osteoarthritis, postherpetic neuralgia (Bernstein et al., 1987), postsurgical pain (including postmastectomy and postamputation pain), rheumatoid arthritis, and other neuropathic pain and complex pain syndromes (Robbins et al., 1998).

Capsaicin has been suggested for refractory pruritus and pruritus associated with renal failure. A small study has suggested that nasal inhalation of capsaicin may be beneficial in nonallergic, noninfectious perennial rhinitis. Poor tolerability may be of issue with larger clinical trials. One study has reported capsaicin's use for urinary urgency. (See *Treating urinary urgency with capsaicin.*) Capsaicin is also increasingly popular as a nonlethal self-defense spray.

Dosage

Because capsaicin is potent, concentrations of topical preparations range from 0.025% to 0.25%. Preparations are most effective when applied t.i.d. or q.i.d., and their duration of action is 4 to 6 hours. Less frequent application typically produces less effective substance P depletion and results in incomplete analgesia.

Adverse reactions

CNS: neuropathy.
EENT: blepharospasm, conjunctival edema, extreme burning pain in eye, hyperemia, lacrimation (ocular complications are rare and usually result from eye rubbing); burning pain in nose, serous nasal discharge, sneezing.
GI: GI discomfort (minimized if seeds are removed from the product before ingestion).
GU: renal dysfunction (when used orally on a regular basis).
Hematologic: deficient coagulability, RBC hemolysis.
Hepatic: hepatic dysfunction (when used orally on a regular basis).
Respiratory: transient ***bronchoconstriction***, cough, and retrosternal discomfort.
Skin: transient erythema, irritation, itching, and stinging without vesicular eruption (diminishes with repeated use).

Interactions

ACE inhibitors: Topical application of capsicum may contribute to the cough reflex. Avoid administration with capsicum.
Anticoagulant and antiplatelet properties: May increase hypocoagulability when used concurrently with such drugs as warfarin and acetylsalicylic acid. Avoid administration with capsicum.
Centrally acting adrenergic agents: May reduce efficacy of antihypertensives such as clonidine and methyldopa. Avoid administration with capsicum.
MAO inhibitors: May promote toxicity (hypertensive crisis) when used together because of catecholamine release. Avoid administration with capsicum.
Sedatives: Concomitant use may cause additive therapeutic and adverse effects. Use together cautiously.

Contraindications and precautions

Contraindicated in patients who are hypersensitive to capsicum or chili pepper products. Also contraindicated in pregnant patients to avoid possible uterine stimulant effects.

Bold italic type indicates that reaction may be life-threatening.

RESEARCH FINDINGS
Treating urinary urgency with capsaicin

In a study of six patients, an intravesical capsaicin injection was shown to reduce urinary urgency, bladder capacity, and the micturition threshold pressure (Dasgupta and Fowler, 1997). Five "hypersensitive bladder" patients experienced resolution or a clinically relevant reduction in urgency, frequency, and pain for up to 16 days posttreatment. The sixth patient had benign prostatic hyperplasia and didn't experience symptomatic improvement. All patients reported adverse reactions that included a feeling of warmth or burning in the urethra after voiding.

The authors suggested that capsaicin induces diuresis through stimulation of the vesicorenal reflex. Increases in urinary levels of sodium and potassium were noted together with increased excretion of prostaglandin E_2.

Special considerations
• The intensity of adverse reactions depends on the dose and concentration.
• After topical application of capsicum to open wounds or injured skin, relief can occur in as little as 3 days but may take 14 to 28 days, depending on the condition that requires analgesia.
• No evidence exists that topical application causes permanent neurologic injury.
• Dose-related (1 to 100 nM) RBC hemolysis associated with significant changes in erythrocyte membrane lipid components as well as acetylcholinesterase activity can occur.
• Instruct the patient to avoid contact with eyes, mucous membranes, and nonintact skin. Direct him to flush the exposed area with cool running water for as long as necessary if incidental contact occurs.
• Caution the patient taking MAO inhibitors or centrally acting adrenergics against using capsicum.
• Advise women to avoid using capsicum during pregnancy or when breast-feeding.
• Instruct the patient not to use other heat applications simultaneously with capsicum.

Points of interest
• More than one-third of its total vitamin C content remains after a chili pepper has been cooked; vitamin C is lost if the pepper is dried.
• Because of its short-term immobilizing effects, capsaicin is used as a humane self-defense spray. The more popular products contain the capsicum oleoresin, which produces immediate blepharospasm, blindness, and incapacitation for up to 30 minutes.

• Peppers are among the most widely consumed spice in the world with an average per-person consumption approaching 50 mg of capsaicin daily in some Southeast Asian countries.

Commentary
Natural capsicum has been used for centuries. Capsaicin, derived from capsicum, has gained widespread popularity as an agent for several potential therapeutic applications. Commercially available capsaicin preparations are effective adjunctive topical analgesics for some pain and pruritic syndromes. Long-term effects of topical application appear benign. For some patients, the initial burning sensation and delayed onset of action may be the most undesirable aspects of its use. The ingestion of capsicum in excess of the amount normally available in food is not recommended.

References
Bernstein, J.E., et al. "Total Capsaicin Relieves Chronic Post-herpetic Neuralgia," *J Am Acad Dermatol* 17:93, 1987.

Capsicum. *Natural Medicines Comprehensive Database.* Stockton, Calif.: Therapeutic Research Faculty, 1999, 197-99.

Dasgupta, P., and Fowler, C.J. "Chillies: From Antiquity to Urology," *Br J Urol* 80:845-52, 1997.

onhealth.com/alternative/resource/herbs/item,15962.asp

Robbins, W.R., et al. "Treatment of Intractable Pain with Topical Large-Dose Capsaicin: Preliminary Report," *Anesth Analg* 86:579-83, 1998.

CARAWAY
CARUM CARVI L., CARVI AETHEROLEUM, CARVI FRUCTUS, KUMMEL, KUMMELOL, OLEUM CARI, OLEUM CARVI

Taxonomic class
Apiaceae

Common trade names
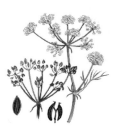

Multi-ingredient preparations: Ajaka, BPC 1973, Cholosum N, Concentrated Caraway Water, Digestozym, Divinal-Bohnen, Enteroplant, Euflat 1, Flatulex, Galloselect N, Gastricard N, Globase, Hevert-Carmin, Lomatol, Majocarmin, Metrophyt-V, Neo-Ballistol, Sanvita Magen, Spasmo Claim, Tirgon

Common forms
Available as capsules, caraway oil, 5% volatile oil, caraway seed, caraway water, powder, coated tablets, film tablets, and tea.

Source
A volatile oil is distilled from dried ripened seeds of *Carum carvi* L., a biennial herb that is native to Europe and Asia. Caraway water is obtained by soaking 1 oz of bruised seeds in 1 pt of cold water for 6 hours.

Chemical components
Caraway oil is chiefly (53% to 63%) composed of a ketone, carvone, an optical isomer also found in spearmint oil. The oil also contains a terpene, D-limonene.

Actions
Caraway was found to relax the tracheal smooth muscle and increase the resting force (contracture) of ileal smooth muscle in guinea pigs (Reiter and Brandt, 1985). Although this herb has been claimed to have a laxative action, this effect was not seen in the guinea pigs.

Another study found that caraway oil may inhibit skin tumors in female mice (Schwaireb, 1993). The oil, either applied topically or taken as a dietary supplement, inhibited croton oil–induced skin tumors as well as resulted in the disappearance of the tumor and a reduction in the incidence, delay in appearance, retardation, and regression of established papillomas. Topical administration appears to be superior to dietary supplementation in producing these effects (Schwaireb, 1993). Human studies have not been performed to assess the efficacy of caraway oil in preventing toxin-induced skin tumors.

Antimicrobial activity has been demonstrated in vitro against *Bacillus, Pseudomonas, Candida,* and *Dermatomyces.*

Reported uses
Caraway oil, an aromatic herb, is used in many pharmaceutical preparations as a flavoring agent. It is claimed to be an effective aid for abdominal distention, bronchitis, colic, constipation, flatulence, hiatal hernia, indigestion, menstrual cramps, mild spastic conditions of the GI tract, and stomach ulcers; a gargle for laryngitis; and a bath additive.

The role of monoterpenes, found in citrus fruits and caraway seed oil, in inhibiting carcinogen activation and preventing carcinogen-induced neoplasm is being evaluated (Wattenberg, 1990). D-Limonene has been shown to inhibit a tobacco-specific carcinogen when administered immediately before carcinogen challenge, but the extent is unknown.

In a small study evaluating the laxative effects of an herbal combination containing caraway, all patients found relief from constipation within the first 2 days. The combination herbal product had no effect on gastric mucosa or ulcer healing rate (Matev et al., 1981). A combination of caraway and peppermint oil was found to decrease or eliminate pain in patients with nonulcer dyspepsia (May et al., 1996). This combination was found to act locally to cause smooth-muscle relaxation in six healthy volunteers (Micklefield et al., 2000).

A 4-week randomized, controlled, double-blind study compared a combination product containing caraway and peppermint oils with cisapride in the relief of symptoms associated with functional dyspepsia. Sixty patients received the combination herbal product (100 mg of caraway oil and 180 mg of peppermint oil) daily and 58 patients received cisapride (30 mg/day). The combination herbal preparation was comparable to cisapride in relieving pain associated with dyspepsia (Madish et al., 1999).

Dosage

For flatulence, the adult dose is 1 to 4 gtt of essential oil in 1 tsp of water or on a lump of sugar P.O., or 1.5 to 6 g of freshly crushed seeds for infusions b.i.d. to q.i.d. between meals. This dose is based on traditional practice.

Adverse reactions

GI: diarrhea, hepatic dysfunction (large doses of the volatile oil taken for extended periods).
GU: renal dysfunction (large doses of the volatile oil taken for extended periods).
Skin: contact dermatitis, mucous membrane irritation.

Interactions

None reported.

Contraindications and precautions

Caraway is contraindicated in patients who are hypersensitive to caraway oil or its components. Avoid using caraway in pregnant patients because of its theoretical relaxant effect on uterine muscle.

Special considerations

• Monitor for diarrhea and efficacy of administration.
• Inform the patient that caraway's efficacy as an antiflatulent or a digestant is largely untested and that other drugs have been widely tested and may be equally as effective or more effective than caraway.
• Advise the patient to check the label carefully to prevent confusing plain and concentrated caraway water.
• Caraway oil should be stored in a glass or metal container and protected from light and moisture.

Points of interest

• Caraway has been used by many civilizations. It is believed to have originated with the ancient Arabs, who called the seed *Karawya.* Dioscorides (A.D. 40 to 90), a Greek physician, recommended that the oil be used by "pale-faced girls," possibly because of its claimed stimulant action.
• Caraway oil is used to flavor such liqueurs as aquavit, Kummel, and L'huile de Venus.
• An old superstition states that caraway has the power of retention, preventing the theft of items that contain the seed. It was used in love potions to keep lovers from losing interest and straying.
• Caraway was traditionally used to improve lactation in breast-feeding mothers.

Commentary

Caraway, an established flavoring agent for many pharmaceutical and food products, has antiflatulent properties. Folklore has produced several therapeutic claims, few of which can be substantiated with clinical trial data. It might have laxative action and may be used to treat nonulcer dyspepsia. Studies performed to evaluate the efficacy of caraway in these roles are not definitive. Further human studies are needed to evaluate caraway's effect on neoplasms and whether it possesses anticancer properties.

When consumed orally for medicinal purposes, caraway has generally been recognized as safe in the United States and is approved for food use up to a maximum of 0.02%.

References

Blumenthal, M., et al., eds. *The Complete German Commission E Monographs: Therapeutic Guide to Herbal Medicines.* Boston: Integrative Medicine Communications, 1998.

Madish, A., et al. "Treatment of Functional Dyspepsia with a Fixed Peppermint Oil and Caraway Oil Combination Preparation as Compared to Cisapride. A Multicenter, Reference-controlled Double-blind Equivalence Study," *Arzneimittelforschung* 49:925-32, 1999. Abstract.

Matev, M., et al. "Use of an Herbal Combination with Laxative Action on Duodenal Peptic Ulcer and Gastroduodenitis Patients with a Concomitant Obstipation Syndrome," *Vutr Boles* 20:48-61, 1981. Abstract.

May, B., et al. "Efficacy of a Fixed Peppermint Oil/Caraway Oil Combination in Non-ulcer Dyspepsia," *Arzneimittelforschung* 46:1149-53, 1996. Abstract.

Micklefield, G.H., et al. "Effects of Peppermint Oil and Caraway Oil on Gastroduodenal Motility," *Phytother Res* 14:20-23, 2000. Abstract.

Reiter, M., and Brandt, W. "Relaxant Effects on Tracheal and Ileal Smooth Muscles of the Guinea Pig," *Arzneimittelforschung* 35:408-14, 1985. Abstract.

Schwaireb, M.H. "Caraway Oil Inhibits Skin Tumors in Female BALB/c Mice," *Nutr Cancer* 19:321-25, 1993.

Wattenberg, L.W. "Inhibition of Carcinogenesis by Naturally Occurring and Synthetic Compounds," *Basic Life Sci* 52:155-66, 1990. Abstract.

CARDAMOM

ALPINIA CARDAMOMUM, AMOMUM CARDAMON, AMOMUM REPENS, CARDAMOMI SEMINA, CARDAMOM SEEDS, CARDAMOMUM MINUS, MALABAR CARDAMOM, MATONIA CARDAMOM

Taxonomic class
Zingiberaceae

Common trade names
None known.

Common forms
Available as dried seeds, whole or powdered, and essential oils.

Source
Cardamom seeds are harvested from the fruits of *Elettaria cardamomum*, a large perennial herb that is native to southern India. The fruits are gathered before they ripen and split because seeds from opened fruits are less aromatic. Seeds yield 4% to 6% of a volatile oil.

Chemical components

The volatile oil is primarily composed of 1,8-cineole and alpha-terpinyl acetate (Baruah et al., 1973). Other components include alpha-pinene, alpha-terpineol, borneol, limonene, linalool, linalyl acetate, and myrcene.

Actions

The few studies that report on the pharmacologic action of cardamom are based on in vitro or animal data. Eugenol, a compound found in cardamom and other spices, significantly inhibits tobacco-induced mutagenicity (Sukumaran and Kuttan, 1995). Cardamom oil, given intraperitoneally, was compared with indomethacin for acute carrageenan-induced edema in male rats. Compared with indomethacin, a lower cardamom dose suppressed edema to a lesser extent, whereas a higher cardamon dose exerted a more potent anti-inflammatory effect.

In one study, cardamom oil halved the *p*-benzoquinone–induced writhing in mice, suggesting a possible analgesic effect, and inhibited the stimulant action of acetylcholine, perhaps explaining its role as an antispasmodic (Al-Zuhair et al., 1996).

Reported uses

Cardamom is a widely used flavoring agent for sweets and coffee and a standard ingredient in curry. Its medicinal use dates back to ancient times. Herbalists recommended it to improve digestion and relieve flatulence. It is also popular in Ayurvedic medicine. When chewed, the seeds have a pleasant taste that may be followed by increased salivation and a warm sensation in the mouth. The herb has been used for bronchitis, colds, and cough and recommended as an appetite stimulant in anorexic patients. Cardamom sprinkled on cooked cereal has been reported to help children with celiac disease who are intolerant to the gluten in grain. Data from human studies cannot be found to support these claims.

Dosage

No human studies support dosing recommendations. Doses listed in other sources are 15 to 30 grains of powder P.O., 1 fluid dram of tincture P.O., and 5 to 30 gtt of fluidextract P.O. Seeds are commonly chewed whole, and the powder is usually sprinkled on food or included in beverages.

Adverse reactions

Skin: contact dermatitis (one case was reported after a confectioner with chronic hand dermatitis had positive patch test reactions to cardamom and terpenoid compounds [Mobacken and Fregert, 1975]).

Interactions

None reported.

Bold italic type indicates that reaction may be life-threatening.

Contraindications and precautions
Avoid using cardamom in pregnant or breast-feeding patients; effects are unknown.

Special considerations
• Ingestion of cardamom beyond amounts commonly found in foods is not recommended.
• Inform the patient of the lack of human trials with cardamom. Instruct him to consult a health care provider if complaints related to GI dysmotility continue despite use of cardamom.
• Advise women to avoid using cardamom during pregnancy or when breast-feeding.

Commentary
Although cardamom has long been claimed to relieve indigestion and flatulence, no clinical trials have tested this effect, and its therapeutic benefit remains unproven. Further study is warranted to evaluate the pharmacologic properties of cardamom, and human data are needed before it can be recommended to treat any medical condition.

References
Al-Zuhair, H., et al. "Pharmacological Studies of Cardamom Oil in Animals," *Pharmacol Res* 34:79-82, 1996.
Baruah, A.K.S., et al. "Chemical Composition of Alleppey Cardamom Oil by Gas Chromatography," *Analyst* 98:168-71, 1973.
Mobacken, H., and Fregert, S. "Allergic Contact Dermatitis from Cardamom," *Contact Dermatitis* 1:175-76, 1975.
Sukumaran, K., and Kuttan, R. "Inhibition of Tobacco-induced Mutagenesis by Eugenol and Plant Extracts," *Mutat Res* 343:25-30, 1995.

CARLINE THISTLE
ARTEMISIA VULGARIS, CARLINA VULGARIS, FELON HERB, MUGWORT, *RADIX CARDOPATIAE*

Taxonomic class
Asteraceae

Common trade names
Multi-ingredient preparations: Blessed Herbs, Chinac Digestive Health Formula, Para-Clens, Phyto Surge

Common forms
Available as a liquid or tea.

Source
Active components are obtained from the seeds, fresh roots, and leaves of *Carlina acaulis.*

Chemical components

The plant contains 0.03% to 0.2% of volatile oil. The main component is cineole; others include alpha-amyrin, alpha- and beta-pinene, beta-sitosterol, fernenol, quebrachitol, sitosterol, tauremisin, tetracosanol, and thujonestigmasterol. Glycosides include rutinosyl-s quercetin as well as 4c-glycosyl flavones, such as carlinoside, homoorientine, orientine, and schaftoside.

Actions

The leaf extract of *Artemisia vulgaris* was found to delay onset of picro-toxin-induced seizures and reduce mortality rates in mice. A plant extract was active against some sarcomas in rats.

Reported uses

Carline thistle is claimed to be effective as an anthelmintic, an anti-epileptic, an antiseptic, an antispasmodic, a colerectic, a diaphoretic, a digestive stimulant, a diuretic, an expectorant, a menstruation aid, a tonic, and a spasmolytic.

Carline thistle is claimed to be effective for asthma, bronchitis, cancerous lesions, chorea, cold, colic, constipation, cramps, diarrhea, dysmenorrhea, epilepsy, fever, gallstones, gastritis, gout, headache, hysteria, inflammation, kidney stones, labor, menstrual problems and irregular periods, nervousness, rheumatism, rickets, tuberculosis, vomiting, worms, and wounds and as a sedative. Anecdotal human data suggest that carline thistle is effective in treating pruritus and atopic dermatitis (Tamuki and Muratsu, 1994; Tezhka et al., 1992).

Possible efficacy as a bladder irrigant was suggested by researchers who used *A. vulgaris* as part of an herbal preparation for continuous bladder irrigation after prostatic adenotomy. They reported decreased bacteremia, blood loss, and purulent inflammation postoperatively (Davidov et al., 1995).

Dosage

No consensus exists.

Adverse reactions

CNS: *seizures* (with overdose).
Musculoskeletal: muscle spasms, myalgia.
Other: allergic reaction.

Interactions

None reported.

Contraindications and precautions

Carline thistle is contraindicated in pregnant patients. The herb is thought to act as an abortificient and a menstrual and uterine stimulant. The effects in breast-feeding patients are unknown. Use cautiously in patients who are hypersensitive to plants in the Asteraceae/Compositae family (common herbs are chrysanthemums, daisies, marigolds, and ragweed), tobacco, honey, or royal jelly.

Bold italic type indicates that reaction may be life-threatening.

Special considerations
• Inform the patient that insufficient data exist to recommend use of carline thistle.
• Caution the patient not to self-treat symptoms of illness before seeking appropriate medical evaluation because this may delay diagnosis of a serious medical condition.
• Advise the patient to consult a health care provider before using herbal preparations because a treatment that has been clinically researched and proved effective may be available.
• Advise women to avoid using carline thistle during pregnancy or when breast-feeding.

Commentary
Anecdotal reports suggest that carline thistle may be effective for treating pruritic skin lesions and atopic dermatitis. Safety of the herb and its components is not supported by the scientific medical literature. Well-designed and controlled human trials are needed before carline thistle can be recommended for any purpose.

References
Davidov, M.I., et al. "Postadenectomy Phytoperfusion of the Bladder," *Urol Nefrol* 5:19-20, 1995.
Tamuki, A., and Muratsu, M. "Clinical Trial of SY Skin Care Series Containing Mugwort Extract," *Skin Res* 36:369-78, 1994. Abstract.
Tezhka, T., et al. "The Clinical Effects of Mugwort Extract on Pruritic Skin Lesions," *Skin Res* 35:303-11, 1992. Abstract.

CASCARA SAGRADA
CALIFORNIAN BUCKTHORN, SACRED BARK

Taxonomic class
Rhamnaceae

Common trade names
Multi-ingredient preparations: Bassoran with Cascara, Bicholax, Cas-Evac, Casvlium, Kondremul with Cascara

Common forms
Available as capsules, bitter and sweet fluidextracts, powders, and dried bark for teas. Cascara sagrada prepared as a tea is not popular because of its extremely bitter taste and the availability of standardized pharmaceutical preparations that perform the same functions.

Source
Cascara sagrada is the dried bark of *Rhamnus purshiana*. It should be aged for at least 1 year before use in medicinal preparations, but 3-year-old bark is preferred for pharmaceutical purposes because it exhibits a milder cathartic activity because of the oxidation of glycosides present in the bark. Cascara sagrada is found in the Pacific Northwest, from Canada to California.

Chemical components

Two types of anthracene compounds—emodin glycosides (*O*-glyco-sides) and aloinlike *C*-glycosides—have been reported. The *C*-glycosides are divided into barbaloin, deoxybarbaloin (chrysaloin), and the cas-carosides. Dried, medicinal-quality cascara bark yields not less than 7% of total hydroxyanthracene derivatives, calculated as cascaroside A, on a dried basis. The cascarosides should make up at least 60% of this total.

Actions

The glycosides found in cascara sagrada are stimulant cathartics that exert their action by increasing the smooth-muscle tone in the wall of the large intestine and have only minor effects on the small intestine. The drug is transformed by intestinal bacteria into substances that in-crease peristalsis in the large intestine and help restore intestinal tone.

Reported uses

Cascara sagrada was traditionally used as a laxative by Native Americans of the Pacific Northwest. In 1990, the FDA released the results of its study on OTC products and placed cascara sagrada in category I (safe and effective) as a laxative (Covington et al., 1996). Dried, aged cascara sagrada bark is widely accepted as a mild and effective treatment for chronic constipation (Morton, 1977).

Dosage

Aromatic fluidextract (sweet cascara): 5 ml P.O.
Extract capsules: 300 mg P.O.
Liquid extract (bitter cascara): 1 to 5 ml P.O.

Adverse reactions

GI: abdominal pain.
EENT: allergic rhinitis.
Respiratory: *IgE-mediated asthma.*
Chronic use or abuse
GI: abdominal cramps, diarrhea, melanosis coli (darkening pigmenta-tion of colonic mucosa), steatorrhea, vomiting.
GU: urine discoloration.
Metabolic: fluid and electrolyte imbalance, vitamin and mineral defi-ciencies.
Musculoskeletal: osteomalacia.
Other: laxative dependency.

Interactions

None reported, but the absorption of some drugs may be diminished.

Contraindications and precautions

Cascara sagrada is contraindicated in pregnant or breast-feeding pa-tients because it crosses the placental barrier, is excreted in breast milk, and increases the risk of diarrhea in a breast-fed infant. Although cas-cara sagrada may be used cautiously during pregnancy, other laxatives (such as bulk-forming and surfactant laxatives) may be preferred.

Bold italic type indicates that reaction may be life-threatening.

Special considerations
- Effective bowel regimens for constipation include temporary pharmacotherapy together with maintaining sufficient fluid intake and hydration, increasing fiber in the diet, eating regular meals, and exercising.
- Patients with chronic constipation (longer than 1 week) should be evaluated by a primary health care provider for underlying causes of obstruction.
- Cascara sagrada appears to be reasonably safe, although the fresher the bark, the higher the risk of adverse reactions. Occupational exposure of pharmacy workers to cascara sagrada has resulted in IgE-mediated asthma and allergic rhinitis (Giavina-Bianchi et al., 1997).
- Inquire about laxative use when taking the drug history.
- Inform the patient that the FDA has determined that cascara sagrada is generally safe and effective.
- Advise women to avoid using cascara sagrada during pregnancy or when breast-feeding.
- Inform the patient that cascara sagrada products are for short-term use.

Points of interest
- Cascara sagrada mostly comes from Oregon, Washington, and southern British Columbia. During the summer, sections of bark are peeled off and rolled into large quills. The bark is then carefully sun-dried so that the inner surface is not exposed to the sun and its yellow color is retained. The drug is then processed into its final form.

Commentary
Cascara sagrada is a mild stimulant laxative that is safe and effective. Although the FDA has approved its use, caution should be used when treating chronic constipation to avoid laxative dependency. Reliable and standardized pharmaceutical forms are preferred because there is no advantage in using the bark as a tea for its medicinal effects. Standardized pharmaceutical products ensure correct dosage and minimize the risk of adverse reactions.

References
Covington, T.R., et al., eds. *Handbook of Nonprescription Drugs,* 11th ed. Washington, D.C.: American Pharmaceutical Association, 1996.

Giavina-Bianchi, P.F., et al. "Occupational Respiratory Allergic Disease Induced by *Passiflora alata* and *Rhamnus purshiana*," *Ann Allergy Asthma Immunol* 79(5):449-54, 1997.

Morton, J.F. *Major Medicinal Plants: Botany, Culture and Uses.* Springfield, Ill.: Charles C. Thomas Pub., Ltd., 1977.

CASTOR BEAN

AFRICAN COFFEE TREE, BOFAREIRA, CARMENCITA, CASTOR OIL PLANT, MEXICO SEED, PALMA CHRISTI, TANGANTANGAN OIL PLANT, WONDER TREE, WUNDERBAUM

Taxonomic class
Euphorbiaceae

Common trade names
Alphamul, Aromatic Castor Oil USP 23, Carmencita, Castor Oil Caps USP 23, Emulsoil, Fleet Castor Oil Emulsion, Neoloid, Purge, Ricino Koki, Unisoil

Common forms
Castor oil emulsion: Alphamul 60% (90 ml, 3,780 ml), Emulsoil 95% (63 ml), Fleet Flavored Castor Oil 67% (45 ml, 90 ml), Neoloid 36.4% (118 ml)
Castor oil liquid: 100% (60 ml, 120 ml, 480 ml)
Purge: 95% (30 ml, 60 ml)

Source
Castor oil is obtained by cold-pressing the seeds of *Ricinus communis,* a perennial herb believed to be native to Africa and India.

Chemical components
Castor oil contains 45% to 50% oil. The oil is a mixture of triglycerides, of which 75% to 90% is ricinoleic acid. The poisonous phytotoxins ricin and ricinine are present in seed cake and oil.

Actions
Castor oil increases peristalsis and laxative action by stimulating the intramural nerve plexus of the small intestinal musculature. It also promotes fluid and ion accumulation in the colon. Castor oil given orally produces one or more stools 2 to 6 hours after ingestion. Ricin is a poisonous protein that disrupts DNA synthesis and protein metabolism, resulting in cell death.

Reported uses
Castor oil is an official USP product used as a laxative and a protectant in hair conditioners as well as in skin creams for treating rash. Application of the oil to an irritated conjunctiva caused by a foreign body provides soothing relief. Castor oil is commonly used to empty the GI tract of gas and feces before proctoscopy or radiographic studies. Topical application of castor oil has also been claimed to dissolve cysts, growths, and warts and to soften bunions and corns. It is also believed to expel worms if used with anthelmintics. No controlled human trials are available to support these claims.

Bold italic type indicates that reaction may be life-threatening.

Dosage
For constipation, 15 to 60 ml of castor oil P.O. daily.

Adverse reactions
CNS: dizziness, fainting.
GI: abdominal cramps and pain.

Large oral doses
GI: colicky pain, nausea, severe purgation, vomiting.

Long-term use
Metabolic: fluid and electrolyte loss.
Skin: allergic reactions (in seed handlers).

Interactions
None reported.

Contraindications and precautions
Avoid using castor bean in pregnant or breast-feeding patients; effects are unknown. Use cautiously in patients with appendicitis, intestinal obstruction, rectal bleeding, and sensitivity to castor oil. Prolonged use of castor oil can result in laxative dependency. Castor oil can also cause malabsorption of fat-soluble vitamins, fluid, and electrolytes.

Special considerations
🐚 **ALERT** Leaves are considered poisonous. Ricin and ricinine can cause toxic symptoms, such as abdominal pain, hepatic and renal injury, irritation of the oral cavity and esophagus, nausea, seizures, and vomiting, and even death (Kinamore et al., 1980). Reversible hepatotoxicity reportedly developed in a 20-month-old infant with no GI symptoms 48 to 72 hours after ingestion of castor beans (Palatnick et al., 2000).
• Castor oil may be refrigerated to improve palatability.
• Inquire about laxative use when taking the drug history.
• Instruct the patient to drink plenty of fluids (6 to 8 glasses) daily.
• Caution the patient to use cascara sagrada for no longer than a few days.
• Advise women to avoid using castor bean during pregnancy or when breast-feeding.

Points of interest
• Castor oil flowers develop into spiny capsules that contain three seeds (also called beans). As they dry, the capsules explode, scattering the seeds.

Commentary
Although castor oil is an official USP product used for its laxative effects, other, more gentle and palatable laxatives exist. Standardized forms of this product are available and recommended over nonstandard herbal preparations. Other uses claimed for this product have little or no supporting clinical evidence.

References

Kinamore, P.A., et al. "Abrus and Ricinus Ingestion: Management of Three Cases," *Clin Toxicol* 17:401-5, 1980.

Palatnick, W., et al. "Hepatotoxicity from Castor Bean Ingestion in a Child," *J Toxicol Clin Toxicol* 38(1):67-69, 2000.

CATNIP

CATARIA, CATMINT, CATNEP, CATRUP, CAT'S-PLAY, CATSWORT, FIELD BALM, NIP

Taxonomic class
Lamiaceae

Common trade names
Multi-ingredient preparations: Catnip, Catnip & Fennel, Catnip & Fennel Extract, Catnip Herb, Catnip Mist

Common forms
Available as capsules (380 mg), elixir, liquid, tincture, and tea.

Source
Obtained from the dried leaves and flowering tops of *Nepeta cataria*, catnip is a perennial herb that is common in Europe and cultivated in the United States.

Chemical components
The major active ingredients in catnip are volatile oils. The primary volatile oils are *cis-trans*-nepetalactone and valeric acid. Nepetalactone is similar in structure to the sedative ingredient found in valerian root. The seeds also contain linolenic, linoleic, oleic acid, and saturated fatty acids. Other chemicals found in *N. cataria* include acetic acid, buteric acid, citral, dipentene, lifronella, limonene, iridoids, tannins, and terpene.

Actions
N. cataria contains volatile oils that produce sedative effects. An alcoholic extract produced a sedative effect in young chicks. Low to moderate doses caused chicks to sleep, whereas higher doses appeared to have a paradoxical effect (Sherry and Hunter, 1979).

The effect of other drugs on catnip-induced pleasures in cats has been conducted (Hatch, 1972). The psychoactive (hallucinogenic) properties of catnip remain controversial.

Reported uses
The principal anecdotal recommendation for catnip is as a tea for insomnia and restlessness. Despite the lack of human clinical trials, the herb is said to be useful also for treating amenorrhea, anemia, bronchitis, colds, diarrhea, dysmenorrhea, fever, flatulence, headaches, hiccups,

---

Bold italic type indicates that reaction may be life-threatening.

RESEARCH FINDINGS
Psychoactive effects of catnip in a toddler

An anecdotal case of altered mental status in a 19-month-old toddler who ingested catnip tea was reported (Osterhoudt et al., 1997). The toddler consumed an unknown quantity of raisins that had been soaked in catnip tea. Three hours later, he became restless and cranky and developed a stomachache. The next day his mother reported that "he looked drugged" and took him to the emergency department. The child's vital signs were as follows: heart rate 199 beats/minute, respiratory rate 28 breaths/minute, blood pressure 131/77 mm Hg, and temperature 99.3° F (37.4° C).

On evaluation, the patient was lethargic but arousable with verbal stimuli. His abdomen was soft with no masses. Cranial nerve function was intact and pain sensation was present. Laboratory values were as follows: leukocytes 7,100/mm³, hemoglobin 12 g/dl, sodium 135 mEq/L, potassium 4.7 mEq/L, carbon dioxide 18 mmol/L, chloride 99 mEq/L, glucose 98 mg/dl, and BUN 7 mg/dl. Urinalysis and urine toxicology screens were negative. A computed tomography brain scan was unremarkable. The toddler was admitted for observation.

Three hours after admission, he continued to be obtunded and responsive only to physical stimuli. A lumbar puncture was then performed with negative results. Six hours after admission, the toddler had a large bowel movement that contained a dozen raisins and some tea leaves. His mental status subsequently improved, and he was discharged the next day. The toddler's symptoms were directly related to his ingestion of catnip and disappeared with the fecal passage of the raisins and tea leaves.

hives, indigestion, infantile colic, and toothaches. Catnip has been used as an antispasmodic, a diaphoretic, a stimulant, and a tonic without scientific data to support these claims. Catnip salve and tea are reported to be folklore remedies for cancer and believed to have psychoactive and euphoric properties when smoked as a cigarette; mind-altering effects can occur after accidental ingestion. (See *Psychoactive effects of catnip in a toddler.*)

Dosage
Human data are lacking.
Tea: Boiling water is poured on 2 tsp of dried leaves and brewed for 10 to 15 minutes.
Tincture: 2 to 4 ml P.O. t.i.d.

Adverse reactions
CNS: headache, malaise.
GI: nausea, vomiting (with large doses).

Interactions
None reported, but concomitant use with barbiturates and other drugs or herbs with sedative properties may cause additive effects. Avoid concomitant use.

Contraindications and precautions
Avoid using catnip in pregnant (uterine stimulant) or breast-feeding patients; effects are unknown. Also avoid use in patients with severe menstrual bleeding or pelvic inflammatory disease because it can induce menstruation.

Special considerations
• Urge the patient to reconsider using catnip as a sleep aid because scientific data supporting this use are lacking. Direct him to consult a health care provider who specializes in treating sleep disorders.
• Advise the patient to notify the prescriber and pharmacist of any herbal or dietary supplement he is taking when filling a new prescription.
• Advise women to avoid using catnip during pregnancy or when breast-feeding.

Points of interest
• *N. cataria* has an aromatic, mintlike odor.
• Most cat owners buy catnip to use in toys. The scent of the catnip—not its consumption—is believed to exert euphoria and sexual stimulation in cats.

Commentary
Although catnip may have sedative effects, human clinical data are lacking. One case report found that catnip altered a toddler's mental status after he consumed a large number of raisins soaked in catnip tea. Further studies are needed to evaluate the safety and efficacy of the herb for the claimed therapeutic uses.

References
Hatch, R.C. "Effects of Other Drugs on Catnip-induced Pleasure Behavior in Cats," *Am J Vet Res* 33:143-55, 1972.
Osterhoudt, K.C., et al. "Catnip and the Alteration of Human Consciousness," *Vet Human Toxicol* 39:373-75, 1997.
Sherry, C.J., and Hunter, P.S. "The Effect of an Ethanolic Extract of Catnip on the Behavior of the Young Chick," *Experientia* 35:237-38, 1979.

CAT'S CLAW

LIFE-GIVING VINE OF PERU, SAMENTO, UNA DE GATO

Taxonomic class
Rubiaceae

Common trade names
Cat's Claw Inner Bark Extract, Vegicaps

Common forms
Capsules and tablets: 25 mg, 150 mg, 175 mg, 300 mg, 350 mg (standard extract); 400 mg, 500 mg, 800 mg, 1 g, 5 g (raw herb)

Also available as cut, dried, or powdered bark, roots, and leaves; teas; and tinctures.

Source
Active components are extracted from the roots, stem bark, and leaves of *Uncaria tomentosa, U. guianensis,* and other species of the woody vine belonging to the Rubiaceae family. The plant is native to the Amazon.

Chemical components
The plant contains oxindole alkaloids, including isopteropodine, pteropodine, isomitraphylline, rhynchophylline, isorynchophylline, and mytraphylline, and indole alkaloidal glucosides, including cadambine, 3-dihydrocadambine, and 3-isodihydrocadambine. Other compounds are quinovic acid glycosides, tannins, proanthocyanidins, polyphenols, catechins (D-catechol), and beta sitosterol.

Actions
Four oxindole alkaloids (isopteropodine, pteropodine, isomitraphylline, and isorynchophylline) have shown immunostimulating properties (increased phagocytotic activity, synthesis of WBCs, and enhanced T-helper cell function) in vitro. Some antitumorigenic activity has also been suggested. A study using rats fed varying concentrations of cat's claw demonstrated a stimulation in lymphocytic proliferation and increased WBC counts compared with controls (Sheng et al., 2000). Another study reported an increase in interleukin-1 and interleukin-6 in rat aveolar macrophages in a dose-dependent manner (Lemaire et al., 1999).

Another alkaloid, rhynchophylline, has been found to inhibit platelet aggregation in rats (Chen et al., 1992) and to inhibit the sympathetic nervous system, reduce the heart rate, decrease peripheral vasculature resistance, and lower blood pressure (Hemingway and Philipson, 1974). Mytraphylline, an alkaloid, has weak diuretic properties. The combined effect of these alkaloids appears to be useful in treating CV disorders, but appropriate studies are lacking.

Another alkaloid, hirsutine, possesses local anesthetic properties and has been shown to inhibit bladder contraction in the guinea pig. High doses of hirsutine inhibited neuromuscular transmission in the rat (Harada and Ozaki, 1976). Both hirsutine and rhynchophylline have shown verapamil-like effects by influencing calcium influx in rabbit aorta strips (Zhang et al., 1987). Other *Uncaria* alkaloids exhibit antiviral activity and antioxidant properties in vitro.

Glycosides found within the bark of cat's claw have been identified as having anti-inflammatory properties. Although questions surface concerning the ability to provide relief in humans, rat studies suggest that cat's claw protects cells against oxidative stress and negates the activation of NF-kappa B (a known inflammatory pathogen; Sandoval et al., 1998).

Reported uses

Cat's claw is claimed to be useful in treating systemic inflammatory diseases (such as arthritis and rheumatism) and inflammatory GI disorders (such as Crohn's disease, diverticulitis, dysentery, gastritis, and ulcerations), but human clinical data confirming these uses are lacking.

South American folk medicine has endorsed cat's claw as a contraceptive. It is anecdotally reported that drinking the tea during menses for 3 consecutive months prevents pregnancy for about 4 years. No scientific support exists for this claim.

Dosage

Usual dosage is 500 to 1,000 mg P.O. t.i.d.

Adverse reactions

CV: hypotension.

Interactions

Antihypertensives: May enhance effects. Avoid administration with cat's claw.

Contraindications and precautions

Cat's claw is contraindicated in patients undergoing skin grafts and organ transplants and in those with coagulation disorders or receiving anticoagulants. Avoid its use in pregnant or breast-feeding patients; effects are unknown.

Special considerations

• Monitor the patient for signs of bleeding, such as petechiae and epistaxis, and for unusual bruising or bleeding gums.
• Recommend another means of contraception if cat's claw is being used for this purpose.
• Advise the patient to rise slowly from a sitting or lying position to avoid dizziness from possible hypotension.
• Instruct the patient to watch for signs of bleeding, especially if anticoagulants are also being taken.
• Advise women to avoid using cat's claw during pregnancy or when breast-feeding.

Points of interest

• Clinical trials are evaluating *Uncaria*'s ability to fight such viruses as herpes simplex, herpes zoster, and HIV.
• About 20 plants are identified as cat's claw in Peru. Botanical verification is needed because some species are considered toxic.
• The alkaloid concentration varies seasonally within cat's claw bark and vines.

Bold italic type indicates that reaction may be life-threatening.

- In the 1970s, preliminary research at the Peruvian National Institute of Health demonstrated promising results for cat's claw in treating children with leukemia.
- The plant gets its name from small thorns at the base of the leaf that resemble feline claws.

Commentary

Although cat's claw may appear to have potential for treating several diseases, more clinical research is needed to determine its efficacy and long-term safety. Research is being conducted for its potential use in treating AIDS, allergic respiratory diseases, GI disorders, leukemia and other cancers, osteoarthritis, and viral infections. Studies on cats with leukemia and immunodeficiency virus are also under way.

References

Chen, C.X., et al. "Inhibitory Effect of Rhynchophylline on Platelet Aggregation and Thrombosis," *Chung Kuo Yao Li Hsueh Pao* 13:126-30, 1992.

Harada, M., and Ozaki, Y. "Effect of Indole Alkaloids from *Gardneria* Genus and *Uncaria* Genus on Neuromuscular Transmission in the Rat Limb In Situ," *Chem Pharm Bull* 24:211, 1976.

Hemingway, S.R., and Philipson, J.D. "Alkaloids from South American Species of *Uncaria* (Rubiaceae)," *J Pharm Pharmacol* 26(suppl):113, 1974.

Lemaire, I., et al. "Stimulation of Interleukin-1 and Interleukin-6 Production in Alveolar Macrophages by the Neotropical Liana, *Uncaria tomentosa* (una de gato)," *J Ethnopharmacol* 64:109-15, 1999.

Sandoval, C.M., et al. "Antiinflammatory Actions of Cat's Claw: The Role of NF-kappaB," *Aliment Pharmacol Ther* 12(12):1279-89, 1998.

Sheng, Y., et al. "Enhanced DNA Repair, Immune Function and Reduced Toxicity of C-MED-100, a Novel Aqueous Extract from *Uncaria tomentosa*," *J Ethnopharmacol* 69(2):115-26, 2000.

Zhang, W., et al. "Effect of Rhyncophylline on the Contraction of Rabbit Aorta," *Chung Kuo Yao Li Hsueh Pao* 8:425-29, 1987.

CELANDINE

CELANDINE POPPY, COMMON CELANDINE, FELONWORT, GARDEN CELANDINE, GREATER CELANDINE, ROCK POPPY, SWALLOW WORT, TETTERWORT, WART WORT

Taxonomic class

Papaveraceae

Common trade names

Multi-ingredient preparations: Bloodroot/Celandine Supreme, Cacau, Celandine Extract, Celandine Tops and Roots, Cytopure, Fennel/Wild Yam Supreme, No. 2040 Headache Remedy, No. 2090 Indigestion Remedy, Venancapsan

Ukrain, a semisynthetic derivative of celandine alkaloids conjugated with thiophosphoric acid, is available only in Europe.

Common forms

Available as extracts, tinctures, and teas and as a prescribed injection in Eastern Europe.

Source

Celandine alkaloids are extracted from the roots and flowering tops of *Chelidonium majus*, a member of the poppy family commonly found in North America, Europe, and Asia. The milky, orange juice from the stems and other parts of the plant has been used for medicinal purposes. Greater celandine *(C. majus)* is not related to the plant known as lesser celandine, *Ranunculus ficaria*.

Chemical components

The main alkaloids from the celandine root are chelidonine and coptisine; more than 30 isoquinoline alkaloids have been detected as secondary metabolites. Other compounds include caffeic acid esters, chelidocystatin, chelidonic acid, chelidoniol, choline, cinnamic acids, flavonoids, histamine, methylamine, other alkaloids, quercetin, rutin, and tyramine.

Actions

Caffeic acid is claimed to have antispasmodic and choleretic activity. Coptisine and caffeoylmalic acid have shown similar spasmolytic activity. Chelidonine has mild central analgesic and strong spasmolytic properties that primarily affect the biliary system (Hiller et al., 1998).

Extracts of celandine inhibit keratinocyte proliferation, suggesting their possible use in treating such skin diseases as warts and psoriasis (Vavreckova et al., 1996). Other researchers found cytotoxic (but not antitumorigenic) activity associated with coptisine chloride and an unidentified alkaloid. Chelidocystatin exhibits proteolytic enzyme (cathepsin, papain) inhibition properties (Rogelj et al., 1998).

Reported uses

Celandine is reported to be useful in treating digestive disorders, eye irritation, and hepatic disease. The plant sap has been used to remove warts, soften calluses and corns, and loosen bad teeth. Chelidonium alkaloids have been used from the late 1800s in cancer treatment. In Europe, they have also been used to treat colonic polyposis and to remove warts, papillomas, condylomas, and nodules. Celandine was found to stimulate the flow of bile and pancreatic enzymes in treating biliary inflammation and obstruction, gallstones, hepatitis, and jaundice. It is also a component of an antiretroviral preparation that may act against the Epstein-Barr and herpes viruses.

One Russian abstract suggests the efficacy of *C. majus* tincture in reducing the recurrence of chronic tonsillitis in children. This information should be viewed as preliminary findings (Khmel'nitskaia et al., 1998).

Ukrain (NSC-631570), a novel, investigational semisynthetic drug obtained from *C. majus* alkaloids, has been demonstrated to possess an-

---

Bold italic type indicates that reaction may be life-threatening.

tineoplastic and immunomodulatory properties. It is thought that the drug may interfere with the metabolism of cancer cells while improving the function of the host immune system (Jagiello-Wojtowicz et al., 1998). A monograph included with Ukrain referred to a claim that a National Cancer Institute study showed drug action against human cancers. However, Ukrain has not been approved by the FDA for use in the United States (Anon., 1997). Ukrain claims to kill cancer cells by inducing apoptosis and inhibiting DNA, RNA, and protein synthesis. It was found to be toxic to malignant cells at levels that are nonlethal to normal cells. This theory has been questioned because the purported host-cellular protection phenomenon is thought to be related to subtherapeutic dosing of Ukrain (Panzer et al., 2000). In a study on women with breast cancer, the drug acted on malignant cells, making them more recognizable to the immune system, and resulting in their rejection (Brzosko et al., 1996). Case reports and studies obtained through MEDLINE document Ukrain's apparent success in treating several types and sites of cancer, including breast, cervical, colorectal, esophageal, ovarian, testicular, and urethral cancers; malignant melanoma; optic nerve astrocytoma; and Kaposi's sarcoma in patients with AIDS.

Dosage

Dosage of celandine extract depends on the product and use. Because the alkaloid content varies, it is not always standardized in available products.

Dosage of Ukrain is determined by the patient's immune status. A single dose is 5 to 20 mg per I.V. injection, depending on tumor mass, speed of growth, extent of the disease, and the patient's immune status. In several published studies, Ukrain injections were given every other day.

Adverse reactions

CNS: dizziness, drowsiness, fatigue, insomnia, restlessness.
CV: hypotension.
GI: *acute cholestatic hepatitis,* elevated liver function test results, nausea, thirst.
GU: polyuria.
Skin: contact dermatitis.
Other: may be embryotoxic (animal studies); tingling, itching, stabbing pains in tumor area.

Interactions

Cardiac glycosides (and Ukrain): May elicit ECG changes. Avoid administration with celandine.
Morphine derivatives and sulfonamides (and Ukrain): May reduce efficacy. Avoid administration with celandine.
Sulfonylureas (and Ukrain): May cause hypoglycemia. Avoid administration with celandine.

Contraindications and precautions

Celandine is contraindicated in children and pregnant or breast-feeding women and for prolonged periods (longer than 2 weeks). Also, herbal supplements and fresh herbs are contraindicated to self-treat serious hepatic and digestive disorders and other organ systems if disease is suspected.

Avoid direct contact with the fresh plant juices (including the milky sap). Also avoid using herb extracts not approved by the FDA for ophthalmic or topical use because blindness, infection, or tissue ulceration can occur.

Special considerations

- Some European patients may receive celandine as a prescription drug.
- Inform the patient that few data exist for using this plant for any indication.
- Caution the patient that celandine may interact with such drugs as analgesics, antibiotics, antidiabetic drugs, and cardiac drugs.

🔺 **ALERT** Caution the patient that the *C. majus* plant must be considered highly toxic. Contact with the sap causes dermatitis, and oral ingestion has been reported to cause abdominal pain, coma, diarrhea, fainting, gastroenteritis, hemorrhagic gastritis, severe stomatitis, vomiting, and even death.

🔺 **ALERT** Mild to severe acute cholestatic hepatitis has been reported in a case series of 10 patients known to have ingested herbal preparations that contained greater celandine. Elevated liver enzyme levels returned to normal in all patients 2 to 6 months after discontinuation of the product (Benninger et al.,1999).

Points of interest

- Ukrain is available by prescription in Europe, but it is not approved for use in the United States. Products available in the United States are manufactured as herbal nutritional supplements or topical herbal treatments and have not undergone FDA testing. The herb should not be used instead of prescribed drugs for diagnosed ailments or considered equivalent to Ukrain for preventing or treating disease.

Commentary

Although substantial evidence exists that celandine extracts can produce several pharmacologic effects, there are many reports of harm, particularly hepatitis, resulting from its ingestion. Because of the serious risk of complications of self-treating GI, hepatic, and ocular diseases and the possibility of dermatologic reactions in areas surrounding hyperkeratotic skin lesions, the use of celandine supplements and topical agents is not recommended. Alternative, more reliable treatment should be sought from a primary health care provider. Ukrain may have an important role in the treatment of cancer and other diseases, but further research is needed before its use in the United States is approved. Patients

---

Bold italic type indicates that reaction may be life-threatening.

interested in Ukrain should try to enroll in compassionate-use protocols or experimental clinical trials after discussing alternatives with their primary care provider or oncologist.

References

Anonymous, "UKRAIN Information for Physicians," Nowicky Pharma. Ukrainian Anticancer Institute, Vienna, Austria. September 1, 1997.

Benninger, J., et al. "Acute Hepatitis Induced by Greater Celandine," *Gastroenterology* 117(5):1234-37, 1999.

Brzosko, W.J., et al. "Influence of Ukrain on Breast Cancer," *Drugs Exp Clin Res* 22:127-33, 1996. Abstract.

Hiller, K.O., et al. "Antispasmodic and Relaxant Activity of Chelidonine, Protopine, Coptisine, and *Chelidonium majus* Extracts on Isolated Guinea-pig Ileum" (Letter), *Plant Med* 64(8):758-60, 1998.

Jagiello-Wojtowicz, E., et al. "Ukrain (NSC-631570) in Experimental and Clinical Studies: A Review," *Drugs Exp Clin Res* 24(5-6):213-19, 1998.

Khmel'nitskaia, N.M., et al. "A Comparative Study of Conservative Treatment Schemes in Chronic Tonsillitis in Children," *Vestn Otorinolaringol* (4):39-42, 1998.

Panzer, A., et al. "The Antimitotic Effects of Ukrain, a *Chelidonium majus* Alkaloid Derivative, Are Reversible In Vitro," *Cancer Lett* 13;150(1):85-92, 2000.

Rogelj, B., et al. "Chelidocystatin, a Novel Phytocystatin from *Chelidonium majus*," *Phytochemistry* 49(6):1645-49, 1998.

Vavreckova, C., et al. "Benzophenanthridine Alkaloids of *Chelidonium majus*. II. Potent Inhibitory Action Against the Growth of Human Keratinocytes," *Planta Med* 62:491-94, 1996.

CELERY

APIUM, CELERY SEED, CELERY SEED OIL, MARSH PARSLEY, SMALLAGE, WILD CELERY

Taxonomic class
Apiaceae

Common trade names
Multi-ingredient preparations: Cachets Lesourd, Dr. Brown's Cel-Ray, Guaiacum Complex, Herbal Diuretic Complex, Rheumatic Pain, Vegetex

Common forms
Available as capsules (450 mg, 505 mg), essential oils, and whole seed.

Source
An oil is obtained by steam distillation of the seeds of *Apium graveolens*, a widely cultivated biennial herb.

Chemical components
Celery is high in minerals, including sodium and chlorine. Celery seed oil contains d-limonene, selinene, and phthalides (3-*n*-butylphthalide, sedanenolide, and sedanonic anhydride). Perillyl alcohol, a monoterpene, has also been isolated from celery oil.

Actions
Some in vitro studies show that the essential oil has fungicidal, hypo-glycemic, and potential anticarcinogenic properties (Hashim et al., 1994). Celery may contain eight anticancer compounds that can detoxi-fy pollutants and cigarette smoke. Two components of celery (3-*n*-butylphthalide and sedanolide) reduced certain tumors in mice. An-other study with rats showed potential cancer reduction; human studies are needed to verify these claims. Perillyl alcohol, which has been isolat-ed from celery oil, has been shown to regress pancreatic, mammary, and liver tumors in animal studies. It exhibits possible application as a chemopreventive for colon, skin, and lung cancers and as a chemother-apeutic for neuroblastoma and prostate and colon cancers. It also in-duces apoptosis in tumor cells without affecting normal cells and can cause tumor cells to revert to a differentiated state. Its exact mechanism of action is unclear, but it appears to act on various cellular substances that control cell growth and differentiation (Belanger, 1998).

Reported uses
Celery is used to flavor food, soap, and gum; has a high fiber content; and is popular with dieters. It is claimed to be useful as an antarthritic, a diuretic for bladder and kidney conditions, a sedative, a spasmolytic, and a urinary antiseptic and for hysteria and nervousness. In the Ori-ent, celery is used as an antiflatulent, an aphrodisiac, a digestive aid, and a diuretic and to stimulate menstrual flow; also, the seeds have been used to treat headaches.

In India and Pakistan, celery is used to treat asthma, bronchitis, cough, fever, flatulence, hiccups, hives, lack of menses, liver and spleen conditions, rheumatism, and urine retention or discharge. The seed tincture is used for heartburn, hives, tension headache, toothache, urine retention, and vomiting. In a small clinical trial of hypertensive pa-tients, celery juice was found to lower blood pressure.

Dosage
No consensus exists.

Adverse reactions
CNS: CNS depression (large doses).
GI: abdominal cramps, diarrhea, nausea, vomiting.
Skin: dermatitis (attributed to allergic reactions to volatile oil), photo-toxic bullous lesions (in celery workers; Birmingham et al., 1961).
Other: hypersensitivity reactions (***anaphylaxis, angioedema***, respirato-ry complaints, and urticaria).

Interactions
None known.

Contraindications and precautions
Avoid the use of celery other than for food purposes in pregnant or breast-feeding patients; effects are unknown.

Bold italic type indicates that reaction may be life-threatening.

Special considerations
• When examining agricultural workers who have skin disorders, consider the possibility of hypersensitivity reactions.
• Advise the patient to limit consumption of celery to amounts commonly found in foods.
• Advise women to avoid using celery other than for food purposes during pregnancy or when breast-feeding.

Points of interest
• Celery tonics and elixirs have been in use since the late 19th century. The ancient Greeks used celery to make wine and served it as an award at athletic games circa 450 B.C.

Commentary
There are several therapeutic claims about celery, but few human trials have been completed. Consumption of quantities beyond that contained in food is not recommended.

References
Belanger, J.T. "Perillyl Alcohol: Applications in Oncology," *Altern Med Rev* 3(6):448-57, 1998.
Birmingham, D.J., et al. "Phytotoxic Bullae Among Celery Harvesters," *Arch Dermatol* 83:73, 1961.
Hashim, S., et al. "Modulatory Effects of Essential Oils from Spices on the Formation of DNA Adduct by Aflatoxin B1 In Vitro," *Nutr Cancer* 21:169-71, 1994.

CENTAURY

BITTER HERB, CENTAUREA, COMMON CENTAURY, EUROPEAN CENTAURY, LESSER CENTAURY, MINOR CENTAURY

Taxonomic class
Gentianaceae

Common trade names
None known.

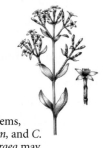

Common forms
Available as the crude herb and liquid.

Source
Active components are extracted from the leaves, stems, and flowers of *Centaurium erythraea, C. umbellatum,* and *C. minus,* which are annual or biennial herbs. *C. erythraea* may be referred to as *Erythraea centaurium.*

Chemical components
Centaury contains numerous compounds, including alkaloids (gentianidine, gentianine, and gentioflavine), monoterpenoids (centapicrin, gentioflavoside, gentiopicroside, iridoids, swertiamarin, and sweroside),

triterpenoids (alpha- and beta-amyrin, brassicasterol, campesterol, crataegolic acid, delta-7 stigmastenol erythrodiol, oleanolic acid, oleanolic lactone, sitosterol, and stigmasterol), phenolic acids (beta-coumaric, caffeic acids, ferulic, *m*- and *p*-hydroxybenzoic acid, protocatechuic, sinapic, syringic, and vanillic), flavonoids, xanthones (demethyleustomin and eustomin), fatty acids (palmitic and stearic acids), alkanes (heptacosane and nonacosane), and waxes.

Actions
Centaury is claimed to have bitter tonic and sedative properties. Gentiopicrin has demonstrated antimalarial properties. The aqueous extract of *C. erythraea* has been shown to have anti-inflammatory activity (Berkan et al., 1991; Mascolo et al., 1987); this anti-inflammatory potency is less than half that of indomethacin.

Two components of centaury (polymethoxylated xanthones), eustomin and demethyleustomin, have demonstrated antimutagenic properties in vitro (Schimmer and Mauthner, 1996).

Reported uses
Claims for centaury stem from traditional use as a bitter tonic to stimulate appetite. Anecdotal information reports that centaury is used for its astringent properties in cosmetics. Ancient Egyptians used this herb to treat kidney stones. The liquid is claimed to be the treatment for the weak-willed and exploited.

Dosage
For most uses, 2 to 4 ml of a liquid extract (1:1 in 25% alcohol) or infusion P.O. t.i.d. The German Commission E suggests 1 to 2 g of the crude herb daily.

Adverse reactions
None reported.

Interactions
None reported.

Contraindications and precautions
Avoid using centaury in pregnant or breast-feeding patients; effects are unknown.

Special considerations
• Urge the patient not to use centaury because little is known about its safety and efficacy.
• Instruct the patient who still wants to use this herb to avoid long-term use because the effects of such usage are unknown.
• Advise women to avoid using centaury during pregnancy or when breast-feeding.

Bold italic type indicates that reaction may be life-threatening.

Points of interest
• Centaury is found in trace quantities in vermouth. Usual concentrations are about 0.0002%, or 2.3 parts per million. Similar quantities occur in some nonalcoholic beverages.

Commentary
Centaury should not be used for any condition because of the lack of safety and efficacy data. No human clinical trial data are available.

References
Berkan, T., et al. "Anti-inflammatory, Analgesic and Antipyretic Effects of an Aqueous Extract of *Erythraea centaurium*," *Planta Med* 57:34-37, 1991.

Mascolo, N., et al. "Biological Screening of Italian Medicinal Plants for Anti-inflammatory Activity," *Phytother Res* 1:28-31, 1987.

Schimmer, O., and Mauthner, H. "Polymethoxylated Xanthones from the Herb of *Centaurium erythraea* with Strong Antimutagenic Properties in *Salmonella typhimurium*," *Planta Med* 62:561-64, 1996.

CHAMOMILE
COMMON CHAMOMILE, ENGLISH CHAMOMILE, GERMAN CHAMOMILE, HUNGARIAN CHAMOMILE, ROMAN CHAMOMILE, SWEET FALSE CHAMOMILE, TRUE CHAMOMILE, WILD CHAMOMILE

Taxonomic class
Asteraceae

Common trade names
Abkit, CamoCare Gold, Chamomile Flowers, Chamomile Tea, Chamomile Organic, Chamomilla, Classic Chamomile, Kamillosan (Germany)

Common forms
Available as candles for aromatherapy, capsules (354 mg, 360 mg), and liquid and in many cosmetic products.

Source
"True chamomile" refers to the German or Hungarian version of chamomile. Pharmacologically active compounds are extracted from dried flower heads of *Matricaria recutita (M. chamomilla)*. Another type of chamomile is Roman or English chamomile, *Chamaemelum nobile (Anthemis nobile)*.

Chemical components
Both kinds of chamomile contain similar compounds. One component of the volatile oil, chamazulene, is formed from natural precursors during steam distillation and constitutes about 0.5% of the flower head. The essential oil mostly consists of alpha-bisabolol, an unsaturated monocyclic sesquiterpene alcohol; other compounds include amyl and isobutyl alcohols, angelic and tiglic acid esters, anthemic acid, anthemol,

apigenin, choline, coumarins, farnesol, germacranolide, heniarin, inositol, luteolin, nerolidol, phenolic and fatty acids, phytosterol, quercetin and associated glycosides, scopoletin-7-glucoside, and umbelliferone.

Actions

The German and Roman chamomiles have similar pharmacologic profiles. In studies with rats, the volatile oil has been found to have antiallergic, antidiuretic, anti-inflammatory, and sedative properties. Some chamomile compounds have been reported to stimulate liver regeneration after oral administration. Others have shown in vitro antitumorigenic activity against human cells. Studies in animals and in vitro models have shown that bisabolol and chamazulene exert anti-inflammatory activity; bisabolol also shows antispasmodic activity. Luteolin and apigenin, two flavonoids in the essential oil, have antispasmodic effects and anti-inflammatory activity similar to those of indomethacin. Chamomile also exhibits some antibacterial and antifungal activity. Bisabolol has shown antiulcerative effects in rats by inhibiting the development of ethanol-, indomethacin-, or stress-induced ulcers (Mann and Staba, 1986). The volatile oil has been reported to lower serum urea levels in rabbits.

Reported uses

Chamomile has been used mainly to aid wound healing and treat stomach disorders, such as abdominal cramps and inflammatory GI conditions. It has also been touted as being useful for insomnia because of its purported sedative properties. Other uses include treatment of eczema, epidermolysis bullosa, eye irritation, hemorrhoids, menstrual disorders, migraine headache, and throat discomfort and as a topical bacteriostatic agent.

Oral chamomile extract can induce a deep sleep in most patients undergoing cardiac catheterization (Mann and Staba, 1986). The extract has also been used as a mouthwash (Fidler et al., 1996).

A therapeutic trial of a topical chamomile product (Kamillosan) suggested that patients with moderate atopic eczema responded slightly better to topical Kamillosan cream than to 0.5% hydrocortisone cream (Patzelt-Wenczler and Ponce-Poschl, 2000). Both products were only marginally better than placebo. The design of this trial is in question because of inadequate blinding of investigators.

Dosage

Chamomile is usually taken as a tea prepared by steeping 1 tbsp (3 g) of the flower head in hot water for 10 to 15 minutes and then taken up to q.i.d. Because of its poor water solubility, only a small amount of the volatile oil is obtained. Tea preparation extracts the hydrophilic flavonoid components. Long-term consumption of low concentrations of the volatile oil in chamomile tea may have a cumulative therapeutic effect.

Adverse reactions

EENT: allergic conjunctivitis.
GI: gastroparesis, vomiting.

Bold italic type indicates that reaction may be life-threatening.

GU: menstrual irregularities.
Skin: contact dermatitis.
Other: *anaphylaxis.*

Interactions
Anticoagulants: May enhance effects. Avoid administration with chamomile.
Other drugs taken concurrently: Potential for decreased absorption of these agents secondary to chamomile's antispasmodic activity in the GI tract. Avoid administration with chamomile.

Contraindications and precautions
Avoid using chamomile in pregnant or breast-feeding patients. It is believed to be an abortifacient, and some of its components have shown teratogenic effects in animals (Habersang et al., 1979). Chamomile may affect menses. Use cautiously in patients who are hypersensitive to the components of the volatile oils and in those at risk for contact dermatitis.

Special considerations
• Caution the patient with a history of plant allergy or known hypersensitivity to ragweed against using chamomile.
• Monitor the patient for bleeding.
• Caution the patient using chamomile that other drugs taken concurrently may not be completely absorbed and thus will be less effective.
🔊 ALERT Advise women to avoid using chamomile during pregnancy or when breast-feeding.

Commentary
Chamomile is well known for its purported anti-inflammatory, antispasmodic, and sedative activities. Limited human data are available to evaluate its clinical efficacy in treating GI disorders and other ailments.

References
Fidler, P., et al. "Prospective Evaluations of a Chamomile Mouthwash for Prevention of 5-FU–Induced Oral Mucositis," *Cancer* 77:522-24, 1996.
Habersang, S., et al. "Pharmacological Studies with Compounds of Chamomile. IV. Studies on Toxicity of Alpha-Bisabolol," *Planta Med* 37:115-23, 1979.
Mann, C., and Staba, E.J. "The Chemistry, Pharmacology, and Commercial Formulations of Chamomile," in *Herbs, Spices and Medicinal Plants: Recent Advances in Botany, Horticulture and Pharmacology,* vol. 1. Arizona: Oryx Press, 1986.
Patzelt-Wenczler, R., and Ponce-Poschl, E. "Proof of Efficacy of Kamillosan Cream in Atopic Eczema," *Eur J Med Res* 19;5(4):171-75, 2000.

CHAPARRAL
CREOSOTE BUSH, GREASEWOOD, *HEDIONDILLA*

Taxonomic class
Zygophyllaceae

Common trade names
None known.

Common forms
Available as capsules, tablets, and teas.

Source
Active components are extracted from the leaves of *Larrea tridentata* or *Larrea divaricata,* desert-dwelling evergreen shrubs that are native to the southwestern United States and Mexico.

Chemical components
Phenolic compounds isolated from *L. tridentata* include nordihyroguaiaretic acid (NDGA) and the related lignans, nor-isoguaiasin, dihydroguaiaretic acid, partially demethylated dihydroguaiartic acid, and 3'-demethoxyisoguaiasin. Younger plants yield more phenolic compounds than older plants.

Actions
The biological activity of chaparral is attributed to NDGA, a lipoxygenase inhibitor that was previously used as a food additive to prevent fermentation and decomposition. Despite studies showing NDGA to have an anticancer effect in vitro, earlier research by the National Cancer Institute found no such effect in vivo (Cunningham et al., 1997; Pavani et al., 1994). Some reports suggest that NDGA may stimulate certain cancers, such as renal cell carcinoma.

NDGA has been shown to inhibit proviral expression and thus may be able to interrupt the life cycle of the causative organism in HIV infections (Gnabre et al., 1995).

Results from an in vitro study of rat hippocampal neurons suggest that NDGA may play a neuroprotective role in Alzheimer's disease (Goodman et al., 1994).

Reported uses
Chaparral tea is derived from the plant leaves. It was widely used by Native Americans as a remedy for bronchitis, colds, pain, and skin disorders. Human clinical trials are lacking to support the claim of anticancer properties.

Dosage
No consensus exists.

Adverse reactions
GI: *hepatotoxicity* (cholestatic hepatitis).
GU: renal cell carcinoma, renal cystic disease.
Skin: contact dermatitis.

Interactions
None reported.

Bold italic type indicates that reaction may be life-threatening.

Contraindications and precautions
Chaparral is contraindicated because of numerous reports of serious hepatotoxicity.

Special considerations
🔺 **ALERT** Hepatotoxicity (cholestatic hepatitis) can occur. Jaundice is characterized with markedly elevated liver function test results. Onset occurs within 3 to 52 weeks after ingestion, and symptoms resolve within 1 to 17 weeks after discontinuing the herb in most cases. Some damage progresses to cirrhosis and acute hepatic failure, requiring transplantation (Shad et al., 1999; Sheikh et al., 1997).
• Monitor the patient who has taken chaparral for fatigue, changes in hepatic function, jaundice, and other signs of hepatotoxicity.
• Caution the patient against using chaparral because of its strong hepatotoxic property.
• Although no known chemical interactions have been reported in clinical studies, consideration must be given to the pharmacologic properties of the herbal product and the potential for exacerbation of the intended therapeutic effect of conventional drugs.

Points of interest
• Chaparral is considered an unsafe herb and was removed by the FDA from its generally recognized as safe list in 1970.
• Anecdotal reports indicate that chaparral tea was used as an anti-cancer agent from the late 1950s to the 1970s.

Commentary
In vitro studies have yielded conflicting results for the use of NDGA, an active component of chaparral, in treating AIDS, Alzheimer's disease, and cancer. Further in vivo and human clinical studies are needed. Because of its strong association with hepatotoxicity, use of this herb is not recommended.

References
Cunningham, D.C., et al. "Proliferative Responses of Normal Human Mammary and MCF-7 Breast Cancer Cells to Linoleic, Conjugated Linoleic Acid and Eicosanoid Synthesis Inhibitors in Culture," *Anticancer Res* 17:197-203, 1997.

Gnabre, J.N., et al. "Inhibition of Human Immunodeficiency Virus Type 1 Transcription and Replication by DNA Sequence-Selective Plant Lignans," *Proc Natl Acad Sci USA* 92:11239-43, 1995.

Goodman, Y., et al. "Nordihydroguaiaretic Acid Protects Hippocampal Neurons Against Amyloid Beta-Peptide Toxicity, and Attenuated Free Radical and Calcium Accumulation," *Brain Res* 654:171-76, 1994.

Pavani, M., et al. "Inhibition of Tumoral Cell Respiration and Growth by Nordihydroguaiaretic Acid," *Biochem Pharmacol* 48:1935-42, 1994.

Shad, J.A., et al. "Acute Hepatitis After Ingestion of Herbs," *South Med J* 92(11):1095-97, 1999.

Sheikh, N.M., et al. "Chaparral-Associated Hepatoxicity," *Arch Intern Med* 157:913-19, 1997.

CHASTE TREE

AGNEAU CHASTE, CHASTEBERRY, GATILLIER, HEMP TREE, KEUSCHBAUM, MONK'S PEPPER, *VITEX AGNUS-CASTUS*

Taxonomic class
Lamiaceae

Common trade names
Estrogentle (combination including chaste tree), Femaprin (premenopausal formula), VAC, Vitex

Common forms
Available as capsules, tinctures, and teas.

Source
Active components are extracted from the dried, ripened fruits and the root bark of *Vitex agnus-castus*.

Chemical components
Several new luteolin-like flavonoids, iridoid glycosides, aucubin, eurostoside, agnuside, some triterpenoids, and an alkaloid, vitricine, have been isolated from the root bark. Both free and conjugated forms of progesterone and hydroxyprogesterone have been isolated from the leaves and flowers. Testosterone and epitestosterone were detected in the flower parts. Androstenedione was extracted from the leaves.

Essential oils contain monoterpenoids and sesquiterpenoids, alpha- and beta-pinene, camphene, cardinene, carophyllene, castine, cineole, citronellol, cymene, eucalyptol, farnesene, ledol, limonene, linalool, myrcene, and sabinene.

Actions
The herb is claimed to have antiandrogenic, anti-inflammatory, antimicrobial, and progesterone-like effects. Recently isolated flavonoids exhibit antineoplastic activity (Hirobe et al., 1997), and studies with rats have shown a hypoprolactinemic effect (Sliutz et al., 1993). Dopaminergic activity has been attributed to the labdan diterpenoids found in the fruit (Hoberg et al., 2000).

Reported uses
Claims for chaste tree include usefulness for several endocrine and female reproductive disorders and hormonal imbalance, including menstrual cycle irregularity, uterine bleeding, ovarian insufficiency, inadequate lactation, and acne. Human data supporting these claims are sparse. A German abstract described a study of women with latent hyperprolactinemia in which prolactin secretion was reduced and both the luteal phase and luteal secretion of progesterone normalized (Milewicz et al., 1993). Clinicians reporting a case of multiple follicular development without pregnancy in the face of deranged serum hor-

---

Bold italic type indicates that reaction may be life-threatening.

mone levels and chaste tree consumption did not advocate the use of the herb to promote normal ovarian function (Cahill et al., 1994).

Although one uncontrolled, open-label study suggested a role for chaste tree in premenstrual syndrome (Loch et al., 2000), more notable information comes from a double-blind, placebo-controlled parallel-group trial conducted in Europe that evaluated *V. agnus-castus* extract for cyclic mastalgia. After a treatment phase that lasted for three consecutive menstrual cycles, intensity of mastalgia was reportedly reduced more rapidly in those who received the extract. Mastalgia during at least 5 days of the cycle was the only inclusion criterion. A visual analogue scale was used to measure response (Halaska et al., 1998).

Dosage
Dosage used in the study by Halaska and colleagues (1998) was 20 mg in capsule form P.O. daily. Other dosages are usually teas or tinctures.

Adverse reactions
CNS: headache.
GI: abdominal pain and cramps, diarrhea.
GU: increased menstrual flow.
Skin: pruritus, rash.

Interactions
None reported.

Contraindications and precautions
Avoid using chaste tree in pregnant or breast-feeding patients; effects are unknown.

Special considerations
• Keep chaste tree's effects in mind if the patient reports increased menstrual flow.
• Advise women to avoid using chaste tree during pregnancy or when breast-feeding or planning pregnancy.
• Inform the patient that most of the information on chaste tree comes from foreign studies, which makes interpretation of results difficult.
• Although no known chemical interactions have been reported in clinical studies, consideration must be given to the pharmacologic properties of the herbal product and the potential for exacerbation of the intended therapeutic effect of conventional drugs.

Points of interest
• A German formulation of chaste tree is indicated for menstrual disorders caused by primary or secondary corpus luteum insufficiency, inadequate lactation, mastodynia, menopausal symptoms, and premenstrual syndrome.
• Postmarketing surveillance in Germany has determined that chaste tree has been discontinued because of adverse reactions only 1% of the time.
• Monks were said to have chewed the leaves of chaste tree to help them maintain their vow of celibacy.

Commentary

It may be worth investigating chaste tree further in disorders specific to women. The lack of data on long-term safety and clinical efficacy precludes conclusive recommendations.

References

Cahill, D., et al. "Multiple Follicular Development Associated with Herbal Medicine," *Hum Reprod* 9:1469-70, 1994.

Halaska, M., et al. "Treatment of Cyclical Mastodynia Using an Extract of *Vitex agnus-castus*: Results of a Double-blind Comparison with a Placebo," *Ceska Gynekol* 63(5):388-92, 1998.

Hirobe, C., et al. "Cytotoxic Flavonoids from *Vitex agnus-castus*," *Phytochemistry* 46:521-24, 1997.

Hoberg, E., et al. "Quantitative High Performance Liquid Chromatographic Analysis of Diterpenoids in agni-casti fructus," *Planta Med* 66(4):352-55, 2000.

Loch, E.G., et al. "Treatment of Premenstrual Syndrome with a Phytopharmaceutical Formulation Containing *Vitex agnus castus*," *J Womens Health Gend Based Med* 9(3):315-20, 2000.

Milewicz, A., et al. "*Vitex agnus-castus* Extract in the Treatment of Luteal Phase Defects Due to Latent Hyperprolactinemia. Results of a Randomized Placebo-Controlled Double-Blind Study," *Arzneimittelforschung* 43:752-56, 1993.

Sliutz, G., et al. "*Agnus castus* Extracts Inhibit Prolactin Secretion of Rat Pituitary Cells," *Horm Metab Res* 25:253-55, 1993.

CHAULMOOGRA OIL

CHAULMOGRA OIL, GYNOCARDIA OIL, HYDNOCARPUS OIL

Taxonomic class

Flacourtiaceae

Common trade names

None known.

Common forms

Available as a topical oil and a salt form of oil for subcutaneous injection.

Source

Active components are extracted from the seeds of *Hydnocarpus wightiana, Hydnocarpus anthelmintica,* and *Taraktogenos kurzii.*

Chemical components

The seeds contain about 50% of the brownish yellow chaulmoogra oil; the remaining components include chaulmoogric acid, fatty acids (palmitic and oleic acids), gorlic acid, and hypnocarpic acid.

Actions

Chaulmoogra oil has demonstrated efficacy against *Mycobacterium leprae* in laboratory experiments and case reports (Levy, 1975). It has also been listed as an antileprotic.

FOLKLORE
Chaulmoogra and leprosy

Throughout the ages, leprosy has been greatly feared. Lepers would be declared legally dead and have their possessions redistributed; in Norway, lepers were forced to wear cowbells around their necks as they walked to warn oncoming pedestrians.

In the 1920s, Joseph Rock, an explorer-botanist, set out to locate a plant he had never seen and knew little about (Dobelis, 1986). After hearing stories of leprosy cures that involved this rare, exotic plant, Rock traveled the globe searching jungles, swamps, mountains, and valleys of the Far East and India until finally obtaining some seeds in an Indian market.

Investigation revealed that the seeds came from a local tree that grew 50 to 60 ft tall and had leathery leaves and large, white flowers. Rock collected a large quantity of the seeds and was able to naturalize the plant in Hawaii. About 20 years later, the active components in the seeds of the chaulmoogra tree provided the elemental materials for synthesizing the first antileprotics.

Reported uses
Folk literature and ancient Hindu and Chinese documents suggest that chaulmoogra oil is an effective treatment for leprosy. (See *Chaulmoogra and leprosy*.)

Dosage
No consensus exists.

Adverse reactions
GI: GI discomfort (with subcutaneous injection).
Skin: calcinosis cutis (forms precipitate under the skin with subcutaneous injection; Ohtaka, 1992).

Interactions
None reported.

Contraindications and precautions
Avoid using chaulmoogra oil in pregnant or breast-feeding patients; effects are unknown.

Special considerations
• Advise the patient who suspects a leprosy diagnosis that more traditional and acceptable forms of antimicrobial therapy exist and that he should seek medical advice from a health care provider experienced in the therapy and care of leprosy.
• Urge the patient not to attempt administration of chaulmoogra oil unless under close supervision of a health care provider experienced in the therapy and care of leprosy.

• Advise women to avoid using chaulmoogra oil during pregnancy or when breast-feeding.

Points of interest
• Despite a decrease in the incidence of leprosy worldwide, as of 1991, there were 6 million cases of leprosy that required treatment (Noordeen, 1991). These cases predominate in Africa, Asia, Latin America, and the Pacific; only a few cases exist in Canada, Europe, and the United States.
• The components of chaulmoogra oil have served as the fundamental structure for synthesis of modern antileprotics.

Commentary
Chaulmoogra oil should be avoided because more accepted, safer therapies for leprosy exist. Its role in the treatment of any disorder, including leprosy, is undetermined.

References
Dobelis, I.N., ed. *Magic and Medicine of Plants.* Pleasantville, N.Y.: Reader's Digest Association, Inc., 1986.

Levy, L. "The Activity of Chaulmoogra Acids Against *Mycobacterium leprae*," *Am Rev Resp Dis* 111:703-5, 1975.

Noordeen, S.K. "A Look at World Leprosy," *Lepr Rev* 62:72-86, 1991.

Ohtaka, K. "Patients with Calcinosis Cutis: National Leprosarium Matsuoka Hoyo-En' Aomori' Japan," *Nippon Rai Gakkai Zasshi* 61:98-101, 1992.

CHICKWEED

MOUSE-EAR, SATIN FLOWER, STAR CHICKWEED, STARWEED, STITCHWORT, TONGUE-GRASS, WHITE BIRD'S-EYE, WINTERWEED

Taxonomic class
Caryophyllaceae

Common trade names
Multi-ingredient preparations: Chickweed formula

Common forms
Available as capsules, the crude herb, liquid extracts (alcohol-free available), oils, ointments, tea bags (caffeine-free), and tinctures.

Source
Components are extracted from the leaves, stems, and flowers of *Stellaria media,* which is native to Europe.

Chemical components
The active components are mainly unknown. Herbal literature lists various components, such as most of the B complex vitamins, calcium, coumarin, flavonoids (rutin), hydroxycoumarin, iron, nitrate salts, saponins, and vitamins A and C.

Actions
None reported. One in vitro animal study isolated two flavonoid components from the herb that possessed antioxidant activity (Budzianowski et al., 1991).

Reported uses
This widely occurring "weed" is commonly prescribed by herbalists as a remedy for both internal and external inflammatory conditions, such as rheumatism and skin disorders (eczema and psoriasis), and for its ability to relieve skin irritation and pruritus. Claims have also been made for chickweed as an antipyretic, an antitussive, and an expectorant as well as an excess-fat reducer because of its mild diuretic and laxative effects.

Chickweed has also been used internally as a "blood cleanser" and as a demulcent for soothing sore throats and stomach ulcers. Externally, it has been used as a poultice to help draw out fluid from abscesses and boils and as an ointment or salve to relieve burns, insect stings and bites, and rashes. Chickweed is claimed to be an excellent emollient for dry, chapped skin and to promote early healing of wounds and cuts, but little evidence exists to support these claims.

Dosage
Traditional uses suggest the following doses:
Capsules: 3 capsules P.O. t.i.d.
Liquid extract: 15 to 30 gtt (diluted) P.O. up to t.i.d.
Ointment: applied liberally to affected areas as needed up to q.i.d.
Tea: several times daily as needed.

Adverse reactions
None reported.

Interactions
None reported.

Contraindications and precautions
Avoid using chickweed in pregnant or breast-feeding patients; effects are unknown.

Special considerations
● Caution the patient about adverse reactions that may occur with nitrates (headache, hypotension, syncope).
🔺 **ALERT** Herbal literature reports one case of nitrate toxicity in grazing farm animals and one case of human paralysis resulting from ingestion of excessive amounts of chickweed. Both reports are attributed to the herb's nitrate content, and the findings remain controversial.
● Although no known chemical interactions have been reported in clinical studies, consideration must be given to the pharmacologic properties of the herbal product and the potential for exacerbation of the intended therapeutic effect of conventional drugs.
● Caution the patient against consuming chickweed because of the lack of clinical data.

• Advise women to avoid using chickweed during pregnancy or when breast-feeding.

Commentary
Despite widespread claims by herbalists of chickweed's potential value for various ailments, clinical evidence supporting these therapeutic applications is insufficient.

References
Budzianowski, J., et al. "Studies on Antioxidative Activity of Some C-glycosyl-flavones," *Pol J Pharmacol* 43:395-401, 1991.

CHICORY

BLUE SAILORS, GARDEN ENDIVE, SUCCORY, WILD SUCCORY

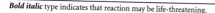

Taxonomic class
Asteraceae

Common trade names
Chicory

Common forms
Available as the crude herb, extracts, root (roasted and unroasted), and teas.

Source
Active components are extracted from the dried roots of *Cichorium intybus*, a biennial or perennial herb that is native to Europe. The leaves of young plants are used as potherbs, whereas the leaves of older plants can be blanched and eaten like celery. The roots can be boiled and eaten with butter or, more commonly, can be roasted and added to coffee or tea for a bitter taste. The roasted, dried root is also used as a coffee substitute.

Chemical components
The flowers contain cichoriin, and the leaves contain carbohydrates, catechol tannins, chicoric acid (dicaffeoyl tartaric acid), flavonoids, glycosides, tartaric acid, and unsaturated sterols and triterpenoids. The roots contain many steam-distillable aromatic compounds. The characteristic aroma of chicory stems from acteophenone. The roots also contain inulin; on roasting, inulin is converted to oxymethylfurfural, which gives off a coffeelike aroma. Chicory also contains maltol, a taste modifier that intensifies the flavor of sugar.

Actions
Chicory is commonly used as a water-soluble or alcoholic extract. The water-soluble fraction is thought to exhibit sedative effects and, therefore, may antagonize the stimulating effects from coffee and tea. Alcohol extracts have demonstrated anti-inflammatory activity (Benoit et al., 1976). Although little information exists regarding chicory use in

RESEARCH FINDINGS
Chicory's dietary fructans

Chicory contains inulin, whose partial hydrolysis yields oligofructose. Both of these compounds are classified as fructans, (beta [2-1] fructo-oligosaccharides), which are specific types of carbohydrate molecules that resist degradation in the stomach to reach the colon, where they are extensively hydrolyzed and fermented by saccharolytic bacteria (Roberfroid, 1999). Inulin and its metabolite, oligofructose, have been shown to promote the growth of seemingly beneficial bacteria known as *Bifidobacteria* in the colon. This ability to stimulate the growth of beneficial bacteria is known as a "probiotic" effect, which may improve bowel function and bowel habits. Animal studies have demonstrated that these dietary chicory fructans may inhibit the development of aberrant crypt foci (ACF), preneoplastic lesions that give rise to colonic adenomas and carcinomas (Reddy, 1999). Inulin appeared to have a more pronounced effect than oligofructose in this regard. Other data suggest an improved ability to absorb calcium and metabolize lipids. Interesting reviews on the subject of functional foods that feature the dietary chicory fructans suggest potential applications in various disease states (Roberfroid and Delzenne, 1998; Roberfroid, 1999). All this awaits confirmation in humans.

humans, several animal studies have shown that it reduces the cardiac rate by an action similar to that of quinidine, suggesting its possible usefulness in treating arrhythmias. Interesting information surrounds the potential application of chicory to reduce the risk of colon cancer. (See *Chicory's dietary fructans.*)

Reported uses
In herbal lore, chicory is primarily touted as a coffee or tea additive because of its ability to antagonize the CNS stimulation brought on by these substances. It has also been used as a coffee substitute because of its coffeelike aroma and taste. In folk medicine, chicory root is used as a diuretic and laxative; human data are lacking for these uses.

Dosage
Little information is available.
Crude herb: 3 g P.O. daily.

Adverse reactions
Skin: contact dermatitis (possibly caused by sesquiterpene lactones; Malten, 1983).

Interactions
None reported.

Contraindications and precautions
There are no known contraindications for chicory. Use it cautiously in patients with cardiac disease because of its potential action on the heart.

Special considerations
• Inquire about chicory use when taking the patient's drug history.
• Advise the patient with cardiac disease to avoid using chicory or to use it cautiously.
• Although no known chemical interactions have been reported in clinical studies, consideration must be given to the pharmacologic properties of the herbal product and the potential for exacerbation of the intended therapeutic effect of conventional drugs.

Points of interest
• Chicory has been shown to take up the fungicide quintozene through its roots, which may lead to colonization with certain bacteria in the soil and subsequent contamination of the plant.

Commentary
Chicory has a long history of traditional use. Because of its flavor and aroma, the root has been used as a substitute for coffee and tea. Unlike coffee, chicory may exhibit sedative properties, which may explain its traditional use in offsetting the stimulant properties of teas and coffee. These claims are unproven. The plant may have some use as an antiarrhythmic, but further studies are needed. Its use as a laxative is also unclear and should be reserved until human trials are completed. Of greatest interest is the potential application of chicory and its dietary fructans, inulin and oligofructose, as colon carcinogenesis inhibitors.

References
Benoit, P.S., et al. "Biological and Phytochemical Evaluation of Plants. XIV. Anti-inflammatory Evaluation of 163 Species of Plants," *Lloydia* 39:160-71, 1976.

Malten, K.E. "Chicory Dermatitis from September to April," *Contact Dermatitis* 9:232, 1983.

Reddy, B.S. "Possible Mechanisms by Which Pro- and Prebiotics Influence Colon Carcinogensis and Tumor Growth," *J Nutr* 129(S-7):1478-82,1999.

Roberfroid, M.B. "Concepts in Functional Foods: The Case of Inulin and Oligo-fructose," *J Nutr* 129(S-7):1398-1401,1999.

Roberfroid, M.B., and Delzenne, N.M. "Dietary Fructans," *Annu Rev Nutr* 18:117-43,1998.

CHINESE RHUBARB

HIMALAYAN RHUBARB, MEDICINAL RHUBARB, RHEI RADIX, RHEI RHIZOMA, RUBARBO, TURKISH RHUBARB

Taxonomic class
Polygonaceae

Bold italic type indicates that reaction may be life-threatening.

Common trade names
Dahuang Liujingao, Extractum Rhei Liquidum

Common forms
Available as tablets and water- and alcohol-based extracts, syrups, and tinctures.

Source
Active components are derived from the dried root bark of *Rheum palmatum*, a large, perennial herb that is native to the mountains of Tibet and northwest China.

Chemical components
Chinese rhubarb contains anthraquinones, stilbenes, and tannins. The anthraquinones occur as glycosides and have been identified as aloe emodin, chrysophanol, emodin, and rhein. Other substances include phenolics (such as catechin, gallic acid, and glucogallin) and sennosides A, B, and C.

Actions
The herb's dramatic purgative or laxative effect is attributable to rhein and sennosides. Sennosides act on the large intestine to increase motility after being degraded by microorganisms in the colon. Increased laxative activity appears to correlate with sennoside content. Anthraquinones exhibit laxative and antimicrobial effects.

Rhubarb extract has been studied in chronic renal failure in the rat (Zhang and El-Nahas, 1996). One study found rhubarb to decrease the severity of proteinuria, decrease BUN levels, and attenuate the severity of glomerulosclerosis.

Rhein and emodin inhibit mitochondrial energy production. This may explain the inhibitory effect of rhubarb extracts on renal growth. Hypermetabolism is implicated in initiation of remnant kidney scarring.

In patients with upper GI bleeding, rhubarb has been found to increase blood vessel constriction and promote hemostasis; the mechanism of this action is unknown (Dong-hai et al., 1980).

Reported uses
Chinese rhubarb has been used medicinally for centuries as an antidiarrheal and a laxative and to treat conjunctivitis, GI bleeding, indigestion, jaundice, menstrual disorders, and traumatic injuries. It has also been used topically to treat burns, scabs, and sores and as an astringent or styptic to stop bleeding.

The combination of an ACE inhibitor, captopril, and Chinese rhubarb was found to be superior to either agent alone in slowing the progression of renal failure (Zhang et al., 1990). Similar results were obtained with rhubarb and other adjuvant drugs. Chinese researchers concluded that such treatments may be used as transitional measures in chronic renal disease before more radical therapies are instituted (Kang et al., 1993).

In patients with GI bleeding, rhubarb was found to help control bleeding, decrease blood loss, reduce the need for clotting agents, resolve fever, increase peristalsis of the colon without affecting the stomach or duodenum, and help eliminate extravasated bleeding.

Rhubarb stalk fiber was studied in hypercholesterolemic men and was shown to lower serum total cholesterol and LDL levels (Goel et al., 1997).

Dosage
Traditional uses suggest the following doses:
For constipation, ½ to 1 tsp P.O. daily of tincture or 1 to 2 tsp P.O. daily of decoction.
For diarrhea, 1 tsp P.O. daily of tincture or decoction.
For upper GI bleeding, 3-g tablets or powder P.O. b.i.d. to q.i.d.
Use lower-strength preparations for older children and patients over age 65.

Adverse reactions
GU: urine discoloration (bright yellow or red).
Skin: contact dermatitis (from handling the leaves).

Interactions
None reported.

Contraindications and precautions
Chinese rhubarb is contraindicated in pregnant or breast-feeding patients, in children under age 2, and in patients with intestinal problems, such as ulcers and colitis. Use of the herb for longer than 2 weeks is contraindicated because it can induce a tolerance in the colon.

Special considerations
• Most of the literature comes from the Orient, making interpretation of published studies difficult.
• Inform the patient that Chinese rhubarb is not the same as rhubarb found in the United States.
• Advise the laboratory that the patient's urine will be bright yellow or red.
• Urge the patient to take Chinese rhubarb for only a short time to avoid such problems as melanosis coli and laxative dependence.
◗ **ALERT** Leaves contain poisonous oxalic acid. Consumption causes abdominal pain, burning in the mouth and throat, diarrhea, nausea, vomiting, and, possibly, seizures and death with ingestion of large amounts.
• Caution the patient against preparing Chinese rhubarb formulations at home to avoid the risk of oxalic acid poisoning. Urge him to keep this plant out of the reach of children and pets.
• Inform the patient that this herb may color the urine bright yellow or red.
• Advise women to stop taking the herb if pregnancy is planned or suspected or if breast-feeding is planned.

Bold italic type indicates that reaction may be life-threatening.

Points of interest
- Chinese rhubarb is officially listed in the Chinese Pharmacopia and was mentioned in the Chinese herbal Pen-King (ca. 2700 B.C.). Rhubarb root is one of the oldest and most common Chinese herbal medicines available. It has also been used in the manufacture of liqueurs and aperitifs.
- Rhubarb species grown in Europe and North America and used for food and medicinal purposes are less potent than Chinese rhubarb.

Commentary
Active medicinal components of Chinese rhubarb suggest its theoretic application as an agent for GI dysmotility. With safety and efficacy data lacking, the herb cannot be recommended for this use.

The use of Chinese rhubarb in renal failure and GI bleeding appears intriguing, but data are from the foreign literature and difficult to interpret. Future studies should probably focus on these aspects of Chinese rhubarb for potential therapeutic application.

References
Dong-hai, J., et al. "Resume of 400 Cases of Acute Upper Digestive Tract Bleeding Treated by Rhubarb Alone," *Pharmacology* 20:128-30, 1980.

Goel, V., et al. "Cholesterol-lowering Effects of Rhubarb Stalk Fiber in Hypercholesteremic Men," *J Am Coll Nutr* 16(6):600-604,1997.

Kang, Z., et al. "Observation of Therapeutic Effect in 50 Cases of Chronic Renal Failure Treated with Rhubarb and Adjuvant Drugs," *J Tradit Chin Med* 13:249-52, 1993. Abstract.

Zhang, G., and El-Nahas, A.M. "The Effect of Rhubarb Extract on Experimental Renal Fibrosis," *Nephrol Dial Transplant* 11:186-90, 1996.

Zhang, J.H., et al. "Clinical Effects of *Rheum* and Captopril on Preventing Progression of Chronic Renal Failure," *Chin Med J* 103:788-93, 1990. Abstract.

CHITOSAN

CHITOSAN ASCORBATE, DEACETYLATED CHITIN, *N*-CARBOXYBUTYL CHITOSAN, *N,O*-SULFATED CHITOSAN, *O*-SULFATED *N*-ACETYLCHITOSAN, SULFATED *N*-CARBOXYMETHYLCHITOSAN, SULFATED *O*-CARBOXYMETHYLCHITOSAN

Common trade names
Chitorich, Chitosan Exofat, Fat Breaker, and Fatsorb.

Common forms
Oral formulations

Source
Chitosan and chitin are nitrogenous polysaccharides that occur naturally in the fungal kingdom, invertebrate animals, some brown algae, and, negligibly, in higher plants (Chobot et al., 1995). It is derived from the powdered shells of marine crustaceans, such as crabs, lobsters,

prawns, and shrimp. Chitosan is a biodegradable, hydrophilic biopolymer that is obtained industrially by hydrolyzing the aminoacetyl groups of chitin.

Chemical components
Chitin is structurally similar to cellulose. Chitosan is a deacetylated chitin.

Actions
Chitosan is proposed to bind to dietary fat, bile acids, and phospholipids, preventing digestion and storage. It has been shown to directly correlate with the inhibition of atherogenesis and the lowering of cholesterol levels in mice, rats, and broiler chickens.

Reported uses
Topically, chitosan has been used to treat periodontitis and to promote tissue regeneration in plastic surgery. Oral chitosan has reportedly been used for weight loss. (See *Chitosan for weight loss.*) A controlled trial was conducted in 80 patients with renal failure on long-term stable hemodialysis; one-half received 30 chitosan tablets (45 mg of chitosan per tablet) three times daily or placebo. Improvement in cholesterol and hemoglobin levels and significant reductions in serum urea and creatinine levels were shown after 4 weeks in chitosan-treated patients (Jing et al., 1997). Patients reported that physical strength, appetite, and sleep had improved after 12 weeks compared with the control group. The mechanisms for these effects are unknown.

Dosage
Clinical trials report using 2 to 3 g/day P.O.

Adverse reactions
GI: constipation, steatorrhea.

Interactions
None known. In theory, the absorption of some drugs may be impaired if administered in proximity to chitosan ingestion.

Contraindications and precautions
Avoid using chitosan in pregnant or breast-feeding patients; effects are unknown. Use cautiously in patients with shellfish allergies. There is a theoretical potential for chitosan to decrease bone mineral content and the absorption of minerals and fat-soluble vitamins.

Special considerations
• Advise the patient to consult a health care provider before using herbal preparations because a treatment that has been clinically researched and proved effective may be available.
• Instruct the patient to notify the prescriber and pharmacist of any herbal or dietary supplement he is taking when filling a new prescription.
• Although no known chemical interactions have been reported in clinical studies, consideration must be given to the pharmacologic proper-

---

Bold italic type indicates that reaction may be life-threatening.

RESEARCH FINDINGS
Chitosan for weight loss

Chitosan is promoted as a remedy to reduce fat absorption, thus enabling weight loss. Two randomized, controlled clinical trials in adults without dietary modifications found no reductions in weight for chitosan-treated patients.

Fifty-one healthy obese women received 3 capsules of microcrystalline chitosan (400 mg twice daily) or placebo (24 women) for 8 weeks before meals (Wuolijoki et al., 1999). Significant reductions in LDL levels were shown at both 4 and 8 weeks ($P > .1$). No differences alterations in serum total cholesterol and HDL levels were seen. There was a slight increase in the serum triglyceride level compared with that seen with placebo. No reductions in weight were seen in either treatment group.

A total of 30 overweight adult patients were evaluated for clinical efficacy of oral chitosan for body weight reduction in the absence of dietary modifications (Pittler et al., 1999). Patients received either 4 capsules of chitosan (n=15; 250 mg deacetylated chitin biopolymer per capsule) or matching placebo (n=15) twice daily for 28 days. A number of dietary markers, including vitamins A, D, K, and E; beta-carotene; total cholesterol; and triglycerides, were assessed. Significant increases were noted for vitamin K levels from baseline to 4 weeks for chitosan- and placebo-treated groups ($P < .05$). Quality of life, assessed using the SF-36 validated questionnaire, was found not to be clinically different between the groups. No differences were noted for systolic blood pressure or body mass index. Mean body weight was not significantly different from baseline to 4 weeks for either chitosan- or placebo-treated patients (71.8 to 72.6 kg and 76.4 to 77.9 kg, respectively). The most reported adverse event in the trial was constipation (6 chitosan-treated patients and 2 placebo-treated patients).

The authors concluded that the use of chitosan in the absence of dietary modifications showed no clinically relevant difference in body weight compared with placebo. When capsules were analyzed after the trial, they were noted to contain 42% chitosan, which was less than the 71% (250 mg) stated by the distributor.

ties of the herbal product and the potential for exacerbation of the intended therapeutic effect of conventional drugs.

Points of interest
• Chitosan is used in the pharmaceutical industry as an excipient (tableting agent) in oral formulations and a vehicle for parenteral drug delivery systems and in manufacturing nasal, ophthalmic, transdermal, and implantable sustained-release delivery systems.

Commentary

The limited human data available investigating the use of chitosan for weight loss have shown minimal effect when no dietary modifications were made. Chitosan has shown some efficacy in improving serum lipid levels and in certain parameters of patients with renal failure. Further investigations into the effects of chitosan are warranted.

References

Chobot, V., et al. "Phytotherapeutic Aspects of Diseases of the Circulatory System. 4. Chitin and Chitosan," *Ceska Slov Farm* 44(4):190-95, 1995.

Jing, S.B., et al. "Effect of Chitosan on Renal Function in Patients with Chronic Renal Failure," *J Pharm Pharmacol* 49(7):721-23, 1997.

Pittler, M.H., et al. "Randomized, Double-blind Trial of Chitosan for Body Weight Reduction," *Eur J Clin Nutr* 53:379-81, 1999.

Wuolijoki, E., et al. "Decrease in Serum LDL Cholesterol with Microcrystalline Chitosan," *Methods Find Exp Clin Pharmacol* 21(5):357-61, 1999.

CHLOROPHYLL

CHLOROPHYLL-A, CHLOROPHYLLIN

Common trade names
Gary Null's Green Stuff

Common forms
Available as capsules, drinks or juices, powders, and tablets.

Source
Dietary sources of chlorophyll include algae, barley grass, chlorella, dark green leafy vegetables, spirulina, and wheat grass. Powders are commonly prepared from the dehydrated juice extracted from vegetables and plants and from unicellular organisms such as spirulina.

Chemical components
Chlorophyll is the green pigment that plants use to convert the sun's energy for photosynthesis. There are several forms of chlorophyll, such as chlorophyll-a. Chlorophyll derivatives, Cp-D and chlorophyllin (a water-soluble derivative of chlorophyll), have also been identified.

Actions
Chlorophyll is claimed to have anti-inflammatory, antioxidant, and wound-healing properties. It is thought to be a natural deodorizer (Chernomorsky and Segelman, 1988).

Preliminary evidence from animal and human cell culture studies suggests that cationic chlorophyll derivatives and chlorophyllin may suppress cancer cell growth (Kobayashi et al., 1996; Chung et al., 1999).

In a mouse-cell model, chlorophyll derivatives (CpD) were found to inhibit Gross leukemia virus, a mouse retrovirus (Lee and Lee, 1990).

Bold italic type indicates that reaction may be life-threatening.

Reported uses

Chlorophyll has been traditionally used as a deodorizer for bad breath and to reduce the odor of urine, feces, colostomy appliances, and infected wounds. Historically, it has been used for GI problems, such as constipation, and to stimulate blood cell formation in anemia.

In a group of geriatric nursing home patients, chlorophyllin was found to be helpful in controlling body and fecal odors, easing chronic constipation and flatulence, and improving morale (Young and Beregi, 1980).

In a trial of 34 patients, chlorophyll-a infusions of 5 to 20 mg/day for 1 to 2 weeks produced favorable symptomatic effects in 23 patients with chronic relapsing pancreatitis (Yoshida et al., 1980).

Dosage

As a deodorant, 100 mg P.O. b.i.d. or t.i.d.

Adverse reactions

None reported.

Interactions

None reported.

Contraindications and precautions

None reported.

Special considerations

- Powders prepared from vegetable juice dehydrated at low temperatures may be preferred.
- Although no known chemical interactions have been reported in clinical studies, consideration must be given to the pharmacologic properties of the herbal product and the potential for exacerbation of the intended therapeutic effect of conventional drugs.
- Advise the patient to consult a health care provider before using herbal preparations because a treatment that has been clinically researched and proved effective may be available.
- Instruct the patient to notify the prescriber and pharmacist of any herbal or dietary supplement he is taking when filling a new prescription.

Points of interest

- Chlorophyll is one of the most important chelates in nature. Other molecules with a similar structure that are involved in biochemical reactions include heme (a component of hemoglobin) and vitamin B_{12}.
- Chlorophyll-a is a green dye (Natural Green 3) used in soaps and cosmetics.

Commentary

Chlorophyll is found in all green plants. Although it is commonly found in the diet and appears to be safe, clinical evidence supporting its use in the treatment of disease is limited. Anecdotal reports and limited evidence suggest that chlorophyll may be effective as an internal deodorant.

References

Chernomorsky, S.A., and Segelman, A.B. "Biological Activities of Chlorophyll Derivatives," *N J Med* 85(8):669-73, 1988.

Chung, W.Y., et al. "Inhibitory Effects of Chlorophyllin on 7,12-dimethylbenz(a)-anthracene-Induced Bacterial Mutagenesis and Mouse Skin Carcinogenesis," *Cancer Lett* 145(1-2):57-64, 1999.

Kobayashi, Y., et al. "Cationic Chlorophyl Derivatives with SOD Mimicking Activity Suppress the Proliferation of Human Ovarian Cancer Cells," *Cancer Biother Radiopharm* 11(3):197-202, 1996.

Lee, M., and Lee, W.Y. "Anti-Retroviral Effect of Chlorophyll Derivatives (CpD-D) by Photosensitization," *Yonsei Med J* 31(4):339-46, 1990.

Yoshida, A., et al. "Therapeutic Effect of Chlorophyll-a in the Treatment of Patients with Chronic Pancreatitis," *Gastroenterol Jpn* 15(1):49-61, 1980.

Young, R.W., and Beregi, J.S. "Use of Chlorophyllin in the Care of Geriatric Patients," *J Am Geriatr Soc* 28(1):46-47, 1980.

CHOCOLATE

CACAO, COCOA AND COCOA BUTTER (THEOBROMA OIL)

Taxonomic class
Sterculiaceae

Common trade names
Various commercial products are available as condiments, flavorings, and foods.

Common forms
Available as cocoa butter, extracts, powder, and syrup.

Source
Cocoa is obtained from the seeds of the cacao tree, *Theobroma cacao*. The tree is native to Mexico but cultivated in many tropical areas, especially western Africa. The crude material (cacao tree and cacao beans) is referred to as cacao, and the processed product is called cocoa. Cacao powder is usually alkalized to improve its color, flavor, and ability to disperse in the process that refines the crude material to cocoa powder. Chocolate is prepared by mixing the cacao powder with sugar, flavoring, and extra cocoa butter fat. Milk chocolate includes milk as an ingredient, whereas dark chocolate does not.

Chemical components
Cocoa powder contains many compounds, including proteins, fats, and alkaloids such as theobromine, caffeine, and tyramine. Cocoa also contains more than 300 volatile compounds, including esters, hydrocarbons, lactones, monocarbonyls, pyrazines, and pyrroles. The main components responsible for its flavor are aliphatic esters, aromatic carbonyls, diketopiperazines, polyphenols, pyrazines, and theobromine. Cocoa butter primarily contains triglycerides, including oleic, palmitic, and stearic acids. About 75% of the fats are monounsaturated.

Bold italic type indicates that reaction may be life-threatening.

Actions

Theobromine and caffeine are both xanthine alkaloids and have similar actions as CNS and cardiac muscle stimulants, diuretics, and smooth-muscle relaxants. Theobromine has the lowest potency of the xanthine alkaloids in exerting these actions, whereas theophylline is the most potent.

In vitro studies of polyphenols in chocolate have demonstrated that they have antioxidant activity. Cocoa phenols also inhibit LDL oxidation. Results of another in vitro study suggest that the polyphenols in chocolate exert immunoregulatory effects (Sanbongi et al., 1997).

Cacao liquor water-soluble polyphenols were evaluated as a treatment for ethanol-induced gastric mucosal lesions in rats (Osakabe et al., 1998) and were found to be as effective as cimetidine or sucralfate in reducing the hemorrhagic lesions. It is theorized that this action may result from the antioxidant and leukocyte-modulating properties of these polyphenols.

A recent study (Planells et al., 1999) showed an improvement in magnesium, calcium, and phosphorus levels in rats that were fed a magnesium-deficient diet supplemented with a 3% cocoa product.

Reported uses

Cocoa extract is an ingredient in alcoholic and nonalcoholic beverages. Cocoa powder and cocoa syrup are used as flavorings in many foods and pharmaceutical products. Cocoa butter is commonly used as a suppository and an ointment base as well as an emollient and a skin protectant in creams, lotions, lipsticks, and soaps. Cocoa butter has also been used to treat wrinkles and prevent stretch marks during pregnancy. No studies have been conducted demonstrating the therapeutic usefulness of any form of cocoa for these indications.

A dose of 330 ml of cacao drink was shown to be effective in assessing gallbladder contractility in volunteers with symptomatic gallstones (Nitsche et al., 1998).

Several studies have suggested that a usual dietary portion of chocolate contains psychoactive doses of caffeine and, probably, theobromine, which may lead to increased well-being, energy, social disposition, and alertness (Mumford et al., 1996).

Dosage

No consensus exists.

Adverse reactions

Skin: acne (controversial).
Other: allergic reaction.

Interactions

MAO inhibitors (phenelzine selegiline, tranylcypromine): Potential severe vasopressor effects. Avoid administration with chocolate.
Theophylline: May inhibit theophylline metabolism. Avoid ingestion of large amounts of cocoa with theophylline.

Contraindications and precautions

Chocolate is contraindicated in known hypersensitivity. Use cautiously in patients on low-sodium diets and those with irritable bowel syndrome.

Special considerations

▲ **ALERT** Ingestion of 1,000 mg or more of theobromine (222 g of dark chocolate) may cause excitement, extrasystoles, headache, insomnia, mild delirium, muscle tremor, nausea, restlessness, and tachycardia. At least two cases of toxicity in canines have been reported: one dog experienced hyperexcitability and seizures and then collapsed and died after eating 2 lb of chocolate chips; two other dogs died suddenly 1 hour after consuming 20 to 30 g of dark chocolate (Stidworthy et al., 1997).

• Restrict cocoa intake in patients with irritable bowel syndrome.

• Instruct the patient with CV disease or special dietary restrictions to minimize consumption of chocolate products because of their high sodium and fat content.

• Caution the patient with arrhythmias or significant CV disease not to ingest large quantities of chocolate products because of the risk of xanthine-induced arrhythmias.

Commentary

Cocoa is used in many cosmetic, food, and pharmaceutical products and is generally considered nontoxic. Although chocolate contains antioxidant flavonoids that may have beneficial CV effects, such flavonoids are also found in other foods. The potential antiulcerative and magnesium-correcting properties of cocoa must be tested in humans before their efficacy and clinical relevancy can be determined.

References

Hertog, M.G.L., et al. "Dietary Antioxidant Flavonoids and Risk of Coronary Heart Disease: The Zutphen Elderly Study," *Lancet* 342:1007-11, 1993.

Mumford, G.K., et al. "Absorption Rate of Methylxanthines Following Capsules, Cola, and Chocolate," *Eur J Clin Pharmacol* 51:319-25, 1996.

Nitsche, R., et al. "Evaluation of a Cacao Drink as a Simple Oral Stimulus to Assess Gallbladder Contraction," *Z Gastroenterol* 36(2):135-41, 1998.

Osakabe, N., et al. "Effects of Polyphenol Substances Derived from *Theobroma cacao* on Gastric Mucosal Lesions Induced by Ethanol," *Biosci Biotechnol Biochem* 62(8):1535-38, 1998.

Planells, E., et al. "Ability of a Cocoa Product to Correct Chronic Mg Deficiency in Rats," *Int J Vitam Nutr Res* 69(1):52-60, 1999.

Sanbongi, C., et al. "Polyphenols in Chocolate, Which Have Antioxidant Activity, Modulate Immune Functions in Humans In Vivo," *Cell Immunol* 177:129-36, 1997.

Stidworthy, M.F., et al. "Chocolate Poisoning in Dogs," *Vet Rec* 141:28, 1997.

Bold italic type indicates that reaction may be life-threatening.

CHONDROITIN

CAS, CHONDROITIN SULFATE A, CHONDROITIN-4-SULFATE,
CHONDROITIN-C, CHONDROITIN-6-SULFATE, CSS

Common trade names
Multi-ingredient preparations: Chondroitin-4 Sulfate, Condrosulf, 100%
CSA, Purified Chondroitin Sulfate, Structum; Osteo-Biflex, Painfree

Common forms
Available as capsules (200 mg, 400 mg), an oral gel, and, in Europe, an
injection.

Source
Chondroitin is extracted from bovine tracheal cartilage.

Chemical components
Chondroitin sulfates are large molecularly sized compounds of glycosaminoglycans and disaccharide polymers composed of equimolar
amounts of D-acetylgalactosamine, D-glucuronic acid, and sulfates in 30
to 100 disaccharide units.

Purified commercial chondroitin preparations contain combinations
of chondroitin-4-sulfate and chondroitin-6-sulfate, which are negatively charged because of carboxylic and dissociated sulfates. Structurally,
chondroitin sulfates are related to the low-molecular-weight hepara-
noid danaproid sodium.

Actions
Because of their large molecular size, chondroitin sulfates are thought
to be poorly absorbed orally (13% absolute bioavailability). They have
been shown to control the formation of new cartilage matrix by stimulating chondrocyte metabolism and synthesis of collagen and proteoglycan.

Chondroitin sulfates are also reported to inhibit the enzymes human
leukocyte elastase and hyaluronidase. High concentrations of human leukocyte elastase are found in the blood and synovial fluid of patients with
rheumatic disease. Chondroitin sulfates also stimulate the production of
highly polymerized hyaluronic acid by synovial cells. Viscosity is subsequently improved and synovial fluid levels return to normal. The ratio of
chondroitin sulfate isomers (chondroitin-4-sulfate and chondroitin-6-
sulfate) in human synovial fluid may serve as a marker for severity of disease in patients with hip osteoarthritis (Yamada et al., 1999).

Reported uses
Chondroitin is claimed to be useful as a dietary supplement in combination with glucosamine sulfate in osteoarthritis and related disorders.
Chondroitin sulfates have been used in ischemic heart disease and hyperlipidemia, as a preservative of corneas for transplantation, and as an
adjunct to eye surgery.

Chondroitin sulfates were first evaluated using parenteral administration (Theodosakis, 1997). Other small trials demonstrated improvement in subjective outcomes, such as use of NSAIDs, visual analogue scales for pain, Lequesne's Index, and patient or physician global assessment after oral administration. More recent information from moderately sized clinical trials seems to support this earlier evidence. Interestingly, chondroitin sulfates may exert beneficial effects in terms of slowing joint space narrowing in osteoarthritis of the knee and hand. (See *Chondroitin sulfate for osteoarthritis.*)

Dosage

The oral dose is based on the patient's weight; chondroitin is usually given in combination with glucosamine sulfate.

Patients who weigh less than 120 lb (54 kg): 1,000 mg of glucosamine sulfate plus 800 mg of chondroitin sulfates P.O.

Patients who weigh between 120 and 200 lb (54 and 91 kg): 1,500 mg of glucosamine sulfate plus 1,200 mg of chondroitin sulfates P.O.

Patients who weigh more than 200 lb: 2,000 mg of glucosamine sulfate plus 1,600 mg of chondroitin sulfates P.O. (Theodosakis, 1997).

The total daily dosage is usually taken with food in divided doses b.i.d. to q.i.d. Studies evaluating chondroitin sulfates alone used doses from 400 mg P.O. b.i.d. or t.i.d. to 1,200 mg P.O. daily as a single dose. The study by Bourgeois and others (1998) suggested that a 1,200-mg/day single dose of chondroitin sulfate was equally as effective as 400 mg t.i.d.

Adverse reactions

CNS: euphoria (reported with use of chondroitin sulfates [Kerzberg et al., 1987]), headache, lack of coordination.

GI: diarrhea, dyspepsia, nausea.

Hematologic: decreased hematocrit, hemoglobin level, platelet and WBC counts, and segmented neutrophils; ***internal bleeding.***

Other: pain at injection site.

Interactions

Anticoagulants: May enhance effects. Avoid administration with chondroitin.

Contraindications and precautions

Avoid using chondroitin in pregnant or breast-feeding patients; effects are unknown. Use cautiously in patients with bleeding disorders because of the risk of anticoagulation.

Special considerations

• Offer additional support, such as intermittent moist heat application and exercise, to the patient with osteoarthritis.

• Instruct the patient to watch for signs of bleeding, especially if he is taking anticoagulants or has a bleeding disorder.

🖤 **ALERT** The risk of internal bleeding may exist because of chondroitin's structural similarity to heparin. Studies in animals found signifi-

---

Bold italic type indicates that reaction may be life-threatening.

RESEARCH FINDINGS
Chondroitin sulfate for osteoarthritis

Several clinical studies were published during the period of 1998 to1999 that evaluated the therapeutic application of chondroitin sulfate ingestion in osteoarthritis (Uebelhart et al., 1998; Bourgeois et al., 1998; Conrozier, 1998; Bucsi and Poor, 1998; Alekseeva et al., 1999). Typically, these studies were randomized, double-blind, placebo-controlled trials that examined the use of chondroitin sulfate at doses of 800 to 1,200 mg/day for knee osteoarthritis. Functional impairment related to osteoarthritis, as evaluated by Lequesne's index, was significantly reduced by 50% in the chondroitin sulfate group (800 mg/day) after 1 year of therapy, compared with the placebo group.

A few of these trials examined chondroitin's effect on disease progression. Use of chondroitin sulfate was associated with stabilization of the medial femorotibial joint space in some patients, whereas placebo-treated patients experienced progressive joint space narrowing. Beneficial effects of chondroitin sulfate over those of placebo were also found in subjects with osteoarthritis of the finger joints. After 3 years, patients receiving chondroitin sulfate (1,200 mg/day) were less likely to progress to what was termed "erosive" finger joints than were those receiving placebo.

Chondroitin sulfate has also been evaluated parallel to NSAIDs in osteoarthritis of the knee. In a study by Morreale and colleagues (1996), a 64.4% decrease in Lequesne Index scores was found in the group receiving the NSAID diclofenac, compared with a 29.7% decrease in the group receiving chondroitin. Mean values for spontaneous pain decreased by 82% for the chondroitin group compared with 36% for the diclofenac group. The difference was statistically significant in favor of chondroitin ($P<.01$). There was a reduction in pain on weight bearing of 53.1% for the chondroitin group compared with a 36.2% reduction in the diclofenac group. Also, analgesic consumption was 20% lower in the chondroitin group; consumption was just 5.2% lower in the diclofenac group. The authors concluded that although NSAID-treated patients showed prompt pain reduction, their symptoms reappeared at the end of the study. In contrast, the chondroitin-treated patients had a slower onset of therapeutic effect, but the effects lasted for up to 3 months after treatment.

Glucosamine, chondroitin sulfate, and manganese ascorbate relieved symptoms of knee osteoarthritis in a randomized, double-blind, placebo-controlled trial of 34 men with degenerative joint disease of the knee and back (Leffler et al., 1999). Symptom relief related to knee osteoarthritis was demonstrated by significant changes in visual analog scales for pain, patient assessment of treatment, summary disease scores, and diary scores.

cantly decreased hematocrit, hemoglobin level, platelet and WBC counts, and segmented neutrophils and reduced aggregation in response to adenosine diphosphate and collagen (McNamara et al., 1996). Bleeding as a result of chondroitin sulfate use in humans has not been reported.

• Advise women to avoid using chondroitin during pregnancy or when breast-feeding.

Points of interest

• Public interest in the combined use of chondroitin sulfates and glucosamine sulfate has risen, especially since the publication of *The Arthritis Cure* (Theodosakis, 1997), which claims that the sulfate combination is "the medical miracle that can halt, reverse, and may even cure osteoarthritis."

Commentary

Although many of the data from older human trials are flawed in study design, new clinical trial evidence for the therapeutic application of chondroitin sulfate in osteoarthritis of the knee is mounting. Aside from symptom relief, of particular interest is the purported beneficial effect in deterring progression of joint space narrowing in both knee and finger osteoarthritis. If this effect continues to be substantiated, chondroitin sulfate will probably become a valuable entity in antarthritic treatment plans. Many questions remain to be answered definitively. Chondroitin sulfate appears to be well tolerated in the short term, but the current body of evidence does not adequately address long-term safety issues. Additional clinical trials in larger patient populations that address optimal dosing of standardized dosage forms and those that compare chondroitin sulfate with other pharmacologic treatments are needed.

References

Alekseeva, L.I., et al. "Structum (Chondroitin Sulfate), a New Agent for the Treatment of Osteoarthrosis," *Ter Arkh* 71(5):51-53, 1999.

Bourgeois, P., et al. "Efficacy and Tolerability of Chondroitin Sulfate 1200mg/day vs Chondroitin Sulfate 3 x 400mg/day vs Placebo," *Osteoarthritis Cartilage* 6(S-A):25-30, 1998.

Bucsi, L., and Poor, G. "Efficacy and Tolerability of Roal Chondroitin Sulfate as a Symptomatic Slow Acting Drug for Osteoarthritis in the Treatment of Knee Osteoarthritis," *Osteoarthritis Cartilage* 6(S-A):31-36, 1998.

Conrozier, T. "Anti-Arthrosis Treatments: Efficacy and Tolerance of Chondroitin Sulfates," *Presse Med* 27(36):1862-65, 1998.

Kerzberg, E.M., et al. "Combination of Glycosaminoglycans and Acetylsalicylic Acid in Knee Osteoarthrosis," *Scand J Rheumatol* 16:377-80, 1987.

Leffler, C.T., et al. "Glucosamine, Chondroitin, and Manganese Ascorbate for Degenerative Joint Disease of the Knee or Low Back: A Randomized, Double-blind, Placebo-controlled Pilot Study," *Mil Med* 164(2):85-91, 1999.

McNamara, P.S., et al. "Hematologic, Hemostatic, and Biochemical Effects in Dogs Receiving an Oral Chondroprotective Agent for Thirty Days," *Am J Vet Res* 57:1390-94, 1996.

Bold italic type indicates that reaction may be life-threatening.

Morreale, P., et al. "Comparison of the Anti-inflammatory Efficacy of Chondroitin Sulfate and Diclofenac Sodium in Patients with Knee Osteoarthritis," *J Rheumatol* 23:1385-91, 1996.

Theodosakis, J. *The Arthritis Cure*. New York: St. Martin's Press, 1997.

Uebelhart, D., et al. "Effects of Oral Chondroitin Sulfate on the Progression of Knee Osteoarthritis: A Pilot Study," *Osteoarthritis Cartilage* 6(S-A):39-46, 1998.

Verbruggen, G., et al. "Chondroitin Sulfate: Structure/Disease Modifying Anti-Arthritis Drug in the Treatment of Finger Joint Osteoarthritis," *Osteoarthritis Cartilage* 6(S-A):37-38, 1998.

Yamada, H., et al. "Levels of Chondroitin Sulfate Isomers in Synovial Fluid of Patients with Hip Osteoarthritis," *J Orthop Sci* 4(4):250-54, 1999.

CHROMIUM

CHROMIUM PICOLINATE, CHROMIUM TRIPICOLINATE, Cr^{3+}

Common trade names
Beer Belly Busters, Body Lean, Chromaslim, Chroma Ultra Chromium Picolinate, Chromax, Chromax II, Chromium Picolinate High Potency, Chromium Picolinate Yeast Free, GTF Chromium Picolinate, Medislim, Perfect Chromium Picolinate, Protecol, The Chromium Picolinate Solution

Common forms
Available in various strengths and dosage forms alone and in combination with vitamin and mineral preparations.

Source
Chromium is found in beer, brewer's yeast, mushrooms, oysters, and some meats (especially kidneys). Some sources recommend a daily chromium intake of 50 to 200 mcg. Only small percentages (0.5% to 2%) of dietary chromium are actually absorbed (Anderson et al., 1988). Absorption does appear to be related to the salt form of chromium ingested, with the picolinate salt being the favored carrier of chromium. Average serum chromium levels in normal subjects range from 0.1 to 0.3 mcg/L (Chavez, 1997).

Chemical components
Chromium in the 3+ oxidation state is an essential trace mineral. It is synthesized endogenously by a pyridine-2-carboxylic acid metabolite of tryptophan. Picolinic acid is a natural ligand that is an isomer of nicotinic acid.

Actions
Studies in animals suggest that chromium is widely distributed in the body and tends to accumulate in tissues, with a mean terminal elimination half-life exceeding 80 days (independent of dose). Early evidence suggests that chromium is necessary in the body for certain biochemical reactions to take place. Most literature appears to link chromium with a role in maintaining adequate glucose homeostasis. Interestingly, patients receiving long-term total parenteral nutrition who eventually de-

veloped glucose intolerance, insulin resistance, weight loss, and other disturbances mimicking syndrome X were reversed with I.V. administration of chromium chloride (Chavez, 1997).

Reported uses

Chromium has been claimed to possess anabolic properties. It has been suggested to be useful for many varied conditions and situations: improving glucose utilization, increasing lean body mass, reducing fat mass, increasing energy, enhancing mood, improving vision, conditioning gums, curing acne, preventing insomnia, curbing addiction, improving psoriasis, preventing osteoporosis, and increasing longevity.

Several studies have pursued a role for chromium in diabetes. It is believed that chromium increases the rate of internalization of insulin within cells by improving cell membrane fluidity. The majority of evidence does suggest that chromium can lower fasting blood glucose levels (Chavez, 1997). However, the most recent randomized, controlled, double-blind trials refute the fact that chromium (220 mcg/day) has any effect on fasting blood glucose or Hgb-A_1C levels (Lee, 1994; Joseph et al., 1999).

Chromium has been evaluated several times for its purported effect on body composition. Several studies suggest that chromium supplementation (200 to 300 mcg/day) for 2 to 3 months produces beneficial changes in body composition. Although not all studies found positive benefits with the same parameters, such changes as increases in lean body mass and body composition index and decreases in body fat and body mass index have been reported (Kaats et al., 1996; Kaats et al., 1992; Bahadori et al., 1995). Again, some additional controlled, double-blind trial evidence is in conflict with the former data (Walker et al., 1998). Even the most recent data, a randomized, placebo-controlled, double-blind trial evaluating the effect of chromium supplementation on resistance training in 18 men, failed to find a benefit of chromium on parameters of muscle size, strength, power development, or lean body mass. Resistance training devoid of chromium supplementation had significant and independent effects on these measurements (Campbell et al., 1999).

Some trials have reported beneficial changes in the lipid profile of patients. Doses in the range of 600 mcg/day appear to produce the most favorable results, although smaller doses also have been evaluated. Patients who are documented to be chromium deficient may be the best candidates for chromium supplementation to improve their lipid profiles.

Although conflicting data exist, a trial of 19 nonobese subjects receiving 1,000 mcg/day of chromium or placebo for 8 weeks failed to identify any significant difference between chromium and placebo in study parameters measuring serum lipid levels, body composition, and insulin sensitivity (Amato et al., 2000).

Dosage

Dosing recommendations vary considerably, depending on the source. No consensus exists. Typically, adults are recommended to receive 200

Bold italic type indicates that reaction may be life-threatening.

to 400 mcg/day. Patients who potentially dispose of more chromium, elderly patients, diabetics, bodybuilders, and patients with hyperlipidemia are suggested to receive as much as 600 mcg/day. Other references suggest no more than 300 mcg/day. Doses used most commonly in clinical trials range from 200 to 400 mcg/day.

Adverse reactions
CNS: cognitive impairment.
GI: diarrhea, epigastric discomfort, flatulence, nausea.
GU: *renal failure* (1,000 mcg/day; Ceruli et al., 1998).
Hematologic: anemia.
Hepatic: *hepatic failure* (1,000 mcg/day; Ceruli et al., 1998).
Musculoskeletal: rhabdomyolysis (Martin and Fuller, 1998).

Interactions
Antacids: May bind dietary chromium, impairing chromium absorption. Stagger doses of both agents to minimize potential interaction.
Antibiotics known to bind cationic compounds (fluoroquinolones, tetracyclines): May bind chromium, decreasing absorption of the antibiotic. Space administration of both drugs or discontinue chromium supplementation during antibiotic therapy.
Vitamin C: May enhance chromium absorption. Consider lower dose of chromium.

Contraindications and precautions
Chromium is contraindicated in patients who are hypersensitive to chromium or the picolinate salt. Avoid consumption of chromium in excess of the RDA during pregnancy.

Special considerations
• Some evidence suggests that most Americans consume less than the RDA of chromium.
• Doses roughly equivalent to 600 mcg/day in humans produced chromosomal damage in Chinese hamster ovary cells (Stearns et al., 1995).
• The American Dietetic Association could not support the use of chromium for diabetics in a 1994 position paper.

Commentary
Clinical trial data evaluating chromium supplementation in diabetes, manipulation of body composition, and cholesterol reduction are fraught with conflict. Many early studies suffer from a small number of subjects, lack of a control group, inadequate description of subjects, missing information, and the use of imprecise or subjective measurements. More recent, rigorously designed and carefully controlled trials have failed to find significant differences that favor chromium supplementation. Chromium's unique pharmacokinetic profile might predispose subjects to acute or chronic chromium intoxication if higher than normal quantities are ingested over a long period. Most studies have been of short duration (less than or equal to 3 months). Subsequently, doses in excess of the RDA (50 to 200 mcg/day) are not recommended.

References

Amato, P., et al. "Effects of Chromium Picolinate Supplementation on Insulin Sensitivity, Serum Lipids, and Body Composition in Healthy, Nonobese, Older Men and Women," *J Gerontol A Biol Sci Med Sci* 55(5):M260-63, 2000.

Anderson, R.A., et al. "Exercise Effects on Chromium Excretion of Trained and Untrained Men Consuming a Constant Diet," *J Appl Physiol* 64:249-52, 1988.

Bahadori, B., et al. "Treatment with Chromium Picolinate Improves Lean Body Mass in Patients Following Weight Reduction," *Int J Obes Relat Metab Disord* 19(S-2):38, 1995. Abstract.

Campbell, W.W., et al. "Effects of Resistance Training and Chromium Picolinate on Body Composition and Skeletal Muscle in Older Men," *J Appl Physiol* 86(1):29-39, 1999.

Ceruli, J., et al. "Chromium Picolinate Toxicity," *Ann Pharmacother* 32:428-31, 1998.

Chavez, M.L. "Chromium Picolinate," *Hosp Pharm* 11:1466-78, 1997.

Joseph, L.J., et al. "Effect of Resistance Training with or Without Chromium Picolinate Supplementation on Glucose Metabolism in Older Men and Women," *Metabolism* 48(5):546-53, 1999.

Kaats, G.R., et al. "The Short Term Therapeutic Efficacy of Treating Obesity with a Plan of Improved Nutrition and Moderate Caloric Restriction," *Curr Ther Res* 51(2):261-74, 1992.

Kaats, G.R., et al. "Effects of Chromium Picolinate Supplementation on Body Composition: A Randomized, Double-masked, Placebo-controlled Study," *Curr Ther Res* 57(10):747-56, 1996.

Lee, N.A. "Beneficial Effect of Chromium Supplementation on Triglyceride Levels in NIDDM," *Diabetes Care* 17(12):1449-52, 1994.

Martin, W.R., and Fuller, R.E. "Suspected Chromium Picolinate-induced Rhabdomyolysis," *Pharmacotherapy* 18(4):860-62, 1998.

Stearns, D.M., et al. "Chromium Picolinate Produces Chromosome Damage in Chinese Hamster Ovary Cells," *FASEB J* 9:1643-48, 1995.

Walker, L.S., et al. "Chromium Picolinate Effects on Body Composition and Muscular Performance in Wrestlers," *Med Sci Sports Exerc* 30(12):1730-37, 1998.

CINNAMON

BATAVIA CASSIA, BATAVIA CINNAMON, CASSIA, CASSIA LIGNEA, CEYLON CINNAMON, CHINESE CINNAMON, CINNAMOMOM, FALSE CINNAMON, PADANG CASSIA, PANANG CINNAMON, SAIGON CASSIA, SAIGON CINNAMON

Taxonomic class
Lauraceae

Common trade names
None known. Various manufacturers produce cinnamon for use as a spice for foods.

Common forms
Available as cinnamon oil, dried bark and leaves, and powder.

Bold italic type indicates that reaction may be life-threatening.

Source
Active components are derived from the dried bark, leaves, and twigs of various species of *Cinnamomum:* Ceylon cinnamon (*C. zeylanicum*), Saigon cinnamon (*C. loureirii*), and others. *C. zeylanicum* grows in Sri Lanka, southeastern India, Indonesia, South America, and the West Indies. Essential oils are removed by steam distillation of the dried bark and leaves.

Chemical components
The main element in the essential oil is cinnamaldehyde. Other components found in smaller amounts include phenols and terpenes (such as eugenol, trans-cinnamic acid, hydroxycinamaldehyde, *O*-methoxycinnamaldehyde, *O*-glucoside, and 3-(2-hydroxyphenol)-propanoic acid), cinnamyl alcohol, tannins, mucilage, procyanidins, and coumarins.

Actions
Eugenol has antiseptic and anesthetic properties. Cinnamic aldehyde has shown fungicidal activity in vitro against such respiratory tract mycoses as *Aspergillus flavus, A. fuigatis, A. midulans, A. niger, Candida albicans, Candida tropicalis, Cryptococcus neoformans,* and *Histoplasma* (Viollon and Chaumont, 1994). *O*-glucoside and 3-(2-hydroxyphenol)-propanoic acid have reportedly demonstrated gastroprotective activity in rats similar to that of cimetidine. Cinnamon extracts have also demonstrated analgesic and antioxidant properties in rodent studies.

Reported uses
Cinnamon oil is widely used in small amounts in detergents, gargles, liniments, lotions, mouthwashes, soaps, toothpaste, and other pharmaceutical products and cosmetics. Claims have been made for cinnamon products as an analgesic, an antidiarrheal, and an antifungal. In Eastern and Western folk medicine, uses for cinnamon include treating abdominal pain, chest pain, chronic diarrhea, colds, female reproductive disorders, hypertension, kidney disorders, and rheumatism.

Cinnamon extracts have demonstrated significant inhibitory effects on strains of *Helicobacter pylori* and its urease, but a pilot study of an alcoholic cinnamon extract was ineffective in eradicating *H. pylori* in 15 subjects after twice-a-day dosing for 4 weeks (Nir et al., 2000).

Dosage
No consensus exists. Most sources cite cinnamon's use as a spice in small quantities only.

Adverse reactions
CV: increased heart rate.
EENT: cheilitis, gingivitis, glossitis, perioral dermatitis, stomatitis.
GI: increased GI motility.
Respiratory: dyspnea.
Skin: facial flushing.
Other: *hypersensitivity reactions* (including contact dermatitis, hand perspiration, post-excitatory state followed by a period of centralized

RESEARCH FINDINGS

Toxic ingestion of cinnamon oil

One case report described acute cinnamon toxicity in a 7-year-old child who had ingested 2 oz of cinnamon oil (Pilapil, 1989). Symptoms of toxicity included burning in the mouth, chest, and stomach; double vision; dizziness; vomiting; and subsequent collapse.

In the emergency department, the child was drowsy and had warm skin, increased bowel sounds, a pulse of 100/minute, and respiration of 20/minute. The child was given 8 oz of milk for toxicity symptoms, followed 15 minutes later with 15 ml of syrup of ipecac. After the child vomited, activated charcoal (120 ml) was administered.

Symptoms of rectal burning, diarrhea, double vision, and abdominal cramps persisted. GI symptoms and drowsiness lasted for 5 hours, after which the patient was asymptomatic. It's unclear from this report whether persistent GI symptoms resulted from cinnamon ingestion or the use of ipecac and activated charcoal.

sedation [drowsiness], second-degree burns), squamous cell carcinoma (Westra et al., 1998).

Interactions
None reported.

Contraindications and precautions
Avoid using cinnamon in excess of amounts normally found in foods in pregnant or breast-feeding women.

Special considerations
• Inform the patient that cinnamon should be used only as a spice. Other uses cannot be recommended because adequate data are lacking.
• Advise the patient that cinnamon or its components can cause allergic reactions, such as skin irritation (including second-degree burns) and stomatitis.
• Toxicity studies in rats suggest that chronic *C. zeylanicum* ingestion (90 days) may cause hepatic damage (reduction in liver weight) and a significant decrease in hemoglobin levels (Shah et al., 1998).
• Urge the patient to report unusual signs or symptoms. Cinnamon toxicity involves the GI tract, CNS, and CV system. (See *Toxic ingestion of cinnamon oil*.)
• Inform the patient that squamous cell carcinoma of the tongue has been linked to prolonged and heavy gum chewing (five packs/day) of cinnamon-flavored gum in one case report (Westra et al., 1998).
🔥 **ALERT** Caution parents that children may use cinnamon products as a recreational drug.

Bold italic type indicates that reaction may be life-threatening.

Points of interest
• Cinnamon extracts inhibit the oxidation of various foodstuffs, suggesting a possible role as a food preservative.

Commentary
Human trials evaluating the efficacy of cinnamon for its proposed uses are lacking. Further studies in animals and humans are needed to determine its safety and efficacy. Ingestion in quantities greater than that for use as a spice cannot be recommended.

References
Nir, Y, et al. "Controlled Trial of the Effect of Cinnamon Extract on *Helicobacter pylori*," *Helicobacter* 5(2):94-97, 2000.

Pilapil, V.R. "Toxic Manifestations of Cinnamon Oil Ingestion in a Child," *Clin Pediatr* 28:276, 1989.

Shah, A.H., et al. "Toxicity Studies in Mice of Common Spices *Cinnamomum zeylanicum* bark and Piper longrum fruits," *Plant Foods Hum Nutr* 52(3):231-39, 1998.

Viollon, C., and Chaumont, J.P. "Antifungal Properties of Essential Oils and Their Main Components upon *Cryptococcus neoformans*," *Mycopathologia* 128:151-53, 1994.

Westra, W.H., et al. "Squamous Cell Carcinoma of the Tongue Associated with Cinnamon Gum Use: A Case Report," *Head Neck* 20(5):430-33, 1998.

CLARY

CLARY OIL, CLARY SAGE, CLEAR EYE, MUSCATEL SAGE, ORVALE, SEE BRIGHT, TOUTE-BONNE

Taxonomic class
Lamiaceae

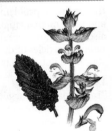

Common trade names
Clary Sea Face Mask

Common forms
Available as an essential oil (5 ml, 10 ml, clear liquid) and bath salts.

Source
The highly aromatic essential oil is steam-distilled from the flowering tops of *Salvia sclarea,* a perennial herb that is native to southern Europe.

Chemical components
The whole plant contains diterpenes (including candidissiol, ferruginol, manool, microstegiol, salvipisone, and sclareol), sesquiterpenes (caryophyllene oxide, spathulenol), alpha-amayrin, beta-sitosterol, flavonoids (including apigenin, luteolin, and 4-methylapigenin), linalyl acetate, linalool, and pionene.

Actions

The pharmacokinetics of clary's major component, diterpene sclareol, has been studied in vivo using a rat model. When given I.V., sclareol was rapidly cleared by biliary excretion; neither sclareol nor its metabolites were excreted in the urine after I.V. or P.O. administration.

The essential oil of clary produced contracture and inhibition of twitch response to nerve stimulation on skeletal muscle, whereas on smooth muscle, it produced contracture with little or no decrease in nerve stimulation (Lis-Balchin and Hart, 1997).

Some diterpenoids and sesquiterpenes extracted from clary have antimicrobial activity against *Staphylococcus aureus, Candida albicans,* and *Proteus mirabilis* (Ulubelen et al., 1994). Another study examining the antimicrobial activity of the essential oil of *S. sclarea* demonstrated only weak inhibitory activity against *S. aureus, Escherichia coli, Streptococcus epidermidis,* and *C. albicans* on local application. Its inhibitory properties increased progressively with contact time (Peana et al., 1999).

Clary is claimed to contain an estrogen-like compound that helps to regulate hormonal balance. Its antispasmodic activity is thought to be caused by nerol, a component of the essential oil. Although the essential oil has also been studied in humans for effects on the CNS and hematopoietic, immune, and enzyme systems, data are difficult to interpret because they were published in foreign journals.

Reported uses

Claimed to have anti-inflammatory, antispasmodic, astringent, euphoric, and sedative properties, clary is also thought to be useful in treating several ailments, including anxiety, decreased libido, depression, digestive and renal problems, menopausal symptoms, menstrual irregularity and pain, mental fatigue, premenstrual syndrome, and sore throat. It is also used in aromatherapy. The mucilaginous seeds have been used to remove particles of dust from the eyes. These claims have not been substantiated in human trials.

Dosage

Traditional uses suggest the following doses:
For anxiety, depression, decreased libido, and mental fatigue:
Baths: add 2 to 10 gtt of essential oil to bath water.
Inhalation: apply 2 gtt of essential oil to a piece of cloth and then inhale.
Massage: apply 2 to 4 gtt of essential oil to 2 tsp of carrier oil or lotion.
For hoarseness, laryngitis, and sore throat, add 3 gtt of essential oil to a glass of water and then rinse mouth and gargle.
For menstrual pain, apply 4 gtt of essential oil to a piece of cloth to be used for warm compresses.

Adverse reactions

CNS: drowsiness, euphoria, headache.
GU: increased menstrual bleeding.

Bold italic type indicates that reaction may be life-threatening.

Interactions
Alcohol: May enhance effects. Discourage use with clary.

Contraindications and precautions
Clary is contraindicated in patients with a history of estrogen-sensitive cancer because of its potential estrogenic effects. Avoid using clary in pregnant or breast-feeding patients; effects (other than with food uses) are unknown.

Special considerations
• Monitor women for increased menstrual bleeding and changes in their menses.
• Inform the patient that therapeutic effects and safety risks are not well documented.
• Advise the patient to avoid hazardous activities until clary's CNS effects are known.
• Instruct the patient to avoid consumption of other CNS depressants, including alcohol, because of purported sedative effects.
• Urge the patient to report unusual symptoms to his health care provider during herbal therapy.
• Advise women to avoid using clary during pregnancy or when breast-feeding.

Points of interest
• In the 16th century, Rhine Valley winemakers added clary to their wines to increase the wines' potency.

Commentary
Despite its many claims of therapeutic usefulness, clary has yet to demonstrate clinical efficacy through controlled animal and human trials. This herb cannot be recommended for use until adequate studies are conducted.

References
Lis-Balchin, M., and Hart, S. "A Preliminary Study of the Effect of Essential Oils on Skeletal and Smooth Muscle In Vitro," *J Ethnopharmacol* 58:183-87, 1997.
Peana, A., et al. "Chemical Composition and Antimicrobial Action of the Essential Oils of *Salvia desoleana* and *S. sclarea*," *Planta Med* 65(8):752-54, 1999.
Ulubelen, A., et al. "Terpenoids from *Salvia sclarea*," *Phytochemistry* 36: 971-74, 1994.

CLOVES
CARYOPHYLLUM, *EUGENIA AROMATICA*, OIL OF CLOVES, OLEUM CARYOPHYLLI

Taxonomic class
Myrtaceae

Common trade names
Dent-Zel-Ite Toothache Relief Drops, Red Cross Toothache Medication

Common forms
Available as drops (85% eugenol), fluid or oil extracts, and mouthwashes and in cigarettes.

Source
Active components are extracted by steam distillation from the dried flower buds of *Syzygium aromaticum* (also called *Eugenia caryophyllata* or *Caryophyllus aromaticus*), an evergreen tree native to Southeast Asia.

Chemical components
The agent is composed primarily of the phenolic substances eugenol and acetyl eugenol. Eugenol constitutes 90% to 95% of the phenolic compounds obtained from the plant and is extracted as a volatile oil. It's chemically known as 2-methoxy-4-(2-propenyl) phenol. Other compounds include a terpene, caryophyllene, and small amounts of alpha-humulene and beta-carophyllene.

Actions
Cloves are reported to have analgesic and antiseptic activity. The primary mechanism for the analgesic activity of cloves is believed to be inhibition of prostaglandin biosynthesis from cyclooxygenase and lipoxygenase blockade by eugenol (Rasheed et al., 1984). Other mechanisms may also exist, such as a reduction in pain perception produced by the phenolic activity of eugenol on nociceptors in dental pulp.

The antiseptic activity of cloves is also related to eugenol. Eugenol has been reported to have antimicrobial activity against various bacteria and *Candida albicans*. The antimicrobial activity of eugenol is poorly described but is thought to be due to a membrane-active antibacterial effect from the phenolic activity of eugenol (Briozzo et al., 1989).

Reported uses
Clove oil has been widely used topically in treating toothache and has been added to mouthwashes as an antiseptic. Some in vitro data have confirmed its anti-inflammatory and antimicrobial activity.

Dosage
Depending on the product being used, doses can vary from 5 to 30 gtt P.O. for the fluidextract to 1 to 5 gtt P.O. for the oil extract and ½ to 1 oz of oral mouth rinses containing clove oil.

Adverse reactions
EENT: hemoptysis, oral tissue sensitivity.
Respiratory: airway epithelium injury, ***bronchospasm,*** high-altitude pulmonary edema accompanied by airway inflammation (associated with clove cigarette smoking; Hackett et al., 1985).
Other: local tissue irritation.

Interactions
None reported.

Bold italic type indicates that reaction may be life-threatening.

Contraindications and precautions
Avoid using topical clove oil because it may further damage dental pulp and supporting periodontium.

Special considerations
• The American Dental Association (ADA) has not accepted clove oil and eugenol as safe and effective nonprescription drugs for toothaches.
• Toothaches or dental pain may signify a more serious problem. Advise the patient to seek professional dental advice regarding such pain. Restrict the application of clove and eugenol to people who are trained in its use, such as dentists.
• Inquire about the use of clove cigarettes (if the patient is a smoker) when taking the patient's history.
• Inform the patient that application of clove oil or eugenol-containing products may further damage viable dental pulp and soft tissue.

Points of interest
• The FDA-appointed advisory review panel on nonprescription drugs has reclassified eugenol to a Category III nonprescription drug (products that have insufficient data available on their use as nonprescription drugs).
• The ADA accepts clove oil and eugenol for professional use only by dentists.
• The German Commission E has approved cloves for use as a local anesthetic and antiseptic.

Commentary
Most clinical data on the use of clove oil or eugenol are obtained from in vitro studies. There are no well-controlled studies in humans evaluating the analgesic and antiseptic properties of clove oil or eugenol. Although data on the effects of clove oil and eugenol on prostaglandin synthesis suggest an analgesic role, further studies are needed.

References
Briozzo, J., et al. "Antimicrobial Activity of Clove Oil Dispersed in a Concentrated Sugar Solution," *J Appl Bacteriol* 66:69-75, 1989.
Hackett, P.H., et al. "Clove Cigarettes and High Altitude Pulmonary Edema," *JAMA* 253:3551-52, 1985. Letter.
Rasheed, A., et al. "Eugenol and Prostaglandin Biosynthesis," *N Engl J Med* 310:50-51, 1984. Letter.

COENZYME Q10
Co-Q10, MITOQUINONE, UBIDECARENONE, UBIQUINONE

Common trade names
Adelir, Co-Q10, Heartcin, Inokiton, Neuquinone, Taidecanone, Ubiquinone, Udekinon

Common forms

Capsules: 10 mg, 30 mg, 60 mg, 100 mg
Tablets: 25 mg, 50 mg, 100 mg, 200 mg

Source

Coenzyme Q10 (2,3 dimethoxy-5 methyl-6-decaprenyl benzoquinone) is an endogenous antioxidant found in small amounts in meats and seafood. It is found in all human cells, but its highest concentrations occur in the heart, kidneys, liver, and pancreas. Coenzyme Q10 is found naturally in the organs of many mammalian species. The "10" in coenzyme Q10 designates the number of isoprene units of the molecular side chain, and this is specific for humanoid ubiquinone. Japan retains all the world's patents for the product and is the major supplier of coenzyme Q10.

Chemical components

Ubiquinones (redox carriers, electron transport shuttles) are lipid-soluble benzoquinones that are involved in electron transport in the cell's mitochondria, where they are most concentrated. Coenzyme Q10 is classified as a fat-soluble quinone with characteristics that are common to many vitamins. It is a unique substance but resembles niacin in general biosynthetic performance. Chemically, its structure resembles that of vitamin K.

Actions

Coenzyme Q10 has antioxidant and membrane-stabilizing properties. It participates in the electron transfer process within the oxidative respiration chain and is part of oxidative phosphorylation. Coenzyme Q10 prevents the depletion of metabolic substrates required for resynthesis of adenosine triphosphate (ATP). Without coenzyme Q10, ATP cannot be regenerated through this pathway. Coenzyme Q10 is a powerful intramembrane antioxidant and free radical scavenger, protecting cell membranes and DNA from oxidative damage. Coenzyme Q10 simply protects tissue from ischemic cellular damage. Studies show that pigs fed diets supplemented with coenzyme Q10 were more likely to be resistant to myocardial ischemia–reperfusion injury (Maulik et al., 2000).

Reported uses

Ubiquinone is marketed to treat several diseases and disorders, including heart failure and ischemic heart disease. The basis for coenzyme Q10 use is that patients with significant heart disease (New York Heart Association [NYHA] classes III and IV) have coenzyme Q10 deficiency relative to normal, healthy people (NYHA classes I and II). (See *Coenzyme Q10 in heart failure.*)

In a preliminary study, 144 patients suffering from acute myocardial infarction appeared to benefit from 28 days of coenzyme Q10 supplementation (120 mg/day) as compared with placebo (Singh et al., 1998). Coenzyme Q10 seemed to decrease the incidence of angina, arrhythmias, and poor left ventricular function and the number of total cardiac

---

Bold italic type indicates that reaction may be life-threatening.

RESEARCH FINDINGS
Coenzyme Q10 in heart failure

In a large, double-blind, placebo-controlled study with coenzyme Q10 and conventional treatment, 651 patients with New York Heart Association (NYHA) class III or IV heart failure demonstrated a significant reduction in hospitalizations (23% versus 37%; Morisco et al., 1993). Episodes of pulmonary edema and cardiac asthma were also lower in the study group than in the control group. The authors concluded that the addition of coenzyme Q10 to conventional therapy significantly reduced hospitalization for decompensated heart failure and the incidence of serious complications in patients with heart failure.

In another investigation of 17 heart failure subjects (Sacher et al., 1997), coenzyme Q10 supplementation reportedly improved functional class by 20% and improved the mean heart failure score by 27%. Other benefits were increased left ventricular ejection fraction, increased cardiac output and stroke volume index, increases in exercise duration and workload, and slight reductions in systolic blood pressure. The authors concluded that coenzyme Q10 enhances cardiac output by exerting a positive inotropic effect on the myocardium besides its vasodilatory effects. The results of this study need be interpreted with caution because of the study's open-label design, lack of a control group, small number of patients, and short duration of therapy.

In 1999, the department of cardiology of Aalborg Hospital in Denmark published their results of a small, randomized, double-blind, controlled, invasive study of 22 patients who were given coenzyme Q10 (100 mg P.O. twice daily; Aalborg Hospital, 1999). Coenzyme Q10 supplementation for 12 weeks was associated with improvements in stroke index (SI), pulmonary artery pressure (PAP), and pulmonary capillary wedge pressure (PCWP) both at rest and during work over those of placebo. Only changes for SI (at rest and work), PAP (at rest), and PCWP (at work) were statistically significant. In contrast, a randomized, double-blind, placebo-controlled study conducted in Baltimore (Khatta et al., 2000) found no benefit in coenzyme Q10 supplementation (200 mg/day) over placebo in measurement of ejection fraction (EF), peak oxygen consumption, or exercise duration in their group of 55 NYHA class III or IV (EF ≤40%) patients who were receiving standard medical therapy.

events (fatal and nonfatal infarction). The investigators noted that early intervention (less than 3 days) was prudent and that larger studies were needed to confirm these results.

Epidemiological evidence exists that high vitamin E doses may reduce the risk of coronary artery disease. Coantioxidants such as coenzyme Q10 may make vitamin E an even more efficient antioxidant for lowering LDL levels (Vasankari et al., 1997).

Randomized, controlled trials fail to support the use of coenzyme Q10 as an ergogenic aid.

Other conditions in which coenzyme Q10 is claimed to be useful include angina pectoris, arrhythmias, Bell's palsy, deafness, diabetes, doxorubicin cardiotoxicity, hypertension, immunodeficiency, mitral valve prolapse, and periodontal disease.

Dosage
Dosages used in clinical trials ranged from 50 to 300 mg P.O. daily.

Adverse reactions
CV: *ischemic tissue damage* (during intense exercise).
GI: anorexia, diarrhea, epigastric discomfort, mild nausea.

Interactions
Oral antidiabetic drugs: May inhibit some coenzyme Q10 enzymes and, thus, inhibit functions of exogenously administered coenzyme Q10. Use together cautiously.
Warfarin: Coenzyme Q10 may diminish response to warfarin. Monitor the patient appropriately.

Contraindications and precautions
Use coenzyme Q10 cautiously in patients who are hypersensitive to coenzyme Q10 or its formulation.

Special considerations
• Caution the patient not to self-treat symptoms of heart disease before seeking appropriate medical evaluation because this may delay diagnosis of a serious medical condition.
• Advise the patient to consult a health care provider before using herbal preparations because a treatment that has been clinically researched and proved effective may be available.
🕭 **ALERT** Caution the patient against performing intense exercise during coenzyme Q10 therapy because damage to ischemic tissue can occur. Some evidence suggests that coenzyme Q10 decreases the time it takes to fatigue muscle.
• Instruct the patient with heart failure to report changes in his condition to his primary health care provider.

Commentary
Despite its apparent usefulness in the symptomatic treatment of heart failure, coenzyme Q10 has not been shown to reduce mortality. Some seemingly positive clinical trial data should be interpreted with caution because of inadequate study design. Comparative trials are needed to evaluate coenzyme Q10 with standard treatments (such as ACE inhibitors, beta blockers, and aspirin) to determine survival rates. Coenzyme Q10 also needs to be further evaluated in the treatment of other diseases before its use can be recommended.

Bold italic type indicates that reaction may be life-threatening.

References

Aalborg Hospital, Department of Cardiology. "Coenzyme Q10 Treatment in Serious Heart Failure," *Biofactors* 9(2-4):1285-89, 1999.

Khatta, M., et al. "The Effect of Coenzyme Q10 in Patients with Congestive Heart Failure," *Ann Intern Med* 132(8):636-40, 2000.

Maulik, N., et al. "Dietary Coenzyme Q 10 Supplement Renders Swine Hearts Resistant to Ischemia-Reperfusion Injury," *Am J Physiol Heart Circ Physiol* 278(4):H1084-90, 2000.

Morisco, C., et al. "Effect of Coenzyme Q10 Therapy in Patients with Congestive Heart Failure. A Long-Term Multicenter, Randomized Study," *Clin Invest* 71:s134-36, 1993.

Sacher, H.L., et al. "The Clinical and Hemodynamic Effects of Coenzyme Q10 in Congestive Cardiomyopathy," *Am J Ther* 4(2-3):66-72, 1997.

Sinatra, S.T., et al. "Coenzyme Q10: A Vital Therapeutic Nutrient for the Heart with Special Application in Congestive Heart Failure," *Conn Med* 65:707-11, 1997.

Singh, R.B., et al. "Randomized, Double-blind, Placebo-controlled Trial of Coenzyme Q10 in Patients with Acute Myocardial Infarction," *Cardiovasc Drug Ther* 12(4):347-53, 1998.

Vasankari, T.J., et al. "Increased Serum and Low-Density-Lipoprotein Antioxidant Potential After Antioxidant Supplementation in Endurance Athletes," *Am J Clin Nutr* 65:1052-56, 1997.

COFFEE

BEAN JUICE, CAFÉ, *COFFEA ARABICA*, ESPRESSO, JAVA, JOE, ROBUSTA COFFEE, SANTOS COFFEE

Taxonomic class
Rubiaceae

Common trade names
Bean Company, Eight o'Clock, Folger's, Maxwell House

Common forms
Available as whole dried or ground beans and freeze-dried or spray-dried crystals (instant coffee). Caffeine is commonly included in allergy medicines, analgesics, cold products, dietary aids, and stimulants.

Source
The fruits of the *Coffea arabica* bush are commonly cultivated for their most popular seeds (referred to as beans after roasting). Grown in semi-tropical areas, other coffee species are also used (*C. canephora, C. robusta*). The chief coffee-growing areas are Central and South America, Africa, Jamaica, and Hawaii. Freshly picked berries are either sun-dried (natural or dry process) or subjected to depulping machines and then dried (washed or wet process). The roasting and blending of other beans gives each coffee its characteristic flavor. Before roasting, caffeine is extracted from green (unripened) beans with organic solvents.

Chemical components

Active components include some B vitamins, caffeine, chlorogenic acid, free amino acids, galactomanan (carbohydrate) protein, trace quantities of niacin, polyamines, tannins, and trigonelline. Coffee oil contains cafestol, cahweol, fatty acids, lanosterol, stearic acids, sterols, and toco-pherols. More than 100 aromatic compounds have been identified in coffee, including some furan derivatives, oxazoles, pyrazines, pyrroles, and various acids.

Actions

Caffeine, a methylxanthine, is responsible for most of coffee's effects. It binds to adenosine receptors in the brain and acts as a stimulant. The normal elimination half-life of caffeine is 3.5 to 4.5 hours, but it can double in pregnancy and last for days in a fetus.

Caffeine increases fatty acid metabolism and the basal metabolic rate and affects metabolism of other drugs. It contains diterpenes that can in-crease cholesterol, LDL, and triglyceride levels. Studies show that the in-crease in lipid levels is caused by boiled, unfiltered coffee. Filtering of cof-fee (with a paper filter) does not produce the same increases in the lipid profile. The proposed mechanisms for increasing the lipid profile are de-creases in cholesterol acyltransferase, cholesterolester transfer protein, and phospholipid transfer protein activity. Unfiltered coffee can also pro-duce negative effects on the CV system by increasing homocysteine levels.

Changes in heart rate and mild blood pressure elevations can also oc-cur acutely (Van Dusseldorp et al., 1989), but chronic use of caffeine shows a tolerance to these effects.

Reported uses

Endurance runners have used coffee to increase fatty acid metabolism and aid exercise tolerance. The effect of coffee on patients with angina was to increase their exercise tolerance and delay time to angina.

Coffee may act as a bronchodilator and was shown to affect pulmo-nary function test results. Twice the dose of coffee would be needed to match the bronchodilating potency of traditional drugs, such as theo-phylline and aminophylline.

Some retrospective studies have reported a possible twofold to three-fold risk reduction in the incidence of Parkinson disease for coffee drinkers. The proposed mechanism for this reduction is by way of ade-nosine receptors, which can also improve motor deficits in primates treated with N-methyl-4-phenyl-1,2,3,6-tetrahydropyridine (MPTP).

Other retrospective studies have shown a one-third risk reduction for developing gallstones in coffee drinkers compared with non–coffee drinkers. Proposed mechanisms are increased cholecystokinin release, gallbladder motility, colonic motility, and bile flow and decreased cho-lesterol crystallization and gallbladder fluid absorption.

Several randomized controlled studies have shown a 10% to 25% risk reduction in colon cancer for coffee drinkers and no increased risk in coffee drinkers who have adenomatous polyps. A critique based on the available evidence surrounding the use of coffee enemas dispels the notion that they may be useful for treating cancer (Green, 1992).

Caffeine was found to help cold sufferers be more alert and lower their general feeling of malaise. Postprandial coffee consumption by elderly patients has been shown to circumvent postprandial hypotension and reduce falls.

Coffee was used to reduce postpartum complications in cows. It lowered the incidence of diarrhea, normalized temperature, and reduced mortality by 75%.

Dosage
No consensus exists. The lethal dose of caffeine is reported to be 10 g.

Adverse reactions
CNS: mild delirium and excitation, headache, insomnia, restlessness; may lower seizure threshold (in patients with refractory psychiatric disorders receiving electroconvulsive therapy).
CV: worsening of CV disease, effects on lipid levels (controversial), extrasystole, increased blood pressure, tachycardia.
EENT: glaucoma (caused by temporary caffeine-induced intraocular pressure).
GI: gastroesophageal reflux disease (GERD), nausea, peptic ulcer disease.
GU: diuresis.
Musculoskeletal: muscle fasciculations (spasms, tremor).

Interactions
None reported.

Contraindications and precautions
Avoid using coffee in pregnant or breast-feeding patients. The infant's heart rate and respiratory rate increase, but long-term effects are unknown.

Special considerations
- Consider coffee intake as a cause in patients who complain of insomnia.
- Inquire about the patient's daily coffee consumption.
- Inform the patient that chronic consumption of coffee can lead to caffeine withdrawal symptoms when it's abruptly discontinued; rebound headaches can occur.
- Advise the patient with hyperlipidemia to minimize consumption of coffee because of adverse effects on lipid profiles, or suggest that he drink only drip-filtered coffee (paper filters may retain a significant portion of lipids that are present in boiled coffee) (Van Dusseldorp et al., 1991).
- Caution the patient with GERD against coffee consumption because coffee can exacerbate the condition.
- Advise women to avoid using caffeine during pregnancy or when breast-feeding.

Points of interest

• Clinical trials dispel the belief that caffeine exacerbates arrhythmias (Graboys et al., 1989) or produces lasting increases in blood pressure (Van Dusseldorp et al., 1989).
• American consumers seem to prefer Colombian and Central American coffee over Brazilian and African varieties.
• In Germany, coffee charcoal (charred outer portion of beans) is used to treat nonspecific acute diarrhea.

Commentary

Coffee is relatively harmless, but some patients may experience adverse pharmacologic reactions from caffeine. A conservative approach may be to limit coffee consumption in patients with gastric diseases, hypercholesterolemia, or hypertension and in pregnant or breast-feeding patients.

References

Graboys, T.B., et al. "The Effect of Caffeine on Ventricular Ectopic Activity in Patients with Malignant Ventricular Arrhythmia," *Arch Intern Med* 149: 637-39, 1989.

Green, S. "A Critique of the Rationale for Cancer Treatment with Coffee Enemas and Diet," *JAMA* 268(22):3224-27, 1992.

Van Dusseldorp, M., et al. "Effect of Decaffeinated Versus Regular Coffee on Blood Pressure," *Hypertension* 14 (5): 563-69, 1989.

Van Dusseldorp, M., el al. "Cholesterol-raising Factor from Boiled Coffee Does Not Pass a Paper Filter," *Arterioscler Thromb* 11(3):586-93, 1991.

COLA TREE

KOLA NUT, KOLANUT

Taxonomic class

Sterculiaceae

Common trade names

Multi-ingredient preparations: Colloidal Energy Formula, Kola Nut, Starter, Ultra Diet Pep

Common forms

Available as nuts and seeds. Extracts of the seeds are available in capsules, fluidextracts, and tablets. Cola nut extract is widely used as a flavoring in carbonated soft drinks in the United States.

Source

Cola nitida and *C. acuminata* are evergreen trees that are native to western Africa, Sri Lanka, and Indonesia. They belong to the sterculia family, which includes cacao, or chocolate. The active components are extracted from the seeds. *C. nitida* has two subspecies, alba and rubra.

Chemical components

Caffeine is the primary component of cola seeds; other notable components include the alkaloid theobromine, significant tannin content, and phenols.

Bold italic type indicates that reaction may be life-threatening.

Actions

Caffeine and theobromine are both methylated xanthines. They act similarly to theophylline by inhibiting phosphodiesterase, which increases intracellular levels of cAMP. Primary effects are bronchodilation, cardioacceleration, CNS stimulation, diuresis, increased blood pressure, and increased gastric acid secretion (Ibu et al., 1986).

Chewing cola nuts tends to increase salivary pH (Gaye et al., 1990), which may contribute to the reduced incidence of tooth decay observed in habitual users. Cola tannins are reported to be carcinogenic. Other studies have shown an extremely high level of methylating activity that is attributed to nitrosamide or nitrosamine formation in subjects who chewed cola nuts, possibly leading to an increased incidence of oral carcinoma (Atawodi et al., 1995). Cola compounds have also shown antibacterial activity (Ebana et al., 1991). In vitro studies of *C. nitida* extract demonstrate an inhibitory effect on luteinizing hormone (LH)-releasing hormone–induced release of LH (Benie et al., 1987).

Intraperitoneal injection of cola nut extract produces varying effects on locomotor (both stimulant and depressive) activity in mice, depending on the dose used (Ajarem, 1990).

Reported uses

Herbal therapy promotes cola as an antidepressant, an antidiarrheal, an aphrodisiac, a cardiac and CNS stimulant, and a diuretic. Human clinical studies are lacking to support these claims. Traditional uses include treatment of diarrhea, dyspnea, heart disease, and several mood and personality disorders. The most common use has been as a CNS stimulant. Studies evaluating the cardiac and CNS effects of caffeine have been performed in animals, but therapeutic implications for humans have not been established. Anecdotally, the bark has been used to treat wounds, and sometimes the root is chewed to clean teeth and freshen the breath. Cola is a common ingredient in weight-loss preparations.

Dosage

Traditional uses suggest the following doses:
Decoctions: 1 to 2 tsp extracted powder boiled in 1 cup of water for 10 to 15 minutes.
Fluidextract: 5 to 40 gtt (¼ to 2 tsp) P.O. up to t.i.d. at meals with juice or water.
Solid extract: 2 to 8 grains (130 to 520 mg) P.O. per dose.

Most commercial preparations are standardized to about 10% caffeine content.

Adverse reactions

CNS: anxiety, excitation, nervousness.
CV: *bradycardia,* hypertension, hypotension, palpitations, tachycardia.
EENT: staining of oral mucosa (bright yellow when cola nuts are chewed; Ashri and Gazi, 1990).
GI: epigastric pain (significant increase in acid secretion; Ibu et al., 1986).

GU: decreased LH release.
Hepatic: *hepatotoxicity* (caused by high tannin content).
Other: allergic reactions; altered brain, kidney, liver, and testicular enzyme activity; may cause *carcinogenesis.*

Interactions

Analgesics, antipyretics: May increase half-life of these drugs. Avoid administration with cola nuts or their extracts.

Contraindications and precautions

Cola nuts and their extracts are contraindicated in pregnant or breast-feeding patients; in those with arrhythmias, hypertension, or peptic ulcer disease; and in patients at risk for stroke. They are also contraindicated in patients who are allergic to chocolate because cross-sensitivity reactions can occur.

Special considerations

• Smokers who chew cola nuts are at increased risk for developing oral carcinoma.
• Monitor the cardiac patient for arrhythmias and changes in blood pressure.
• Urge the patient to report changes in mood or behavior.
• Advise the patient who is allergic to chocolate to avoid cola nuts and their extracts.
• Advise women to avoid using cola nuts and their extracts during pregnancy or when breast-feeding.

Points of interest

• According to the German Commission E monograph, cola nut is therapeutically useful for mental and physical fatigue.

Commentary

The contribution of the cola tree to the Western economy is assured because it is the primary source of caffeine for carbonated soft drinks. Small amounts of cola nut extract are probably harmless and would be equivalent to a strong cup of coffee or the standard dose of OTC caffeine products. Other components whose activities have not been fully investigated may contribute to unidentified toxicity.

Although caffeine and theobromine in cola nuts have useful CNS and respiratory system effects, single-ingredient medications that have a standardized dose and known adverse effects are preferred. Additional research is needed to develop complete adverse effect and toxicity profiles and to identify new antimicrobial activities.

References

Ajarem, S. "Effects of Fresh Kola-nut Extract (*Cola nitida*) on the Locomotor Activities of Male Mice," *Acta Physiol Pharmacol Bulg* 16(4):10-15, 1990.
Ashri, N., and Gazi, M. "More Unusual Pigmentations of the Gingiva," *Oral Surg Oral Med Pathol* 70(4):445-49, 1990.

Atawodi, S.E., et al. "Nitrosatable Amines and Nitrosamide Formation in Natural Stimulants: *Cola acuminata, C. nitida,* and *Garcinia cola,*" *Food Chem Toxicol* 33:625-30, 1995.

Benie, T., et al. "Natural Substances Regulating Fertility. Effect of Plant Extracts in the Ivory Coast Pharmacopoeia on the Release of LH by Hypophyseal Cells in Culture," *CR Seances Soc Biol Fil* 181(2):163-67, 1987.

Ebana, R.U., et al. "Microbiological Exploitation of Cardiac Glycosides and Alkaloids from *Garcinia kola, Borreria ocymoides, Kola nitida,* and *Citrus aurantifolia,*" *J Appl Bacteriol* 71:398-401, 1991.

Gaye, F., et al. "Experimental Study of Variations of Salivary pH Affected by Chewing Cola," *Dakar Med* 35:148-55, 1990.

Ibu, J.O., et al. "The Effect of *Cola acuminata* and *Cola nitida* on Gastric Acid Secretion," *Scand J Gastroenterol* 124(Suppl):39-45, 1986.

COLOSTRUM

BOVINE COLOSTRUM, BOVINE IMMUNOGLOBULIN CONCENTRATE (BIC), HYPERIMMUNE BOVINE CONCENTRATE (HBC), IMMUNIZED BOVINE COLOSTRUM (IIBC)

Common trade names
Bioenervi, Lactobin

Common dosage forms
Available in capsules (liquid or powder), cream, dry powder, liquid, and tablets (500 mg).

Source
Colostrum is the thick, yellowish fluid secreted by the mammary glands immediately after birth. It contains immune factors and growth factors for the neonate as well as other nutrients. Bovine colostrum contains the same types of ingredients as human colostrum except with higher levels of immune and growth factors. For this reason, cattle are the source for commercially produced colostrum.

Chemical components
Colostrum contains several immune factors (such as immunoglobulin [Ig]A, IgD, IgE, IgG, and IgM) and specific immunity (antibodies) to diseases acquired by the mother that are potentially transferable to other mammals. The levels of IgA, IgG, IgG_2, and IgM in bovine colostrum are about 100 times higher than in normal milk. Colostrum also contains cytokines, glycoproteins (such as trypsin and protease inhibitors), lactalbumins, lactoferrin, leukocytes, lysozyme, vitamins, and other immune factors. Specific insulin-like growth factors (such as IgF-I and IgF-II) are abundant, which stimulates cell growth and tissue repair.

Actions
Bovine colostrum has been used to transfer antibodies, growth and immune factors, and specific immunity to certain disease states to other

mammals. Animal studies have suggested that growth factors and immune factors are transferable between mammals.

Reported uses

A Finnish study of human athletes taking bovine colostrum supplementation demonstrated an increase in the serum IgF-I level during strength and speed training (Mero et al., 1997). The results of several studies have showed that colostrum from cows immunized against rotavirus prevented or decreased the severity of diarrheal episodes in children (Davidson et al., 1989; Ebina et al., 1992; Mitra et al., 1995; Sarker et al., 1998). It has also been shown that oral anticholera toxin bovine colostral immunoglobulins are ineffective in treating patients with active cholera diarrhea (McClead et al., 1988). Other studies have evaluated the use of bovine colostrum for *Escherichia coli* and *Cryptosporidium parvum* infections (Huppertz et al., 1999; Greenberg et al., 1996). Unsubstantiated claims for colostrum include its use as an antiaging agent, an anticancer agent, an antiviral, a dietary supplement, a digestive aid, a growth or regeneration agent, an immune system stimulant, and a skin repair agent.

Dosage

Dosage varies with the product. No standard dosing is available. A popular dose used in some trials is 10 g/day.

Adverse reactions

GI: elevated liver enzyme levels (Greenberg et al., 1993).

Interactions

None reported.

Contraindications and precautions

Avoid using colostrum in pregnant or breast-feeding patients; effects are unknown.

Special considerations

• No reactions were documented in patients with milk allergy.
• Urge the patient to notify the prescriber and pharmacist of any herbal or dietary supplement he is taking when filling a new prescription.

Points of interest

• The bulk of research on colostrum has used fresh colostrum (free of fat and lactose). A few studies have used dried colostrum or compared different preparations of colostrum (Zaremba et al., 1993; Greenberg et al., 1996).
• A major factor in selecting a colostrum product is quality. Because the immune and growth factors are easily destroyed by heat, proper manufacturing procedures are imperative. No independent assays or standards for quality and production are available.

Bold italic type indicates that reaction may be life-threatening.

Commentary

Animal research constitutes the bulk of the literature on colostrum. Although initial information is promising, further study in human trials is needed. Standardization of colostrum products is needed to ensure quality of growth and immune factors. Evidence to support claims is lacking.

References

Davidson, G.P., et al. "Passive Immunization of Children with Bovine Colostrum Containing Antibodies to Human Rotavirus," *Lancet* 2(8665):709-12, 1989.

Ebina, T., et al. "Passive Immunizations of Suckling Mice and Infants with Bovine Colostrum Containing Antibodies to Human Rotaviruses," *J Med Virol* 38(2):117-23, 1992.

Greenberg, P., et al. "A Preparation of Bovine Colostrum in the Treatment of HIV-positive Patients with Chronic Diarrhea," *Clin Invest* 71(1):42-45, 1993.

Greenberg, P., et al. "Treatment of Severe Diarrhea Caused by *Cryptosporidium parvum* with Oral Bovine Immunoglobulin Concentrate in Patients with AIDS," *JAIDS* 13:348-54, 1996.

Huppertz, H., et.al. "Bovine Colostrum Ameliorates Diarrhea in Infection with Diarrheagenic *Escherichia coli*, Shinga-toxin Producing *E. coli*, and *E. coli* Expressing Intimin and Hemolysin," *J Pediatr Gastroenterol Nutr* 29:452-56, 1999.

McClead, R.E., et al. "Orally Administered Bovine Colostral Anti-Cholera Toxin Antibodies: Results of Two Clinical Trials," *Am J Med* 85:6:811-16, 1988.

Mero, A., et al. "Effects of Bovine Colostrum Supplementation on Serum IGF-I, IgG, Hormone, and Saliva IgA During Training," *J Appl Physiol* 83:4:1144-51, 1997.

Mitra, A.K., et al. "Hyperimmune Cow Colostrum Reduces Diarrhoea Due to Rotavirus: A Double-Blind, Controlled Clinical Trial," *Acta Paediatr* 84(9):996-1001, 1995.

Sarker, S.A., et.al. "Successful Treatment of Rotavirus Diarrhea in Children with Immunoglobulin from Immunized Bovine Colostrum," *Pediatr Infect Dis J* 17:1149-54, 1998.

Zaremba, W., et.al., "Efficacy of a Dried Colostrum Powder in the Prevention of Disease in Neonatal Holstein Calves," *J Dairy Sci* 76:3:831-36, 1993.

COLT'S FOOT

ASS'S FOOT, BULLSFOOT, COUGHWORT, FARFARA, FIELDHOVE, FILUIS ANTE PATREM, FOALSWORT, HALLFOOT, HORSEHOOF, KUANDONG HUA, PAS DÍANE

Taxonomic class
Asteraceae

Common trade names
Phytostyle Holding Spray (hair spray)

Common forms
Available as extract, syrup, tea, and tincture.

Source

Active components are extracted from dried leaves, flowers and, sometimes, roots of *Tussilago farfara,* a low-growing perennial herb that commonly occurs in Europe, England, Canada, and the northern United States.

Chemical components

The plant contains many compounds, including carotenoids, flavonoids, dihydride alcohol, a glucoside, mucilage, phytosteol alcohol, senecionine, senkirine, tannins, pyrrolizidine alkaloids, terpene alcohol, and tussilagone.

Actions

The components of *T. farfara* have different pharmacologic effects. Mucilage supplies the demulcent effect of colt's foot. L-652,469 acts as a calcium channel blocker and an inhibitor of platelet activation factor, a component in the asthma process, in rabbits and humans (Hwang et al., 1987). In studies with animals, tussilagone showed a pressor effect similar to that of dopamine but without the tachyphylaxis (Li et al., 1988). Other studies have found anti-inflammatory and gram-negative antibacterial activity.

Senkirine is thought to cause hepatotoxicity in animals. Urinary bladder papilloma was also observed (Hirono et al., 1976). Pyrrolizidine alkaloids are known to be carcinogenic.

Reported uses

Colt's foot was first used 2,000 years ago in Asia and Europe primarily for asthma, bronchitis, and cough. Although some recommend that colt's foot be smoked for respiratory relief, heat destroys the mucilage that provides colt's foot's demulcent effects. No human trials have evaluated these claims.

Dosage

Traditional uses suggest the following doses:
Dried herb: 0.6 to 2.9 g P.O. by decoction.
Liquid extract (1:1 in 25% alcohol): 0.6 to 2 ml P.O. t.i.d.
Syrup (liquid extract 1:4 in syrup): 2 to 8 ml P.O. t.i.d.
Tea: 1 to 3 tsp of dried flowers or leaves in 1 cup of boiling water P.O. t.i.d.
Tincture (1:5 in 45% alcohol): 2 to 8 ml P.O. t.i.d.

Adverse reactions

CNS: fever.
CV: increased blood pressure.
GI: diarrhea, loss of appetite, nausea, vomiting.
Respiratory: upper respiratory tract infection.
Skin: jaundice.

Bold italic type indicates that reaction may be life-threatening.

Interactions
Antihypertensives: May antagonize hypotensive effects. Avoid administration with colt's foot.

Contraindications and precautions
Colt's foot is contraindicated in patients with hepatic disease. Also avoid its use in pregnant or breast-feeding patients because of its potential for carcinogenicity and abortifacient effects. Use cautiously in patients who are hypersensitive to other members of the composite family, such as chamomile and ragweed, because cross-sensitivity can occur. Also use colt's foot cautiously in hypertensive patients because of its pressor effect.

Special considerations
● Monitor blood pressure of the patient taking colt's foot.
● Inform the patient that data regarding colt's foot's safety and efficacy profiles are insufficient.
● Assess the patient for jaundice.
● Advise women to avoid using colt's foot during pregnancy or when breast-feeding.
● Instruct the patient to report unusual symptoms while taking this or other herbal supplements.
● Urge the patient to avoid colt's foot if he is allergic to chamomile or ragweed.

Points of interest
● Colt's foot was once used as a flavoring agent in candy.
● A few plants of different genera have been commonly referred to as "coltsfoot."

Commentary
The little information available about colt's foot is based on animal research and, therefore, difficult to extrapolate to humans. Colt's foot's CV effects and carcinogenic potential as well as the risk of an allergic reaction should be considered before use. Because data are lacking, the use of colt's foot cannot be recommended. The FDA has classified this herb as of "undefined safety," and Canada has banned its use.

References
Hirono, J., et al. "Carcinogenic Activity of Coltsfoot, *Tussilago farfara*," *Jpn J Cancer Res* 67:125-29, 1976.

Hwang, S., et al. "L-652,469 as a Dual Receptor Antagonist of Platelet Activating Factor and Dihydropyridines from *Tussilago farfara*," *Eur J Pharmacol* 141:269-81, 1987.

Li, Y.P., et al. "Evaluation of Tussilagone: A Cardiovascular-Respiratory Stimulant Isolated from Chinese Herbal Medicine," *Gen Pharmacol* 19:261-63, 1988.

COMFREY

ASS EAR, BLACK ROOT, BLACKWORT, BONESET, BRUISEWORT, CONSOLIDA, CONSOUD ROOT, GUM PLANT, HEALING HERB, KNITBACK, KNITBONE, SALSIFY, SLIPPERY ROOT, WALLWORT, YALLUC

Taxonomic class
Boraginaceae

Common trade names
Wise Woman Comfrey Salve. Several combination products are available, including Alticort, Atri-Res, Black Ointment, C&F Formula, Comfrey/Aloe Capsules, Comfrey and Fenugreek, EB5 Footcare Formula, EB5 Toning Formula, #483 Oxox Cell Activator, Goldenseal Salve, H-Complex, Heal-All Salve, Kytta-Plasma f, Kytta-Salbe F, Liniment Virtue, Muco-Plex, Mucoplex, Mustard Salve, Pain-Less Rub, Plantain Salve, Procomfrin, Respa-Herb, Simicort, Super Salve, T-ANEM, T-ASMA, T-BC, T-BF, Traumaplant, T-SLC, and T-ULC.

Common forms
Comfrey is available as a blended plant extract also known as "green drink," homeopathic preparations, a poultice or liniment, a tea (dried leaf and whole root), and a topical cream or ointment and in bulk roots or leaves, capsules, elixir, mucilaginous decoctions, powder, and tincture. Pyrrolizidine alkaloid (PA)–free comfrey preparations are also available. Commercial root preparations are available, but they are not recommended for internal or external use because of their high concentration of PAs. Comfrey is available in combination products in veterinary medicine for topical treatment of muscle strains and ruptures and for oral administration as an antidiarrheal.

Source
An oil is extracted from the leaves and roots of *Symphytum officinale*, a member of the borage family. Comfrey is a perennial herb that grows in temperate regions, including western Asia, North America, and Australia.

Chemical components
Comfrey contains a few compounds that show medicinal activity. Mucilage, a mucopolysaccharide of fructose and glucose, is concentrated in the root up to 29%. Allantoin, asparagine, beta-sitosterol, consolicine, consolidine, isobanerenol, lithospermic acid, PAs (up to 0.7% in dried root materials), rosmarinic acid, silicic acid, stigmasterol, symphytocynoglossin, tannins, and triterpenoids (including symphytoxide A) are also found in the plant.

Actions
Mucilage is reported to possess demulcent properties by forming a protective film to soothe irritation and inflammation. Allantoin is claimed

---

to be a cell-growth stimulator, accounting for comfrey's ability to stimulate wound healing and tissue regeneration. Tannin provides the astringent properties and rosmarinic acid imparts anti-inflammatory properties. The triterpenoid symphytoxide A is reported to possess hypotensive activity.

Reported uses

The application of comfrey is limited to claims for healing wounds. Historically, comfrey was used for several internal ailments, such as ulcers of the bowel, stomach, liver, and gallbladder, but because the alkaloids are converted to toxic metabolites by liver enzymes after being ingested, internal use is no longer recommended.

External application of comfrey products is not considered as dangerous as oral administration. Externally, it is used for bruises and sprains and to promote bone healing.

The anti-inflammatory effects of comfrey were analyzed in 41 patients with musculoskeletal rheumatism. Twenty patients were treated with a PA-free ointment and the remainder received placebo for 4 weeks. Significant improvement was reported with the ointment compared with placebo in patients with epicondylitis and tendovaginitis, but no difference was found in patients with periarthritis (Petersen et al., 1993).

Dosage

The oil from the leaves and roots can be incorporated in creams and ointments or used in a compress. Ointments and other external preparations are typically made with 5% to 20% comfrey. Comfrey should be applied topically on unbroken skin for less than 10 days or a maximum of 6 weeks per year in amounts at or below a daily dosage of 100 mcg of the unsaturated PAs.

Although comfrey has been used as a tea or taken in capsule form, it is not recommended for internal use because of its toxicity.

Adverse reactions

CNS: chills, fever.
GI: abdominal pain, diarrhea, hematemesis, poor appetite, vomiting.
Hepatic: *hepatotoxicity.*
Skin: exfoliative dermatitis, jaundice.
Other: weight loss, *cancer* (several animal studies report hepatocellular adenomas and urinary bladder tumors caused by PAs in comfrey [Hirono et al., 1978]), *death.*

Interactions

Eucalyptus: May increase the risk of PA toxicity because of enzyme induction by eucalyptus. Avoid administration with comfrey.
Other PA-containing herbs: May increase risk of toxicity. Herbs that contain PAs include agrimony, alkanna, alpine ragwort, borage, colt's foot, dusty miller, golden ragwort, goundsel, gravel root, ground's tongue, hemp, petasties, and tansy ragwort. Avoid administration with comfrey.

Contraindications and precautions
Internal use of comfrey is contraindicated because of hepatotoxicity. Because PAs are teratogenic and excreted in breast milk of animals, comfrey is contraindicated in pregnant or breast-feeding patients and in young children. It is also contraindicated in patients who are hypersensitive to comfrey and in those with a history of hepatic disease.

Special considerations
• Caution the patient not to use the root for medicinal purposes.
• Instruct the patient to apply the mature leaves externally on intact skin for only a limited period; caution him not to use the leaves on open wounds.
• Monitor wound appearance and size if the patient is taking comfrey to promote healing.
• Assess for signs and symptoms of hepatotoxicity.
• Comfrey either alone or in combination has been reported to cause abdominal pain, chills, death, diarrhea, exfoliative dermatitis, fever, hematemesis, jaundice, poor appetite, vomiting, and weight loss (U.S. FDA, 1998).
ALERT Several studies report on hepatic veno-occlusive disease caused by PAs in the plant (Mattocks, 1980).
• Caution the patient against consuming comfrey.
• Advise the patient to try commercially available antiseptic ointments and creams before attempting to use comfrey to promote wound healing.
• Advise women to avoid using comfrey during pregnancy or when breast-feeding.

Points of interest
• Comfrey has been used since the time of the ancient Greeks and Romans. In the Middle Ages, it was commonly applied as a poultice for treating broken bones, giving rise to the common names of boneset, knitback, and knitbone.
• The botanical genus name, *Symphytum*, originates from the Greek physician Disocorides some 2,000 years ago and is derived from the Greek word *sympho,* meaning to unite. The common name, comfrey, is derived from the Latin *confirmare,* which means to heal or unite.

Commentary
Although comfrey has a long history of therapeutic claims for several ailments, it is potentially hepatotoxic and thus should not be consumed. Anecdotal reports and animal studies suggest medicinal benefit for wound healing. Commercially available topical antiseptic agents are probably safer and more effective.

References
Awang, D.V.C. "Comfrey," *Can Pharm J* 120:101-4, 1987.
Awang, D.V.C., and Kindack, D.G. "Atropine as Possible Contaminant of Comfrey Tea" (Letter), *Lancet* 2:44, 1989.
Bach, N., et al. "Comfrey Herb Tea-induced Hepatic Veno-occlusive Disease," *Am J Med* 87:97-99, 1989.

Bold italic type indicates that reaction may be life-threatening.

Hirono, I., et al. "Carcinogenic Activity of *Symphytum officinale*," *J Natl Cancer Inst* 61(3):865-69, 1978.

Mattocks, A.R. "Toxic Pyrrolizidine Alkaloids in Comfrey" (Letter)," *Lancet* 11:1136-37, 1980.

McDermott, W.V., and Ridker, P.M. "The Budd-Chiari Syndrome and Hepatic Veno-occlusive Disease," *Arch Surg* 125:525-27, 1990.

Petersen, G., et al. "Anti-inflammatory Activity of a Pyrrolizidine Alkaloid–free Extract of Roots of *Symphytum officinale*," *Planta Med* 59(Suppl):A703-4, 1993.

Ridker, P.M., and McDermott, W.V. "Comfrey Herb Tea and Hepatic Veno-occlusive Disease," *Lancet* 1:657-58, 1989.

Ridker, P.M., et al. "Hepatic Veno-occlusive Disease Associated with the Consumption of Pyrrolizidine-containing Dietary Supplements," *Gastroenterology* 88:1050-54, 1985.

U.S. Food and Drug Administration. The Special Nutritionals/Adverse Event Monitoring System Web Report Search Results for Comfrey (1998, October 20). Available from http://vm.cfsan.fda.gov/%7Edms/aems.html.

Weston, C.F.M., et al. "Veno-occlusive Disease of the Liver Secondary to Ingestion of Comfrey," *Br Med J (Clin Res Ed)* 295:183, 1987.

Yeong, M.L., et al. "Hepatic Veno-occlusive Disease Associated with Comfrey Ingestion," *J Gastroenterol Hepatol* 5:211-14, 1990.

CONDURANGO

CONDOR-VINE BARK, CONDURANGO BARK, CONDURANGO BLANCO, EAGLE VINE, GONOLOBUS CONDURANGO TRIANA, MARSEDENIA CONDURANGO

Taxonomic class
Asclepiadaceae

Common trade names
Conduran, Condurango, Condurango Bark

Common forms
Available as dried or powdered bark, liquid extract, and tincture.

Source
Condurango is the dried bark of *Marsedenia condurango,* a member of the milkweed family that is native to Ecuador and other parts of South America.

Chemical components
Condurango contains tannin, small quantities of a strychnine-like alkaloid, caoutchouc, conduragin, condruit, essential oil, phytosterin, resin, sitosterol, and condurangoglycoside (an aglycone). Other components of the bark include catteic acid, chlorogenic acid, cichorin, *p*-coumaric acid, coumarin, esculetin, flavonoids, 7-hydroxycoumarin, neochlorogenic acid, and vanillin.

Actions
Tannic acid has local astringent properties that act on the GI mucosa; it also forms insoluble complexes with some heavy metal ions, alkaloids,

and glycosides. Tannic acid has also been shown to have antiulcerative and antisecretory effects within the GI tract.

Saponin glycosides, referring to condurangoglycoside, have a bitter taste and are irritating to the mucous membranes. In humans, they are generally nontoxic after oral ingestion, but they act as potent hemolytics when given I.V. Coumarin is converted to 7-hydroxycoumarin by the cytochrome P-450 2A6 enzyme system (Klaassen, 1996). Although coumarin is considered a less active anticoagulant than warfarin, doses of 4 g have been shown to decrease sympathetic nerve activity. The presence of a strychnine-like compound may also contribute to the herb's proposed uses because strychnine (from the dried ripe seed of *Strychnos Nux-vomica*) has been used medicinally as a bitter.

Reported uses

Condurango is mainly used as an appetite stimulant, an astringent, and a bitter and promotes functional stomach activity. Its bark is claimed to relax the nerves of the stomach, thus making it suitable for tension- or anxiety-induced indigestion. The herb has also been suggested for use as an analgesic, a diuretic, a hemostatic, and a tonic.

In the late 1800s, condurango was considered a cure in the early stages of cancer of the breast, epithelium, esophagus, face, lips, neck, pylorus, skin, stomach, and tongue and for lymphadenomas. Although human studies are lacking, two glycosides were isolated from condurango bark and found to have antitumorigenic activity against sarcoma-180 and Ehrlich cancers in rats (Hayashi et al., 1980). Natives of South America have used condurango to treat chronic syphilis.

Dosage

Tincture: 1 to 2 ml P.O. t.i.d.

Adverse reactions

CNS: CNS stimulation (stiff neck and facial muscles, restlessness, excitable reflexes, ***seizures)***.
Hepatic: hepatic dysfunction.
Other: increased urine output, sweating, vertigo, and visual disturbances have occurred after ingestion of 12 g of bark.

Interactions

Drugs using the CYP2A6 enzyme system (carbamazepine, paroxetine, ritonavir, sertraline): Altered metabolism of these drugs because coumarin also uses this pathway. Avoid administration with condurango.
Iron-containing products, alkaloid-related substances (atropine, scopolamine), medicinal glycosides (digoxin): Absorption prevented when used with condurango. Avoid concomitant use.

Contraindications and precautions

Condurango is contraindicated in patients with a history of seizures or other CNS disorders and in pregnant or breast-feeding patients. Use cautiously in patients with hepatic disease and those who are taking drugs that are metabolized by the cytochrome P-450 2A6 enzyme sys-

---

Bold italic type indicates that reaction may be life-threatening.

tem. Parenteral administration of tannic acid has been used as an experimental hepatotoxin.

Special considerations
- Instruct the patient to discontinue condurango immediately if liver transaminase levels become elevated or muscle stiffness or rigidity, excitable reflexes, or seizures occur.
- A change in the therapeutic levels of other concurrent drugs can occur because of competition for metabolism through the cytochrome P-450 2A6 enzyme system.
- Urge the patient to report symptoms of hepatic dysfunction (fever, jaundice, right upper quadrant pain) and other adverse reactions immediately.
- **ALERT** Inform the patient that poisoning from conduragin ingestion is possible because the bark compound is believed to be a violent toxin.
- **ALERT** Seizures resulting in paralysis have occurred after conduragin ingestion and overdoses of bark itself.
- Caution the patient to avoid hazardous activities, such as driving, until tolerance to the herb is known.
- Advise women to avoid using condurango during pregnancy or when breast-feeding.

Commentary
Human studies are lacking. Antitumorigenic activity was reported in rats (Hayashi et al., 1980). Excessive amounts of condurango are not recommended because of the risk of adverse effects on the liver, interactions with drugs metabolized through the cytochrome P-450 2A6 enzyme system and, possibly, stimulant effects on the CNS.

References
Hayashi, K., et al. "Antitumor Active Glycosides from Condurango Cortex," *Chem Pharm Bull* 28:1954-58, 1980.
Klaassen, C.D. *Casarett and Doull's Toxicology: The Basic Science of Poisons*, 5th ed. New York: McGraw-Hill Book Co., 1996.

CORIANDER
CHINESE PARSLEY, CILANTRO, ORIANDER

Taxonomic class
Apiaceae

Common trade names
None known.

Common forms
Available as a crude extract of the fruits, essential oils for aromatherapy, and seeds.

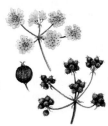

Source
Active components are obtained by steam distillation of an

essential oil from the dried ripe fruits of *Coriandrum sativum*. The varieties commonly used are *C. sativum* var. *vulgare* and *C. sativum* var. *microcarpum*. Fruits of coriander are often incorrectly referred to as seeds.

Chemical components
Fruits contain a volatile oil. Major components of the oil include alpha pinene, anethole, borneol, camphene, camphor, carvone, caryophyllene oxide, coriandrol, elemol, geraniol, geranyl acetate, limonene, monoterpene hydrocarbons, para cymene, phellandrene, and terpinene. Other components in fruit include oleic, petroselinic, and linolenic acids; sitosterols, triacontanol, tricosanol, tricontane, octadecenoic acid, proteins, starch, sugars, coumarins, psoralen, angelicin, scopoletin, and umbelliferone; flavonoid glycosides (quercetin 3-glucuronide, isoquercetin, coriandrinol, rutin); tannins; chlorogenic and caffeic acids.

Generally, the composition of the leaves is similar to that of the fruit, except that there is less volatile oil and more protein; ascorbic acid is also present in the leaves.

Actions
Coriander has been reported to possess several potentially beneficial pharmacologic effects. These effects have been shown in animal and laboratory models and include antibacterial, antifungal, cytotoxic, larvicidal, and lipolytic activity and hypoglycemic effects (Gray and Flatt, 1999).

Coriander oil was observed in vitro to suppress the formation of DNA adducts by acting on microsomal enzymes and may signal a potential use as an anticarcinogen (Hashim et al., 1994). Aqueous extracts of fresh coriander produced a dose-dependent anti-implantation effect but failed to produce complete infertility in rats (Al-Said et al., 1987).

Reported uses
Coriander is commonly used with other ingredients as a flavoring agent. The fruits are used extensively in all types of food dishes. In Oriental cooking, coriander is referred to as Chinese parsley; in Spanish cooking, the leaves are called cilantro. It is also popular as a flavoring agent in beverages, frozen dairy desserts, candy, puddings, gelatins, and relishes. The oil is used in creams, lotions, and perfumes (maximum 0.6%) and sometimes added to tobacco. Coriander is claimed to be effective as an anthelmintic and antarthritic and in enhancing the functional activity of the stomach. No human trials have examined these claims.

Dosage
No consensus exists.

Adverse reactions
GI: fatty infiltration of liver.
Skin: allergic reactions to the essential oils.

Bold italic type indicates that reaction may be life-threatening.

Interactions
Hypoglycemic drugs: Increased hypoglycemic effect. Monitor blood glucose levels closely during coriander use.

Contraindications and precautions
Avoid using coriander in pregnant or breast-feeding patients; effects are unknown.

Special considerations
• Inform the patient that insufficient evidence exists to support coriander's use for medicinal purposes.
• Advise the patient not to ingest more of this herb than that commonly found in foodstuffs because of potential untoward pharmacologic effects.
• Advise women to avoid using coriander during pregnancy or when breast-feeding.

Points of interest
• The highest reported levels of coriander in foodstuffs are 0.52% (fruits) in meat products and 0.12% (oil) in alcoholic beverages.

Commentary
Coriander is most appropriately used as a flavoring agent. No human data exist concerning its efficacy for other purposes.

References
Al-Said, M.S., et al. "Post-coital Antifertility Activity of the Seeds of *Coriandrum sativum* in Rats," *J Ethnopharmacol* 21:165-73, 1987.

Gray, A.M., and Flatt, P.R. "Insulin-releasing and Insulin-like Activity of the Traditional Anti-diabetic Plant *Coriandrum sativum*," *Br J Nutr* 81(3):203-9, 1999.

Hashim, S., et al. "Modulatory Effects of Essential Oils from Spices on the Formation of DNA Adduct by Aflatoxin B_1 In Vitro," *Nutr Cancer* 21:169-75, 1994.

CORKWOOD

CORKWOOD TREE, PITURI

Taxonomic class
Solanaceae

Common trade names
None known.

Common forms
Available as an extract of the corkwood tree (leaves and stems) in liquid and tablets.

Source
The active ingredients are extracted from the leaves, stems, and root bark of *Duboisia myoporoides*, which is native to Australia.

Chemical components
The corkwood tree is a rich source of alkaloids and has been used as a commercial source of scopolamine. The major alkaloids found in young leaves and stems are scopolamine and valtropine; other alkaloids—hyoscyamine, trigloyl tropine, and valeroidine—occur in lesser quantities. Alkaloids extracted from older leaves and stems include acetyl tropine, apohyoscine, butropine, hyoscyamine, isoporoidine, noratropine, poroidine, scopolamine, tropine, valeroidine, and valtropine. The young root and bark of the tree yield apohyoscine, atropine, hyoscyamine, scopolamine, tropine, valeroidine, and valtropine. Similar alkaloids are found in old root and bark samples. Nicotine and nornicotine have also been reported in the leaves (Coulsen and Griffin, 1967, 1968).

Actions
Scopolamine and the other alkaloids found in corkwood are antimuscarinics or muscarinic-cholinergic blockers and exhibit a wide range of pharmacologic effects. When taken in therapeutic doses, scopolamine may cause drowsiness and a dreamlike state. Larger doses can result in excitement or restlessness and hallucinations. These antimuscarinics may also affect heart rate, reduce gastric and salivary secretions and GI motility, and cause mydriasis and blurred vision because of cycloplegia.

Reported uses
The corkwood tree was principally used as a main source of scopolamine and atropine before the availability of other commercial sources.

Scopolamine is commonly used to prevent motion-induced nausea and vomiting, and atropine has limited use in treating GI motility disturbances. It has been reported that corkwood leaves are cured, rolled into a quid, and chewed by native Australians for their stimulant effects and used in hunting to stun animals. Extracts of the leaves have been used medicinally as a substitute for atropine. Quids are chewed to ward off hunger, pain, and tiredness. Alkaloids from the plant are used as a therapeutic substitute for atropine.

Dosage
No consensus exists.

Adverse reactions
CNS: disorientation, drowsiness, euphoria, excitation (in high doses), fatigue, hallucinations (in high doses).
CV: alterations in heart rate.
EENT: blurred vision, cycloplegia, dry mouth.
GI: constipation.
GU: urine retention.
Skin: dry skin.

Interactions
Amantadine, beta blockers, digoxin, tricyclic antidepressants and other drugs with anticholinergic or anticholinergic-like effects: Increased anticholinergic-like effects. Avoid administration with corkwood.

Bold italic type indicates that reaction may be life-threatening.

RESEARCH FINDINGS

Hyoscine poisoning from corkwood

In 1981, four case reports described accidental and occupational exposure to the corkwood tree or leaves, resulting in clinical hyoscine poisoning. During the harvesting of commercially grown trees in Australia, exposure to the dust and leaf particles led to mydriasis and cycloplegia ("cork-eye") in workers. Exposure of several hours resulted in dry mouth, facial flushing, delirium, depression, irrational behavior, or withdrawal. This syndrome has been described as being "corked up" (Pearn, 1981).

Ingestion of a mixture of boiled corkwood leaves and coffee has been shown to cause hallucinations and intoxication-like behavior. Dilated pupils have been noted in children at schools near commercial corkwood tree farms. No specific treatments were described and patients recovered after several hours of nonexposure to corkwood.

Contraindications and precautions

Corkwood and its products are contraindicated in patients who are hypersensitive to antimuscarinics; in those with CV disease, glaucoma, myasthenia gravis, obstructive GI conditions, obstructive uropathy or renal disease, or other conditions that may be exacerbated by antimuscarinics; and in pregnant or breast-feeding patients.

Special considerations

• Adverse reactions from corkwood alkaloids are related to their antimuscarinic action. (See *Hyoscine poisoning from corkwood.*)
• Consider exposure to corkwood if the patient manifests pupillary, vision, or behavioral changes.
• Advise the patient who is already receiving anticholinergic-like drugs to avoid taking corkwood because of the risk of increased anticholinergic effects.
• Caution the patient who may be at risk for disease exacerbation or adverse effects from anticholinergic drugs against using corkwood.
• Advise women to avoid using corkwood during pregnancy or when breast-feeding.

Commentary

Although corkwood leaves and stems have been used for medicinal purposes, primarily as an atropine substitute, no clinical studies of the plant have been undertaken. Antimuscarinic toxicity has been reported after occupational or accidental exposure, with absorption through the mucous membranes and upper respiratory tract. Medicinal use of the plant is not recommended.

References

Corkwood Tree. Natural Medicines Comprehensive Database. Therapeutic Research Faculty, Stockton, Calif., 1999, 294-95.

Coulsen, J.F., and Griffin, W.J. "The Alkaloids of *Duboisia myoporoides*. I. Aerial Parts," *Planta Med* 15:459-66, 1967.

Coulsen, J.F., and Griffin, W.J. "The Alkaloids of *Duboisia myoporoides*. II. Roots," *Planta Med* 16:174-81, 1968.

Pearn, J. "Corked Up: Clinical Hyoscine Poisoning with Alkaloids of the Native Corkwood, *Duboisia*," *Med J Aust* 2:422-23, 1981.

COUCH GRASS

Agropyron, cutch, dog-grass, durfa grass, quack grass, quick grass, scotch quelch, *Triticum*, twitch, twitch grass, wheat grass, witch grass

Taxonomic class
Poaceae

Common trade names
Multi-ingredient preparations: Aqua-Lim, Chromolite 3, Cybergenetics Quick Trim Complex 1, Diuplex, Diutrate, Doctor's Choice for Heart Health, Herbal Diuretic, More than a Diet, Pro-Guard, Thermojetics Cell-U-Loss

Common forms
Available most commonly in multi-ingredient capsules and tablets; also available as dried rhizome, liquid extract, and tincture.

Source
Medicinal preparations of couch grass are composed of the rhizome of *Agropyron repens*, also known as *Triticum repens*, *Graminis rhizoma*, *Elymus repens*, and *Elytrigia repens*. Less frequently, the roots, short stems and, sometimes, seeds of this hearty weed are used medicinally. This herb should not be confused with *Cynodon dactylon*, also known as couch grass or dog's tooth.

Chemical components
Couch grass contains acid malates, flavonoids (including tricin), fructose, glucose, inositol, lactic acid, levulose, mannitol, mucilage, pectin, saponins, and triticin, a carbohydrate similar to inulin. The volatile oil contains agropyrene (95%), carvacrol, carvone, *p*-cymene and sesquiterpenes, fixed oil, menthol, menthone, phenolcarboxylic acid, silicates, silicic acid, thymol, trans-anethole, and vanillin monoglucoside. Even though potentially genotoxic anthraquinones have been detected in couch grass, these constituents are not believed to present a danger when the herb is consumed in small amounts (Mueller et al., 1999).

Actions
Couch grass has mild diuretic and, because of its mucilage component, demulcent properties. Rodent studies have also reported sedative and

---

Bold italic type indicates that reaction may be life-threatening.

weak anti-inflammatory activity. Because of the presence of agropyrene, the essential oil has demonstrated antimicrobial effects.

Reported uses
Couch grass is approved by the German Commission E for flushing-out therapy (use of a mild diuretic with copious fluid intake) for inflammatory disorders of the urinary tract and for helping to prevent kidney and bladder stones. Commonly reported uses include treatment of benign prostatic hyperplasia, bladder and kidney stones, premenstrual syndrome, prostatitis, and urinary tract infections. Other uses in folk medicine include treatment of chronic skin disorders, gout, and rheumatic complaints and alleviation of bronchial irritation. Juice prepared from the roots of the plant has been used for treating jaundice and other hepatic disorders. In Germany, couch grass seeds are placed in a hot, moist pack and applied to the abdomen to soothe peptic ulcer disease.

Dosage
Traditional uses suggest the following doses:
Dried rhizome: 6 to 9 g P.O. in divided doses t.i.d. (may also be prepared as a tea or decoction)
Liquid extract (1:1 in 25% alcohol): 4 to 8 ml P.O. t.i.d.
Tincture (1:5 in 40% alcohol): 5 to 15 ml P.O. t.i.d.

Adverse reactions
Metabolic: electrolyte depletion.
Skin: contact dermatitis.

Interactions
Potassium-depleting diuretics: May contribute to hypokalemia. Do not use together.

Contraindications and precautions
Avoid using couch grass in pregnant or breast-feeding patients; effects are unknown. Couch grass grain may become contaminated with ergot, and poisoning from tainted preparations is possible. Patients with edema caused by cardiac or renal insufficiency should not undergo flushing-out therapy.

Special considerations
• Caution the patient about the risk of ergot poisoning from using contaminated couch grass preparations.
• Urge the patient not to self-treat symptoms of infection or inflammation before seeking appropriate medical evaluation because this may delay diagnosis of a serious medical condition.
• Advise the patient to consult a health care provider before using herbal preparations because a treatment that has been clinically researched and proved effective may be available.
• Advise women to avoid using couch grass during pregnancy or when breast-feeding.

Points of interest
• Couch grass extracts have been used as flavoring agents for foods and beverages and the plant's roots have been roasted and ground into flour during times of famine. Animals have likewise benefitted from use of couch grass. Dogs will seek out and chew couch grass leaves to induce emesis when they are ill (hence the nickname dog grass). The grass has long been used as a food for grazing animals.

Commentary
Couch grass is listed as generally regarded as safe in the United States when consumed in the amounts present in foodstuffs. A MEDLINE search of the medicinal use of couch grass yielded a single rat study with negative results (Grases et al., 1995). Although the herb is probably safe when taken in limited quantities, insufficient clinical testing has been performed to determine its safety and efficacy when used medicinally for any of its reported indications.

References
Grases, F., et al. "Effect of *Herniaria hirsuta* and *Agropyron repens* on Calcium Oxalate Urolithiasis Risk in Rats," *J Ethnopharmacol* 45:211-14, 1995.

Mueller, S.O., et al. "Occurrence of Emodin, Chrysophanol and Physcion in Vegetables, Herbs and Liquors. Genotoxicity and Anti-Genotoxicity of the Anthraquinones and of the Whole Plants," *Food Chem Toxicol* 37:481-91, 1999.

COWSLIP

AMERICAN COWSLIP, ARTETYKE, ARTHRITICA, BUCKLES, CREWEL, DRELIP, FAIRY CAPS, HERB PETERPAIGLE, KEYFLOWER, KEY OF HEAVEN, MAY BLOB, MAYFLOWER, OUR LADY'S KEYS, PAIGLE, PALSYWORT, PASSWORD, PEAGLES, PETTY MULLEINS, PLUMROCKS

Taxonomic class
Primulaceae

Common trade names
None known.

Common forms
Available as dried flowers and liquid extracts.

Source
Active components are derived from the flowers of *Primula veris,* which is native to the mountains of western North America.

Chemical components
Cowslip contains many compounds, including carbohydrates (galactose, glucose, xylose, and others); flavonoids (apigenin, luteolin, kaempferol, quercetin); phenols (primulaveroside and primveroside); primin; several flavones (dimethoxyflavones, monomethoxyflavones, penta

---
Bold italic type indicates that reaction may be life-threatening.

methoxyflavones, and trimethoxyflavones); a quinone; saponins; tannins; silicic acid; and a volatile oil.

Actions
Cowslip is claimed to have antispasmodic, diuretic, expectorant, and sedative properties. Saponins are not well absorbed orally but cause GI irritation.

Studies with animals have suggested that saponins in cowslip produce both hypotensive and hypertensive effects (Cebo et al., 1976). In vitro studies suggest that the saponins inhibit prostaglandin synthetase, imparting weak anti-inflammatory and analgesic effects (Cebo et al., 1976). Flavonoids may be responsible for anti-inflammatory and antispasmodic activity. Tannins typically exhibit astringent properties.

Reported uses
The claims that cowslip is effective as a sedative-hypnotic to treat insomnia, hysteria, and anxiety associated with restlessness and irritability are based on traditional folklore medicine and animal studies. Human clinical trials have been conducted only with combination products that contain cowslip.

Dosage
Traditional uses suggest the following doses:
Dried flowers: 1 to 2 g P.O. as an infusion t.i.d.
Liquid extract (1:1 solution in 25% alcohol): 1 to 2 ml P.O. t.i.d.

Adverse reactions
GI: diarrhea, nausea, severe GI irritation, vomiting.
Hematologic: hemolysis.
Hepatic: *hepatotoxicity* (possibly caused by tannin content).
Skin: contact dermatitis (primin is a potential contact allergen).

Interactions
Antihypertensives: May interfere with therapy. Avoid administration with cowslip.
Diuretics: May enhance effects. Avoid administration with cowslip.
Sedatives: May enhance effects of other sedatives. Avoid administration with cowslip.

Contraindications and precautions
Avoid using cowslip in pregnant or breast-feeding patients; effects are unknown.

Special considerations
• Monitor the patient for allergic reactions, adverse GI reactions, and hepatotoxicity.
♠ ALERT Severe GI irritation can occur. Raw cowslip leaves are thought to cause severe GI symptoms and may compromise heart function.
• Inform the patient that the safety of cowslip has not been established.

•Advise women to avoid using cowslip during pregnancy or when breast-feeding.

Commentary
Little information is available regarding cowslip's chemical and pharmacologic properties. Because safety data are lacking, large doses and prolonged use of cowslip are not recommended.

References
Cebo, B., et al. "Pharmacologic Properties of Saponin Fraction from Polish Crude Drugs," *Herb Pol* 22:154-62, 1976.

CRANBERRY
BOG CRANBERRY, ISOKARPALO (FINLAND), MARSH APPLE, MOUNTAIN CRANBERRY, PIKKUKARPALO (FINLAND), SMALL CRANBERRY

Taxonomic class
Ericaceae

Common trade names
Multi-ingredient preparations: Cranberry Power, Cranberry Whole Fruit, Cran Relief, Cran-Tastic

Common forms
Capsules: 475 mg, 500 mg
Juices: usually 10% to 20% pure
   Also available as powdered concentrates of varying strengths, tablets, and tea.

Source
Cranberries are trailing evergreen shrubs that grow in various climates, most notably in acidic bogs, from Tennessee to Alaska. The juice and powdered concentrate of *Vaccinium macrocarpon, Vaccinium oxycoccos,* and *Vaccinium erythrocarpum* are made from whole berries (fruit); the skins and seeds are then screened out.

Chemical components
Cranberry juice contains many compounds, some of which are considered active. Benzoic, citric, malic, and quinic acids are present. Benzoic and quinic acids break down and form hippuric acid found in urine. Carbohydrates, especially fructose and oligosaccharides, are considered active ingredients for antibacterial activity. Anthocyanin and proanthocyanidins are also found in cranberry. The berries are a minor source of ascorbic acid.

Actions
Studies in mice and humans have demonstrated cranberry's ability to irreversibly interfere with bacterial adherence to uroepithelial surfaces (P-fimbriae; Ahuja et al., 1998). In vitro studies using extracts of *Vaccinium*

Bold italic type indicates that reaction may be life-threatening.

fruits (blueberries and cranberries) have shown possible antitumorigenic activity and inhibition of LDL oxidation (Wilson et al., 1998).

Reported uses

Cranberry has been proposed as a nonantibiotic treatment to prevent urinary tract infections (UTIs) and has a 100-year history of being used to prevent recurrent UTIs. Mice given cranberry juice as a water supply demonstrated that bacterial adherence was significantly inhibited in urine (Sobota, 1984). Human clinical trials have also been promising. (See *Cranberry juice and urinary tract infection,* page 242.)

Although Europeans have proposed cranberry as an anticancer drug, well-designed trials are lacking. Cranberry has been proposed to help urostomy patients with skin irritations from urine and as a deodorant for incontinence. It has also been used in drug overdose cases to help with urinary excretion of phencyclidine.

Dosage

Most studies gave patients between 10 and 16 oz of juice P.O. daily or 1 or 2 capsules of concentrate P.O. daily.

Adverse reactions

GI: diarrhea (if excessive quantities are ingested).

Interactions

No significant drug interactions reported. Cranberry has the potential to enhance elimination of some drugs excreted in urine by changing the pH of the urine.

Contraindications and precautions

Use cranberry cautiously in patients with benign prostatic hyperplasia and urinary obstruction.

Special considerations

- Counsel the diabetic patient who is prone to UTIs to use sugar-free versions, thus minimizing carbohydrate load.
- Advise the patient to drink sufficient fluids to ensure adequate urine flow.
- Inform the patient of other beneficial strategies to prevent recurrent UTIs, such as practicing good hygiene, emptying the bladder often, and avoiding foods containing baking soda or baking powder.
- Urge the patient to notify his primary health care provider if signs of an unresolving UTI (fever, suprapubic pain, painful urination, urinary bleeding) develop, continue, or worsen.

Points of interest

- The ability of cranberry juice to prevent UTI was noted in 1840 by German scientists who found hippuric acid in the urine of people who consumed the fruit juice. For 100 years, the acidifying and bacteriostatic action of hippuric acid was thought to be caused by antibacterial action.

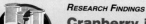

RESEARCH FINDINGS

Cranberry juice and urinary tract infection

Many urinary tract infections (UTIs) are caused by enteric flora, and about one-half are caused by *Escherichia coli*. The bacterium uses surface pili (fimbriae) to attach to carbohydrate structures on the uroepithelial cell lining of the urinary tract. The most common fimbriae types are a mannose-sensitive type I fimbriae and the P fimbriae.

Extracts of *Vaccinium* fruits have been found to inhibit *E. coli* adhesion (Ofek et al., 1996). Cranberry juice has two chemical components that can affect the ability of the bacteria to adhere to the cell lining. Fructose, found in many fruit juices, inhibits mannose-sensitive type I fimbriae. A large-molecular-weight compound similar to the Tumms-Harefall glycoprotein inhibits P fimbriae. Only blueberries and cranberries of the *Vaccinium* type contain both fructose and the large-molecular-weight compound.

Because about 25% of isolates have different adhesion characteristics, future studies that include S-type fimbriae will help to clarify cranberry's true role in the treatment of UTI.

One clinical trial involved 153 women (Avorn et al., 1994). Patients drank 300 ml of juice daily for 6 months. The placebo drink was similar in taste and color to the actual juice. Results showed the presence of bacteria in the urine in 28% of the placebo group compared with 15% in the cranberry group. Antibiotics were needed for 16 members of the placebo group but for only 8 of the cranberry group. Bacteriuria persisted in just 25% of the patients taking cranberry juice compared with almost 100% of the placebo group.

Another trial sought to determine the effect of cranberry prophylaxis on rates of bacteriuria and overt UTI in children with neurogenic bladder receiving intermittent catheterization (Schlager et al., 1999). This double-blind, crossover comparison of 15 children tested cranberry concentrate versus placebo for 6 months (3 months each). At trial end, the frequency of bacteriuria was essentially the same in each group. Also, three clinically evident UTIs were documented in each group. No significant difference was seen in acidification of the urine. Despite reasonable theoretical evidence suggesting potential beneficial effects of cranberry juice in preventing UTIs, clinical trial data have failed to confirm such an effect. A review of the available literature surrounding the treatment of UTIs failed to support cranberry for this therapy predominantly because few trial data met the investigators' inclusion criteria for the review (Jepson et al., 2000).

Bold italic type indicates that reaction may be life-threatening.

During the 1960s, it was found that the hippuric acid concentration was too low to be bacteriostatic and another explanation was pursued.

• Cranberry is one of the more frequently used alternative remedies by patients of a health maintenance organization in central Texas.

Commentary

For acute UTI, appropriate antibacterials remain the mainstay of treatment. Despite interesting anecdotal and reasonable theoretical evidence for cranberry, clinical trial evidence does not support its use for the prevention or treatment of UTIs. Additional clinical trial information is warranted before clinicians can rely on this "functional" fruit juice.

References

Ahuja, S., et al. "Loss of Fimbrial Adhesion with the Addition of *Vaccinum macrocarpon* to the Growth Medium of P-fimbriated *Escherichia col," J Urol* 159(2):559-62, 1998.

Avorn, J., et al. "Reduction of Bacteriuria and Pyuria After Ingestion of Cranberry Juice," *JAMA* 271:751-54, 1994.

Jepson, R.G., et al. "Cranberries for Treating Urinary Tract Infection," *Cochrane Database Syst Rev* (2):CD001322, 2000.

Ofek, I., et al. "Anti-*Escherichia coli* Adhesion Activity of Cranberry and Blueberry Juices," *Adv Exp Med Biol* 408:179-83, 1996.

Schlager, T.A., et al. "Effect of Cranberry Juice on Bacteriuria in Children with Neurogenic Bladder Receiving Intermittent Catheterization," *J Pediatr* 135(6):698-702, 1999.

Sobota, A.E. "Inhibition of Bacterial Adherence by Cranberry Juice: Potential Use for the Treatment of Urinary Tract Infections," *J Urol* 131:1013-16, 1984.

Wilson, T., et al. "Cranberry Extract Inhibits Low Density Lipoprotein Oxidation," *Life Sci* 62(24):PL381-86, 1998.

CREATINE MONOHYDRATE

CREATINE

Common trade names

Multi-ingredient preparations: Advanced Genetics, ATP Advantage, Bio-Tech, Champion's Choice, GNC Pro Performance Labs, ISP Nutrition, Joe Weider, Labrada, Metaform, MMUSA Xtra Advantage, Muscle Tribe, Nature's Best, Universal Nutrition, VitaLife Sport Products

Common forms

Available in effervescent powder, gum, liquid (serum, 2,500 mg [2.5 g] per dose), powder (1 tsp contains 5 g), and tablets (2.5 g, 5 g).

Source

Creatine is found in such dietary sources as red meat, milk, and fish. The human body also synthesizes endogenous creatine in the kidneys, liver, and pancreas.

Chemical components

Creatine is an amino acid that's synthesized from arginine and glycine. The highest levels of creatine are found in skeletal muscle, mostly in the form of creatine phosphate. High levels also occur in cardiac and smooth muscle, brain, kidneys, and spermatozoa; data suggest that creatine amounts in muscle vary.

Actions

Ingestion of creatine monohydrate increases cellular levels of creatine and creatine phosphate, which maintains high intracellular levels of adenosine triphosphate (ATP), the principal energy source for muscle contraction. As ATP stores become depleted, muscle fatigue ensues. Regeneration of ATP stores at a rate similar to that of ATP hydrolysis may delay onset of muscle fatigue. The phosphate from creatine phosphate is transferred to adenosine diphosphate, restoring ATP and releasing free creatine. Creatine phosphate also transfers ATP equivalents from within the mitochondria to the cytoplasm, where ATP is needed for cellular metabolism.

Studies of oral absorption of creatine show that it increases the plasma creatine pool. Low doses of creatine monohydrate produced only a moderate rise in plasma creatine levels, whereas higher doses resulted in a larger increase. Repeated dosing maintained plasma levels. Oral supplementation also significantly increased total creatine content of skeletal muscle, with the greatest changes in those subjects who had low initial total creatine content (Harris et al., 1992).

Reported uses

Creatine is used to enhance exercise performance. It's been shown to improve short-term or intermittent high-intensity exercise performance, such as weightlifting and short-distance running.

Creatine continues to be studied in relation to many other types of exercise, including isokinetic torque; isometric force; arm, cycle, and kayak ergometer performance; high-intensity prolonged exercise; and endurance tasks at lower intensity both inside and outside the laboratory (Graham and Hatton, 1999). Positive results with the use of creatine have been difficult to replicate consistently, sample sizes have generally been small, subjects range from highly trained athletes to sedentary individuals, and various doses and sources of creatine have been used in the clinical trials.

An interesting preliminary study of patients with muscular dystrophies suggests some value of creatine in improving daily activities (Walter et al., 2000).

Dosage

The amount of creatine ingested in a nonvegetarian diet is 2 g/day P.O. The recommended dose to achieve an ergogenic effect is a loading dose of 15 to 20 g/day P.O. taken for the first 5 days and then 5 to 10 g/day P.O. as a maintenance dose. Other dose recommendations are 5 to 30 g/day P.O. or 2 to 4 g P.O. as a long-term supplement. Most clinical tri-

---

Bold italic type indicates that reaction may be life-threatening.

als have used a dose of 20 to 25 g/day P.O. for 5 days and then measured exercise performance. Because creatine is a low-molecular-weight compound and readily excreted by the kidneys, ingestion of doses over 20 g/day P.O. is not valuable.

Adverse reactions
GI: abdominal pain, bloating, diarrhea.
GU: renal dysfunction.
Musculoskeletal: muscle spasms.
Other: dehydration, weight gain (perhaps caused by water rather than increased muscle mass).

Interactions
Caffeine: May reduce or abolish ergogenic effect of creatine. Avoid administration with creatine.
Glucose: May increase creatine storage in muscle. Increase in muscle creatine accumulation because of carbohydrate ingestion may result from a stimulatory effect of insulin on muscle creatine transport. Avoid administration with creatine.

Contraindications and precautions
Avoid using creatine in pregnant or breast-feeding patients; effects are unknown. Use cautiously in patients with renal disease.

Special considerations
● Monitor young athletes for overuse or abuse of creatine.
● Urinary excretion of creatine does not indicate declining renal function. It correlates with the increase in muscle creatine storage seen during creatine supplementation and reflects the increased rate of muscle creatine degradation to creatinine. Renal dysfunction associated with creatine use has been reported (Pritchard and Kaira, 1998; Koshy et al., 1999). In both cases, renal function normalized after creatine supplementation was discontinued.
● Urge the patient with renal disease to avoid creatine supplements.
● Athletes participating in a resistance-training program may benefit from creatine supplementation because it allows them to complete workouts at a higher level of intensity and strength.
● Creatine is not on the International Olympic Committee's drug list, but some consider it in a gray zone between doping and substances allowed to enhance performance.
● Advise the patient to avoid long-term (more than 30 days) use of creatine until effects are known.
● Instruct the patient to discontinue supplementation or to take smaller daily doses if muscle spasms occur. Increased intracellular water content can lead to muscle spasms and tightened muscles. Athletes should avoid combinations of diuretics along with creatine supplements in an effort to control the water weight.
● Inform the patient that creatine is useful only for exercise that is intense and of short duration or when short bursts of strength are need-

ed, as in weightlifting and sprinting.
- Advise the parents of athletes who may take this agent about its action, potential adverse effects, and proper use.
- The FDA recommends that a health care provider be consulted before creatine is used.

Points of interest

- Low-dose supplementation for 30 days results in increased total muscle creatine stores at a much lower rate than aggressive and higher loading doses. Most creatine uptake appears to occur during the first few days. The kidneys readily excrete creatine not retained by tissues. Because the storage of and response to creatine are varied, 20% to 30% of patients may not respond to creatine supplementation.
- A single 5-g dose of oral creatine monohydrate is equivalent to the creatine content of about 2.4 lb (1 kg) of uncooked steak.
- Responses to a national poll of professional athletes indicated that the use of creatine is greatest with football players, with baseball players being the second largest group of professional athletes who consume creatine.

Commentary

Although studies have shown that creatine supplementation improves high-intensity intermittent exercise performance, its use in enhancing aerobic exercise or endurance exercise performance is unclear and probably insignificant. Improvement in strength is probably related to an increase in the rate of phosphocreatine resynthesis from creatine stores during recovery between short-duration, high-intensity exercise. Physical strength improvements, although statistically significant, are generally minor and beneficial only to the highly trained athlete who is engaged in specific intermittent activities. Most other forms of exercise, such as low-intensity longer-duration workouts, have revealed negative results (Williams and Branch, 1998).

Because the normal creatine content of muscle varies, response to creatine supplementation also varies. It appears that patients who start with low creatine levels benefit more from supplementation than those with higher baseline creatine levels. The long-term safety of creatine is unknown. If creatine was held to FDA drug-testing standards, it would be in phase 2 of clinical trials and not yet generally available to the public (Fillmore et al., 1999). Until further trials are conducted, use of creatine cannot be recommended.

References

Earnest, C.P., et al. "The Effect of Oral Creatine Monohydrate Ingestion on Anaerobic Power Indices, Muscular Strength, and Body Composition," *Acta Physiol Scand* 153:207-9, 1995.

Fillmore, C.M., et al. "Nutrition and Dietary Supplements," *Phys Med Rehabil Clin North Am* 10(3):673-703, 1999.

Graham, A.S., and Hatton, R.C. "Creatine: A Review of Efficacy and Safety," *J Am Pharm Assoc* 39:803-10, 1999.

Bold italic type indicates that reaction may be life-threatening.

Greenhaff, P.L., et al. "Influence of Oral Creatine Supplementation of Muscle Torque During Repeated Bouts of Maximal Voluntary Exercise in Man," *Clin Sci* 84:565-71, 1993.

Harris, R.C., et al. "Elevation of Creatine in Resting and Exercised Muscle of Normal Subjects by Creatine Supplementation," *Clin Sci* 83:367-74, 1992.

Koshy, K.M., et al. "Interstitial Nephritis in a Patient Taking Creatine," *N Engl J Med* 19:814-15, 1999.

Kreider, R.B., et al. "Effects of Creatine Supplementation on Body Composition, Strength, and Sprint Performance," *Med Sci Sports Exer* 30:73-82, 1998.

Pritchard, N.R., and Kaira, P.A. "Renal Dysfunction Accompanying Oral Creatine Supplements," *Lancet* 351:1252-53, 1998.

Vandenberghe, K., et al. "Long-term Creatine Intake Is Beneficial to Muscle Performance During Resistance Training," *J Appl Physiol* 83:2055-63, 1997.

Walter, M.C., et al. "Creatine Monohydrate in Muscular Dystrophies: A Double-blind, Placebo-controlled Clinical Study," *Neurology* 54(9):1848-50, 2000.

Williams, M.H., and Branch, J.D. "Creatine Supplementation and Exercise Performance: An Update," *J Am Coll Nutr* 17(3):216-34, 1998.

CUCUMBER

WILD COWCUMBER

Taxonomic class
Cucurbitaceae

Common trade names
None known.

Common forms
Available as seeds and juice and used as an ingredient in many cosmetics and soaps.

Source
Several active components are derived from the seeds and fruits of *Cucumis sativus,* a low-growing annual vegetable that is native to northern India.

Chemical components
The cucumber plant is composed mainly of water. The seeds and leaves contain compounds that inhibit trypsin and chymotrypsin. Seeds contain cucurbitin (a glycoside), a fatty oil, proteins, and resin.

Actions
The raw juice is reported to have mild diuretic activity, and the seeds possess mild diuretic properties in animals. The soothing topical effects of the plant can probably be attributed to its water content.

Reported uses
Some sources claim that cucumber is nature's best diuretic. This claim is not based on human clinical trials but on anecdotal evidence (Liener, 1980). Cucumber is high in potassium and has been used to correct both high and low blood pressure but without clinical verification.

Cucumber has been used in topical products to soothe irritated skin and is included in face-cleansing cosmetics. The seeds are reported to have cooling and anthelmintic properties.

Dosage
Traditional uses suggest the following doses:
As a cosmetic, the juice is extracted and applied topically.
As a diuretic, 1 to 2 oz of ground seed is steeped in water and then consumed.

Adverse reactions
None reported, but fluid and electrolyte losses are possible.

Interactions
Diuretics: May enhance effects of fluid and electrolyte loss of these drugs. Avoid administration with cucumber.

Contraindications and precautions
Avoid using cucumber except as food in pregnant or breast-feeding patients; effects are unknown.

Special considerations
• Monitor serum electrolyte levels periodically if large quantities of cucumber are consumed.
• Inform the patient about the lack of clinical data on this plant.
• Advise the patient that proven and safe diuretics are available.
• Advise women to avoid using cucumber, except as a food, during pregnancy or when breast-feeding.

Points of interest
• Cucumbers have a long and distinguished history. They originated in northern India, where they were domesticated more than 3,000 years ago. History records a few noteworthy cucumber fanatics, including the Roman emperor Tiberius, who ate some daily; his gardeners were ordered to find ways to grow them out of season. Even Columbus included them in his experimental gardens on Hispaniola (Haiti) during his second voyage, in 1494.

Commentary
Few clinical data substantiate medicinal or therapeutic claims for cucumber. Standardized, safe, and effective diuretics eliminate the need to use cucumber for this purpose.

References
Liener, I.E. *Toxic Components of Plant Foodstuffs.* London: Academic Press, 1980.

Bold italic type indicates that reaction may be life-threatening.

CUMIN
CUMIMUM CYMINUM, CUMINO AIGRO (HOT CUMIN)

Taxonomic class
Apiaceae

Common trade names
None known.

Common Forms
Available as an oil, a powder, and an ingredient in
curry powder.

Source
Cumin is a small annual, herbaceous plant that
is indigenous to northern Egypt. Today it is cultivated mostly in countries along the Mediterranean. Active
components are extracted from ripe fruit and ripe, dried fruit.

Chemical components
Cumin contains beta-pinenes, cuminaldehyde, p-cymene, gamma-
terpenes, 1-3-p-menthandial, petroselic acid, and palmitic acid.

Actions
Cumin is claimed to have antimicrobial, blood-clotting, estrogenic, and
mutagenic effects. In a powder suspension formulation, it may inhibit
mycelium growth and toxin production. Dried cumin extract may inhibit (in vitro) arachidonic acid–induced platelet aggregation. Acetone
extracts of cumin may increase protein and alkali phosphates in the en-
dometrium (Gruenwald et al., 1998). In rats, cumin was observed to
decrease the activity of beta-glucuronidase and mucinase, which may
have protective effects on the colon (Nalini et al., 1998).

Reported uses
Cumin has analgesic, carminative, and stimulant effects. It has been
used as an antispasmodic, an aphrodisiac, and a diuretic. It has also
been reported to treat GI problems, headaches, and rheumatic illnesses.
Cumin also may produce abortive effects. No human trials have examined these claims.

Dosage
Average single dose is 300 to 600 g (5 to 10 fruits) of drug (Gruenwald
et al., 1998).

Adverse reactions
GU: abortifacient effects (Gruenwald et al., 1998).

Interactions
None reported.

Contraindications and precautions

Avoid use of cumin in pregnant or breast-feeding patients because it may possess abortive effects; other effects are unknown.

Special considerations

• Caution the patient not to self-treat symptoms of stomach problems, headaches, or arthritis before seeking appropriate medical evaluation because this may delay diagnosis of a serious medical condition.
• Advise the patient to consult a health care provider before using herbal preparations because a treatment that has been clinically researched and proved effective may be available.
• Although no known chemical interactions have been reported in clinical studies, consideration must be given to the pharmacologic properties of the herbal product and the potential for exacerbation of the intended therapeutic effect of conventional drugs.
◤ ALERT   Caution the patient who is pregnant or breast-feeding to avoid cumin because it may produce abortive effects.

Points of interest

• Cumin was used medicinally in Europe during the Middle Ages but has now been replaced by caraway seed, which has a more agreeable flavor. It has been used in veterinary medicine and as an ingredient in curry powder.

Commentary

Because no clinical data support cumin's several therapeutic claims, it cannot be recommended for any use.

References

Gruenwald, J., et al., eds. *PDR for Herbal Medicines*. Montvale, N.J.: Medical Economics Company, Inc., 1998.
Nalini, N., et al. "Influence of Spices on the Bacterial (Enzyme) Activity in Experimental Colon Cancer," *J Ethnopharmacol* 62:15-24, 1998.

CYCLADOL

ACHOCCHA, CAIGUA, CAIHUA, KORILA, WILD CUCUMBER

Taxonomic class

Cucurbitaceae

Common trade names

Caigua, Cycladol, Cycladin

Common forms

Available as capsules (300 mg) and powder.

Source

Cyclanthera pedata, or caigua, as it is commonly referred to in its native land of Peru and other parts of South America, is an annual plant. The immature fruit and shoots have been cultivated for centuries.

Chemical components
The primary active ingredients of *C. pedata* are largely undescribed.

Actions
The fruit of *C. pedata* is claimed to possess hypoglycemic, hypotensive, and lipid-lowering effects.

Reported uses
Cycladol is claimed to be valuable for treating hyperlipidemia and as a weight loss agent. Dehydrated caigua has been studied for its ability to affect the lipid profile in one small study of premenopausal and post-menopausal women (Gustavo et al., 1995). Eighteen premenopausal and 24 postmenopausal Peruvian women participated in a 12-week study intended to characterize the differences in lipid profiles that exist beween premenopausal and postmenopausal women and to examine the potential effects of escalating doses of Cycladin (dehydrated caigua) on lipid parameters. Treatment with 600-mg (6 x 100 mg) capsules daily reduced serum cholesterol level (22%), reduced serum LDL level (33%), and increased serum HDL level (more than 33%) compared with baseline. Data from the trial suggest that doses less than 600 mg of Cycladin daily had no effect on lipid parameters. Triglycerides weren't reduced by any dose of caigua. Despite rather dramatic results, any conclusions drawn from this trial must be considered preliminary because of the small number of subjects, short duration of the trial, differences in baseline demographics between groups, and other questionable aspects of its study design.

Dosage
Dosing is not agreed on. Some manufacturers of caigua suggest doses of 6 capsules daily P.O. as a single dose (6 capsules $\times$ 300 mg = 1,800 mg/day) in the morning before breakfast. Note that the clinical trial (Gustavo et al., 1995) used 6 capsules daily of 100 mg (600 mg/day) dehydrated caigua capsules.

Adverse reactions
None reported.

Interactions
Antidiabetic drugs and insulin: May increase hypoglycemic effects when used concurrently. Monitor blood glucose level intensively.
Antihypertensives: May increase hypotensive effects. Monitor blood pressure closely during concomitant use.

Contraindications and precautions
Cycladol is contraindicated in pregnant or breast-feeding patients; effects are unknown.

Special considerations
● Some dosing recommendations suggested by manufacturers do not match those from the solitary clinical trial.

- Inform the patient that no data exist to support caigua's beneficial effects on long-term outcomes (such as survival, myocardial infarction, stroke).
- Advise the patient to consult a health care provider before using herbal preparations because a treatment that has been clinically researched and proved effective may be available.
- Monitor blood pressure and blood glucose level in patients with hypertension or diabetes mellitus.

Points of interest

- The plant family to which *C. pedata* belongs consists of about 100 genera and several hundred species. Considerable genetic diversity exists within the family that has allowed numerous species to adapt to climates as varied as tropical and subtropical regions, arid deserts, and temperate locations and to extreme elevations, such as the Peruvian Andes.

Commentary

The dramatic changes in cholesterol levels (22% to 33%) cited by the Gustavo trial approximate or exceed reductions demonstrated with some of the most effective lipid-lowering drugs, especially when one considers the sensational elevations in HDL levels (greater than 33%). If these effects are consistently proven to be valid, then caigua or components of *C. pedata* may evolve into a welcome addition to the cholesterol-lowering armamentarium. These results are preliminary. Large-scale randomized, controlled trials that examine patient outcomes would be welcome evidence to caigua's benefit. Until then, patients should be counseled to remain on allopathic medicines that have proven long-term benefits in terms of reductions in mortality and CV or cerebrovascular events.

References

Gustavo, F., et al. "Serum Lipid and Lipoprotein Levels in Post-menopausal Women: Short-course Effect of Caigua," *Menopause* 2(4):225-34, 1995.

DAFFODIL

DAFFYDOWN-DILLY, FLEUR DE COUCOU, LENT LILY,
NARCISSUS, PORILLON

Taxonomic class
Amaryllidaceae

Common trade names
None known.

Common forms
None known.

Source
Active components are derived from powders or extracts of the flowers of *Narcissus pseudonarcissus* of the narcissus family, common in Europe and the United States.

Chemical components
A crystalline alkaloid, narcisssine, has been isolated from daffodil bulbs and is identical to lycorine, isolated from *Lycoris radiata*. Other alkaloids (masonin and homolycorin) and a lectin known as *N. pseudonarcissus* agglutinin (NPA) have also been found in the bulbs. Crystals of calcium oxalate have been noted in plant sap.

Actions
Daffodil preparations have astringent properties. Narcissine (lycorine) acts as an emetic. In one study, extracts containing masonin and homolycorin were found to induce delayed hypersensitivity in guinea pigs. NPA binds to alpha$_2$-macroglobulin and to glycoprotein 120 of the HIV in vitro. NPA is inhibitory to HIV-1, HIV-2, and cytomegalovirus (CMV) infections in vitro. NPA also inhibits rabies virus attachment to susceptible cells and rubella virus multiplication in vitro (Balzarini et al., 1991).

Reported uses
Historically, preparations made from boiled daffodil bulbs were used as an emetic. Plasters made from the bulbs were used locally for burns, joint pain, strains, and wounds. The powdered flowers have been used as an emetic. Infusions or syrups have been used in pulmonary congestion.

NPA is used in biochemical research for its ability to bind with glycoconjugates that occur on such viruses as HIV-1 and HIV-2, simian immunodeficiency virus, CMV, rabies, and rubella. It has also been used to develop novel enzyme-linked immunoassays for quantitation of envelope glycoprotein 120 on HIV (Balzarini et al., 1991).

Dosage
Some sources suggest 1,300 mg of powdered flowers or 130 to 195 mg of extract P.O. as an emetic.

Adverse reactions
CV: *CV collapse.*
EENT: hypersalivation, miosis.
GI: nausea, vomiting.
Respiratory: *respiratory collapse.*
Skin: contact dermatitis (Gude et al., 1988).

Interactions
None reported.

Contraindications and precautions
Daffodil flowers and bulbs are poisonous. Ingestion of even small quantities can lead to rapid death. Avoid using daffodil in pregnant or breast-feeding patients; effects are unknown.

Special considerations
◆**ALERT** Narcissine (lycorine) causes eventual collapse and death by paralysis of the CNS. Accidental poisoning by daffodil bulbs has been reported in Switzerland, Germany, Finland, Sweden, the Netherlands, Britain, and the United States.
• Caution the patient against consuming any part of this plant.
• Caution the patient to keep plant parts out of the reach of children and pets.
• Advise the female patient to avoid using daffodil during pregnancy or when breast-feeding.

Points of interest
• Daffodil bulbs have been mistaken for onions in cases of accidental poisonings.

Commentary
In vitro studies showing the inhibitory effects of a daffodil-derived lectin on HIV and CMV infections indicate potential in biochemical research and in the development of new immunoassays for these viruses; however, there is insufficient evidence for future therapeutic use. Therapeutic claims are anecdotal and not based on controlled human trials. Daffodil plants are toxic, and caution should be used when handling them. This plant is not recommended for internal use.

References
Balzarini, J., et al. "Alpha-(1,3)- and Alpha-(1-6)-mannose Specific Plant Lectins Are Markedly Inhibitory to Human Immunodeficiency Virus and Cytomegalovirus Infections In Vitro," *Antimicrob Agents Chemother* 35:410-16, 1991.

Bold italic type indicates that reaction may be life-threatening.

Gude, M., et al. "An Investigation of the Irritant and Allergenic Properties of Daffodils (*Narcissus pseudonarcissus* L., Amaryllidaceae). A Review of Daffodil Dermatitis," *Contact Dermatitis* 19:1-10, 1988.

DAISY

BAIRNWORT, BRUISEWORT, COMMON DAISY, DAY'S EYE

Taxonomic class
Asteraceae

Common trade names
None known.

Common forms
None known.

Source
Several chemical compounds are derived from the fresh or dried flowers and leaves of *Bellis perennis*, a common perennial herb.

Chemical components
The flower heads contain saponins, tannin, organic acids, an essential oil, bitter principle, flavones, and mucilage.

Actions
Daisy is claimed to have anti-inflammatory and astringent properties.

Reported uses
The Iroquois Indians used the daisy as a GI aid. It has also been used as a mild analgesic, an antidiarrheal, an antispasmodic, an antitussive, an astringent, and an expectorant. When used as an infusion, daisy was reported to treat arthritis, catarrh, diarrhea, hepatic and renal disorders, and rheumatism and to act as a blood purifier. Few data are available to support these claims.

The plant also has reportedly been used externally in compresses and bath preparations for treating skin disorders, wounds, and bruises (Launert, 1981).

Dosage
Traditional uses suggest the following doses:
Infusion: 1 tsp of dried herb steeped in boiling water for 10 minutes and taken t.i.d.
Tincture: 2 to 4 ml P.O. t.i.d.

Adverse reactions
None reported.

Interactions
None reported.

Contraindications and precautions
Avoid using daisy in pregnant or breast-feeding patients; effects are unknown.

Special considerations
• Although daisy has been used as food in some parts of the world, pharmacologic effects are largely undocumented. Use with caution.
• Monitor the patient taking this herb for adverse effects.
• Although no known chemical interactions have been reported in clinical studies, consideration must be given to the pharmacologic properties of the herbal product and the potential for exacerbation of the intended therapeutic effect of conventional drugs.
• Advise the female patient to avoid using daisy during pregnancy or when breast-feeding.

Commentary
Although the daisy has a long history of anecdotal safety, no clinical data exist to substantiate the claims for medicinal purposes. Moreover, its chemical components have not been well described. Subsequently, medicinal use of daisy cannot be recommended.

References
Launert, E. *The Hamlyn Guide to Edible and Medicinal Plants of Britain and Northern Europe.* London: Hamlyn Publishing Group Ltd., 1981.

DAMIANA

DAMIANA HERB, DAMIANA LEAF, HERBA DE LA PASTORA, MEXICAN DAMIANA, MIZIBOC, OLD WOMAN'S BROOM, ROSEMARY

Taxonomic class
Turneraceae

Common trade names
Damiana liqueur, Damiana Root, Damiania

Common forms
Available as a capsule, extract, powder, tea, tincture, or tonic.

Source
Damiana comes from the leaves of the Mexican shrub *Turnera diffusa*. It is also found in the southwestern United States, the Caribbean, South Africa, and South America. The plant is aromatic and has a pleasant taste.

Chemical components
Studies indicate that damiana contains a volatile oil that has an odor similar to that of chamomile that primarily consists of 1,8-cineol and pinenes. Other compounds include thymol, sesquiterpenes, gonzali-

---

Bold italic type indicates that reaction may be life-threatening.

tosin (a cyanogenic glycoside), a bitter element, resin, tannins, gum, mucilage, starch, and, possibly, caffeine.

Actions
The pharmacologic activity of the plant is unknown. No active components have been identified as the basis for damiana's alleged aphrodisiac and hallucinogenic effects.

Reported uses
Damiana has traditionally been used as an aphrodisiac. It was available in the United States in the 1870s as a tincture and used as an aphrodisiac to "improve the sexual ability of the enfeebled and aged." It may increase pelvic secretions. Some information suggests that drinking damiana as a tea or smoking the leaves can produce a euphoric and relaxed state, similar to the effects of marijuana (Lowry, 1984). It has been used to treat bedwetting, atonic constipation, nervous dyspepsia, and headaches and to boost and maintain mental and physical capacities. Damiana has also reportedly been used as an antidepressant, a diuretic, a mild purgative, and a tonic.

Dosage
Some sources suggest the following doses:
Dried leaf: 2 to 4 g P.O. t.i.d.
Powdered herb: 18 g in a 500-ml decoction P.O. (taken as a tea) t.i.d.
Tincture: up to 2.5 ml P.O. t.i.d.

Adverse reactions
CNS: hallucinations.
GU: irritation of urethral mucosa (may contribute to illusion of aphrodisiac effects).
Hepatic: hepatic dysfunction (large amounts, caused by tannin content).

Interactions
Antidiabetics: May interfere with effects of these drugs. Monitor blood glucose levels closely.

Contraindications and precautions
Damiana is contraindicated in pregnant or breast-feeding patients; effects are unknown.

Special considerations
• Monitor the patient for hepatotoxicity if large amounts of damiana are ingested.
• Observe the patient taking damiana who experiences hallucinations; rule out other drugs that may cause similar effects.
🔺 **ALERT** Tetanus-like seizures resulting in symptoms similar to those of rabies or strychnine poisoning have occurred with damiana overdoses (200 g).

• Inquire about the reason for consumption of damiana; suggest available alternatives and assist the patient in consulting a health care provider.

• Advise the female patient to avoid using damiana during pregnancy or when breast-feeding.

• Advise the patient to avoid hazardous activities until damiana's CNS effects are known.

Commentary
Although damiana is claimed to have aphrodisiac and hallucinogenic effects, evidence to support these claims is lacking. A detailed review of damiana's history indicates that claims of its use stem from a hoax.

References
Gruenwald, J., et al. *PDR for Herbal Medicines.* Montvale, N.J.: Medical Economics Company, Inc., 1998.

Jellin, J.M., et al. *Natural Medicines Comprehensive Database.* Stockton, Calif.: Therapeutic Research Faculty, 1999.

Lowry, T.P. "Damiana," *J Psychoactive Drugs* 16:267-68, 1984.

DANDELION
LION'S TOOTH, PRIEST'S-CROWN

Taxonomic class
Asteraceae

Common trade names
Dandelion

Common forms
Available as capsules, extracts, root, and teas.

Source
Active components are obtained from the leaves and roots of *Taraxacum officinale* or *T. laevigatum,* common low-growing weeds that are native to Europe and Asia and naturalized worldwide.

Chemical components
Dandelions contain many compounds, including caffeic, parahydroxyphenylacetic, chlorogenic, linoleic, linolenic, oleic, and palmitic acids; minerals such as potassium, iron, silicon, magnesium, sodium, zinc, manganese, copper, and phosphorus; resins, taraxasterol, taraxacin, taraxacum, taraxerin, taraxerol, and terpenoids; and vitamins A, B, C, and D. Other compounds include carotenoids (taraxanthin), choline, inulin, pectin, phytosterols, sugars, and triterpenes.

Actions
Taraxacum, a dandelion compound, increases gastric and salivary juice secretions, stimulates the release of bile from the gallbladder and liver, and acts as a mild laxative. Also, a leaf extract was found to exert a

---
Bold italic type indicates that reaction may be life-threatening.

stronger diuretic effect in rats and mice than did a root extract (Racz-Kotilla et al., 1974). An anti-inflammatory effect has also been shown for dandelion root extract in an animal model (Mascolo et al., 1987).

Dandelion is considered a liver and kidney tonic because of its choleretic effects and ability to directly stimulate contraction of the gallbladder, thus releasing stored bile.

Extracts of dandelion markedly inhibited the growth of cancer cells, perhaps by its resemblance to tumor polysaccharides such as lentinan. Also in the United States, antibodies to active polypeptides in tumor-induced mouse ascites fluid were produced from dandelion.

Reported uses

Dandelion is claimed to possess antirheumatic, bile-stimulating, diuretic, and laxative properties. Herbalists recommend its use for hepatic and gallbladder disorders, cholecystitis, digestive complaints, and constipation and when diuresis may be indicated (premenstrual syndrome, weight loss, heart failure, and hypertension). Results obtained from human and animal studies showed improvement in jaundice, hepatic congestion, gallstones, hepatitis, and bile duct inflammation.

Dandelion's milky sap has been used externally for removing corns, calluses, and warts. The plant is one of nine herbal ingredients of a British proprietary preparation that has been used to treat viral hepatitis.

In a small group of patients, dandelion root was used successfully to treat chronic, nonspecific colitis, bringing relief from abdominal pain, constipation, and diarrhea.

Dosage

Some sources suggest the following doses:
Dried leaf: 4 to 10 g P.O. by infusion t.i.d.
Dried root: 2 to 8 g P.O. by infusion or decoction t.i.d.
Fluidextract (1:1 in 25% alcohol): 4 to 8 ml P.O. (1 to 2 tsp) t.i.d.
Juice of root: 4 to 8 ml P.O. t.i.d.
Tincture of root (1:5 in 45% alcohol): 5 to 10 ml P.O. t.i.d.

Adverse reactions

GI: blockage of GI or biliary tract, gallbladder inflammation, gallstones.
Skin: contact dermatitis (in allergic patients), photosensitivity.

Interactions

Antidiabetic drugs: May enhance effects, promoting hypoglycemia. Avoid administration with dandelion.
Antihypertensives: May have additive or synergistic hypotensive effect. Avoid administration with dandelion.
Diuretics: May potentiate fluid and electrolyte losses. Avoid administration with dandelion.
Quinolone antibiotics: Because of high mineral content, absorption of quinolones is decreased (Zhu et al., 1999). Administer interacting drug doses 2 or more hours apart.

Contraindications and precautions
Avoid using dandelion in pregnant or breast-feeding patients; effects are unknown.

Special considerations
• Monitor intake and output and serum electrolyte levels in patients taking dandelion and diuretics together.
• Monitor blood glucose level in diabetic patient taking dandelion. Adjust therapy as needed.
• Instruct the patient taking dandelion with an antihypertensive to watch for symptoms of an exaggerated hypotensive effect (orthostatic hypotension, dizziness, syncope); advise him to rise slowly from a sitting or lying position if orthostatic hypotension develops.
• Advise the diabetic patient to monitor blood glucose levels more carefully because hypoglycemia can occur.
• Advise the female patient to avoid using dandelion during pregnancy or when breast-feeding.
• Advise the patient to use sunscreen when outdoors.

Points of interest
• Sometimes dandelion root is roasted and used as a coffee substitute. The flowers are used to make wine and schnapps. The plant is also commonly used as a food, mainly in soups and salads.
• Dandelion contains more vitamin A than carrots.

Commentary
Dandelion is a well-known herbal remedy and a natural food item. Scientific data are lacking to justify its reported therapeutic uses. The plant has been used in foods for several years without adverse effects. It cannot be recommended in amounts larger than what is normally present in foods or drinks.

References
Mark, K.A., et al. "Allergic Contact and Photoallergic Contact Dermatitis to Plant and Pesticide Allergens," *Arch Dermatol* 135(1):67-70, 1999.
Mascolo, N., et al. "Biological Screening of Italian Medicinal Plants for Anti-inflammatory Activity," *Phytotherapy Res* 1:28-29, 1987.
Racz-Kotilla, E., et al. "The Action of *Taraxacum officinale* Extracts on the Body Weight and Diuresis of Laboratory Animals," *Planta Med* 26(3):212-17, 1974.
Zhu, M., et al. "Effects of *Taraxacum mongolicum* on the Bioavailability and Deposition of Ciprofloxacin in Rats," *J Pharm Sci*, 88(6):632-34, 1999.

DEVIL'S CLAW

GRAPPLE PLANT, WOOD SPIDER

Taxonomic class
Pedaliaceae

Common trade names
Multi-ingredient preparations: Devil's Claw, Devil's Claw Capsule, Devil's Claw Secondary Root, Devil's Claw Vegicaps

Common forms
Capsules: 200 mg, 420 mg, 499 mg, 510 mg, 750 mg
   Also available as extracts, teas, and tinctures.

Source
The drug is extracted from the roots and secondary tubers of *Harpagophytum procumbens*, a member of the pedalia family.

Chemical components
The major active ingredient in devil's claw is harpagoside. Other compounds include harpagide, procumbide, stigmasterol, beta sitosterol, fatty acids, aromatic acids, triterpenes, sugars, gum resins, and flavonoids.

Actions
Harpagoside possesses anti-inflammatory properties. Unlike conventional NSAIDs that alter arachidonic acid metabolism, devil's claw's anti-inflammatory effects are not produced by this mechanism. Harpagoside was found to produce negative chronotropic and positive inotropic effects by altering the mechanisms that regulate calcium influx in smooth muscles. Reduced blood pressure and heart rate as well as antiarrhythmic activity have been reported in animals. In contrast, harpagide possesses negative chronotropic and inotropic properties. A study using rats evaluated the efficacy of the plant in reducing edema of the hind foot and found no effect on the edema and insignificant alteration of prostaglandin synthetase activity.

Reported uses
Devil's claw has been used as an antarthritic, antirheumatic, and appetite stimulant. Despite one finding of an anti-inflammatory effect, studies have failed to replicate this finding (Whitehouse et al., 1983).
   Other therapeutic claims, which lack scientific support, include treatment of allergies, arteriosclerosis, boils, climacteric problems, dysmenorrhea, GI disturbances, headaches, heartburn, renal and hepatic disorders, lumbago, malaria, neuralgia, nicotine poisoning, and skin cancer.

Dosage
For decreased eicosanoid production: 2,000 mg P.O. daily (Moussard et al., 1992).
For appetite stimulation: 1.5 g (root)/day.

Adverse reactions
CNS: headache.
EENT: loss of taste, tinnitus.
Other: weight loss.

Interactions

Antiarrhythmics: Devil's claw has chronotropic and inotropic effects. Use cautiously in patients taking both agents.

Antidiabetic drugs: Increased hypoglycemic effect. Monitor blood glucose level.

Antihypertensives: Increased hypotensive effects. Monitor blood pressure.

Warfarin: Potentiated hypoprothrombinemic effects of warfarin. Monitor patient more intensively for signs of bleeding and excessive INR elevations.

Contraindications and precautions

Devil's claw is contraindicated in patients with gastric or duodenal ulcers. It is also contraindicated in pregnant patients because it may stimulate uterine contractions; alleged abortive properties of devil's claw remain controversial. Use cautiously in patients with diabetes or cardiac disorders.

Special considerations

• Monitor heart rate and rhythm of patients taking antiarrhythmics concurrently with devil's claw.

• Advise the patient taking the drug for anti-inflammatory effect that many OTC and prescription anti-inflammatories exist that have known risks and benefits.

• Urge the female patient taking devil's claw to report if pregnancy is planned or suspected.

• Advise the female patient to avoid using devil's claw during pregnancy or when breast-feeding.

Points of interest

• The common name devil's claw comes from the plant's unique fruits, which are covered with hooks to facilitate their spread by animals.

Commentary

Evidence for devil's claw's anti-inflammatory effect is scanty. Larger and well-designed human clinical studies are needed to evaluate its efficacy and safety for treating arthritis. No clinical data support its use for the other disorders described. Other anti-inflammatory products (such as NSAIDs) are readily available.

References

Moussard, C., et al. "A Drug in Traditional Medicine, Harpagophytum procumbens: No Evidence for NSAID-Like Effect on Whole Blood Eicosanoid Production in Humans," *Prostaglandins Leuko Essent Fatty Acids* 46:283-86, 1992.

Whitehouse, L.W., et al. "Devil's Claw (Harpagophytum procumbens): No Evidence for Anti-inflammatory Activity in the Treatment of Arthritic Disease," *Can Med Assoc J* 129:249-51, 1983.

DHEA AND DHEA-S

DEHYDROEPIANDROSTERONE AND SULFATED
DEHYDROEPIANDROSTERONE

Taxonomic class
Dioscoreaceae

Common trade names
Multi-ingredient preparations: Born Again's DHEA Eyelift Serum,
DHEA Men's Formula, DHEA with Antioxidants 25 mg, DHEA with
Bioperine 50 mg

Common forms
Capsules: 5 mg, 25 mg, 50 mg
Cream: 4 oz (with other vitamins and herbs)
Tablets (timed-release): 15 mg

Source
Steroid precursors found in members of the yam family have been used
to produce dehydroepiandrosterone (DHEA). Most commercially available DHEA is produced in Europe and China.

Aside from its occurrence in certain plants, the neurosteroid hormone DHEA (5-androsten-3beta-ol-17-one) and DHEA-S are secreted
exclusively by the zona reticularis of the adrenal gland (in response to
adrenocorticotropin) in women; small quantities are also secreted from
the testes. DHEA-S, the most abundant circulating steroid hormone of
the two, is the hydrosteroid sulfatase metabolite of DHEA.

DHEA concentrations are highest in the brain, with lesser concentrations in the plasma, spleen, kidneys, and liver (in descending order).

Chemical components
DHEA (5-androsten-3beta-ol-17-one) and DHEA-S have structural origins that result from a cholesterol nucleus. Pregnenolone is the immediate precursor to DHEA, which is converted from pregnenolone by 17,20-desmolase. DHEA serves as a substrate in which to synthesize half the
endogenous androgens in men and most of the estrogens in women.
DHEA has a shorter half-life (1 to 3 hours versus 10 to 20 hours, respectively) and is less highly bound to albumin than DHEA-S.

Actions
A comprehensive review by Kroboth and colleagues (1999a) provides
more detail on the complex effects, clinical trials (up to 1999), and metabolic pathway of DHEA and DHEA-S.

In humans, serum levels of DHEA peak at age 20 and again at age 40
and then decline dramatically to about 20% to 30% of maximum by
age 70 to 80. Documentation of this age-related decline in DHEA levels
has led to suggestions that exogenous DHEA supplementation could result in a "fountain of youth" effect. Some preliminary evidence suggests
that DHEA-S may be a marker for Alzheimer's disease (Hillen et al.,

2000) and erectile dysfunction (Reiter et al., 2000). Several physiologic effects have been ascribed to DHEA, including its conversion into androgens and estrogens and its ability to raise serum levels of insulin-like growth factor 1, a mediator of human growth hormone. The degree of androgenic versus estrogenic effect of DHEA appears to depend on the patient's hormonal milieu. DHEA has been shown to reduce luteinizing hormone through direct pituitary inhibition (Labrie et al., 1997). In men, DHEA has also been reported to increase levels of several immune cell types (Khorram et al., 1997). Several aspects of disease have been shown to influence DHEA and DHEA-S serum levels, including age, gender, serious illness, burns, and acute exercise (Kroboth et al., 1999a).

Reported uses
Numerous claims for health benefits with regular DHEA use have been touted in the scientific and lay press. They include immune system enhancement; antidiabetogenic, antineoplastic, and antiatherosclerotic effects; osteoporosis prevention; treatment for certain autoimmune conditions; and a general antiaging effect. Seemingly positive benefits in animal studies have generally met with mixed results or less when similar studies have been conducted in humans.

At least two trials have suggested that DHEA supplementation promotes a greater sense of well-being (Morales et al., 1994; Cawood and Bancroft, 1996). Questions have been raised about study design in these trials. A Cochrane Database Review determined that evidence supporting this kind of effect is limited. The review also pointed out that essentially no evidence exists supporting DHEA supplementation as a nootropic (enhances cognitive function) agent (Huppert et al., 2000).

Two placebo-controlled trials argue against any potential anabolic effect from DHEA supplementation (Wallace et al., 1999; Brown et al., 1999).

Small trials have been conducted evaluating DHEA supplementation in light of its effects on sleep, diet and body composition, SLE, HIV infection (Kroboth et al., 1999a), menopausal symptoms (Barnhart et al., 1999), and anorexia nervosa (Gordon et al., 1999). All work in these areas is considered preliminary.

Dosage
Various doses have been used in human studies. Doses have ranged from 50 to 1,600 mg daily. It has been suggested but not agreed on that serum levels of DHEA-S should be checked periodically during exogenous replacement and the dose adjusted to youthlike levels (3,600 ng/ml for men and 3,000 ng/ml for women). DHEA has been administered by various routes, including I.V., subcutaneous, transdermal, and vaginal.

Adverse reactions
CNS: aggressiveness, fatigue, headache, insomnia, irritability.
EENT: nasal congestion.
GI: elevated liver function test results.

Bold italic type indicates that reaction may be life-threatening.

Hematologic: slightly decreased hemoglobin level and RBC count.
Skin: hirsutism.
Other: gynecomastia.

Interactions

This list presents information from reports of drugs and their potential effect on endogenous DHEA or DHEA-S serum levels; however, the absolute effect on these levels may or may not be similar when exogenous DHEA is ingested in combination with the interacting drug.

Alprazolam: May increase endogenous serum levels of DHEA. DHEA-S concentrations were not changed (Kroboth et al., 1999b). Evaluate the need for combination therapy.

Calcium channel blockers: Increases endogenous serum DHEA and DHEA-S levels in obese, hypertensive men (Kroboth et al., 1999a). Monitor the patient and adjust dose as needed.

Carbamazepine, dexamethasone: Decreases endogenous serum levels of DHEA-S (Kroboth et al., 1999a; Osran et al., 1993). Monitor the patient and adjust dose as needed.

Insulin (exogenous): Decreases serum levels of DHEA and DHEA-S in men (Nestler and Kahwash, 1994). Monitor the patient and adjust dose as needed.

Insulin-sensitizing drugs (metformin, other oral hypoglycemics): May increase serum DHEA and DHEA-S levels (Kroboth et al., 1999a). Monitor the patient and adjust dose as needed.

Although not documented, DHEA may interact with other exogenous androgen or estrogen hormone therapies. Monitor the patient taking both of these agents.

Contraindications and precautions

DHEA is contraindicated in patients with benign prostatic hyperplasia, estrogen-responsive tumors (such as those of the breast and uterus), or prostate cancer because of DHEA's potential for promoting growth of these tumors. Avoid using DHEA in pregnant or breast-feeding patients; effects are unknown.

Special considerations

🔺**ALERT** Patients older than age 40 should be aggressively screened for hormonally sensitive cancers before taking DHEA.

- Monitor the patient for excessive hair growth.
- Instruct the patient to report mood or behavioral changes.
- Advise women to avoid using DHEA during pregnancy or when breast-feeding.
- Monitor the male patient for breast enlargement.

Commentary

Many claims for DHEA use are based on in vitro or animal studies; moreover, nonprimate mammals do not produce significant amounts of endogenous DHEA, so using them in clinical studies may be erroneous. Although declining DHEA levels in humans may be assumed to act as a marker for aging and degenerative diseases, inconclusive evidence exists that exogenous DHEA replacement will prevent or be therapeutic for such conditions. Long-term safety data for DHEA use in humans are also lacking. Larger, more comprehensive trials are needed to determine a role for this agent.

References

Barnhart, K.T., et al. "The Effect of Dehydroepiandrosterone Supplementation to Symptomatic Perimenopausal Women on Serum Endocrine Profiles, Lipid Parameters, and Health-related Quality of Life," *J Clin Endocrinol Metab* 84(11):3896-902, 1999.

Brown, G.A., et al. "Effect of Oral DHEA on Serum Testosterone and Adaptions to Resistance Training in Young Men," *J Appl Physiol* 87(6):2274-83, 1999.

Cawood, E.H.H., and Bancroft, J. "Steroid Hormones, the Menopause, Sexuality and Well-being of Women," *Psychol Med* 26:925-36, 1996.

Gordon, C.M., et al. "Changes in Bone Turnover Markers and Menstrual Function After Short-term Oral DHEA in Young Women with Anorexia Nervosa," *J Bone Miner Res* 14(1):136-45, 1999.

Hillen, T., et al. "DHEA-S Plasma Levels and Incidence of Alzheimer's Disease," *Biol Psychiatry* 47(2):161-63, 2000.

Huppert, F.A., et al. "Dehydroepiandrosterone Supplementation for Cognition and Well-being," *Cochrane Database Syst Rev* (2):CD000304, 2000.

Khorram, O., et al. "Activation of Immune Function by Dehydroepiandrosterone (DHEA) in Age-Advanced Men," *J Gerontol A Biol Med Sci* 52(1):M1-M7, 1997.

Kroboth, P.D., et al. "DHEA and DHEA-S: A Review," *J Clin Pharmacol* 39:327-48, 1999a.

Kroboth, P.D., et al. "Alprazolam Increases Dehydroepiandrosterone Concentrations," *J Clin Psychpharmacol* 19(2):114-24, 1999b.

Labrie, F., et al. "Physiologic Changes in Dehydroepiandrosterone Are Not Reflected by Serum Levels of Active Androgens and Estrogens But of Their Metabolites," *J Clin Endocrinol Metab* 82:2403-9, 1997.

Morales, A.J., et al. "Effects of Replacement Dose of Dehydroepiandrosterone in Men and Women of Advancing Age," *J Clin Endocrinol Metab* 78:1360-67, 1994.

Nestler, J.E., and Kahwash, Z. "Sex-specific Action of Insulin to Acutely Increase Metabolic Clearance Rate of Dehydroepiandrosterone in Humans," *J Clin Invest* 94:1484-89, 1994.

Osran, H., et al. "Adrenal Androgens and Cortisol in Major Depression," *Am J Psychiatry* 150:806-9, 1993.

Reiter, W.J., et al. "Serum Dehydroepiandrosterone Sulfate Concentrations in Men with Erectile Dysfunction," *Urology* 55(5):755-58, 2000.

Wallace, M.B., et al. "Effects of Dehydroepiandrosterone vs Androstenedione Supplementation in Men," *Med Sci Sports Exerc* 31(12):1788-92, 1999.

Wolkowitz, O.M., et al. "Dehydroepiandrosterone Treatment of Depression," *Biol Psychiatry* 41:311-18, 1997.

DILL

DILL SEED, DILLWEED

Taxonomic class
Apiaceae

Common trade names
Atkinson & Barker's Gripe Mixture, Concentrated
Dill Water BPC 1973, Neo, Neo Baby Mixture, Nurse
Harvey's Gripe Mixture, Woodward's Gripe Water

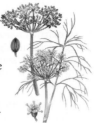

Common forms
Available as dill oil, distilled or concentrated dill water, and dried fruits.

Source
All parts of the plant are used, but most products use the dried ripe
fruit, seeds, or flowers of *Anethum graveolens,* a member of the carrot
family.

Chemical components
Dill plants contain volatile oil (carvone, d-limonene, eugenol, and an-
theole), flavonoids (including kaempferol, quercetin, and isorhamnetin), coumarins, xanthone derivatives, triterpenes, phenolic acids,
proteins, fixed oil, myristicin, dillapiole, paraffins, and phellandrene.

Actions
Dill is believed to have antiflatulent, antispasmodic, aromatic, lactogenic, and soporific actions.

Reported uses
Dill is a common ingredient in "gripe water," used to relieve flatulence
and colic in infants. It is also used in breast-feeding patients and in cattle to help promote the flow of milk (Morton, 1981). The oil has been
used for its antifoaming and antiflatulent action to improve appetite
and digestion. The seeds have been used to treat abdominal pain, halitosis (on chewing), and hiccups and to strengthen the nails when the
hands are soaked in a decoction. No controlled human studies support
these claims. One Bulgarian study concluded that dill oil has weak choleretic effects and should be used with other drugs for benefit (Gruncharov and Tashev, 1973).

Dosage
Some sources suggest the following doses:
Concentrated dill water: 0.2 ml P.O. t.i.d.
Dill oil: 0.05 to 2 ml P.O. t.i.d.
Distilled dill water: 2 to 4 ml P.O. t.i.d.
Dried fruits: 1 to 4 g P.O. t.i.d.

Adverse reactions
None reported.

Interactions
None reported.

Contraindications and precautions
Dill weed is contraindicated in patients who require a low-salt diet because of its high sodium content. Use cautiously in patients with plant allergies because dill has allergenic components that may demonstrate cross-sensitivity in some people.

Special considerations
• Periodically monitor serum electrolyte levels, particularly sodium, in patients who take dill.
• Inform the patient that the potentially beneficial effects of dill remain unproved and the safety profile is unknown.
• Recommend that the patient seek medical advice before taking the herb.
• Reinforce the importance of a low-sodium diet in patients who require it.

Points of interest
• The name dill is believed to have originated from the Norse word *dilla* (to lull) because of its sedative and antiflatulent properties.
• In the Middle Ages, dill was used by magicians in their potions and magic spells and was grown in gardens as a charm against witchcraft and enchantments.

Commentary
Clinical data for dill are extremely limited. No trial data from the United States support its use for flatulence or colic in infants or as a stimulant for milk flow, although this appears to be the primary medicinal claim in the herbal literature. More studies are needed to determine the effects of dill in children and adults.

References
Gruncharov, V., and Tashev, T. "The Choleretic Effect of Bulgarian Dill Oil in White Rats," *Eksp Med Morfol* 12:155-61, 1973.
Morton, J.F. *Atlas of Medicinal Plants of Middle America: Bahamas to Yucatan.* Springfield, Ill.: Charles C. Thomas Publisher, 1981.

DOCK, YELLOW

CHIN CH'IAO MAI, CURLED OR CURLY DOCK, GARDEN
PATIENCE, HUALTATA, HUMMAIDH, KIVIRCIK LABADA,
NARROW DOCK, NIU SHE T'OU, OSEILLE MARRON
(SAUVAGE), SHEEP SORREL, SOUR DOCK, SURALE DI
BIERDJI, YELLOW DUCK

Taxonomic class
Polygonaceae

Common trade names
Multi-ingredient preparations: Detox, LC Tone, Rumex Crispus

Common forms
Available in capsules (470 mg, 500 mg), liquid, root, and tea.

Source
A dried extract is prepared from the roots of *Rumex crispus*, a common
and troublesome perennial weed that is native to Europe and Asia.
Dock has become naturalized in the United States and grows along
roadsides and in gravelly soils of pastures and meadows.

Chemical components
The primary component of the dried root of *R. crispus* is chrysophanic
acid; others include rumicin, emodin (oxymethylanthraquinone), calcium oxalate, oxalic acid, brassidinic acid, tannins, and volatile oils. The
stems, leaves, and fruit also contain anthraquinones and oxalic acid. Loss
of activity has occurred if the root is boiled for an extended period.

Actions
Rumex species have been studied in vitro and in vivo in animals and
found to have both anti-inflammatory and antiviral effects. The anti-
itch effect of the leaves of *R. nepalensis* is believed to be caused by the
antibradykinin, anticholinergic, and antihistaminic properties of the
plant (Aggarwal et al., 1986).

An in vitro study of sheep seminal vesicles noted that aqueous and
A root extract of *R. hastatus* was found to inactivate the herpes simplex virus; antiviral activity against poliovirus and Sindbis virus was
unaffected (Taylor et al., 1996). Extracts of the *R. crispus* fruit also
showed significant inhibitory activity against HIV reverse transcriptase
(el-Mekkawy et al., 1995).

An in vitro study of sheep seminal vesicles noted that aqueous and
ethanolic extracts of *R. sagittatus* root significantly inhibited cyclooxygenase activity.

Reported uses
Dock root is said to be an astringent and a cathartic. It has been used to
treat syphilis and cutaneous eruptions, particularly of the scrofulous
type. Some *Rumex* species were known for curing intermittent fevers
and others have been used in chronic hepatic congestion and dyspepsia.

An ointment made by boiling the root in vinegar has been used to treat glandular swellings and various skin diseases, such as scabies. Bruising and applying the fresh root is a popular antidote to the rash induced by stinging nettle. Other claimed uses include diuresis and symptomatic treatment of tonsillitis and sore throat. No human trials have evaluated these claims.

Dosage

Most in vitro studies reported pharmacologic activity of *Rumex* species in concentrations ranging from 25 to 100 mcg/ml. Doses tested clinically ranged from 2.5 to 5 mg P.O. as a single dose.

Adverse reactions

GI: abdominal pain, diarrhea, nausea, vomiting.
Metabolic: hypocalcemia.

Interactions

None reported.

Contraindications and precautions

Rumex species are contraindicated as a laxative in pregnant women because of the presence of anthraquinones, which have stimulant effects that may lead to miscarriage. They are also contraindicated in patients with renal dysfunction or failure, type 1 or 2 diabetes, hepatic disease, and severe electrolyte imbalances because of the possibility of oxalic acid precipitation in the renal tubules. (See *Toxicity of* Rumex crispus.)

Use cautiously in patients with alcoholic disease, new-onset diabetes, heart failure, hypoalbuminemic disease states, malnutrition, or recent thyroid or parathyroid surgery. Also use with caution in patients who are concurrently taking drugs known to cause hypocalcemia (such as calcitonin, carbonic anhydrase inhibitors, loop and potassium-sparing diuretics, mithramycin, and phenytoin).

Special considerations

• Monitor serum calcium levels and for signs of hypocalcemia.
• **ALERT** Severe hypocalcemia and metabolic acidosis with resultant death may follow consumption of excessive quantities of dock.
• Advise the patient to report sudden onset of abdominal pain, nausea, and vomiting.
• Inform the patient to use small portions of dock for culinary purposes, if at all.
• Advise the patient not to use dock as a replacement for antivirals to treat herpes or HIV infection.
• Inform the patient with continued allergy or allergic response despite herbal use to notify his health care provider.
• Urge the patient to watch for symptoms of hypocalcemia (confusion, fatigue, muscle spasms, perioral paresthesia, and seizures).
• Instruct women taking the herb to report planned or suspected pregnancy.

Bold italic type indicates that reaction may be life-threatening.

RESEARCH FINDINGS

Toxicity of *Rumex crispus*

Although only a few cases of *Rumex* poisonings have been identified in humans, fatal incidents dating back to 1949 have been identified in animals (Panciera et al., 1990). The most recent case in humans involved fatal poisoning caused by *Rumex crispus* ingestion (Farr et al., 1989). A 53-year-old patient with type 1 diabetes for 10 years went to the emergency department with symptoms of vomiting and diarrhea after ingesting 500 to 1,000 g of this plant in a sorrel soup.

The patient was dehydrated with moderate metabolic acidosis. Laboratory values were as follows: liver enzyme levels more than three times the upper limit of normal (AST 8,000 IU/L, ALT 12,000 IU/L); total serum calcium level 6.3 mg/dl, with an ionized calcium of 2.3 mg/dl; serum creatinine level 5.3 mg/dl (534 mmol/L); BUN level 100 mg/dl (18.5 mmol/L); PT ratio 3.14; and fibrinogen 1.2 mg/ml.

The patient lapsed into a coma and exhibited respiratory depression and multiorgan failure. Initially, calcium gluconate was given for the hypocalcemia and sodium bicarbonate, for the metabolic acidosis, followed by hemodialysis for the renal insufficiency. Shortly after hemodialysis, the patient experienced arrhythmias that progressed to ventricular fibrillation. The patient died 72 hours after ingesting the plant.

Autopsy revealed birefringent crystals in the kidneys and liver, confirmed later to be calcium oxalate crystals. Other findings included liver necrosis and centrilobular vascular stasis with portal lymphocytic infiltration, necrosis of the proximal and distal convoluted tubules of the kidneys, severe lung edema, and pulmonary congestion. These findings were consistent with *R. crispus* toxicity.

Other family members who had also ingested the plant recovered uneventfully in a few days. The mean lethal dose of oxalic acid in adults is 5 to 30 g. This patient ingested about 6 to 8 g of oxalic acid from the sorrel soup.

● Advise women to avoid using dock during pregnancy or when breast-feeding.

Points of interest
● Dock is cultivated in Europe as a vegetable or salad. It is also a popular Himalayan antidote for rash caused by stinging nettles.

Commentary
All clinical data on *Rumex* are from in vitro studies on animals. This herb has mild to moderate antipruritic effects. Although it reduces the size of inflammatory wheal reactions, the mechanism is unknown. Be-

cause of the risk of poisoning, available antihistamine or antiallergy products are recommended instead of the herb.

References
Aggarwal, M., et al. "Effect of *Rumex nepalensis* Extracts on Histamine, Acetylcholine, Carbachol, Bradykinin, and PGs Evoked Skin Reactions in Rabbits," *Ann Allerg* 56:177-82, 1986.

el-Mekkawy S., et al. "Inhibitory Effects of Egyptian Folk Medicines on Human Immunodeficiency Virus (HIV) Reverse Transcriptase," *Chem Pharm Bull (Tokyo)* 43:641-48, 1995. Abstract.

Farr, M., et al. "Fatal Oxalic Acid Poisoning from Sorrel Soup," *Lancet* 23:1524, 1989. Letter.

Panciera, R., et al. "Acute Oxalate Poisoning Attributable to Ingestion of Curly Dock *(Rumex crispus)* in Sheep," *J Am Vet Med Assoc* 196:1981-90, 1990.

Taylor, R.S., et al. "Antiviral Activities of Medicinal Plants of Southern Nepal," *J Ethnopharmacol* 53:97-104, 1996.

DONG QUAI

CHINESE ANGELICA, DRY-KUEI, **FP3340010/FP334015/FT334010**, TANG-KUEI, WOMEN'S GINSENG

Taxonomic class
Apiaceae

Common trade names
Dong Kwai, Dong Quai Capsules, Dong Quai Fluid Extract

Common forms
Raw root: 4.5 to 30 g (boil or soak in wine)
Tablet (fluidextract): 0.5 g
Also available as capsules, powders, teas and, in some countries, injectable forms.

Source
Active components are obtained from the roots of dong quai (*Angelica polymorpha* var. *sinensis*), a fragrant perennial umbelliferous herb that is native to China, Korea, and Japan.

Chemical components
The volatile oils extracted from the root contain *n*-butylphthalide, cadinene, carvacrol, dihydrophthalmic anhydride, folinic acid, isosafrole, ligustilide, nicotinic acid, safrole, succinic acid, uracil, and vitamin B_{12}. Coumarin derivatives identified in dong quai include bergapten, imperatorin, osthole, oxypeucedanin, and psoralen. Ferulic acid has also been found.

Actions
Dong quai alters uterine activity in female rabbits. The volatile oil has an inhibitory action on the uterus, whereas the nonvolatile and water-

and alcohol-soluble components have stimulatory action.

Studies conducted in rats showed increases in metabolism, oxygen use by the liver, and glutamic acid and cysteine oxidation; these actions may be attributed to vitamin B_{12} and folinic acid that occur in the herb's root.

Dong quai extracts, especially alcoholic extracts, were also found to exert quinidine-type effects, prolong the refractory period, and correct atrial fibrillation in animals. Other studies in rats showed that these extracts may prevent atherosclerosis, expand coronary arteries, and increase coronary blood flow. Some coumarins are known to act as vasodilators. Although studies in animals have shown that the volatile oil exerts vasodilatory action to lower blood pressure, the duration of action is short.

Reported uses

Dong quai is recommended by Western herbalists for many gynecologic disorders, including dysmenorrhea, excessive fetal movement, menstrual irregularities, chronic pelvic infection, and premenstrual syndrome. Most claims are based on data from animal studies or small, uncontrolled human trials, but in a double-blind, placebo-controlled trial of 71 postmenopausal women, dong quai alone was found not to produce estrogen-like responses in endometrial thickness or vaginal maturation and not to be useful in managing postmenopausal symptoms (Hirata et al., 1997). In traditional Chinese medicine, dong quai is used in combination with other herbs to relieve dysmenorrhea and other disorders. Kotani and colleagues (1997) evaluated such an herbal preparation including dong quai in 41 women with dysmenorrhea and found it effective in diminishing symptoms. Because an NSAID was allowed on an as-needed basis, it is difficult to determine the effect of the herbal preparation. Other reported uses include treatment of Buerger's disease, constipation, headache, hepatitis, hepatocirrhosis, herpes zoster, hypertension, malaria, neuralgia, pyogenic infection, Raynaud's disease, chronic rhinitis, sepsis, toothache, and ulcerous diseases or abscess. None of these uses has been evaluated clinically.

Dosage

Dosage forms, strengths, and extraction forms vary. In a placebo-controlled study evaluating the estrogenic effects of dong quai on endometrial thickness in postmenopausal women, 500-mg capsules taken P.O. t.i.d. (equivalent to 0.5 mg/kg of ferulic acid), for a total daily dose 4.5 g of root, were used.

Adverse reactions

GI: diarrhea.
Hematologic: *bleeding.*
Skin: increased photosensitivity (psoralens in herb may cause severe photodermatitis).
Other: fever.

Interactions
Anticoagulants, antiplatelets: May enhance effects. Avoid administration with dong quai (Page et al., 1999; Shimizu et al., 1991).

Contraindications and precautions
Safrole, a component of the volatile oil, is carcinogenic and not recommended for ingestion. Dong quai is contraindicated in pregnant or breast-feeding patients because its chemical components may cause fetal harm. Traditional Chinese texts advise against using dong quai in the presence of an acute infection.

Special considerations
- Monitor the patient for potential bleeding.
- Ask why the patient is using dong quai and suggest that he seek a health care provider to address these concerns.
- Caution the patient that some of the herb's components have been shown to increase the risk of some cancers.
- Instruct the patient who becomes photosensitive to use sunblock and to wear adequate clothing and sunglasses.
- Caution the patient against using dong quai for its yet unproven estrogenic effects.
- Advise women to report planned or suspected pregnancy and to avoid using this herb during pregnancy or when breast-feeding.

Commentary
Despite numerous therapeutic claims for dong quai, only a few controlled clinical trials and animal-based studies are available to support its use to treat dysmenorrhea. Most claims regarding dong quai are unsubstantiated and need additional investigation. Dong quai appears to have more than 18 active chemical components, many of which exert widely divergent pharmacologic effects. Some components are carcinogens, and adverse effects of others are unknown. Extensive testing of individual components is needed before dong quai can be regarded as safe or effective.

References
Hirata, J.D., et al. "Does Donq Quai Have Estrogenic Effects in Postmenopausal Women? A Double-Blind Placebo-Controlled Trial," *Fertil Steril* 68:981-86, 1997.

Kotani, N., et al. "Analgesic Effect of a Herbal Medicine for Treatment of Primary Menstrual Dysmenorrhea: A Double-blind Study," *Am J Chinese Med* 25:205-12, 1997.

Page, R.L., and Lawrence, J.D. "Potentiation of Warfarin by Dong Quai," *Pharmacotherapy* 19(7):870-76, 1999.

Shimizu, M., et al. "Evaluation of *Angelica radix* (Touki) by the Inhibitory Effect on Platelet Aggregation," *Chem Pharm Bull* 39:2046-48, 1991.

Bold italic type indicates that reaction may be life-threatening.

E

ECHINACEA

American coneflower, black sampson, black susans, cock-up-hat, comb flower, coneflower, echinacea care liquid, hedgehog, Indian head, Kansas snakeroot, Missouri snakeroot, narrow-leaved purple coneflower, purple coneflower, purple Kansas coneflower, red sunflower, scurvy root, snakeroot

Taxonomic class
Asteraceae

Common trade names
Multi-ingredient preparations: Coneflower Extract, Echinacea, Echinacea Angustifolia Herb, Echinacea Care Liquid, Echinacea Fresh Freeze-Dried, Echinacea Glycerite, Echinacea Herb, Echinacea Herbal Comfort Lozenges, Echinacea Purpurea

Common forms
Capsules: 125 mg, 355 mg (85 mg herbal extract powder), 470 mg (whole root), 500 mg
Tablets: 335 mg
   Also available as candles, glycerite, hydroalcoholic extracts, fresh-pressed juice, lollipops, lozenges, teas, and tinctures.

Source
Echinacea dietary supplements are obtained from the dried rhizomes and roots of *Echinacea angustifolia* or *E. pallida* and from the fresh juice of the roots or above-ground parts of *E. purpurea.*

Chemical components
Echinacea contains alkylamides, caffeic acid derivatives, polysaccharides, essential oils, and other constituents, including polyacetylene flavonoids and glycoproteins. The plant contains three classes of compounds that exhibit nonspecific immunostimulatory activity: alkylamides, chicoric acids and related glycosides, and high-molecular-weight polysaccharides. The concentration of the pharmacologically active constituents varies, depending on many factors, including the species and plant part used, growing conditions, and extractive process.

Actions
Extract of echinacea stimulates phagocytosis and increases respiratory cellular activity and mobility of leukocytes. No single component appears to be responsible for the immunostimulating activity, although

the caffeic acid derivatives and high-molecular-weight polysaccharides in echinacea stimulate phagocytosis. The alkylamides in the plant are reported to exert local anesthetic and anti-inflammatory effects. Some of these compounds also have insecticidal activity (Jacobson, 1967). Caffeoyl conjugates in the plant stimulate the production of properdin and interferon and activate adrenal cortex activity. In vitro studies using the fresh-pressed juice of the aerial portion of *E. purpurea* and the aqueous extract of the roots inhibited herpes infections, influenza, and vesicular stomatitis virus.

The extract of echinacea can reduce the growth of *Trichomonas vaginalis* and reduces recurrence of *Candida albicans* infections (Combest and Nemecz, 1997). Intraperitoneal administration of purified arabinogalactan in rats caused activation of macrophages against *Leishmania enrietti*. Arabinogalactan stimulated macrophages to produce tumor necrosis factor, interleukin-1, and interferon beta-2. The lipid-soluble compound 1,8 pentadecadiene exhibits direct antitumorigenic activity (Combest and Nemecz, 1997).

The extract has inhibited edema in rats and inflammation in mice. In vitro studies indicate that the polyphenols from echinacea protect collagen against free radical attack.

Reported uses

Echinacea is claimed to be useful as a wound-healing agent for abscesses, burns, eczema, varicose ulcers of the leg, and other skin wounds and as a nonspecific immunostimulant for the supportive treatment of upper respiratory tract and urinary tract infections. Two small studies have demonstrated that parenteral administration of purified Echinacin (not available in the United States) may be beneficial as an immunotherapeutic agent in combination with standard chemotherapeutic drugs in the treatment of colorectal and hepatocellular cancers (Lersch et al., 1990, 1992). Several groups of investigators have attempted to define a role for echinacea in the prevention or treatment of colds. (See *Echinacea and the common cold.*)

Dosage

Some sources suggest the following doses:
Capsules containing the powdered herb: equivalent to 900 mg to 1 g P.O. t.i.d.; doses can vary.
Expressed juice: 6 to 9 ml P.O. daily.
Tea: 2 tsp (4 g) of coarsely powdered herb simmered in 1 cup of boiling water for 10 minutes. Avoid this method of administration because some active compounds are water-insoluble.
Tincture: 0.75 to 1.5 ml (15 to 30 gtt) P.O. two to five times daily. The tincture has been given as 60 gtt P.O. t.i.d.

Adverse reactions

Other: allergic reactions, ***anaphylaxis*** (Mullins, 1998).

Bold italic type indicates that reaction may be life-threatening.

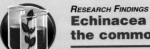

RESEARCH FINDINGS
Echinacea and the common cold

A number of clinical trials testing echinacea attempted to identify a role for echinacea in the treatment and prevention of upper respiratory tract infections (URIs). The evidence conflicts with earlier information. Interestingly, all studies differed as to the echinacea preparations they studied and the dosing regimens they used.

One study suggesting a benefit of echinacea studied three dosage forms of echinacea against placebo in 246 adult volunteers who had caught a common cold (Brinkeborn et al., 1999). The primary efficacy endpoint was the change in a 12-symptom "complaint index" derived from the doctor's record. At trial completion, two formulations of echinacea appeared to fare better than the other treatments for URI. Another randomized, controlled, double-blind trial suggesting benefit used a mixed herbal combination that included *Echinacea radix* (Henneicke-von Zepelin et al., 1999). Although somewhat subjective, primary efficacy parameters (patient's estimation of intensity of illness, 10-point cold scale, general well-being color scale) appeared to favor the herbal combination product over placebo for URI treatment.

Three modest-sized randomized, controlled, double-blind studies failed to identify a statistically significant difference between echinacea prevention remedies and placebo for outcome variables such as incidence of URIs, number of days until the first URI, and duration of URI (Melchart et al., 1998; Turner et al., 2000; Grimm and Muller, 1999). Despite several trials with positive results, a review of the available clinical trial information failed to find sufficient evidence to recommend echinacea for either prevention or treatment of URIs (Melchart et al., 2000).

Interactions
None reported.

Contraindications and precautions
Echinacea is contraindicated in patients with severe illnesses, including autoimmune diseases, collagen diseases, HIV infection, leukemia, multiple sclerosis, or tuberculosis, and in those who are hypersensitive to plants belonging to the daisy family. Avoid use in pregnant or breast-feeding patients; effects are unknown.

Special considerations
🔥 **ALERT** Many tinctures contain significant concentrations of alcohol (ranging from 15% to 90%) and may not be suitable for children, alco-

holic patients, patients with hepatic disease, or those taking disulfiram or metronidazole.

ALERT Echinacea should not be used for longer than 8 weeks; therapy lasting 10 to 14 days is probably sufficient. Urge the patient not to delay treatment for an illness that does not resolve after taking this herb.

• Echinacea might adversely influence fertility. In vitro studies have demonstrated echinacea's interference with spermatozoa enzymes (Ondrizek et al., 1999). This finding remains to be proven.

• Advise the pregnant or breast-feeding patient to avoid using echinacea.

Commentary
The evidence for echinacea appears to be conflicting. More human clinical trial information is needed before a role for echinacea in the treatment or prophylaxis of disease can be defined. It is unknown which *Echinacea* species and which dosage forms are most valuable.

References
Brinkeborn, R.M., et al. " Echinaforce and Other Echinacea Fresh Plant Preparations in the Treatment of the Common Cold. A Randomized, Placebo-controlled, Double-blind Clinical Trial," *Phytomedicine* 6(1):1-6, 1999.

Combest, W.L., and Nemecz, G. "Echinacea," *U.S. Pharmacist* October, 126-32, 1997.

Grimm, W., and Muller, H.H. "A Randomized Controlled Trial of the Effect of Fluid Extract of *Echinacea purpurea* on the Incidence and Severity of Colds and Respiratory Infections," *Am J Med* 106(2):138-43, 1999.

Henneicke-von Zepelin, H., et al. "Efficacy and Safety of a Fixed Combination Phytomedicine in the Treatment of the Common Cold: Results of a Randomized, Double-blind, Placebo-controlled, Multi-centre Study," *Curr Med Res Opin* 15(3):214-17, 1999.

Jacobson, M. "The Structure of Echinacein, the Insecticidal Component of American Coneflower Roots," *J Org Chem* 32:1646-47, 1967.

Lersch, C., et al. "Stimulation of the Immune Response in Outpatients with Hepatocellular Carcinomas by Low Doses of Cyclophosphamide (LDCY), *Echinacea purpurea* Extracts (Echinacein), and Thymostimulin," *Arch Gescwulstforsch* 60:379-83, 1990.

Lersch, C., et al. "Nonspecific Immunostimulation with Low Doses of Cyclophosphamide (LDCY), Thymostimulin, and *Echinacea purpurea* Extract (Echinacein) in Patients with Far Advanced Colorectal Cancers. Preliminary Results," *Cancer Invest* 10:343-48, 1992.

Melchart, D., et al. "Echinacea Root Extracts for the Prevention of Upper Respiratory Tract Infections: A Double-blind, Placebo-controlled Randomized Trial," *Arch Fam Med* 7(6):541-45, 1998.

Melchart, D., et al. "Echinacea for Preventing and Treating the Common Cold," *Cochrane Database Syst Rev* 2:CD000530, 2000.

Mullins, R.J. "Echinacea-associated Anaphylaxis," *Med J Aust* 168(4):170-71, 1998.

Ondrizek, R.R., et al. "Inhibition of Human Sperm Motility by Specific Herbs Used in Alternative Medicine," *J Assist Reprod Genet* 16(2):87-91, 1999.

Turner, R.B., et al. "Ineffectiveness of Echinacea for Prevention of Experimental Rhinovirus Colds," *Antimicrob Agents Chemother* 44(6):1708-9, 2000.

ELDERBERRY

ANTELOPE BRUSH (*SAMBUCUS TRIDENTATA*), BLACK ELDER (*SAMBUCUS NIGRA*), BLUE ELDERBERRY (*SAMBUCUS CAERULEA*), BORETREE, COMMON ELDER (*SAMBUCUS CANADENSIS*), DANEWORT (*SAMBUCUS EBULUS*), DWARF ELDER, ELDER, EUROPEAN ELDER, PIPE TREE, RED ELDERBERRY, RED-FRUITED ELDER (*SAMBUCUS PUBENS*, *SAMBUCUS RACEMOSA*), *SAMBUCUS*, SWEET ELDER

Taxonomic class
Caprifoliaceae

Common trade names
Elderberry Power, Elder Flowers

Common forms
Available as ointments and aqueous solutions of the bark and leaves as well as oils, ointments, and wine; all are derived from the berries.

Source
Several species of *Sambucus* produce elderberries. Most of the literature refers to *S. nigra* and *S. canadensis,* although other species with similar chemical components exist. The flowers and berries are used most often; the inner bark and leaves contain most of the potentially toxic compounds.

Chemical components
The flowers of *S. nigra* contain flavonoid glycosides, a cyanogenic glycoside (sambunigrine), essential oils, mucilage, tannins, and organic acids. Fruit from the elder (*S. nigra*) contains organic pigments (anthocyanins), amino acids, sugar, rutin, and a substantial amount of vitamin C (36 mg per 100 g of fruit). The elder leaves contain 3.5% rutin. The inner bark of the elder also consists of baldrianic acid. Other species contain additional compounds.

Actions
Elder has traditionally been used to treat diabetes, although studies in mice indicate that the agent exerts no effects on glucose control (Swanston-Flatt et al., 1989). This plant has shown activity against *Salmonella typhi* and *Shigella dysenteriae* and limited activity against *Shigella flexneri.* A branch tip extract of the red elder (*Sambucus racemosa*) was found to have strong in vitro antiviral activity against respiratory syncytial virus. No studies in humans or animals have been reported.

A recent study (Yesilada et al., 1997) indicated that *S. nigra* was somewhat active against the production of inflammatory cytokines in vitro, giving some merit to folklore suggesting that the plant is effective in the treatment of fever, infections, and rheumatism. Elderberries have been reported to have antispasmodic, diaphoretic, diuretic, laxative, and sedative activity. The cyanogenic glycosides contained in the elder plants release cyanide when hydrolyzed, as when they are chewed; this effect might eventually explain some of the purported actions of this plant. Anthocyanins have been detected in human plasma after oral administration of an elderberry extract (Cao and Prior, 1999).

Reported uses

Elder has been used as an insect repellent, with sprays of the flowers placed in horses' bridles. The powder of dried elder flowers has been added to water and dabbed on the skin as a mosquito repellent. The herb has been used as a weight-loss agent and to treat colds, "dropsy," insomnia, migraine headaches, renal disorders, and rheumatism. Clinical support for these uses in humans is lacking.

Mixed with sage, lemon juice, vinegar, and honey, elder has also traditionally been used as a gargle. With peppermint and honey in a hot drink, elder is said to be able to treat a cold, inducing diaphoresis to "sweat out" an illness. Elderberry juice has been used in hair dye and scented ointments. Other reported uses include treatment of asthma, burns, cancer, chafing, edema, epilepsy, gout, headache, hepatic disease, measles, neuralgia, psoriasis, syphilis, and toothache and for wound healing, although no scientific data support such uses.

Dosage

No consensus exists.

Adverse reactions

GI: diarrhea (from berries of the *S. ebulus* and leaves of any species), vomiting (with ingestion of excessive amounts of *S. racemosa* berries).

Interactions

None reported.

Contraindications and precautions

Berries of the dwarf elder species (*S. ebulus*) are contraindicated. Because all green parts of the elder plant are poisonous, avoid consumption of the leaves and stems. Avoid using elderberry in pregnant and breast-feeding patients. Use elderberry products cautiously because of the risk of cyanide toxicity.

Special considerations

• Monitor fluid intake and output of patients who experience adverse GI reactions from elderberry.
• The dwarf elder (*S. ebulus*) is regarded as particularly poisonous. Large doses can cause diarrhea, vertigo, and vomiting (signs of cyanide toxicity).
🕭 **ALERT** Cyanide poisoning can result from ingesting the bark, roots, leaves, and unripe berries of the elder plant. Children making pipes or peashooters from the hollowed shafts of the elder can suffer cyanide poisoning. Ingestion of 60 mg of cyanide has caused death in humans. Emesis and gastric lavage are recommended for known elder plant ingestion. Amyl nitrate, sodium nitrate, and sodium thiosulfate can also be used when cyanide toxicity is suspected.

Bold italic type indicates that reaction may be life-threatening.

• Instruct the patient to keep this plant out of the reach of children and pets and to have the telephone number for the nearest poison control center readily available.

• Advise the female patient to avoid using elderberry during pregnancy or when breast-feeding.

Commentary

The use of elderberry products as cathartics is not recommended because of the risk of cyanide toxicity. Numerous other laxatives and cathartics exist whose safety and efficacy are well established. Because safe and effective anti-inflammatory drugs are also available for treating rheumatism and other conditions for which elderberries have been used, elderberry use for these conditions is not recommended. There is insufficient evidence to support use of this herbal product for medicinal applications.

References

Cao, G., and Prior, R.L. "Anthocyanins Are Detected in Human Plasma After Oral Administration of an Elderberry Extract," *Clin Chem* 45(4):574-76, 1999.

Swanston-Flatt, S.K., et al. "Glycaemic Effects of Traditional European Plant Treatments for Diabetes. Studies in Normal and Streptozotocin Diabetic Mice," *Diabetes Res* 10:69-73, 1989.

Yesilada, E., et al. "Inhibitory Effects of Turkish Folk Remedies on Inflammatory Cytokines: Interleukin-1$_{alpha}$, Interleukin-1$_{beta}$ and Tumor Necrosis Factor Alpha," *J Ethnopharmacol* 58:59-73, 1997.

ELECAMPANE

AUNEE, ELFDOCK, ELFWORT, HORSEHEAL, SCABWORT, VELVET DOCK, WILD SUNFLOWER

Taxonomic class

Asteraceae

Common trade names

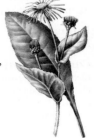

Multi-ingredient preparations: Blood Sugar Blues, Cough-eze Syrup, Digestease, HAS Original Formula, Lung-Mend

Common forms

Available as capsules, fluidextract, powdered root preparations, and topical product.

Source

Active ingredients of elecampane are extracted from the dried rhizome and roots of 2- to 3-year-old *Inula helenium* plants.

Chemical components

The main constituents in *I. helenium* are inulin, helenin, volatile oils, and a mixture of sesquiterpene lactones—primarily alantolactone, alantol, and alantic acid.

Actions

Claims for *I. helenium* include anthelmintic, antiseptic, bactericidal, diaphoretic, diuretic, and expectorant activities. Anecdotal animal data suggest that the agent exerts relaxant effects on tracheal and ileal smooth muscles (Reiter and Brandt, 1985) and antiparasitic activity against the liver fluke *Clonorchis sinensis* (Rhee et al., 1985). It failed to demonstrate in vitro antiviral activity against the tick-borne encephalitis virus (Fokina et al., 1991). Specific pharmacokinetic and pharmacodynamic data are not available. In vitro data indicate activity against *Mycobacterium tuberculosis.*

Reported uses

I. helenium is claimed to be effective in treating asthma, bronchitis, cough, diarrhea, nausea, and pulmonary disease. It is also claimed to be useful as an antiseptic, an appetite stimulant, a bactericidal agent against *M. tuberculosis,* a diuretic, and an agent to treat dyspepsia. Medical data regarding the efficacy of *I. helenium* are largely anecdotal and derived from animal research. Anecdotal human reports suggest possible use as a snake venom antidote. Randomized, placebo-controlled human trials using *I. helenium* have not been conducted.

Dosage

Some sources suggest the following doses:
Dried root: 2 to 3 g P.O. t.i.d.
Extract: 3 g of dried root in 20 ml of alcohol and 10 ml of water P.O. t.i.d.
Fresh root: 1 or 2 tbsp P.O. t.i.d.

Adverse reactions

CNS: paralysis (large oral doses).
GI: GI upset (large oral doses).
Skin: contact dermatitis.

Interactions

None reported.

Contraindications and precautions

Elecampane is contraindicated in pregnant and breast-feeding patients. Use cautiously in patients with a history of atopy, in those prone to contact dermatitis, or in those who are hypersensitive to the Asteraceae family (common herbs include ragweed, chrysanthemums, marigolds, and daisies).

Special considerations

• Several case reports suggest that elecampane is highly allergenic when applied topically. The mechanism is thought to involve degranulation of mast cells. The identified toxin is SL alantolactone.
• Monitor for signs of an allergic reaction in patients who are prone to hypersensitivity reactions.

Bold italic type indicates that reaction may be life-threatening.

• Inform the patient that allergic reactions can occur when elecampane is handled. Advise him to take precautions (wear gloves, long sleeves) if he is likely to handle the herb.
• Inform the patient that no scientifically proven therapeutic use is associated with elecampane.

Points of interest
• In France and Switzerland, elecampane root is one of the substances used in the preparation of absinthe, a popular cordial at the turn of the century.
• Helen of Troy is said to have carried elecampane when she was abducted from Sparta by the Trojans.

Commentary
Elecampane has been used as a medicinal product for many centuries in Europe and Asia. The presence of volatile oils suggests that the herb might be effective as an expectorant, but the lack of animal or human data limits its usefulness for this purpose. Elecampane appears to be safe and well tolerated, but medical supervision is recommended. Data supporting the use of *I. helenium* suggest some efficacy as an antiseptic and mild GI stimulant, but the lack of well-designed human trials prevents recommendation for its use.

References
Cantrell, C.L., et al. "Antimycobacterial Eudesmanolides from *Inula helenium* and *Rudbeckia subtomentosa*," *Planta Med* 65(4):351-55, 1999.

Fokina, G.I., et al. "Experimental Phytotherapy of Tick-Borne Encephalitis," *Vopr Virusol* 36:18-21, 1991. Abstract.

Lamminpaa, A., et al. "Occupational Allergic Contact Dermatitis Caused by Decorative Plants," *Contact Dermatitis* 34(5):330-35, 1996.

Natural medicines comprehensive database. www.naturaldatabse.com.

Pazzaglia, M., et al. "Contact Dermatitis Due to a Massage Liniment Containing *Inula helenium* Extract," *Contact Dermatitis* 33(4):267, 1995.

Reiter, M., and Brandt, W. "Relaxant Effects on Tracheal and Ileal Smooth Muscles of the Guinea Pig," *Arzneimittelforschung* 35:408-14, 1985. Abstract.

Rhee, J.K., et al. "Alterations of *Clonorchis sinensis* EPG by Administration of Herbs in Rabbits," *Am J Chin Med* 13:65-69, 1985. Abstract.

EPHEDRA

BRIGHAM TEA, CAO MA HUANG (CHINESE EPHEDRA), DESERT TEA, EPITONIN, HERBA EPHEDRAE, HERBAL, JOINT FIR, MA HUANG, MAHUUANGGEN (ROOT), MEXICAN TEA, MORMON TEA, MUZEI MU HUANG (MONGOLIAN EPHEDRA), NATURAL ECSTACY, POPOTILLO, SEA GRAPE, SQUAW TEA, TEAMSTER'S TEA, YELLOW ASTRINGENT, YELLOW HORSE, ZHONG MA HUANG (INTERMEDIATE EPHEDRA)

Taxonomic class
Ephedraceae

Common trade names
Multi-ingredient preparations: Herbal Fen-Phen, Power Trim, Ultimate Energizer, Up Your Gas

Common forms
Available as crude extracts of root and aerial parts, powders, tablets (about 7 mg), and teas.

Source
There are many species of ephedra, the most common being *Ephedra sinica* (ma huang) and *E. nevadensis.* Other forms include *E. trifurca, E. equisetina,* and *E. distachya.* The ephedras are evergreen plants with a pinelike odor. Pharmaceutical properties result from components in the seeds and stems.

Chemical components
The primary active ingredient is the alkaloid ephedrine. Not all ephedra species contain ephedrine, but of those that do, most contain 0.5% to 2.5% alkaloids. *E. equisetina* contains the most ephedrine, whereas the American species, *E. nevadensis* and *E. trifurca,* lack the agent. Other alkaloids commonly found in ephedra species include methylephedrine, methylpseudoephedrine, pseudoephedrine, norpseudoephedrine (cathine), norephedrine, ephedine, ephedroxane, and pseudoephedroxane. Other compounds include a volatile oil (varies in components, depending on source), ephedrans, catechin, gallic acid, tannins, flavonoids, inulin, dextrin, starch, pectin and some common plant acids, sugars, and trace minerals. The root contains ephedradines, feruloylhistamine, moakonine, and mahuannins. The woody stems contain the alkaloids, which are almost always absent from the fruit and root.

Actions
Most of ephedra's activity stems from the ephedrine component, which produces amphetamine-like actions. Ephedrine acts as a CNS stimulant, produces mydriasis, enhances myocardial contraction and increases heart rate, causes bronchodilation, decreases GI motility, and stimulates peripheral vasoconstriction with an associated elevation in blood

---

Bold italic type indicates that reaction may be life-threatening.

pressure. Pseudoephedrine is similar in adrenergic activity but less potent than ephedrine. It also possesses stronger diuretic properties than ephedrine. A Chinese abstract reports that the agent can preserve renal function and correct certain electrolyte imbalances in rats (Wang and Hikokichi, 1994). *E. altissima* yields several mutagenic *N*-nitrosamines in vitro. The significance of this finding is unclear. Transitorine, a component of *E. transitoria,* has demonstrated antibacterial properties against some common bacteria (Al-Khalil et al., 1998).

Reported uses
Ephedra has been used in Chinese medicine for several years for arthralgia, bronchial asthma, chills, colds, coughs, edema, fever, flu, headaches, and nasal congestion. In the West, it is commonly used for its CNS stimulant properties ("natural ecstasy") and as an appetite suppressant ("natural fen-phen"). There is little debate that the vasoconstrictive effects of ephedra (primarily from ephedrine and pseudoephedrine) may be useful in conditions marked by edematous tissues and congested membranes. Standardized pharmaceuticals that contain pseudoephedrine or phenylpropanolamine are preferred to crude ephedra products.

Dosage
American species of ephedra (*E. nevadensis* and *E. trifurca*) that do not contain ephedrine alkaloids are used for teas. Herbalists typically recommend placing ½ oz of dried branches in 1 pt of boiling water and steeping this mixture for 10 to 20 minutes.

Adverse reactions
CNS: anxiety, confusion, dizziness, headache, insomnia, nervousness, psychosis, restlessness, *seizure, CVA.*
CV: *arrhythmias, cardiac arrest, hypersensitivity myocarditis* (Zaacks et al., 1999), *myocardial infarction.*
GI: constipation (caused by tannin content).
GU: urine retention, uterine contractions.
Skin: exfoliative dermatitis.

Interactions
Beta blockers: May increase sympathomimetic effects on vasculature from unopposed alpha agonist effect, increasing risk of hypertension. Avoid administration with ephedra.
Ephedra alkaloids, MAO inhibitors: May increase risk of hypertensive crisis. Avoid administration with ephedra.
Phenothiazines: May block alpha effects of ephedra, causing hypotension and tachycardia. Avoid administration with ephedra.
Theophylline: May increase risk of GI and CNS adverse effects. Avoid administration with ephedra.

Contraindications and precautions
Ephedra is contraindicated in pregnant patients because of the risk of uterine stimulation and in diabetic patients because of its hyperglyce-

RESEARCH FINDINGS

Variability in products containing ma huang

Toxicity from ephedra alkaloids does not appear to result from differences in bioavailability of the ephedra alkaloids contained in ma huang (dietary supplement) products. A cross-over pharmacokinetic study of 10 subjects that examined three brands of botanical ephedrine products found little difference in absorption between the synthetic version of ephedrine and its "natural" ancestor (Gurley et al., 1998a). The same group of lead investigators discovered considerable variability in the ephedra alkaloid content (range 1.08 to 13.54 mg) of nine commercially available products after HPLC analysis. One product demonstrated lot-to-lot variability of more than 135% (Gurley et al., 1998b). In a related work, Gurley and colleagues cited lot-to-lot variations in specific ephedra alkaloids for 20 different ephedra products. One particular product exhibited variations of (-)-ephedrine, (+)-pseudoephedrine, and (-)-methylephedrine of more than 180%, 250%, and 1,000%, respectively. Many products exhibited discrepancies between the label claim for ephedra alkaloid content and the actual alkaloid content of more than 20% (Gurley et al., 2000).

mic effects. Use cautiously in patients with arrhythmias, angina and other cardiac disorders, hypertension, and prostatic enlargement and in those with a history of cerebrovascular disease.

Special considerations
◆ **ALERT** The FDA advises people using the herb to take less than 8 mg every 6 hours and no more than 24 mg daily. They further advise that ephedra products not be used for more than 7 consecutive days.
• Some ephedra-related adverse effects appear to be dose-related.
• Closely monitor younger patients taking ephedra for adverse reactions. Many of the heart attacks, seizures, and strokes reported to the FDA occurred in previously healthy young adults.
◆ **ALERT** The FDA has found more than 800 cases, including 17 deaths, from adverse reactions associated with ephedrine products.
• Monitor the patient for behavioral or mood changes.
• Recommend standard pharmaceutical formulations of ephedrine and pseudoephedrine for patients with a valid need for these compounds. (See *Variability in products containing ma huang.*)
• Advise the patient with cardiac disease, diabetes, hypertension, or prostatic enlargement to avoid using ephedra.
• Advise the diabetic patient to monitor his blood glucose level closely.

Bold italic type indicates that reaction may be life-threatening.

- Caution the patient to watch for adverse reactions (especially chest pain, dizziness, fainting, palpitations, and shortness of breath), and advise him to quickly seek medical attention if they occur.
- Some herbal mixtures may contain ma huang or ephedra as one of many ingredients. The alkaloids contained in ma huang may be considered "banned substances" within specific guidelines put forth by collegiate, Olympic, or professional sports committees for competitive play.
- Advise the patient to take less than 8 mg of ephedra every 6 hours and not to exceed 24 mg daily. Also, stress that it is not wise to use the product for more than 7 consecutive days.
- Urge the patient to avoid ephedra combination products that contain caffeine or guarana.

Points of interest
- The FDA has issued warnings against the use of ephedra as an appetite suppressant and advises that ingestion more than the recommended amount can result in heart attack, seizure, stroke, or death. The FDA prohibits the marketing of ephedrine with other CNS stimulants, such as caffeine and yohimbine.

Commentary
Unquestionably, the principal components in some ephedra species can play a valid role in medicine, especially in the treatment of edema and congestion. With standardized formulations of the active constituents available OTC and because of the dramatic variability in ephedra content seen with dietary supplements, the ingestion of the herbal product seems unwarranted.

References
Al-Khalil, S., et al. "Transitorine, a New Quinoline Alkaloid from *Ephedra transitoria*," *J Nat Prod* 61(2):262-63, 1998.

Gurley, B.J., et al. "Ephedrine Pharmacokinetics After the Ingestion of Nutritional Supplements Containing *Ephedra sinica* (ma huang)," *Ther Drug Monit* 20(4):439-45, 1998a.

Gurley, B.J., et al. "Ephedrine-type Alkaloid Content of Nutritional Supplements Containing *Ephedra sinica* (ma huang) as Determined by High Performance Liquid Chromatography," *J Pharm Sci* 87(12):1547-53, 1998b.

Gurley, B.J., et al. "Content Versus Label Claims in Ephedra-containing Dietary Supplements," *Am J Health System Pharm* 15;57(10):963-69, 2000.

Wang, G.Z., and Hikokichi, O. "Experimental Study in Treating Chronic Renal Failure with Dry Extract and Tannins of Herbal Ephedra," *Chin J Stomatol* 14:485, 1994.

Zaacks, S.M., et al. "Hypersensitivity Myocarditis Associated with Ephedra Use," *J Toxicol Clin Toxicol* 37(4):485-89, 1999.

EUCALYPTUS

FEVER TREE, GUM TREE, TASMANIAN BLUE GUM

Taxonomic class
Myrtaceae

Common trade names
Eucalyptamint, Eucalyptus Oil

Common forms
Available as aromatherapy room spray, bath salts, leaves, lotion, and oil.

Source
The herb is extracted from the leaves of the *Eucalyptus globulus* plant.

Chemical components
The eucalyptus plant contains several chemicals, including eucalyptrin, hyperoside, quercetin, quecitrin, tannins, and associated acids. The primary constituent of the volatile oil is eucalyptol (1,8-cineole).

Actions
Eucalyptus has hypoglycemic activity in rabbits, but its mechanism of action is unknown. Eucalyptus produces a stimulant effect on nasal temperature receptors. It is also a counterirritant and increases cutaneous blood flow (Hong et al., 1991). It has been shown to exert antifungal, anti-inflammatory, and antimicrobial effects (Pattnaik et al., 1996; Santos et al., 1997; Egawa et al., 1977). Cineole has demonstrated inhibitory effects on tumor necrosis factor-α, specific interleukins, thromboxanes, and leukotrienes (Juergens et al., 1998).

Reported uses
The herb was first used more than 100 years ago to relieve nasal congestion. When inhaled eucalyptus was evaluated in human patients, the changes in nasal resistance were similar to those of breathing air alone (Burrow et al., 1983). Russian literature supports the use of eucalymine, a eucalyptus-based product, for the therapy of some sinusitis.

Dosage
For topical use, 30 ml oil is mixed with 500 ml of water.
For various uses, typical oral dosages include 0.05 to 0.2 ml (eucalyptol), 0.05 to 0.2 ml (eucalyptus oil), or 2 to 4 g (fluidextract).

Adverse reactions
CNS: delirium, dizziness, ***seizures*** (eucalyptus oil is a powerful convulsant).
EENT: miosis.
GI: epigastric burning, esophagitis (Sharara, 2000), nausea, vomiting.
Musculoskeletal: muscle weakness.
Respiratory: ***cyanosis.***

Interactions
None reported.

Contraindications and precautions
Eucalyptus oil is contraindicated in patients receiving hypoglycemic therapy and in pregnant or breast-feeding patients.

Bold italic type indicates that reaction may be life-threatening.

Special considerations

⚫ ALERT CNS, GI, and respiratory reactions can occur even with low doses.

⚫ ALERT Several sources suggest that eucalyptus oil is extremely toxic if ingested. Even topical application has produced toxicity in a 6-year-old girl, who presented with ataxia, slurred speech, muscle weakness, and progression to unconsciousness after widespread application of eucalyptus oil for urticaria (Darben et al., 1998).

- Advise the patient that the herb should be diluted before internal or external use.
- Instruct the patient to keep eucalyptus out of the reach of children and pets.
- Advise the pregnant or breast-feeding patient to avoid using eucalyptus.

Commentary

Although eucalyptus is widely consumed, few clinical data support its claims. Data on the herb's antifungal and antimicrobial effects have not been evaluated in humans or animals; therefore, its use cannot be recommended. Eucalyptus oil should be kept out of the reach of children because of its potential for severe CNS and GI toxicity.

References

Burrow, A., et al. "The Effects of Camphor, Eucalyptus, and Menthol Vapors on Nasal Resistance to Airflow and Nasal Sensation," *Acta Otolaryngol* 96:157-61, 1983.

Darben, T., et al. "Topical Eucalyptus Oil Poisoning," *Australas J Dermatol* 39(4):265-67, 1998.

Egawa, H., et al. "Antifungal Substances Found in Leaves of Eucalyptus Species," *Specialia* 15:889-90, 1977.

Hong, C., et al. "Effects of a Topically Applied Counterirritant (Eucalyptamint) on Cutaneous Blood Flow and on the Skin and Muscle Temperature," *Am J Phys Med Rehabil* 70:29-33, 1991.

Juergens, U.R., et al. "Inhibition of Cytokine Production and Arachadonic Acid Metabolism by Eucalyptol (1,8-cineole) in Human Blood Monocytes In Vitro," *Eur J Med Res* 3(11):508-10, 1998.

Pattnaik, S., et al. "Antibacterial and Antifungal Activity of Ten Essential Oils In Vitro," *Microbios* 86:237-46, 1996.

Santos, F., et al. "Mast Cell Involvement in the Rat Paw Oedema Response to 1,8-cineole, the Main Constituent of Eucalyptus and Rosemary Oils," *Eur J Pharmacol* 331:253-58, 1997.

Sharara, A.I. "Lozenge-induced Esophagitis," *Gastrointest Endosc* 51(5):622-23, 2000.

EYEBRIGHT

MEADOW EYEBRIGHT, RED EYEBRIGHT

Taxonomic class

Scrophulariaceae

Common trade names
None known.

Common forms
Available as capsules, infusion, and lotion and in eye makeup remover.

Source
Eyebright comes from *Euphrasia officinalis* (common name eyebright), an annual plant that grows to about 1 ft and is mainly found in Europe. Eyebright is odorless and has a bitter, salty taste.

Chemical components
Eyebright is composed of carbohydrates, iridoide monoterpenes, tannins, alkaloids, lignans, sterols, phenolic acids, caffeic acids, aucubin, flavonoid glycosides, amino acids, and a volatile fraction.

Actions
None of the plant's constituents exert significant therapeutic effect. Despite the claim that caffeic acid exerts bacteriostatic properties, this effect has not been scientifically documented. A study using extracts of *E. officinalis* in vitro revealed that eyebright exerts a significant cytotoxic effect (Trovato et al., 1996).

Reported uses
Eyebright has been claimed to be useful as a lotion or through internal consumption in the treatment of blepharitis and conjunctivitis. Other reported indications include eye fatigue, styes, disorders of muscular and nervous origin, cough, and hoarseness. No clinical trials have examined these claims.

Dosage
Traditional uses suggest the following doses:
For ophthalmic use, soak a pad in an infusion and apply to the eyes as a compress. As an eyewash, 5 to 10 gtt of tincture in water.
For oral consumption, an infusion can be prepared by steeping the plant in boiling water.

Adverse reactions
CNS: confusion, headache, insomnia, weakness.
EENT: nasal congestion, photophobia, redness and swelling of lid margins, sneezing, toothache, *violent pressure in the eyes with tearing, vision disturbances.*
GI: constipation.
GU: polyuria.
Respiratory: dyspnea.
Skin: pruritus, sweating.

Interactions
None reported.

Bold italic type indicates that reaction may be life-threatening.

Contraindications and precautions
Avoid using eyebright in pregnant or breast-feeding patients; effects are unknown.

Special considerations
- Monitor for adverse reactions, particularly during ophthalmic use.
- Advise the patient that this herb should not be used to treat ophthalmic conditions because of the risk of infection.
- Advise the patient to avoid using eyebright because of the risk of cytotoxic effects.
- Instruct the patient to report changes in vision and eye swelling, redness, or discharge.
- Advise the patient to wear sunglasses and avoid bright light.

Points of interest
- The plant has been used since the Middle Ages to treat bloodshot and irritated eyes. Its use for these conditions evolved because the flowers, which have spots and stripes, resemble bloodshot eyes.

Commentary
No evidence exists that eyebright is effective as an ophthalmic agent. The risk of ophthalmic infection is high with this product because preparations may not be sterile. Thus, eyebright cannot be recommended for use.

References
Gruenwald, J., et al. *PDR for Herbal Medicines.* Montvale, N.J.: Medical Economics Company, Inc., 1998.

Jellin, J.M., et al. *Natural Medicines Comprehensive Database.* Stockton, Calif.: Therapeutic Research Faculty, 1999.

Trovato, A., et al. "In Vitro Cytotoxic Effect of Some Medicinal Plants Containing Flavonoids," *Boll Chim Farm* 135:263-66, 1996.

FALSE UNICORN ROOT

BLAZING STAR, FAIRYWAND, HELONIAS DIOICA, STARWORT

Taxonomic class
Liliaceae

Common trade names
Multi-ingredient preparations: #22 F+ Female Plus, Alertis Compound, Atri-Fem-Reg, Atri-FM-H, Change-O-Life Formula, Cycla-Action, False Unicorn-Squaw Vine Virtue, Fem-H, Fem-mend Formula, Femtone, Femtrol, O.U.T (ovarian uterine tonic), Pregnancy-6 Formula, T-5W, T-endo, T-miss, Wild Yam–False Unicorn–Virtue

Common forms
Available as dried roots, chopped for decoction, liquid, and tincture and as a component of tablets used for menopausal symptoms.

Source
The drug is extracted from the root system of *Chamaelirium luteum* in autumn. The plant is native to North America, generally harvested from the wild, and seldom cultivated. It should not be confused with unicorn root *(Aletris farinosa)*.

Chemical components
The key constituents of false unicorn root are diosgenin and other steroidal saponins, the glycosides chamaelirin and helonin, and stearic and linoleic acids.

Actions
Claims for the pharmacologic activity of *C. luteum* include diuretic effects, uterine and ovarian tonic effects, and genitourinary stimulant activity. The steroidal saponins are claimed to stimulate the uterus, but animal studies fail to support any uterine stimulant effect.

Reported uses
False unicorn root has traditionally been promoted for menstrual and uterine problems, including ovarian cysts, menopause, threatened miscarriage, and vomiting from pregnancy, and to normalize hormones after contraceptive use. The presence of steroidal saponins in the drug is claimed to be effective as a uterine tonic in amenorrhea and dysmenorrhea, in hepatic dysfunction, and as a stimulant in genitourinary weakness (Grieve, 1996). It has also been used for digestive problems and as

an anthelmintic. No published clinical trials or other clinical evidence is available to support these claims.

Dosage
Traditional uses suggest the following doses:
For menopausal symptoms, 5 to 10 gtt of tincture P.O. four to six times daily. Or, if using a decoction, ½ cup P.O. b.i.d.

Adverse reactions
GI: nausea, vomiting (with oral consumption of large amounts of the herb).

Interactions
None reported.

Contraindications and precautions
Avoid using false unicorn root in pregnant or breast-feeding patients; effects are unknown. Also avoid its use in patients with infectious or inflammatory GI conditions.

Special considerations
• Inform the patient that reported beneficial effects of false unicorn root may take months to appear.
• Although no known chemical interactions have been reported in clinical studies, consideration must be given to the pharmacologic properties of the herbal product and the potential for exacerbation of the intended therapeutic effect of conventional drugs.
• Caution the patient not to self-treat symptoms of gynecologic problems before seeking appropriate medical evaluation because this may delay diagnosis of a serious medical condition.
• Advise the patient to consult a health care provider before using herbal preparations because a treatment that has been clinically researched and proved effective may be available.

Points of interest
• False unicorn root was listed as a uterine tonic and a diuretic in the U.S. National Formulary from 1916 to 1947.

Commentary
There is no documented evidence that false unicorn root is effective for conditions that affect the uterus and ovaries. The lack of animal and human data to support its claims and the unknown risks associated with its use limit its usefulness. This product cannot be recommended because of the lack of efficacy for any therapeutic indication.

References
Grieve, M. *A Modern Herbal.* New York: Barnes & Noble, Inc., 1996.

FENNEL

ANETH FENOUIL, BITTER FENNEL, BRONZE *FOENICULUM
VULGARE* "RUBRUM," CAROSELLA, COMMON FENNEL,
FENCHEL, FENOUIL, FENOUILLE, FINOCCHIO, FLORENCE
FENNEL, FUNCHO, GARDEN FENNEL, HINOJO, LARGE
FENNEL, SWEET FENNEL, WILD FENNEL

Taxonomic class
Apiaceae

Common trade names
Bitter Fennel, Fennel Herb Tea, Sweet Fennel

Common forms
Capsules: 455 mg
Volatile oil in water: 2% (Sweet Fennel), 4% (Bitter Fennel)
   Also available as essential oil, seeds, teas, and tinctures.

Source
Fennel oil is usually obtained from the seeds of *Foeniculum vulgare*. The
plant is native to Europe and now also found in parts of Asia and Egypt.
The root of this plant is also considered useful.

Chemical components
The seeds of *F. vulgare* contain 2% to 6% volatile oil, 20% fixed oil
(composed of petroselinic acid, oleic acid, and linoleic acid), and high
concentrations of tocopherols. Other components of the seeds include
flavonoids, umbelliferone, kaempferols, stigmasterol, proteins, sugars,
vitamins, and minerals. The herb has a high potassium and calcium
content. The volatile oil consists of anethol, fenchone, estragole, limonene, camphene, and alpha-pinene. Other components of the herb include monoterpene hydrocarbons, sabinene, alpha-phellandrene, myrcene, terpinenes, terpinolene, fenchyl alcohol, anisaldehyde, and myristicin apiole.

Actions
Fennel and its volatile oil are reported to have antiflatulent and stimulant properties. Fennel oil with methylparaben has been shown to inhibit the growth of *Salmonella enteriditis* and, to a lesser extent, *Listeria
monocytogenes* (Fyfe et al., 1997). The oil inhibited the twitch response
in smooth muscle and tracheal and ileal muscles in guinea pigs (Lis-
Balchin and Hart, 1997). Aqueous fennel extracts increase ciliary function of frog epithelium. An acetone extract of fennel seeds produced an
estrogenic effect on the genital organs of male and female rats (Malini
et al., 1985).
   Anethole has been found to inhibit tumor necrosis factor–induced
cellular responses (Chainy et al., 2000), and it is theorized that this action may suppress both inflammation and carcinogenesis. Further studies are needed to determine the clinical significance of this finding.

Bold italic type indicates that reaction may be life-threatening.

Reported uses
Despite fennel's claims to increase milk secretion, promote menses, facilitate birth, and increase libido, human data are lacking. Fennel has also been used historically to treat colic, indigestion, and irritable bowel syndrome.

Dosage
Traditional uses suggest the following doses:
For GI complaints, 0.1 to 0.6 ml P.O. daily of the oil, or 5 to 7 g daily of the fruit.
Tea: 2 to 3 g of fennel seeds steeped in 8 oz of water.
Tincture: 2 to 4 ml P.O. t.i.d.

Adverse reactions
CNS: *seizures.*
GI: nausea, vomiting.
Respiratory: pulmonary edema (rare).
Skin: contact dermatitis, photodermatitis.
Other: tumors (an essential oil component, estragole, has caused tumors in animals).

Interactions
Ciprofloxacin: Fennel significantly decreased the bioavailability of ciprofloxacin when administered concurrently in rats (Zhu et al., 1999); further studies are needed to determine the extent of this effect in humans. Maintain adequate dosing interval.

Contraindications and precautions
The use of fennel is not recommended in patients with estrogen-dependent cancers because anethole and other terpenoids found in fennel are believed to possess estrogen-like activity (Albert-Puleo, 1980).

Also avoid its use in pregnant patients. Use cautiously in patients who are hypersensitive to other members of the Apiaceae family, such as celery, carrots, and mugwort.

Special considerations
• Inform the patient that this herb cannot be recommended for any use because of insufficient evidence.
• Inform the patient that the long-term risks of fennel use are unknown.
• Advise the patient to avoid sun exposure if photodermatitis occurs.
• Advise the pregnant or breast-feeding patient to avoid using fennel.
🕭 **ALERT** The fennel plant may be mistaken for poison hemlock, which contains the strong narcotic coniine. Ingestion of a small amount of hemlock causes vomiting, paralysis, and death. Inform the patient who may attempt to harvest this plant in the wild to avoid mistakenly retrieving poison hemlock.

Points of interest
• Fennel is used as a flavoring in liquors, baked goods, meat products, snacks, and gravies, and as a food. The highest concentration of fennel

oil in foods cannot exceed 0.119%. In soaps, lotions, and perfumes, the maximum is 0.4%.

Commentary

Because of a lack of clinical data, fennel cannot be recommended as treatment for any condition, although possibilities exist for further study.

References

Albert-Puleo, M., "Fennel and Anise as Estrogenic Agents," *J Ethnopharm* 2(4):337-44, 1980.

Chainy, G.B., et al. "Anethole Blocks Both Early and Late Cellular Responses Transduced by Tumor Necrosis Factor: Effect on NF-kappaB, AP-1, JNK, MAPKK, and Apoptosis," *Oncogene* 19(25):2943-50, 2000.

Fyfe, L., et al. "Inhibition of *Listeria monocytogenes* and *Salmonella enteriditis* by Combinations of Plant Oils and Derivatives of Benzoic Acid: The Development of Synergistic Antimicrobial Combinations," *Int J Antimicrob Agents* 9:195-99, 1997.

Lis-Balchin, M., and Hart, S. "A Preliminary Study of the Effect of Essential Oils on Skeletal and Smooth Muscle In Vitro," *J Ethnopharmacol* 58:183-87, 1997.

Malini, T., et al. "The Effects of *Foeniculum vulgare* Mill Seed Extract on the Genital Organs of Male and Female Rats," *Indian J Physiol Pharmacol* 29:21, 1985.

Zhu, M., et al. "Effect of Oral Administration of Fennel (*Foeniculum vulgare*) on Ciprofloxacin Absorption and Disposition in the Rat," *J Pharm Pharmacol* 52(12):1391-96, 1999.

FENUGREEK

BIRD'S-FOOT, FENIGREEK, GREEK HAY, GREEK HAY SEED, TRIGONELLA

Taxonomic class

Fabaceae

Common trade names

Fenugreek Seed, Fenu-Thyme

Common forms

Available as a crude drug, extracts in liquid and spray, dried forms, a poultice, seeds in a dried powder or capsules, tablets, and teas.

Source

Fenugreek, or *Trigonella foenum-graecum*, is native to countries on the eastern shores of the Mediterranean. The plant is cultivated in India, Egypt, Morocco, and, occasionally, England. The medicinally active component of fenugreek is found exclusively in the seeds, which are contained in sicklelike pods comprising 10 to 20 brown seeds.

Chemical components

The seeds contain saponins (diosgenin, tigogenin, gitogenin, trigogenin, yamogenin, neotigogenin, fenugreekine, neogitogenin, smilagenin), alkaloids (trigonelline, gentianine, carpaine, choline), proteins, and amino acids (lysine, tryptophan, 4-hydroxyisoleucine, histidine, and arginine). Other components include coumarin, mucilage fiber, vitamins (including nicotinic acid), minerals, and lipids.

Actions

Hypocholesterolemic activity in rats and dogs has been attributed to the fiber and saponin components of the seeds. Nicotinic acid, in unknown amounts in the seeds, is thought to contribute to lowering cholesterol levels. Most studies report a reduction of total cholesterol and triglyceride levels, but the extent of reduction varied.

Fenugreek has been shown to exert hypoglycemic effects in rabbits, rats, and dogs. The saponin fenugreekine and the amino acid 4-hydroxyisoleucine have been reported to possess hypoglycemic effects (Broca et al., 1999, 2000; Sauvaire et al., 1998). Fenugreekine may also possess antihypertensive, antiviral, cardiotonic, and diuretic properties.

Aqueous and alcoholic extracts of fenugreek have shown a stimulant action on the uterus of guinea pigs, especially late in pregnancy. Aqueous extracts have also been found to increase heart rate and exert antiinflammatory and diuretic activity in animals (Newall et al., 1996). Fenugreek extracts may decrease calcium oxalate deposition in the kidneys (Ahsan et al., 1989).

The effects of fenugreek seed extract on serum thyroid hormone levels were studied in rats and mice. The findings suggest that fenugreek supplementation decreased serum triiodothyronine (T_3) levels and T_3-T_4 ratio but increased serum thyroxine (T_4) levels and body weight (Panda et al., 1999).

Reported uses

Fenugreek has traditionally been used to treat anorexia, constipation, dyspepsia, gastritis, and other related GI conditions. Topical formulations have been used for leg ulcers, myalgia, gout, wounds, and lymphadenitis. Additional claims include use as an antidiabetic agent and as a treatment for cellulitis and tuberculosis. These claims await verification from clinical trials.

Dosage

Traditional uses suggest the following doses:
Powdered drug: 50 g to ¼ L of water applied topically.
Seeds: 1 to 6 g P.O. t.i.d.

Adverse reactions

Hematologic: *bleeding*, bruising.
Metabolic: hypoglycemia.
Skin: allergic reactions (Patil et al., 1997).

Interactions

Anticoagulants: May increase hypoprothrombinemic effect of these drugs. Avoid administration with fenugreek.
Antidiabetic drugs: May increase glucose-lowering effects. Dosage adjustments may be needed during herbal treatment.

Other oral drugs: Decreased absorption. Separate administration of doses by at least 2 hours.

Contraindications and precautions
Avoid using fenugreek in pregnant patients because of the risk of oxytocic action.

Special considerations
◤ **ALERT** Monitor coagulation studies and blood glucose levels in patients at high risk, especially in those who consume large quantities of the plant.
- Monitor the patient for signs of bleeding.
- Advise the patient to report loss of efficacy of other drugs.
- Instruct the patient to self-monitor blood glucose levels until the fenugreek's hypoglycemic effects are known.
- Teach the patient how to recognize the signs and symptoms of hypoglycemia.
- Instruct the patient to report unusual bleeding or bruising.
- Advise the patient taking fenugreek for its effects on blood glucose and serum cholesterol levels that other effective pharmacologic agents with known morbidity and mortality data exist.

Points of interest
- In the United States, fenugreek is categorized by the FDA as generally recommended as safe at concentrations below 0.05%.
- The taste and odor of fenugreek resemble those of maple syrup. In the past, fenugreek was added to liquid medicinals to mask their taste. A child receiving fenugreek tea was noted to have urine that smelled like maple syrup. This symptom mimics one found in a rare hereditary metabolic disorder, branched-chain hyperaminoaciduria, otherwise known as maple syrup urine disease.

Commentary
Although fenugreek may hold promise for use in diabetes or hypercholesterolemia, data regarding dosage, efficacy, and safety have not been established for humans or compared with existing pharmacologic agents with proven beneficial effects. Large-scale clinical trials evaluating morbidity and mortality are needed before the herb can be recommended.

References
Ahsan, S.K., et al. "Effect of *Trigonella foenum-graecum* and *Ammi majus* on Calcium Oxalate Urolithiasis in Rats," *J Ethnopharmacol* 26:249, 1989.
Broca, C., et al. "4-Hydroxyisoleucine: Experimental Evidence of Its Insulintropic and Antidiabetic Properties," *Am J Physiol* 227(4):617-23, 1999.
Broca, C., et al. "4-Hydroxyisoleucine: Effects of Synthetic and Natural Analogues on Insulin Secretion," *Eur J Pharmacol* 390(3):339-45, 2000.
Newall, C.A., et al. *Herbal Medicines. A Guide for Health-Care Professionals.* London: The Pharmaceutical Press, 1996.
Panda, S., et al. "Inhibition of Triiodothyronine Production by Fenugreek Seed Extract in Mice and Rats," *Pharmacol Res* 40(5):405-9, 1999.

Patil, S.P., et al. "Allergy to Fenugreek (*Trigonella foenum graecum*)," *Ann Allergy Asthma Immunol* 78(3):297-300, 1997.

Ravikumar, P., and Anuradha, C.V. "Effect of Fenugreek Seeds on Blood Lipid Peroxidation and Antioxidants in Diabetic Rats," *Phytother Res*, 13(3):197-201, 1999.

Sauvaire, Y., et al. "4-Hydoxyisoleucine," *Diabetes* 47(2):206-11, 1998.

FEVERFEW

ALTAMISA, BACHELORS' BUTTON, CHAMOMILE GRANDE, FEATHERFEW, FEATHERFOIL, FEBRIFUGE PLANT, MIDSUMMER DAISY, MUTTERKRAUT, NOSEBLEED, SANTA MARIA, WILD CHAMOMILE, WILD QUININE

Taxonomic class
Asteraceae

Common trade names
Feverfew, Feverfew Glyc, Feverfew Power, Tanacet

Common forms
Available as capsules (pure leaf, 380 mg; leaf extract, 250 mg), liquid, and tablets. The leaves are commonly used to make infusions or teas.

Source
Feverfew, a plant from Europe naturalized in the United States and Canada, bears yellow-green leaves and yellow flowers from July to October. The leaves of the plant are usually dried or used fresh in teas and extracts. The most commonly cited botanical name is *Chrysanthemum parthenium*, synonymous with *Tanacetum parthenium*. *Matricaria parthenium*, *Leucanthemum parthenium*, and *Pyrethrum parthenium* are also used to refer to the plant.

Chemical components
The leaves and flowering tops of feverfew contain many monoquiterpenes and sesquiterpenes as well as sesquiterpene lactones (chrysanthemolide, chrysanthemonin, 10-epi-canin, magnoliolide, and parthenolide), reynosin, santamarin, tanaparthins, and other compounds. Parthenolide may be absent or occur in variable amounts, depending on geographic and other variables. Interestingly, melatonin has been found in significant quantities in both the feverfew plant and commercial feverfew products. Fresh green feverfew leaf contains 2.45 mcg/g of melatonin, whereas the freeze-dried leaf contains 1.61 mcg/g of melatonin (Murch et al., 1997).

Actions
The main active ingredients are the sesquiterpene lactones, particularly parthenolide, which inhibits serotonin release by human platelets in vitro. This may be the mechanism of action for feverfew's purported efficacy in treating migraine headaches (Groenewegen and Heptinstall, 1990). Parthenolide also inhibits serotonin release (Heptinstall et al., 1992) and has demonstrated significant cytostatic activity toward mouse fibrosar-

coma (MN-11) and human lymphoma (TK6; Ross et al., 1999). Extracts of feverfew contain several chemicals that inhibit activation of polymorphonuclear leukocytes and the synthesis of prostaglandins and leukotrienes (by way of inhibition of the cyclooxygenase and 5-lipoxygenase pathways; Williams et al., 1999). In murine studies, anti-inflammatory and antinociceptive effects have been documented for both feverfew extract and parthenolide (Jain and Kulkarni, 1999).

Reported uses
Although the initial enthusiasm for feverfew has waned, plant preparations are again becoming increasingly popular for use in migraine prophylaxis and as an antipyretic. (See *Feverfew and migraine prophylaxis.*) A detailed and systematic review of all trials of feverfew for migraine prevention published before mid-1998 failed to find sufficient evidence to support the use of feverfew in this regard (Vogler et al., 1998).

Feverfew is also claimed to be useful for treating asthma, insect bites, menstrual problems, threatened miscarriage, psoriasis, rheumatism, stomachache, and toothache. These uses have not been assessed in human trials.

Dosage
For migraine prophylaxis, 25 mg of freeze-dried leaf extract P.O. daily; 50 mg of leaf P.O. daily with food; or 50 to 200 mg of aerial parts of plant P.O. daily.
For migraine treatment, average dose of 543 mcg P.O. parthenolide daily.

Adverse reactions
EENT: mouth ulcers (common with teas and whole-herb preparations). **Other:** *hypersensitivity reactions,* post-feverfew syndrome (withdrawal syndrome characterized by moderate to severe pain, joint and muscle stiffness, and anxiety; Johnson et al., 1985).

Interactions
None reported.

Contraindications and precautions
Feverfew is contraindicated in pregnant or breast-feeding women.

Special considerations
• Monitor for allergic reaction.
• Monitor for mouth ulcers. Encourage the patient to exercise proper oral hygiene.
• Feverfew potency is often based on the parthenolide content in the preparation, which is variable.
• Instruct the patient not to withdraw the herb abruptly but to taper its use gradually because of the risk of post-feverfew syndrome.
• Inform the patient that several other strategies for migraine treatment and prophylaxis exist and that they should be attempted before taking products with unknown benefits and risks.

Bold italic type indicates that reaction may be life-threatening.

RESEARCH FINDINGS
Feverfew and migraine prophylaxis

The efficacy of feverfew for migraine prophylaxis has been assessed in a randomized, double-blind, placebo-controlled clinical trial (Murphy et al., 1988). The study included 76 patients with classic or common migraine headaches for longer than 2 years and at least one attack monthly. All other migraine treatments were discontinued before the trial began. After a 1-month, single-blind, placebo run-in period, the patients were randomized to receive one capsule daily of either placebo or feverfew for 4 months. At that time, the patients were crossed over to the other treatment arm of the study. Patients recorded the number, duration, and severity of each migraine attack. Working days missed, nausea, vomiting, and visual or neurologic effects were noted in their diaries.

Of the 76 patients enrolled, 59 patients completed the trial. The number of attacks during feverfew treatment was reduced by 24% compared with placebo. There was no significant difference in the duration of migraine attacks between the herb and placebo. Nausea and vomiting were reduced significantly with feverfew treatment. The number of working days missed with herbal therapy was 68, whereas that for placebo was 76.

At the end of the study but while still blinded to the therapy received, 59% of patients reported that the feverfew treatment period was more effective; only 24% chose placebo. No significant differences between the two treatments were noted in 17% of patients.

• Encourage the patient to promptly report unusual symptoms, such as mouth sores and skin ulcerations.
• Commercial feverfew products are likely to contain small amounts of melatonin.

Points of interest
• The concentration of parthenolide in the leaves and flowering tops is highest during the summer, before the seeds are set, and drops rapidly thereafter. This has been offered as an explanation for the difference in parthenolide levels between brands of feverfew capsules and tablets.
• The Health Protection Branch of the Canadian government has proposed a standard that formulations contain a minimum of 0.2% parthenolide.

Commentary
Although feverfew has been shown to be effective for migraine prophylaxis in at least two clinical trials, further studies are needed to define bet-

ter dosage guidelines and specific drug interactions and mechanisms of action. For patients in whom standard drug therapy has failed, feverfew may be an agent that can prevent migraine attacks. Although standardized feverfew preparations with dosages based on free parthenolide content have the best experimental support, no consensus on use exists. The presence of melatonin in feverfew and other botanicals emphasizes the need for complete biochemical characterization of herbal medicinals.

References

Groenewegen, W.A., and Heptinstall, S. "A Comparison of the Effects of an Extract of Feverfew and Parthenolide, a Component of Feverfew, on Human Platelet Activity In Vitro," *J Pharm Pharmacol* 43:553-57, 1990.

Heptinstall, S., et al. "Parthenolide Content and Bioactivity of Feverfew (*Tanacetum parthenium* [L.] Schultz-Bip.). Estimation of Commercial and Authenticated Feverfew Products," *J Pharm Pharmacol* 44:391-95, 1992.

Jain, N.K., and Kulkarni, S.K. "Antinociceptive and Anti-inflammatory Effects of *Tanacetum parthenium* Extract in Mice and Rats," *J Ethnopharmacol* 68(1-3):251-59, 1999.

Murch, S.J., et al. "Melatonin in Feverfew and Other Medicinal Plants," (Letter) *Lancet* 350:1598-99, 1997.

Murphy, J.J., et al. "Randomised, Double-Blind, Placebo-Controlled Trial of Feverfew in Migraine Prevention," *Lancet* 2:189-92, 1988.

Ross, J.J., et al. "Low Concentrations of the Feverfew Component Parthenolide Inhibit In Vitro Growth of Tumor Lines in a Cytostatic Fashion," *Planta Med* 65(2):126-29, 1999.

Vogler, B.K., et al. "Feverfew as a Preventive Treatment for Migraine: A Systematic Review," *Cephalgia* 18(10):704-8, 1998.

Williams, C.A., et al. "The Flavonoids of *Tanacetum parthenium* and *T. vulgare* and Their Anti-inflammatory Properties," *Phytochemistry* 52(6):1181-82, 1999.

FIG

MORACEAE

Taxonomic class
Moraceae

Common trade names
None known.

Common forms
Extract of fruit or leaves and extract from the latex of leaves and stem.

Source
Active components are obtained from the fruit, leaves, or latex of *Ficus carica*, a deciduous tree that is indigenous to Asia Minor (western Asia), Syria, and Iran. It is cultivated in many subtropical regions.

Chemical components
Figs contain about 50% fruit sugars (mainly glucose), flavonoids, vitamins, and enzymes, as well as citric and malic acids. The latex from the leaves and stems contains an enzymatic protein called ficin.

Bold italic type indicates that reaction may be life-threatening.

Actions
Fig tree latex has been investigated as a possible anthelmintic in mice (Amorin et al., 1999). The results were disappointing, with no significant anthelmintic properties and a high degree of toxicity. The focus of fig tree research has been on its hypoglycemic and hypolipidemic effects. An extract of fig tree leaves was shown to have mild hypoglycemic effects in streptozocin-diabetic rats (Perez et al., 1996). Fig tree leaf extract also had mild hypolipidemic effects in streptozocin-diabetic rats (Dominguez et al., 1996). Animal studies have also been completed in diabetes treatment.

Reported uses
The dried fruit has been used as a gentle laxative for mild constipation. The pulp of the fruit is claimed to relieve pain and inflammation, although no studies support this claim. The roasted fruit has also been claimed to treat tumors, swellings, and gum abscesses. Figs have been purported to have mild expectorant properties, once again without clinical support. The stem latex was used as an anthelmintic in the late 1800s, but toxicity and lack of efficacy led to diminished use. Fig leaf extract has been reported to decrease blood glucose levels in diabetic patients. Serraclara and others (1998) conducted a trial in 10 diabetic patients. Eight patients completed the trial, and it was found that the four who had taken the fig leaf extract had lower blood glucose levels than the four who took a commercial tea extract.

Dosage
As a laxative, one or two fruits taken as needed.
In the diabetes trial, a decoction (boiling one 13-g sachet of leaf for 15 minutes and then filtering) was taken every morning before the insulin dose.

Adverse reactions
GI: *GI bleeding* (if stem latex is ingested).
Skin: photosensitivity.

Interactions
None reported.

Contraindications and precautions
Oral ingestion of leaf and stem latex may cause severe GI bleeding. Safety in pregnant or breast-feeding women has not been evaluated, and its use is not recommended.

Special considerations
• Advise the patient to consult a health care provider before using herbal preparations because a treatment that has been clinically researched and proved effective may be available.
• Monitor the patient for GI bleeding.
• Instruct the patient to report intestinal bleeding or dark stools to health care provider.

- Advise the patient to take precautions with exposure to sunlight.
- Although no known chemical interactions have been reported in clinical studies, consideration must be given to the pharmacologic properties of the herbal product and the potential for exacerbation of the intended therapeutic effect of conventional drugs.
- Urge the patient to notify the prescriber and pharmacist of any herbal or dietary supplement he is taking when filling a new prescription.

Commentary
Ingestion of the fruit appears to be safe but offers little therapeutic benefit except as a mild laxative. Its use in diabetes needs further investigation in controlled clinical human trials before it can be recommended for this indication, and its role in lowering lipid levels is awaiting human trials. Overall, fig tree fruit and leaf extract appears safe, but the latex from the stem must be used cautiously. There are not enough data to recommend any therapeutic use of fig tree.

References
Amorin, A., et al. "Anthelmintic Activity of the Latex of *Ficus* Species," *J Ethnopharmacology* 64:255-58, 1999.

Dominguez, E., et al. "Hypolipidemic Activity of *Ficus carica* Leaf Extract in Streptozocin-Diabetic Rats," *Phytother Res* 10:526-28, 1996.

Perez, C., et.al. "A Study on the Glycemic Balance in Streptozocin-Diabetic Rats Treated with an Aqueous Extract of *Ficus carica* (Fig Tree) Leaves," *Phytother Res* 10:82-83, 1996.

Serraclara, A., et al. "Hypoglycemic Action of an Oral Fig-leaf Decoction in Type-I Diabetic Patients," *Diabetic Res Clin Prac* 39:19-22, 1998.

FIGWORT

CARPENTER'S-SQUARE, COMMON FIGWORT, ROSE-NOBLE, SCROFULA PLANT, SQUARE STALK, STINKING CHRISTOPHER, THROATWORT

Taxonomic class
Scrophulariaceae

Common trade names
None known.

Common forms
Available as a compress, liquid extract, soak, tincture, wash, or whole herb.

Source
Figwort is most commonly derived from *Scrophularia nodosa* and *Scrophularia ningpoensis*. Medicinal components are removed from the dried leaves and flowers. The root has also been used, principally in China.

Chemical components
Figwort consists of the amino acids alanine, isoleucine, leucine, lysine, phenylalanine, threonine, tyrosine, and valine. It also contains flavo-

---

Bold italic type indicates that reaction may be life-threatening.

noids (diosmetin, diosmin, acacetin rhamnoside, iridoids, aucubin, acetylharpagide, harpagide, harpagoside, isoharpagoside, procumbid, and catalpol), caffeic acid, cinnamic acid, ferulic acid, sinapic acid, and vanillic acid. Also present are saponins, cardioactive glycosides, phytosterols, essential fatty acids, and aspargine.

Actions
Figwort appears to possess antibacterial and anti-inflammatory properties, although the mechanism of action has not been described. Aucubin and catalpol exert cathartic action in rodents (Inouye et al., 1974). Figwort is related to foxglove, which contains digitalis-like glycosides and contains chemicals that strengthen the force of cardiac contraction and slow the heart rate.

Reported uses
Figwort is believed to be useful for eczema, psoriasis, pruritus, and other chronic skin conditions. Additional claims involve the agent's use as an anti-inflammatory, a cardiac stimulant, and an agent for GI disorders. No human trials have investigated these claims.

Dosage
Traditional uses suggest the following doses:
Infusion: 2 to 8 g of dried herb P.O.
Liquid extract: 2 to 8 ml P.O.
Tincture: 2 to 4 ml P.O.
   Dosage frequency is unknown.

Adverse reactions
CV: *asystole, bradycardia,* heart block.
GI: diarrhea, nausea, vomiting.

Interactions
Beta blockers, calcium channel blockers, cardiac glycosides: May increase cardiac effects of these drugs. Avoid administration with figwort.

Contraindications and precautions
Avoid using figwort in pregnant and breast-feeding patients; safety has not been established. Use it cautiously in patients with underlying heart disease or in those at risk for arrhythmias.

Special considerations
• Monitor heart rate and rhythm.
• Inform the patient that scientific evidence supporting use of figwort is lacking.
• Instruct the patient to immediately report changes in heart rate, lightheadedness, weakness, and shortness of breath.
• Caution the patient with underlying heart disease or at risk for arrhythmias against using figwort.
• Advise the pregnant or breast-feeding patient to avoid using figwort.

Points of interest
- Figwort is not known to be a component of any food.
- The chemical components of figwort resemble those of devil's claw (*Harpagophytum procumbens*).

Commentary
Literature supporting any use of this plant is lacking. Figwort should not be used by any patient, especially one with heart disease.

References
Inouye, H., et al. "Purgative Activities of Iridoid Glucosides," *Planta Med* 25:285-88, 1974.

FLAX

FLAXSEED, LINSEED, LINT BELLS, LINUM

Taxonomic class
Linaceae

Common trade names
Barlean's Flax Oil, Barlean's Vita-Flax, Flaxseed

Common forms
Available as capsules, powder, softgel capsules (1,000 mg), oil, and seeds.

Source
Flaxseed is the soluble fiber mucilage obtained from the fully developed seed of *Linum usitatissimum* and is sometimes used in poultices.

Chemical components
Flaxseed and flaxseed oil (linseed oil) are rich (30% to 45%) in unsaturated fatty acids, including linolenic, linoleic, and oleic acids. About 3% to 6% of the plant contains soluble fiber mucilage consisting of galactose, arabinose, rhamnose, xylose, galactuonic, and mannuronic acids. Seed chaff and leaves contain cyanogenic glycosides, linamarin, linustatin, and nicolenustatin. Linamarase can potentiate cyanide release from linamarin. The plant also contains 25% protein. Some products contain additional essential fatty acids, fiber, vitamins, and minerals.

Actions
Flaxseed is a rich source of plant lignans and is reported to have weak antiestrogenic, estrogenic, and steroidlike activity. Diets high in flaxseed may lower the risk of breast and other hormone-dependent cancers, but this premise awaits clinical confirmation (Thompson et al., 1997). A review focuses on the therapeutic potential of these phytoestrogens found in flaxseed (and soybeans) and the epidemiological, laboratory, and clinical evidence surrounding application for their use (Brzezinski and Debi, 1999).

Bold italic type indicates that reaction may be life-threatening.

Flaxseed supplementation in 28 postmenopausal women significantly increased urinary excretion of certain estrogen metabolites in a linear, dose-repsonse manner (Haggans et al., 1999).

In humans, linolenic acid decreases total cholesterol and LDL levels. One study in humans noted a decrease in thrombin-mediated platelet aggregation (Bierenbaum et al., 1993).

Reported uses

Flax has been used for constipation, functional disorders of the colon resulting from laxative abuse, irritable bowel syndrome, and diverticulitis. Externally, flax has been made into a poultice and used to treat areas of local inflammation.

Flaxseed muffins were evaluated for their potential in treating hyperlipidemia (Jenkins et al., 1999). A randomized, crossover trial was conducted of 29 patients with hyperlipidemia who ingested either flaxseed muffins (50 g of partially defatted flaxseed per day) or wheat bran muffins (control) for two 3-week treatment periods. Also, all subjects followed NCEP step II diets. On average, the flax muffins reduced total cholesterol levels by 4.6%, LDL levels by 7.6%, apolipoprotein B levels by 5.4%, and apolipoprotein A_1 levels by 5.8% (all $P \leq .001$), while having no effect on HDL levels, as compared with the control group.

Another study determined that linolenic acid supplement, derived from flax, arginine, and yeast RNA, improved weight gain in some patients with HIV infection (Suttman et al., 1996).

Dosage

For all systemic uses, 1 to 2 tbsp of oil or mature seeds daily P.O. in divided doses b.i.d. or t.i.d. Average dose is 1 oz of oil or mature seeds daily.

For topical use, 30 to 50 g of flax meal applied as a hot, moist poultice or compress as needed.

Adverse reactions

GI: diarrhea, flatulence, nausea.

Other: *anaphylaxis.*

Interactions

Laxatives, stool softeners: May increase laxative actions of flax. Avoid administration with flax.

Oral drugs: May diminish absorption of oral drugs. Separate doses by at least 2 hours.

Contraindications and precautions

Flaxseed is contraindicated in pregnant or breast-feeding patients because its hormonal effects may cause teratogenicity or spontaneous abortion. Avoid its use in patients with prostate cancer or suspected or actual ileus.

Special considerations

ALERT Immature seedpods are especially poisonous. All parts of the plant contain cyanogenic nitrates and glucosides, particularly linamarin. Overdose symptoms include but are not limited to shortness of breath, tachypnea, weakness, and unstable gait, progressing to paralysis and seizures.

• Monitor for potential toxicity related to oral ingestion of flax; cyanosis is a symptom of flax toxicity.

• Encourage the patient to drink plenty of fluids to minimize the risk of flatulence.

• Instruct the patient to refrigerate flaxseed oil to prevent breakdown of the essential fatty acids.

• Inform the patient that other cholesterol-lowering therapies exist that have been proven to improve survival and lower the risk of cardiac disease; flax has no such clinical support.

• Instruct the patient not to ingest immature seeds and to keep flax out of the reach of children and pets.

• Inform the patient that the long-term risks of flax use are unknown.

• Encourage the patient to report decreased effects of other drugs being taken.

Points of interest

• Flax has been used as a source of fiber for weaving and clothing for more than 10,000 years. Linseed oil, derived from flax, has been used in paints and varnishes and as a waterproofing agent. Flaxseed cakes are used as a food source for cattle.

Commentary

Supplementation of flax as a source of omega-3 fatty acids and its value in the treatment of inflammatory diseases warrant further investigation. Of particular interest are the phytoestrogens contained in flaxseed and their potential for therapeutic application in breast cancer, lipid disorders, and postmenopausal conditions. The potentially toxic components (cyanogenic nitrates) and the potential mutagenic effect of flax require further study to determine if its long-term safety profile would offset any potential benefit on morbidity and mortality. Additional clinical trial data are needed before definitive recommendations for its consumption can be made.

References

Bierenbaum, M.L., et al. "Reducing Atherogenic Risk in Hyperlipidemic Humans with Flax Seed Supplementation: A Preliminary Report," *J Am Coll Nutr* 12:501, 1993.

Brzezinski, A., and Debi, A. "Phytoestrogens: The Natural Selective Estrogen Receptor Modulators?" *Eur J Obstet Gynecol Reprod Biol* 85(1):47-51, 1999.

Dobelis, I.N., ed. *Magic and Medicine of Plants*. Pleasantville, N.Y.: The Reader's Digest Association, Inc., 1986.

Haggans, C.J., et al. "Effect of Flaxseed Consumption on Urinary Estrogen Metabolites in Postmenopausal Women," *Nutr Cancer* 33(2):188-95, 1999.

Bold italic type indicates that reaction may be life-threatening.

Jenkins, D.J., et al. "Health Aspects of Partially Defatted Flaxseed, Including Effects on Serum Lipids, Oxidative Measures, and Ex Vivo Androgen and Progestin Activity: A Controlled Crossover Trial," *Am J Clin Nutr* 69(3):395-402, 1999.

Suttman, U., et al. "Weight Gain and Increased Concentrations of Receptor Proteins for Tumor Necrosis Factor After Patients with Symptomatic HIV Infection Received Fortified Nutrition Support," *J Am Diet Assoc* 96:565-69, 1996.

Thompson, L.U., et al. "Variability in Anticancer Lignan Levels in Flaxseed," *Nutr Cancer* 27:26-30, 1997.

FUMITORY

EARTH SMOKE, HEDGE FUMITORY, WAX DOLLS

Taxonomic class
Fumariaceae

Common trade names
Elusan Digest

Common forms
Capsules.

Source
Fumitory comes from the leaves and aerial parts of the *Fumaria officinalis* plant, which is native to Europe and North Africa but is also grown in Asia, North America, and Australia.

Chemical components
Fumitory contains many alkaloids, including protopine (also known as fumarine, an isoquinoline derivative), aurotensine, coridaline, cryptopine, stylopine, cryptocavine, sinactine, *n*-methylsinactine sanquinarine, and bulbocapnine.

Fumitory also contains fumaric acid salts (fumaricine, fumariline, fumaritine), phlobaphene, yellow dye, flavonoids, quercetin and isoquercetin-related compounds, benzophenanthridines, chlorogenic acids, caffeic and fumaric acids, mucilage, resinous substances, and other compounds.

Actions
In animals, fumitory extracts exhibit antibacterial action, vasodilating properties, antispasmodic activity on smooth muscle, positive inotropic effects, a moderate hypotensive effect, modulation of bile flow, and inhibition of biliary calculus formation. Also, the predominant alkaloid, protopine, has antihistaminic and sedative effects at low doses and stimulatory and convulsive activity at higher doses (Preininger, 1975). Cryptopine and protopine, when isolated, exert negative chronotropic effects in vitro.

Reported uses
Various therapeutic claims have been made for fumitory, including as a treatment for dermatologic eruptions (milk crust, eczema, and scabies)

and as a diuretic and a laxative. None of the data supporting these claims have been published in English. Clinical case reports and animal studies have suggested the usefulness of fumitory in treating functional diseases of the biliary system, although no placebo-controlled studies have been conducted (Hentschel et al., 1995). A Russian report noted that injections of fumitory alkaloids were effective in resolving myocardial ischemia and arrhythmias caused by reversible coronary blood flow disorders (Gorbunov et al., 1980).

Dosage
Traditional uses suggest the following doses:
Dried herb: 2 to 4 g P.O. t.i.d., or a tea with 2 to 4 g of the dried herb P.O. t.i.d.
Liquid extract (1:1 in 25% alcohol): 2 to 4 ml P.O. t.i.d.
Tincture (1:5 in 45% alcohol): 1 to 4 ml P.O. t.i.d.

Adverse reactions
CNS: sedation, ***seizures*** (at high or toxic doses).
CV: ***bradycardia***, hypotension.
EENT: elevated intraocular pressure.

Interactions
Antihypertensives: May increase hypotensive effect. Avoid administration with fumitory.
Beta blockers, calcium channel blockers, digoxin, other drugs that slow the heart rate: May cause bradycardia, heart block, or asystole. Avoid administration with fumitory.

Contraindications and precautions
Fumitory is contraindicated in patients with glaucoma, in those at risk for seizures, and in pregnant or breast-feeding patients.

Special considerations
• Monitor intraocular pressure in patients who are at risk for glaucoma.
• Monitor heart rate and blood pressure.
• Inform the patient who is at risk for seizures that although not reported in humans, studies with animals suggest that high doses or prolonged use of fumitory or protopine may exacerbate seizure disorders.
• Encourage the patient to report light-headedness, weakness, shortness of breath, and changes in heart rate.
• Advise the pregnant or breast-feeding patient to avoid using fumitory.
• The German Commission E considers *F. officinalis* approved for the indication of "colicky pain affecting the gallbladder and biliary system, together with the gastrointestinal tract."

Commentary
Fumitory has not been systematically evaluated in humans. Data from studies with animals are limited. Safety and efficacy for any use remain unproven.

Bold italic type indicates that reaction may be life-threatening.

References

Gorbunov, N.P., et al. "Pharmacological Correction of Myocardial Ischemia and Arrhythmias in Reversible Coronary Blood Flow Disorders and Experimental Myocardial Infarct in Dogs," *Kardiologiia* 20:84-87, 1980.

Hentschel, C., et al. "*Fumaria officinalis* (fumitory)—Clinical Applications," *Fortschr Med* 113:291-92, 1995.

Preininger, V. "The Pharmacology and Toxicology of the Papaveraceae Alkaloids," in *The Alkaloids XV.* Edited by Manske, R.H.F. London: Academic Press, 1975.

GALANGAL

Alpinia officinarum, China root, Chinese ginger, colic root, East Indian root, galanga, kaempferia galanga, rhizoma galangae

Taxonomic class
Zingiberaceae

Common trade names
Galangal Oil, Low John the Conqueror Root Extract

Common forms
Oil and root extracts.

Source
Alpinia consists of the dried root of *Alpinia officinarum,* a native of eastern and southeastern Asia. The plant has been grown in Hainan (southern China) and coastal areas around Pak-hoi.

Chemical components
The active ingredients of the root are the volatile oil (consisting of cineol, eugenol, sesquiterpenes, and isomerides of cadinene) and resin (containing kaempferide, galangol, galangin, alpinin, and starch).

Actions
The galangal root is thought to contain inhibitors against prostaglandin biosynthesizing enzyme. Traditionally, galangal is used for its aromatic, carminative, and diaphoretic activities.

    A. galanga is reported to have antifungal activity, and studies in mice show an antitumorigenic effect (Morita and Itokawa, 1988; Qureshi et al., 1992). The chemical component of *A. galanga,* acetoxychavicol acetate, is thought to have antifungal activity (Janssen and Scheffer, 1985). There is some interest in the use of galangal extract as a food additive because it has been shown to extend shelf life by improving the oxidative stability of minced beef (Cheah and Gan, 2000).

Reported uses
Well-controlled clinical trials in humans are lacking. Therapeutic studies have been conducted only in animals. Galangal has been used in Saudi medicine as an antirheumatic.

Dosage
Usual dose is 1 g P.O.

Adverse reactions
GI: diarrhea, nausea, vomiting.

Interactions
None reported.

Contraindications and precautions
Galangal is contraindicated in patients in whom pregnancy is planned or suspected and in those with chronic GI disorders.

Special considerations
• Advise the patient to consult a health care provider before taking galangal.
• Although no known chemical interactions have been reported in clinical studies, consideration must be given to the pharmacologic properties of the herbal product and the potential for exacerbation of the intended therapeutic effect of conventional drugs.
• Urge women to report planned or suspected pregnancy.

Points of interest
• Galanga is related to ginger both botanically and pharmacologically.

Commentary
There is little well-documented evidence that galangal is effective in rheumatic disorders or fungal infections. The lack of animal and human data to support its claims and its risks limits its use. Galangal cannot be recommended for use in humans.

References
Cheah, P.B., and Gan, S.P. "Antioxidative/Antimicrobial Effects of Galangal and Alpha-tocopherol in Minced Beef," *J Food Prot* 63(3):404-7, 2000.
Janssen, A., and Scheffer, J.J. "Acetoxychavicol Acetate, an Antifungal Component of *Alpinia galanga*," *Planta Med* 51:507, 1985.
Morita, H., and Itokawa, H. "Cytotoxic and Antifungal Diterpenes from the Seeds of *Alpinia galanga*," *Planta Med* 54:117, 1988.
Qureshi, S., et al. "Toxicity Studies on *Alpinia galanga* and *Curcuma longa*," *Planta Med* 58:124, 1992.

GALANTHAMINE
GALANTHAMINE HYDROBROMIDE

Taxonomic class
Liliaceae

Common trade names
Galantamine, Jilkon, Lycoremine, Nivalin, Reminyl

Common forms
Ampules: 5 mg
Tablets (coated): 5 mg, 10 mg

Source

Galanthamine can be isolated from the bulbs of the common snow-drop, *Galanthus nivalis,* and daffodils *(Narcissus* spp.). It is also available as a synthetic chemical.

Chemical components

Galanthamine is a water-soluble alkaloid.

Actions

Galanthamine is a selective, competitive acetylcholinesterase inhibitor. The drug inhibits erythrocyte acetycholinesterase more effectively than brain acetylcholinesterase. It is nearly 100% bioavailable and crosses the blood-brain barrier. Galanthamine is hepatically metabolized into *O*-demethylgalanthamine glucuronide, *N*-demethylgalanthamine, and epigalanthamine.

O-Demethylgalanthamine is 10 times more selective as an acetylcholinesterase inhibitor than galanthamine itself. About 25% of a dose of galanthamine is excreted unchanged (Bachus, 1999). In animal models, the agent attenuates drug- and lesion-induced cognitive deficits (Bores et al., 1996). One trial in Wistar rats suggested that parenteral galanthamine improved speed of learning, short-term memory, and spatial orientation of the rats under conditions of prolonged alcohol intake (Iliev et al., 1999).

In healthy male volunteers, galanthamine reversed central anticholinergic syndrome induced by I.V. scopolamine (Baraka and Harik, 1977).

Reported uses

Galanthamine has been used to reverse neuromuscular blockade and, in some countries, for myasthenia gravis and postpolio paralysis.

Preliminary clinical trials of galanthamine with Alzheimer's patients have provided mixed results. In one placebo-controlled trial of 95 patients with mild to moderate Alzheimer's disease, clinical evaluation indicated significantly less deterioration in patients receiving galanthamine after 10 weeks of treatment (Kewitz et al., 1994). In another trial, galanthamine did not provide any benefit (Dal-Bianco et al., 1991). More recently, two large, randomized, multicenter trials have examined galanthamine supplementation versus placebo in mild to moderate Alzheimer's disease. Tariot and colleagues (2000) found statistically significant benefits favoring galanthamine at both 16 and 24 mg/day doses after 5 months of therapy when evaluating Alzheimer's patients through common standardized assessment scales that measure cognition and functional and behavioral symptoms. The 12-month trial by Raskind and colleagues (2000) mirrors these findings. Galanthamine supplementation in patients with Alzheimer's disease is approved in Austria but not in the United States. Other drugs with similar mechanisms of action have been approved in the United States for Alzheimer's disease.

Bold italic type indicates that reaction may be life-threatening.

Dosage
For Alzheimer's disease, initially 5 mg P.O. t.i.d., increased to 30 to 40 mg/day. Dosage should reduce acetylcholinesterase activity by 35% to 60%.

Adverse reactions
CNS: agitation, dizziness, light-headedness, sleep disturbances.
GI: abdominal pain, diarrhea, nausea, vomiting.

Interactions
Drugs metabolized by way of CYP450 2D6: Significant galanthamine metabolism occurs through this pathway. Galanthamine metabolism may be inhibited by drugs that use the CYP450 2D6 enzyme (fluoxetine, quinidine, paroxetine; Bachus, 1999). Avoid administration with galanthamine or monitor appropriately if unavoidable.
MAO inhibitors: May cause hypertensive crisis. Do not use together.
Organophosphate fertilizers that inhibit acetylcholinesterase: Use with galanthamine may be harmful. Avoid administration with galanthamine.

Contraindications and precautions
Galanthamine is contraindicated in patients with bradycardia, diabetic crisis, epilepsy, hyperkinesia, severe hypotonia, recent myocardial infarction, Parkinson's disease, and obstructions to the digestive, respiratory, or urinary tract.

Special considerations
- Advise the patient to seek medical advice before taking galanthamine.
- Inform the patient that other, conventional and accepted treatment regimens are available.
- Urge the patient to avoid hazardous activities until CNS effects of galanthamine are known.
- Inform the patient who may be at risk for organophosphate fertilizer exposure to avoid using galanthamine.

Points of interest
- A report in 1983 suggested that the common snowdrop was probably the antidote used by Odysseus to counter the effects of Circe's poisonous drugs in Homer's epic poem *The Odyssey.* If this is true, this was the first recorded use of galanthamine to reverse central anticholinergic intoxication (Plaitakis and Duvoisin, 1983).

Commentary
There is significant support for the use of galanthamine in Alzheimer's disease. Modulation of acetylcholine receptor function appears to be a contemporary approach toward Alzheimer's disease therapy. Based on galanthamine's mechanism of action, its efficacy and safety might be considered somewhat more predictable. Additional studies evaluating efficacy and safety are needed to define its precise role in treating this disease. Meanwhile, supervised use of galanthamine might be considered only on an individual basis for patients with significant Alzheimer's dis-

ease who have not responded to the available substantiated allopathic therapies, provided reliable, standardized dosage forms are obtainable.

References

Bachus, R. "The O-Demethylation of the Antidementia Drug Galanthamine Is Catalysed by Cytochrome p450 2D6," *Pharmacogenetics* 9(6):661-68, 1999.

Baraka, A., and Harik, S. "Reversal of Central Anticholinergic Syndrome by Galanthamine," *JAMA* 238:2293-94, 1977.

Bores, G.M., et al. "Pharmacological Evaluation of Novel Alzheimer's Disease Therapeutics: Acetylcholinesterase Inhibitors Related to Galanthamine," *J Pharmacol Exp Ther* 277:728-38, 1996.

Dal-Bianco, P., et al. "Galanthamine Treatment in Alzheimer's Disease," *J Neural Transm Suppl* 33:59-63, 1991.

Kewitz, H., et al. "Galanthamine, a Selective Nontoxic Acetylcholinesterase Inhibitor Is Significantly Superior over Placebo in the Treatment of SDAT," *Neuropsychopharmacology* 10 (Suppl Part 2):130, 1994.

Iliev, A., et al. "Effect of Acetylcholinesterase Inhibitor Galanthamine on Learning and Memory in Prolonged Alcohol Intake Rat Model of Acetylcholine Deficit," *Methods Find Exp Clin Pharmacol* 21(4):297-301, 1999.

Plaitakis, A., and Duvoisin, R.C. "Homerís Moly Identified as *Galanthus nivalis* L.: Physiologic Antidote to Stramonium Poisoning," *Clin Neuropharmacol* 6:1-5, 1983.

Raskind, M.A., et al. "Galanthamine in AD: A 6-Month Randomized, Placebo-controlled Trial with a 6-Month Extension. The Galanthamine USA-1 Study Group," *Neurology* 54(12):2261-68, 2000.

Tariot, P.N., et al. "A 5-Month Randomized, Placebo-controlled Trial of Galanthamine in AD. The Galanthamine USA-10 Study," *Neurology* 54(12):2269-76, 2000.

GAMMA BUTYROLACTONE

4-BUTANOLIDE, BUTYROLACTONE, 4-BUTYROLACTONE, BUTYROLACTONE GAMMA, DIHYDRO-2(3H)-FURANONE, 2(3H)-FURANONE DIHYDRO, TETRAHYDRO-2-FURANONE

Common trade names

Blue Nitro, Firewater, Gamma G, GBL, GH Revitalizer, Insom-X, Invigorate, Longevity, Remforce, Renewtrient, Revivarant

Common forms

Liquid and powder.

Source

Gamma butyrolactone occurs naturally in humans and decreases in concentration with age. Gamma hydroxybutyric acid (GHB) is converted to gamma butyrolactone in the stomach by gastric acid after oral administration. GHB is a short-chain fatty acid metabolite of gamma aminobutyric acid (GABA), which is found in all body tissues, with the highest concentration in the brain.

Chemical components
Gamma butyrolactone is chemically related to both GHB and 1,4-butanediol (BD).

Actions
When ingested orally, gamma butyrolactone is converted to GHB in the stomach. GHB is distributed rapidly within the body and easily crosses the blood-brain barrier. It is then converted to succinic semialdehyde and then to succinic acid or, possibly, GABA by way of Krebs' cycle. GHB is a naturally occurring inhibitory neurotransmitter and has the highest concentration in the basal ganglia. It is thought to be involved in sleep cycle mediation, temperature regulation, cerebral glucose metabolism and blood flow, memory, and emotion. At low doses, GHB decreases dopaminergic activity, and at high doses, it can stimulate dopamine release. Complete GHB function and metabolism are complex and incompletely understood.

Reported uses
Many claims have been made for gamma butyrolactone. It has been promoted to induce sleep, enhance sexual activity, build muscle, release growth hormone, cause weight loss, and relieve depression and stress. No human clinical trials support these observations.

GHB is approved as an anesthetic in some countries, and FDA approval is pending for its use as an investigational drug to treat narcolepsy.

Dosage
No dosing regimen is available.

Adverse reactions
CNS: aggression, agitation, amnesia, anxiety, CNS depression, *coma,* combativeness, confusion, euphoria, hypothermia, *seizures,* unconsciousness.
CV: *bradycardia,* tachycardia.
GI: vomiting.
Musculoskeletal: hypotonia, myoclonus.
Respiratory: slow respiratory rate.
Skin: sweating.

Interactions
Alcohol: Increased effects of alcohol. Avoid administration with gamma butyrolactone.
CNS depressants: Increased effects of CNS depressants. Avoid administration with gamma butyrolactone.

Contraindications and precautions
Gamma butyrolactone is considered unsafe. The use of products that contain gamma butyrolactone has been associated with more than 55 cases of serious adverse reactions and at least 1 death. Together, gamma butyrolactone, GHB, and BD account for more than 122 case reports of serious illnesses and at least 3 deaths reported to the FDA.

Special considerations

ALERT On March 13, 2000, GHB was classified by the FDA as a Schedule I controlled substance. Because gamma butyrolactone is a precursor to GHB, according to the FDA, it can be treated as a Schedule I controlled substance if it is intended for human consumption.

• On January 21, 1999, the FDA issued a warning about products that contain gamma butyrolactone and asked manufacturers to issue a recall. This action was initiated because of the emergence of GHB and gamma butyrolactone as drugs of abuse, most notably as "date rape" drugs, because of their euphoric and sedative effects.

• Gamma butyrolactone has been advertised on the Internet and in health food stores and bodybuilding magazines. With the FDA implications, manufacturers have been renaming their products and substituting BD for gamma butyrolactone. Ingesting this drug can be just as dangerous as ingesting gamma butyrolactone and produces the same serious adverse effects. There have also been reports of potential GHB abusers making their own product by mixing gamma butyrolactone, water, and sodium hydroxide. This type of "kitchen chemistry" is popular among adolescents and young adults and can lead to serious injury because of the unknown amount of each ingredient.

ALERT Gamma butyrolactone is associated with many of the same adverse effects as GHB. Comatose events and at least one death have been documented with the use of gamma butyrolactone. Effects of GHB are dose-related, with short-term amnesia and hypotonia at 10 mg/kg; drowsiness and sleep at 20 to 30 mg/kg; and bradycardia, bradypnea, a hypnotic state, nausea, and vomiting at 50 to 70 mg/kg. Higher doses cause seizures and cardiopulmonary depression. Adverse reactions usually resolve within 4 to 6 hours but may take 3 to 4 days. Supportive treatment with a focus on airway protection is recommended for GHB toxicity. One study advocates the use of physostigmine, 2 mg I.V., as an antidote for GHB (Henderson and Holmes, 1976).

Points of interest

• Gamma butyrolactone, as a solvent, can be used in the production of pesticides, herbicides, and plant growth regulators. It is also an ingredient in commercial floor strippers. This solvent can be combined with water and sodium hydroxide to create GHB.

Commentary

Few studies have been conducted on the use of gamma butyrolactone in humans. GHB has been investigated and found to be unsafe in the public forum. Although the FDA has allowed GHB to have investigational status, it is still considered an unapproved and illegal drug. Because gamma butyrolactone is a precursor to GHB, it has been given the same restrictions. Gamma butyrolactone, GHB, and BD cannot be recommended for any use. Because of the multiple case reports of serious injury and even death, it is best to avoid these dietary supplements.

Bold italic type indicates that reaction may be life-threatening.

References

Anonymous. "Internet Sale of Gamma Butyrolactone (GBL)," *WHO* 13(1):22, 1999.

Food and Drug Administration. "FDA Warns About Products Containing Gamma Butyrolactone or GBL and Asks Companies to Issue a Recall." Rockville, Md., U.S. Department of Health and Human Services, Public Health Service, Food and Drug Administration, 1999. Talk paper T99-5. Available at http://www.fda.gov/bbs/topics/ANSWERS/ANS00937.html.

Food and Drug Administration. "Report Serious Adverse Events Associated with Dietary Supplements Containing GBL, GHB, or BD." 1999. Available at http://www.vm.cfsan.fda.gov/~dms/mwgblghb.html.

Food and Drug Administration. Import Alert IA664. 2000. Available at http://www.fda.gov/ora/fiars/ora_import_ia664l.html.

"Gamma Hydroxybutyrate Use—New York and Texas, 1995-1996," *JAMA* 277(19):1511, 1997.

Henderson, R.S., and Holmes, C.M. "Reversal of the Anaesthetic Action of Sodium Gamma-hydroxybutyrate," *Anaesth and Intensive Care* 4(4):351-54, 1976.

LoVecchio, F., et al. "Butyrolactone-induced Central Nervous System Depression After Ingestion of RenewTrient, a 'Dietary Supplement,'" *N Engl J Med* 339(12):847-48, 1998. Letter.

Smith, S.W., et al. "Adverse Events Associated with Ingestion of Gamma Butyro-lactone—Minnesota, New Mexico, and Texas, 1998-1999," *MMWR* 48(7):137-140, 1999.

Tunnicliff, G. "Sites of Action of Gamma-hydroxybutyrate (GHB)—A Neuroactive Drug with Abuse Potential," *Clin Toxicol* 35(6):581-90, 1997.

Viswanathan, S., et al. "Revivarant (Gamma-butyrolactone) Poisoning," *Am J Emerg Med* 18(3):358-59, 2000. Letter.

GARCINIA

GARCINIA INDICA, GARCINIA CAMBOGIA, GARCINIA HANBURYI, HCA, HYDROXYCITRIC ACID, MALABAR TAMARIND

Taxonomic class
Clusiaceae

Common trade names
None known.

Common forms
Capsules, chewing gum, powders, snack bars, and tablets.

Source
Garcinia cambogia and related *Garcinia* spp. are indigenous to Southeast Asia and India and produce a small, pumpkin-shaped fruit. This fruit is considered to be one of the richest sources of hydroxycitric acid (HCA).

Chemical components
HCA is a fruit extract with a chemical composition similar to that of citric acid. Citric acid is a common compound in citrus fruits.

Actions

Studies in animals and in vitro models have suggested that HCA is a potent competitive inhibitor of the extramitochondrial enzyme adenosine triphosphate-citrate (pro-3S)-lyase. This inhibitory action apparently suppresses de novo fatty acid synthesis, reduces food intake, increases hepatic glycogen synthesis, and decreases weight gain (Heymsfield et al., 1998).

Reported uses

Early studies on the application of HCA were contradictory and suffered from poor study design and small sample sizes. A more recent double-blind, randomized, controlled trial evaluated 135 overweight men and women in an outpatient weight-control research facility (Heymsfield et al., 1998). After 12 weeks of either 1,500 mg/day of HCA (given as *G. cambogia* extract 3,000 mg—50% HCA) or placebo before each meal, both groups had lost a significant amount of weight compared with baseline ($P<.001$). When compared against each other, neither group fared better. The investigators concluded that *G. cambogia* failed to produce any significant weight or fat mass loss beyond that of placebo.

Dosage

Information on appropriate dosing is scarce. One trial used 1,500 mg/day (2 capsules t.i.d.) of HCA as 3,000 mg of *G. cambogia* extract P.O. 10 minutes before meals.

Adverse reactions

None reported.

Interactions

None reported.

Contraindications and precautions

Garcinia is contraindicated in patients who are hypersensitive to *Garcinia* spp. and in pregnant or breast-feeding patients.

Special considerations

• Inform the patient that diet and exercise are still the hallmarks to weight loss and weight control.
• Consider referring the patient to a registered dietitian or an exercise physiologist or both.
• Inform the patient about new breakthroughs in weight loss products. However, these drugs are typically reserved for the morbidly obese.

Points of interest

• Scientific investigation into the actions and effects of HCA began as early as the 1960s.

Commentary

G. cambogia and other *Garcinia* species are noteworthy as rich sources of HCA. Despite interesting animal and in vitro data suggesting weight-reducing properties, modern-day human clinical trials have failed to support the use of garcinia or HCA for weight loss purposes

References

Heymsfield, S.B., et al. "*Garcinia cambogia* (Hydroxycitric Acid) as a Potential Antiobesity Agent. A Randomized, Controlled Trial," *JAMA* 280:1596-1600, 1998.

GARLIC

AIL, ALLIUM, CAMPHOR OF THE POOR, DA-SUAN, KNOBLAUNCH, LA-SUAN, NECTAR OF THE GODS, POOR MAN'S TREACLE, RUSTIC TREACLE, STINKING ROSE

Taxonomic class
Liliaceae

Common trade names
Comfey Mullein Garlic Syrup, Garlic, Garlic Go, Garlic-Power, Garlic Time, Garlique, Heart Aid, Kwai, Kyolic, Lashan, Lashuna, Odorless Garlic Tablets, One a Day Garlic, Rasonam, Sapec

Common forms
Dried powder: 400 to 1,200 mg
Fresh bulb: 2 to 5 g
Tablets (allicin total potential): 2 to 5 mg
Tablets (garlic extract): 100 mg, 320 mg, 400 mg, 600 mg
   Also available as an antiseptic oil, fresh extract, freeze-dried garlic powder, and garlic oil (essential oil).

Source
Garlic, or *Allium sativum,* is one of the most extensively researched and published medicinal plants. The fresh garlic bulb is usually dried, crushed into a powder, and then compressed to produce a tablet. The tablet form is the most commonly used commercial preparation of garlic. Raw whole cloves have similar effects.

Chemical components
Garlic is made up of more than 23 constituents, including alliin, *s*-methyl-l-cysteine sulfoxide, various enzymes (alliinase, peroxidase, myrosinase), ajoenes, proteins, lipids, amino acids, phosphorus, potassium, and zinc. Also isolated are minor concentrations of selenium, vitamins A and C, calcium, magnesium, sodium, iron, manganese, and B complex vitamins. Garlic has the highest sulfur content of the *Allium* species; several sulfur-containing compounds occur in the volatile oil. Alliin, which is enzymatically converted to allicin, gives garlic its characteristic odor when the clove is crushed and ground. Allicin is believed to be the active ingredient.

Actions

Garlic and its components are being investigated for several uses, but the most commonly studied areas are its potential antithrombotic, lipid-lowering, antitumorigenic, and antimicrobial effects. Cholesterol-lowering effects have been well documented in animals and humans. Garlic lowers total cholesterol, triglyceride, and LDL levels and increases HDL levels. One study reported a mean reduction of 6% in total cholesterol levels and 11% in LDL levels (Jain et al., 1993).

Garlic has documented hypoglycemic activity in rabbits; hypotensive properties in animals and humans; and amebicidal, antibacterial, antifungal, antiviral, insecticidal, and larvicidal activities in several in vitro and in vivo models. A component in garlic oil, methylallyltrisulphide, has been linked with inhibition of adenosine diphosphate–induced platelet aggregation (Makheja et al., 1979). An allicin derivative, ajoene, has also been shown to inhibit platelet aggregation. These effects on the platelets are reported to last only a few hours (Boullin, 1981). The antiplatelet effect was again confirmed with aged garlic extract (Steiner and Lin, 1998).

In Chinese studies, garlic has been shown to decrease nitrosamine (a type of carcinogen) and nitrite accumulation. Garlic extract was found to significantly prolong survival in mice injected with virulent cancer cells (Pareddy and Rosenberg, 1993). Also, garlic oil has been shown to be beneficial in rodents with GI hypermotility disorders.

Two studies examined garlic's potential to protect LDL from oxidation (Byrne et al., 1999; Munday et al., 1999). The thinking behind these experiments is that if garlic is found to inhibit LDL oxidation, then it may be valuable in preventing the development and progression of atherosclerotic plaques, thereby reducing CV risk. The study by Munday and colleagues evaluated doses of raw garlic (6 g), aged garlic extract (2.4 g), and DL-alpha-tocopherol acetate (0.8 g) for 7 days in human subjects. The subjects who received aged garlic or alpha-tocopherol, but not raw garlic, were significantly more resistant to LDL oxidation than those who did not receive supplements. This finding conflicts with the study by Byrne and colleagues, who found no change in susceptibility of LDL oxidation in a randomized, double-blind, placebo-controlled trial of 31 moderately hypercholesterolemic subjects who received garlic tablets (Kwai, 900 mg/day) for 6 months. In a related study, Koscielny and colleagues (1999) detected a slight (5% to 18%) reduction in atherosclerotic plaque volume in subjects who ingested high doses of garlic powder over a 48-month period. Some subjects actually experienced plaque regression. Although intriguing, the results of these studies must be viewed as preliminary.

Reported uses

There are many claims for garlic's use, from warding off evil spirits to healing wounds and curing infections. A few human trials have documented garlic's ability to improve serum lipid profiles. Such studies have been small compared with those evaluating other cholesterol-

---

Bold italic type indicates that reaction may be life-threatening.

RESEARCH FINDINGS
Garlic as a lipid-lowering agent

Several trials have attempted to document the efficacy of garlic to reduce serum lipid levels. One placebo-controlled, randomized trial studied the effects of a commercial brand of garlic tablet (Kwai) in 20 patients with documented serum cholesterol levels of 220 mg/dl or higher for 12 weeks (Jain et al., 1993); patients with triglyceride levels over 400 mg/dl were excluded from the study. After 6 weeks, no significant differences in lipid levels were detected, but after 12 weeks, both serum total cholesterol and LDL levels were lower by 6% and 11%, respectively, compared with placebo.

Another positive trial investigated a dose of 4 capsules daily of an ethyl acetate extract of 1 g of garlic for 3 months in 30 patients with coronary artery disease (Bordia et al., 1998). Small but significant reductions in total cholesterol and triglyceride levels with elevations in HDL levels were seen.

Three later trials evaluated garlic preparations in adult hypercholesterolemic outpatients. In one trial, 5 mg of a steam-distilled garlic oil product given twice a day produced insignificant results in lipoprotein parameters compared with placebo (Berthold et al., 1998). In another trial, similar results in both the treatment (900 mg/day garlic) and the placebo groups were obtained (Isaacsohn et al., 1998). In the third randomized, controlled, double-blinded investigation (Superko and Krauss, 2000), 50 moderately hypercholesterolemic subjects showed no significant changes in plasma levels of major lipoproteins after receiving 900 mg/day of garlic therapy for 90 days compared with placebo.

Most clinical trials do not support garlic therapy to reduce cholesterol levels. Whether this inconsistency might be related to the selection of one particular dosage form of garlic over another or to subtherapeutic dosing is unknown.

lowering agents and have not evaluated garlic's effect on morbidity and mortality or shown greater reductions in cholesterol than with other agents, such as the statins—atorvastatin, lovastatin, simvastatin. (See *Garlic as a lipid-lowering agent.*) In one study, high allicin doses significantly lowered diastolic blood pressure but tended to produce only slightly lower systolic blood pressure (McMahon et al., 1993).

The antimicrobial properties of garlic have been reported anecdotally. Garlic extract has been used on wounds as recently as World War II. Despite reports of inhibited bacterial growth in vitro, its low potency prohibits garlic from becoming a useful clinical agent.

Ajoene, an organic trisulphuric isolate of garlic, has been found to be equally as effective as terbinafine (1%) cream in treating superficial dermatophyte infections (tinea cruris, tinea corporis) when used as a topical gel (0.6% ajoene) in a randomized evaluation of 60 soldiers (Ledezma et al., 1999).

Preliminary pilot studies with AIDS patients suggest that garlic extract may reduce morbidity. It may also be useful for treating asthma, constipation, diabetes, heavy metal poisoning, and inflammation, but there is little, if any, evidence to support these claims.

Dosage
It has been suggested that garlic products be standardized to assure the amount of active ingredient (thought to be allicin) in each form. A German product containing 600 mg of dried garlic powder corresponds to a 1.3% alliin component and a 0.6% allicin release.

For lipid-lowering action, 600 to 900 mg/day P.O., or an average of 4 g of fresh garlic or 8 mg of garlic oil daily.

Adverse reactions
CNS: dizziness.
Metabolic: hypothyroidism.
GI: GI complaints, irritation of mouth and esophagus, nausea, vomiting.
Skin: contact dermatitis, garlic odor, other allergic reactions (***asthma, anaphylaxis***, rash), sweating.

Interactions
Anticoagulants: Increased risk of bleeding. Do not use together.
Antiplatelets: May increase effects of antiplatelet therapy. Monitor the patient.

Contraindications and precautions
Garlic is contraindicated in patients who are hypersensitive to garlic or other members of the Lilaceae family, in those with GI disorders such as peptic ulcer and gastroesophageal reflux disease, and in pregnant patients because of its oxytocic effects.

Special considerations
🔊 **ALERT** Chronic use or large doses of garlic may lead to decreased hemoglobin production and lysis of RBCs.
• Monitor CBC of the patient who is taking high-dose or long-term garlic.
• Advise the patient that cholesterol-lowering drugs are commonly used for hypercholesterolemia because of their proven survival data and effectiveness in lowering cholesterol levels more than garlic.
• Instruct the patient to watch for and report signs of bleeding (bleeding gums, easy bruising, tarry stools, petechiae) if garlic supplements are taken with hemostatics.
• Urge the patient to report adverse reactions promptly.

Points of interest
• In Germany, garlic products are a major OTC sales item.
• Fresh and powdered garlic are commonly used as spices. The FDA states that garlic oil, extract, and oleoresin are generally regarded as safe.

Bold italic type indicates that reaction may be life-threatening.

● The value of commercial preparations that are odorless or deodorized is questionable because the beneficial properties of garlic appear to lie with the chemical constituents that give garlic its characteristic odor.

Commentary

Garlic is one of the oldest and most revered herbals, with references to its medicinal value dating back thousands of years. Although beneficial effects on the lipid profile have been described, most of the data do not support a role for garlic in reducing cholesterol levels. Whether this controversy in the data might be explained by the choice of one particular dosage form of garlic over another remains to be seen. Intriguing information exists with respect to atherosclerotic plaque volume reduction and regression, but it is quite preliminary.

It is not known whether or not garlic ingestion reduces mortality from coronary artery disease or stroke. Other allopathic drugs are available that do produce greater and more reliable reductions in cholesterol levels along with proven survival benefits. If garlic is to be recommended for its cholesterol-lowering action, it should be used as only a portion of a comprehensive cholesterol-lowering program under the direction of a health care provider.

Additional indications for garlic, such as hypertension, GI motility disorders, and AIDS, await sufficient clinical confirmation.

References

Berthold, H.K., et al. "Effect of a Garlic Oil Preparation on Serum Lipoproteins and Cholesterol Metabolism. A Randomized Controlled Trial," *JAMA* 279:1900-02, 1998.

Bordia, A., et al. "Effect of Garlic on Blood Lipids, Blood Sugar, Fibrinogen and Fibrinolytic Activity in Patients with Coronary Artery Disease," *Prostaglandins Leukot Essent Fatty Acids* 58(4):257-63, 1998.

Boullin, D.J. "Garlic as a Platelet Inhibitor," *Lancet* 1:776, 1981. Letter.

Byrne, D.J., et al. "A Pilot Study of Garlic Consumption Shows No Significant Effect on Markers of Oxidation or Sub-fraction Composition of Low-density Lipoprotein Including Lipoprotein(a) After Allowance for Non-compliance and the Placebo Effect," *Clin Chim Acta* 285(1-2):21-33, 1999.

Isaacsohn, J.L., et al. "Garlic Powder and Plasma Lipids and Lipoproteins. A Multicenter, Randomized, Placebo-controlled Trial," *JAMA* 158:1189-94, 1998.

Jain, A.K., et al. "Can Garlic Reduce Levels of Serum Lipids? A Controlled Clinical Study," *Am J Med* 94:632, 1993.

Koscielny, J., et al. "The Antiatherosclerotic Effect of *Allium sativum*," *Atherosclerosis* 144(1):237-49, 1999.

Ledezma, E., et al. "Ajoene in the Topical Short-term Treatment of Tinea Cruris and Tinea Corporis in Humans. Randomized Comparative Study with Terbinafine," *Arzneimittelforschung* 49(6):544-47, 1999.

Makheja, A.N., et al. "Inhibition of Platelet Aggregation and Thromboxane Synthesis by Onion and Garlic," *Lancet* 1:781, 1979. Letter.

McCrindle, B.W., et al. "Garlic Therapy in Children with Hypercholesteremia," *Arch Pediatr Adolesc Med* 152(11):1089-94, 1998.

McMahon, F.G., et al. "Can Garlic Lower Blood Pressure? A Pilot Study," *Pharmacotherapy* 13:406, 1993.

Munday, J.S., et al. "Daily Supplementation with Aged Garlic Extract, But Not Raw Garlic, Protects Low Density Lipoprotein Against In Vitro Oxidation," *Atherosclerosis* 143(2):399-404, 1999.

Pareddy, S.R., and Rosenberg, J.M. "Does Garlic Have Useful Medicinal Purposes?" *Hospital Pharmacist Report* 8:27, 1993.

Steiner, M., and Lin, R.S. "Changes in Platelet Function and Susceptibility of Lipoproteins to Oxidation Associated with Administration of Aged Garlic Extract," *J Cardiovascular Pharmacol* 31(6):904-8, 1998.

Superko, H.R., and Krauss, R.M. "Garlic Powder, Effect on Plasma Lipids, Postprandial Lipemia, Low Density Lipoprotein Particle Size, High Density Lipoprotein Subclass Distribution and Lipoprotein(a)," *J Am Coll Cardiol* 35(2):321-26, 2000.

GENTIAN

BITTERROOT, FELTWORT, GALL WEED, PALE GENTIAN, STEMLESS GENTIAN, YELLOW GENTIAN

Taxonomic class
Gentianaceae

Common trade names
Angostura Bitters (a proprietary cocktail flavoring that contains an alcoholic extract of stemless gentian)

Common forms
Available as stemless gentian extract or tea. Other products include compound gentian infusion BP 1993, concentrated compound gentian infusion BP 1993, and gentian root low alcohol (liquid).

Source
Gentian is extracted from the roots and rhizome of 2- to 5-year-old *Gentiana lutea* L. plants during the summer months. The bitterness of the product is related to the speed with which the plant is dried: slow drying reduces the bitterness. Stemless gentian is extracted from the entire plant of *G. acaulis* L.

Chemical components
Gentian contains several bitter compounds, including gentiopicrin, gentiin, gentiamarin, gentisin (also called gentianin or gentianic acid), gentisic acid, and gentianose.

Actions
The ingestion of bitter substances before eating has been thought to improve appetite and aid digestion by stimulating the release of gastric juices and bile. Gentian is most often used as part of an alcoholic beverage. It is difficult to separate the effects of gentian and alcohol because in moderate amounts, alcohol has similar effects (Dombek, 1993).

Reported uses
Bitters, such as gentian, have been used for centuries for mild to moderate digestive disorders, including colic, flatulence, heartburn, irritable bowel syndrome, and loss of appetite.

Bold italic type indicates that reaction may be life-threatening.

Increased salivary flow was observed in patients who were given, among others, an herbal extract combination that contained gentian (Borgia et al., 1981). Similar results were noted in another study by the same researchers using patients with mild GI disturbances (constipation, dyspepsia, and loss of appetite). No adverse effects were noted. The therapeutic efficacy of gentian cannot be determined, however, because of incomplete patient information and because gentian was not compared in a single-ingredient product. Both gentian and stemless gentian are approved for use in foods. Extracts of stemless gentian are used in foods, cosmetics, and some smoking cessation products (Dombek, 1993). It has been reported to be active against *Plasmodium* malaria and has been used for malarial fevers (Osol, 1973).

Dosage
The dosage is not well documented.
Tea: ½ tsp of coarsely powdered gentian root boiled in ½ cup (120 ml) of water for 5 minutes. This mixture is strained and then taken 30 minutes before meals. If this tea is strong and unpalatable, the amount of herb may be reduced. This decoction can be taken up to q.i.d.

Adverse reactions
CNS: headache.
GI: nausea, vomiting (with overdose).

Interactions
None reported.

Contraindications and precautions
Gentian is contraindicated in patients who are pregnant and in those with severe hypertension.

Special considerations
• Brewing gentian as a tea is the best way to take the herb.
• Monitor blood pressure in hypertensive patients taking gentian.
• Caution the patient against collecting the herb in the wild (Garnier et al., 1985) because the nonflowering form of *G. lutea* may be difficult to distinguish from the toxic white hellebore.

Points of interest
• Gentian is no longer listed in the USP but is still included in European pharmacopoeias, including the British Pharmacopoeia.
• The German Commission E has reported that the constituents of gentian stimulate the taste buds and increase the release of saliva and gastric secretions. The herb is regarded as a tonic.
• The dye gentian violet is a separate chemical entity and is not derived from plants that contain gentian.
• Gentian is a flavoring agent in vermouth.
• The toxic white hellebore (*Veratrum album*) usually grows near gentian. One report noted acute *Veratrum* alkaloid poisoning in people

who consumed homemade gentian wine that was accidentally contaminated with *Veratrum* (Garnier et al., 1985).

Commentary

Gentian-containing products have long been used as bitter tonics. Anecdotal reports and evidence from one small clinical trial that used a combination product suggest that a small amount of the herbal extract, usually mixed with alcohol, can act as an appetite stimulant and digestive aid. The other claims for gentian are poorly documented; use of the herb cannot be recommended.

References

Borgia, M., et al. "Pharmacological Activity of an Herb Extract: A Controlled Clinical Study," *Curr Ther Res* 29:525-36, 1981.

Garnier, R., et al. "Acute Dietary Poisoning by White Hellebore (*Veratrum album*). Clinical and Analytical Data. A Propos of 5 Cases," *Ann Med Intern* 36:125-28, 1985.

Dombek, C. ed. "Gentian," in *The Lawrence Review of Natural Products.* St. Louis, Mo.: Facts and Comparisons, 1993.

Osol, A., ed. *The United States Dispensatory,* 27th ed. Philadelphia: Lippincott-Raven Pubs., 1973.

GINGER

ZINGIBER

Taxonomic class

Zingiberaceae

Common trade names

Multi-ingredient preparations: Cayenne Ginger, Gingerall, Ginger Ease, Ginger Peppermint Combo, Ginger Power, Ginger Root Alcohol Free, Ginger Trips, Low Alcohol Misty Ginger Blend

Common forms

Capsules, liquid, powder: 100 mg, 465 mg
Extract: 250 mg
Root: 530 mg
Tablets (chewable): 67.5 mg
   Also available as teas.

Source

Ginger (*Zingiber officinale*) is a perennial that grows in India, Jamaica, and China. The plant produces green-purple flowers that resemble orchids. The rhizome (root) is found underground and usually the most valued part of the plant.

Chemical components

The root contains both volatile and nonvolatile compounds. The nonvolatile constituents, which include the gingerols and gingerol-like compounds, are thought to be responsible for ginger's flavor, aromatic

---

properties, and any pharmacologic activity. The volatile oil contains zingiberol, zingeberene, curcumene, farnesene, bis-abolene, sesquiphellandrene, and several monoterpenes (linalool, borneol, neral, geraniol, and others). Other compounds present are zingibain (a proteolytic enzyme), oleoresins, fats, waxes, carbohydrates, vitamins, and minerals.

Actions

Human studies have shown that ginger inhibits platelet aggregation induced by adenosine diphosphate and epinephrine (Lumb, 1994; Verma et al., 1993). Other studies have demonstrated a lack of effects on platelet aggregation (Janssen et al., 1996). Ginger extracts have documented anti-inflammatory effects in rodent models (Suekawa et al., 1986). Specific components of ginger produce varying CV effects. Methanolic extracts of ginger have shown positive inotropic effects in a guinea pig model.

Other studies in animals have suggested that components in ginger may be gastroprotective against various chemical insults and stressors. The GI protective action is postulated to be promoted by increased mucosal resistance and potentiation of the defensive mechanism against chemicals or alterations in prostaglandins, providing more protective effects. A study of acetone extracts in mice found them to have similar stimulatory effects on GI motility as those seen with metoclopramide and domperidone (Yamahara et al., 1990).

Reported uses

Claims for ginger include its use as an antiemetic, an anti-inflammatory useful for arthritis treatment, an antioxidant, an antitumorigenic drug, a CV stimulant, and a GI protectant and as a therapy for microbial and parasitic infestations.

The antiemetic effects of ginger have been extensively studied in humans for morning, motion, and sea sickness and for postoperative nausea and vomiting; most findings provided support for this action. (See *Ginger's antiemetic and antivertigo effects,* pages 330 and 331.) Doses and duration of therapy varied considerably with each study. The antiemetic properties of ginger probably result from local effects on the GI tract rather than the CNS. Increased gastric peristalsis has been shown in animals, but any mechanism in humans is considered speculative.

Ginger has provided relief from pain and swelling in patients with muscle discomfort, osteoarthritis, or rheumatoid arthritis (Srivastava and Mustafa, 1992). A proposed mechanism is that it inhibits prostaglandin, thromboxane, and leukotriene biosynthesis.

Dosage

Dosage forms and strength vary with each disease state.
As an antiemetic, studies used 500 to 1,000 mg of powdered ginger P.O., or 1,000 mg of fresh ginger root P.O.

RESEARCH FINDINGS
Ginger's antiemetic and antivertigo effects

Most research focuses on ginger's potential application as an agent to prevent nausea and vomiting from noxious stimuli of various origins.

Provocation stimulus testing

One of the first controlled studies of ginger as an anti–motion sickness agent mimicked seasickness by spinning 36 blindfolded, sea-sickness-prone subjects for up to 6 minutes in a motor-driven chair. Dimenhydrinate (100 mg), powdered whole ginger root (940 mg), or chickweed was given to the subjects before their spin (Mowrey and Clayson, 1982). No one in the chickweed or dimenhydrinate group was able to remain in the chair for the full 6 minutes. Subjects in the ginger root group averaged 5.5 minutes in the chair, whereas those given dimenhydrinate or chickweed averaged 3.5 and 1.5 minutes, respectively. Although the results of this study are intriguing, the study design of the trial has been questioned.

Grontved and Hentzer (1986) studied the effects of powdered ginger root on vertigo and nystagmus in eight healthy volunteers upon caloric stimulation of the vestibular system in a randomized, double-blind crossover, placebo-controlled manner. After consumption of 1,000 mg of powdered ginger root or 1,000 mg of lactose (placebo), subjects lay supine in a dark room. The vestibular system was challenged with 111.2° F (44° C) water for 40 seconds. Test results showed that ginger root reduced vertigo significantly better than did placebo ($P<.05$).

Another trial using a rotating chair failed to support the application of either powdered ginger or whole ginger root in doses of 500 to 1,000 mg for the prevention of motion sickness (Stewart et al., 1991). Ginger was compared with scopolamine and placebo in 28 healthy human volunteers. Although ginger had minor effects on the gastric response to motion sickness, the investigators concluded that these effects were insufficient to count ginger as an anti–motion sickness agent.

Seasickness

Grontved and colleagues in 1988 examined powdered ginger root versus placebo in prevention of seasickness in 80 "unseasoned" Danish naval cadets. When their ship met with heavy seas, 40 of the cadets received 1,000 mg of powdered ginger root and the other 40 received 1,000 mg of lactose in a randomized, double-blind manner. Each cadet recorded sweating, nausea, vertigo, and vomiting on a scorecard every hour for 4 hours after their dose. The first 3 hours revealed no significant differences in the comparative data for total symptom scores. At hour 4, a significant difference was found favoring ginger root over placebo for total symptom score ($P<.05$).

Bold italic type indicates that reaction may be life-threatening.

Ginger's antiemetic and antivertigo effects *(continued)*

Postoperative nausea and vomiting

Powdered ginger root was compared with metoclopramide and placebo in a trial evaluating the incidence of postoperative nausea and vomiting. In this study (Bone et al., 1990), 60 gynecologic surgery patients were given ginger (1,000 mg P.O.), metoclopramide (10 mg I.V.), or placebo 1.5 hours before their operations in a randomized, double-blind manner. After evaluation, incidences of nausea and intensity of nausea favored both active treatment groups over placebo.

Hyperemesis gravidarum

In another study that evaluated ginger's antiemetic potential, ginger (250 mg P.O. four times a day) was compared with placebo for 4 days in 30 pregnant women who were suffering from hyperemesis gravidarum. A statistically significant percentage of women appeared to prefer treatment with ginger over that with placebo, as demonstrated by patient-reported symptom scores (Fisher-Rasmussen et al., 1990).

Summary of trials evaluating ginger for antiemetic and antivertigo effects

Investigators	Trial	Results	Limitations
Mowrey and Clayson (1982)	Motion sickness provocation testing	+	No mention of randomization; lacks descriptions for inclusive or exclusive criteria; another herbal agent used as placebo
Grontved and Hentzer (1986)	Motion sickness provocation testing	+ / -	Small sample size; lacks descriptions for inclusive or exclusive criteria; no mention of concomitant drugs
Grontved et al. (1988)	Seasickness	+ / -	Subjective outcome measurements; reporting bias suspected by investigator; no mention of concomitant drugs
Bone et al. (1990)	Postoperative nausea and vomiting	+	Subjective measurements used
Stewart et al. (1991)	Motion sickness provocation testing	-	Few limitations; sample size = 28 subjects
Fisher-Rasmussen et al. (1990)	Hyperemesis gravidarum	+	Subjective measurements used

Adverse reactions
CNS: CNS depression (with overdose).
CV: *arrhythmias* (with overdose).
GI: heartburn.

Interactions
Anticoagulants: Increased risk of bleeding. Avoid administration with ginger.

Contraindications and precautions
Ginger is contraindicated in pregnant patients; effects are unknown. Some components of ginger have been determined to be mutagenic, whereas others appear to exert an antimutagenic effect. The net effect of these components is unknown (Nagabhushan and Amonkar, 1987; Nakamura and Yamamoto, 1983; Unnikrishnan and Kuttan, 1988). Use only under medical supervision in patients receiving anticoagulants because it may affect bleeding time by inhibiting platelet function.

Special considerations
• Advise women to avoid excessive use of ginger during pregnancy.
• Instruct the patient to watch for signs of bleeding when taking ginger.
• No consensus exists with respect to dosing and monitoring.

Commentary
Although some data support the use of ginger as an antiemetic in humans, results from several trials have conflicted. Recommendation of ginger for use as an antiemetic, an anti-inflammatory, or a gastroprotective agent, before long-term, controlled, pharmacologic studies of its constituents have been conducted, is premature. Pregnant women should probably avoid excessive consumption of ginger until the effects of all its constituents are understood.

References
Bone, M., et al. "The Effect of Ginger Root on Post-operative Nausea and Vomiting After Major Gynecological Surgery," *Anesthesia* 45:669-71, 1990.

Fisher-Rasmussen, W., et al. "Ginger Treatment of Hyperemesis Gravidarum," *Eur J Obstet Gynecol Reprod Biol* 38:19-24, 1990.

Grontved, A., and Hentzer, E. "Vertigo-reducing Effect of Ginger Root," *ORL* 48:282-86, 1986.

Grontved, A., et al. "Ginger Root Against Seasickness. A Controlled Trial on the Open Seas," *Acta Otolaryngol* 105:45-49, 1988.

Holtman, S., et al. "The Anti-motion Sickness Mechanism of Ginger. A Comparative Study with Placebo and Dimenhydrinate," *Acta Otolaryngol* 108:168-74, 1989.

Janssen, P.L., et al. "Consumption of Ginger Does Not Affect Ex Vivo Platelet Thromboxane Production in Humans," *Eur J Clin Nutr* 50(11):772-74, 1996.

Kawai, T., et al. "Anti-emetic Principles of *Magnolia obovata* Bark and *Zingiber officinale*," *Planta Med* 60(1):17-20, 1994.

Lumb, A. "Effect of Dried Ginger on Platelet Function," *Thrombosis Haemostasis* 71(1):110-111, 1994.

Meyer, K., et al. "*Zingiber officianale* (Ginger) Used to Prevent 8-MOP Associated Nausea," *Derm Nursing* 7(4):242-44, 1995.

Mowrey, D.B., and Clayson, D.E. "Motion Sickness, Ginger and Psychophysics," *Lancet* 1:655-57, 1982.

Nagabhushan, M., and Amonkar, A. "Mutagenicity of Gingerol and Shogaol and Antimutagenicity of Zingerone in Salmonella/Microsomal Assay," *Cancer Letters* 36:221-23, 1987.

Nakamura, H., and Yamamoto, T. "The Active Part of the [6]-Gingerol Molecule in Mutagenesis," *Mutat Res* 122(2):87-94, 1983.

"Pharmacologic Studies of Antimotion Sickness Actions of Ginger," (Chinese) *Chung Kuo Chung His I Chieh Ho Tsa Chih* 12(2):70, 1992.

Phillips, S., et al. "*Zingiber officinale* (Ginger)—An Antiemetic for Day Case Surgery," *Anaesthesia* 48:715-17, 1993a.

Phillips, S., et al. "*Zingiber officinale* Does Not Affect Gastric Emptying Rate. A Randomized, Placebo-controlled, Crossover Trial," *Anaesthesia* 48(5):393-95, 1993b.

Sharma, S.S., et al. "Antiemetic Efficacy of Ginger Against Cisplatin-induced Emesis in Dogs," *J Ethnopharmacol* 57(2):93-96, 1997.

Srivastava, K.C., and Mustafa, T. "Ginger (*Zingiber officinale*) in Rheumatism and Musculoskeletal Disorders," *Med Hypotheses* 39:342-48, 1992.

Stewart, J.J., et al. "Effects of Ginger on Motion Sickness Susceptibility and Gastric Function," *Pharmacology* 42(2):111-20, 1991.

Suekawa, M., et al. "Pharmacological Studies on Ginger IV Effect of [6]-Shogaol on the Arachidonic Cascade," *Nippon Ya Kruigaku Zasshi* 88(4):263-69, 1986.

Unnikrishnan, M., and Kuttan, R. "Cytotoxicity of Extracts of Spices to Cultured Cells," *Nutr Cancer* 11(4):251-57, 1988.

Verma, S., et al. "Effect of Ginger on Platelet Aggregation in Man," *Indian J Med Res* 98:240-42, 1993.

Yamahara, J., et al. "GI Motility Enhancing Effects of Ginger and Its Active Constituents," *Chem Pharm Bull* 38:430-31, 1990.

GINKGO

EGB 761, GBE, GBE 24, GBX, GINKGO BILOBA, GINKOGINK, LI 1370, ROKAN, SOPHIUM, TANAKAN, TEBOFORTAN, TEBONIN

Taxonomic class
Ginkgoaceae

Common trade names
Multi-ingredient preparations: Bioginkgo 24/6, Bioginkgo 27/7, Cardio Ginko Power, Gincosan, Ginexin Remind, Ginkai, Ginkgoba, Ginkgo Go!, Ginkgold, Ginkgo Phytosome, Ginkgo Power, Ginkoba, Ginkocure, Ginko Sharp Herb Tea

Common forms
Available as ginkgo biloba extract in capsules, nutrition bars, sublingual sprays (standardized to contain 24% flavone glycosides and 6% terpenes), and tablets and as concentrated alcoholic extract of fresh leaf.
Capsules, tablets: 30 mg, 40 mg, 60 mg, 120 mg, 260 mg, 420 mg
Sublingual sprays: 15 mg/spray, 40 mg/spray

Ginkgo biloba extract (24% standardized extract) bound to phosphatidylcholine is available as 80-mg capsules.

Source

Ginkgo biloba extract is obtained from the leaves of the *Ginkgo biloba* tree, formerly *Salisburia adiantifolia*. The tree is also known as the maidenhair tree and the kew tree. The extract is produced by a complex, multistep process that concentrates the active constituents and removes the potentially toxic ginkgolic acid.

Chemical components

Ginkgo biloba extract is composed of a complex mixture of polar and nonpolar compounds. The extract contains various flavonol and flavone glycosides, 20-carbon diterpene lactones (including ginkgetin, ginkgolic acid, and isoginkgetin), 20-carbon diterpene lactone derivatives termed ginkgolides (of which ginkgolide A, B, C, J, and M have been identified), and a 15-carbon sesquiterpene termed bilobalide. Other isolated compounds include ascorbic acid, catechin, iron-based superoxide dismutase, *p*-hydroxybenzoic acid, 6-hydroxkynurenic acid, protocatechuic acid, shikimic acid, sterols including sitosterol, and vanillic acid.

Actions

Ginkgo biloba extract produces arterial and venous vasoactive changes that increase tissue perfusion and cerebral blood flow. The physiologic effects are attributed to the extract's ability to produce arterial vasodilation, inhibit arterial spasms, decrease capillary permeability, reduce capillary fragility, decrease blood viscosity, and reduce erythrocyte aggregation. These effects are probably caused by stimulation of prostaglandin biosynthesis or by indirect vasoregulatory effects on catecholamines (Nemecz and Combest, 1997; Princemail et al., 1989). Ginkgo biloba extract also acts as an antioxidant (Bastianetto et al., 2000; Kobuchi et al., 1997); ginkgolide B is reported to be a potent inhibitor of platelet activating factor (Koltai et al., 1991) and has been reported to offer potential neuroprotection by inhibiting MAO (Sloley et al., 2000), although some data suggest that ginkgo biloba administration does not cause MAO inhibition in the human brain (Fowler et al., 2000).

Gingko biloba was shown to inhibit angiogenesis in a rat model of experimental retinopathy (Juarez et al., 2000).

Reported uses

Ginkgo biloba extract has been studied for the treatment of cerebrovascular disease and peripheral vascular insufficiency. (See *Use of ginkgo for dementia.*) Other studies have evaluated the use of extract or isolated constituents for such disorders as arrhythmias, asthma, hearing loss, impotence secondary to serotonin reuptake inhibitors, peripheral arterial disease, premenstrual syndrome, senile macular degeneration, and vestibular disorders. Ginkgo biloba has also also been investigated for the treatment of glaucoma.

Bold italic type indicates that reaction may be life-threatening.

RESEARCH FINDINGS
Use of ginkgo for dementia

At least two studies indicate that ginkgo may benefit patients with dementia. A 52-week multicenter, randomized, double-blind, placebo-controlled trial (LeBars et al., 1997) followed 309 outpatients with mild to severe dementia from Alzheimer's disease or multi-infarct dementia. Patients were randomly given placebo or ginkgo, 120 mg daily, and assessed using the Alzheimer's Disease Assessment Scale-Cognitive Subscale (ADAS), the Geriatric Evaluation by Relative's Rating Instrument (GERRI), and the Clinical Global Impression of Change (CGIC). A small statistically significant treatment difference in favor of ginkgo was noted through improved ADAS and GERRI scores. CGIC test scores did not change. The authors concluded that ginkgo improved cognitive and social functioning for 6 to 12 months in many patients.

A similar trial of 216 patients with Alzheimer's disease or multi-infarct dementia showed that ginkgo, 240 mg daily, improved various symptoms (Kanowski et al., 1996). In this 24-week study, patients benefited if scores in at least two of the three functional tests increased. Patients with cardiac or hepatic disease, chronic renal failure, and type 1 diabetes were excluded from the study. The safety and efficacy of ginkgo biloba extract in these populations, therefore, have not been evaluated.

Wettstein (2000) compared the available cholinesterase inhibitors for dementia (donepezil, metrifonate, rivastigmine, tacrine) with ginkgo biloba and determined that, with the exception of tacrine, all were equally effective in treating mild to moderate Alzheimer's dementia.

Ginkgo biloba extract is claimed to improve mental alertness and overall brain function; evidence for this use is not substantiated in well-controlled clinical trials.

Dosage
For dementia syndromes, 120 to 240 mg P.O. in divided doses b.i.d. or t.i.d. *For peripheral arterial disease, tinnitus, and vertigo,* 120 to 160 mg P.O. in divided doses b.i.d. or t.i.d. Doses as high as 320 mg/day have also been studied. Most studies reported a minimum duration of 4 to 6 weeks of therapy was required before positive effects were noted.

Use of crude, dried leaf preparations or extemporaneous preparation of the leaves as a tea is not recommended because of insufficient quantity of active ingredients.

Adverse reactions
CNS: headache, *seizures* (with excessive ingestion of ginkgo seeds by children—more than 50 seeds), *subdural hematoma.*

EENT: hyphema.
GI: diarrhea, flatulence, nausea, vomiting.
Hematologic: *bleeding.*
Skin: contact hypersensitivity reactions, dermatitis if contact with fruit occurs.

Interactions

Anticoagulants, antiplatelets: Use ginkgo biloba extract with caution because of its effect on platelet activating factor. Carefully monitor patients who are taking anticoagulants or antiplatelet drugs.

There is one report of the onset of coma in a patient with Alzheimer's disease that was induced by the combination of gingko biloba and low-dose trazodone (Galluzzi et al., 2000).

Contraindications and precautions

Ginkgo is contraindicated in patients who are hypersensitive to ginkgo preparations, in pregnant patients, and in children. Use cautiously in patients who are taking anticoagulants.

Special considerations

• Advise the patient to report bleeding or bruising.
• Instruct the patient to keep seeds out of the reach of children because of the risk of seizures from ingestion.
• Advise the patient to avoid contact with the fruit pulp or seed coats because of the risk of contact dermatitis. The fruit pulp and seed coats contain ginkgolic acid and bilobin, which are structurally related to the urushiols found in cashew nut shells, mango fruit rind, and poison ivy. More potent preparations may cause irritation or blistering of skin or mucus membranes if applied externally.

Points of interest

• Standardized ginkgo biloba extract is among the leading prescriptions in Germany and France but is available only as a dietary supplement in the United States. Ginkgo was the third-best-selling herbal product in health food stores in the United States in 1997.
• Ginkgo is considered an "effective substance for the treatment of peripheral arterial occlusive disease," according to the Federal German Drug Law (1996). The same reference reports that ginkgo's efficacy is similar to that of pentoxifylline and just as variable.
• Ginkgo has been approved in Germany for treating dementia.
• Ginkgo biloba extract preparation bound to phosphatidylcholine is claimed to increase the absorption and incorporation of ginkgo into biological membranes. There is no published support of this claim.
• The seeds, reported to be edible, are sold at oriental shops and usually boiled before consumption to remove toxic components.

Commentary

Ginkgo might be best characterized as a mild to moderate vasoactive agent. Most of the clinical data are from animal or uncontrolled studies; many of these trials were flawed and used small sample size, lacked ob-

---

Bold italic type indicates that reaction may be life-threatening.

jective outcome measurements, had incomplete descriptions of patient characteristics and inadequate descriptions of the randomization process, and were of short duration. The most convincing preliminary human trial data seem to suggest a role for ginkgo in dementia and peripheral vascular disease, but further studies are needed to define its specific role in therapy. Few studies compare ginkgo with standard-of-care treatments or other controls. Allergic reactions have been reported primarily with exposure to the whole ginkgo plant or contact with the fruit pulp. The potential for such reactions warrants discriminate use in patients who have a history of hypersensitivity reactions. The potential for drug interactions with antithrombotics and antiplatelet drugs requires diligence in monitoring.

References

Bastianetto, S., et al. "The Ginkgo Biloba E (Egb 761) Protects and Rescues Hippocampal Cells Against Nitric Oxide-induced Toxicity: Involvement of Its Flavonoid Constituents and Protein Kinase C," *J Neurochem* 74(6): 2268-77, 2000.

Fowler, J.S., et al. "Evidence That Gingko Biloba Extract Does Not Inhibit MAO A and B in Living Human Brain," *Life Sci* 66(9):PL141-46, 2000.

Galluzzi, S., et al. "Coma in a Patient with Alzheimer's Disease Taking Low Dose Trazodone and Gingko Biloba," *J Neurol Neurosurg Psychiatry* 68(5):679-80, 2000. Letter.

Juarez, C.P., et al. "Experimental Retinopathy of Prematurity: Angiostatic Inhibition by Nimodipine, Gingko-biloba, and Dipyridamole, and response to Different Growth Factors," *Eur J Ophthalmol* 10(1):51-59, 2000.

Kanowski, S., et al. "Proof of Efficacy of the Ginkgo Biloba Special Extract EGB 761 in Outpatients Suffering from Mild to Moderate Primary Degenerative Dementia of the Alzheimer Type of Multi-Infarct Dementia," *Pharmacopsychiatry* 29:47-56, 1996.

Kobuchi, H., et al. "*Ginkgo biloba* Extract (EGB 761): Inhibitory Effect of Nitric Oxide Production in the Macrophage Cell Line RAW 264.7," *Biochem Pharmacol* 53:897-903, 1997.

Koltai, M., et al. "Platelet Activating Factor (PAF). A Review of Its Effects, Antagonists and Possible Future Clinical Implications: Part 1," *Drugs* 42:9-29, 1991.

LeBars, P.L., et al. "A Placebo-controlled, Double-Blind Randomized Trial of an Extract of Ginkgo Biloba for Dementia," *JAMA* 278:1327-32, 1997.

Nemecz, G., and Combest, W.L. "Ginkgo Biloba," *US Pharmacist* 22:144-51, September 1997.

Princemail, J., et al. "Superoxide Anion Scavenging Effect and Superoxide Dismutase Activity of *Ginkgo biloba* Extract," *Experientia* 45:708-12, 1989.

Sloley, B.D., et al. "Identification of Kaempferol as a Monoamine Oxidase Inhibitor and Potential Neuroprotectant in Extracts of Ginkgo Biloba Leaves," *J Pharm Pharmacol* 52(4):451-59, 2000.

Wettstein, A. "Cholinesterase Inhibitors and Gingko Extracts—Are They Comparable in the Treatment of Dementia? Comparison of Published Placebo-controlled Efficacy Studies of at Least 6 Months' Duration," *Phytomedicine* 6(6):393-401, 2000.

GINSENG

AMERICAN GINSENG, ASIATIC GINSENG, CHINESE GINSENG,
FIVE-FINGERS, G115, JAPANESE GINSENG, JINTSAM,
KOREAN GINSENG, NINJIN, ORIENTAL GINSENG, SCHINSENT,
SENG AND SANG, TARTAR ROOT, WESTERN GINSENG

Taxonomic class
Araliaceae

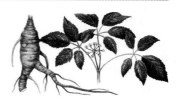

Common trade names
Multi-ingredient preparations: Bio
Star, Cimexon, Energy Rise, Fast
Lane Herb Tea, Gincosan, Ginsana,
Ginsatonic, Ginseng Action, Neo
Ginsana

Common forms
No standards exist for ginseng despite availability of chromatographic
assays for ginsenosides and ginseng polysaccharides.
Capsules: 100 mg, 250 mg, 500 mg
Extract: 2 oz root extract (in alcohol base)
Root powder: 1 oz, 4 oz
Tea bags: 1,500 mg ginseng root
   Also available as a cream, eye gel, nutrition bar, and oil. The root is
available in bulk by the pound.

Source
The most common species is *Panax quinquefolius*, commonly known as
American or Western ginseng. Sought after most commonly for its root,
the plant's other characteristics (wild or cultivated) and the shapes of
the root make it more valuable. Traditionally, ideal plants are at least 6
years old. *Panax ginseng* is known as the Asian, Korean, or Japanese ginseng. Asian ginseng usually undergoes treatment, such as drying and
curing, before it is sold; the American variety undergoes less manipulation and carries less distinction.

Chemical components
Ginseng is composed primarily of ginsenosides, also known as panaxosides. About 12 major panaxosides have been isolated but are found in
only minute quantities and are difficult to purify on a large scale. Other
components of the plant isolated for pharmacologic effects include a
volatile oil, beta-elemine, sterols, flavonoids, peptides, vitamins (B_1, B_2,
B_{12}, panthotenic acid, nicotinic acid, and biotin), fats, polyacetylenes,
minerals, enzymes, and choline.

Actions
Several pharmacologic effects have been noted that vary with dose and
duration of treatment. The panaxosides, found in the root, are thought
to be the pharmacologically active agents. Although they are similar in

---

Bold italic type indicates that reaction may be life-threatening.

structure, sometimes these compounds exert opposing pharmacologic effects. For example, ginsenoside Rb-1 has analgesic, anticonvulsant, antipsychotic, and CNS depressant effects; stress ulcer–preventing action; and acceleration of glycolysis and nuclear RNA synthesis. Ginsenoside Rg-1 has antifatigue, CNS stimulating, hypertensive, and stress ulcer–aggravating activities. These opposing features form the basis for the theory that ginseng serves to "balance bodily functions."

Another example of these opposing actions is that Rg and Rg-1 enhance cardiac performance, whereas Rb depresses cardiac function. Other ginsenosides have shown antiarrhythmic activity similar to that of verapamil and amiodarone. Oral ginseng was found to reduce cholesterol and triglyceride levels, decrease platelet adhesiveness, impair coagulation, and increase fibrinolysis in cholesterol-fed rats. Ginsenosides may reduce stress by acting on the adrenal gland.

Hypoglycemic activity in rodents has been documented, but the mechanism of action has not been proved (Suzuki and Hikino, 1989). Extracts of ginseng have shown antioxidant activity on human erythrocytes in a laboratory model and prevented the development of morphine tolerance in rats. Some studies in animals have documented ginseng's anti-inflammatory and antiviral activities and its hepatoprotective effects at low doses (destruction at high doses) in a rat model, whereas others found that tumors in mice were suppressed by components of ginseng (Yun and Choi, 1990).

Reported uses

Ginseng is popularly claimed to minimize or reduce thymus gland activity. Other claims include its use as an antidepressant, an aphrodisiac, a demulcent (soothes irritated or inflamed internal tissues and organs), a diuretic, a sedative, and a sleep aid. Short-term use of the herb may improve concentration, healing, stamina, stress resistance (adaptogenic), vigilance, and work efficiency; long-term use is claimed to improve well-being in elderly patients with debilitated or degenerative conditions. Few claims have supporting data from animal studies and fewer still have data from human studies.

Although studies conducted in humans were mostly small and poorly designed, results suggest that ginseng has several beneficial effects. Improvement in appetite, emotional lability, sleep, and work efficiency in animals and humans indicates the ginseng's ability to enhance physical and mental performance. Ginseng may also indirectly exhibit corticosteroid-like effects.

Ginseng decreased fasting blood glucose and hemoglobin A_{1C} levels in both diabetic and nondiabetic patients such that some diabetics were free of insulin therapy for the duration of the study (Sotaniemi et al., 1995). The herb has also been shown to be beneficial in patients with hepatic dysfunction, hyperlipidemia, and impaired cognitive function. (See *Ginseng's effect on cognitive function,* page 340.)

RESEARCH FINDINGS
Ginseng's effect on cognitive function

A few studies have been performed to determine ginseng's claim of improved psychomotor performance and cognitive functions.

One randomized, double-blind, placebo-controlled study of 32 healthy male volunteers (aged 20 to 24) was performed to evaluate the effect of standardized ginseng extract (Ginsana) on psychomotor performance. Patients were given ginseng (100 mg) or placebo twice daily for 12 weeks and evaluated at baseline and at 11 weeks. A favorable effect was shown in attention, logical deduction, and sensory and motor perception within the same person (acting as his control) at baseline and 11 weeks. Results were only slightly in favor for ginseng for mathematical reasoning (D'Angelo et al., 1986).

Another randomized, double-blind, placebo-controlled trial evaluated ginseng's effects on cognitive function. The 112 subjects were randomized to receive standardized ginseng or inactive placebo. The primary outcome was the change in score on each cognitive test, evaluated both at baseline and at 8 weeks. Safety was also evaluated by questioning the subjects. Results demonstrate a tendency to faster simple reaction times and better abstract thinking in the ginseng-treated group—the only statistically significant finding (Sorensen and Sonne, 1996).

A third clinical trial evaluated the cognitive effects of a ginkgo and ginseng combination in healthy volunteers with neurasthenic complaints. This 90-day, double-blind, placebo-controlled parallel study group involved 64 patients (aged 40 to 65), who were randomly assigned to receive 80, 160, or 320 mg of the combination or placebo twice daily and assessed at baseline and at days 1, 30, and 90. Cognitive outcomes measured were basic memory skills, accuracy and speed of response, and immediate and delayed word and picture recognition. Although well tolerated, the adverse reactions most often reported included dizziness, somnolence, and increased frequency of urination. The only significant finding occurred 1 hour after the 320-mg dose, in which cognitive improvement was seen on day 90. A larger dose and shorter dosing interval may be necessary (Wesnes et al., 1997).

One study suffered from a small sample size. Baseline demographics and characteristics differed significantly between groups in some cases and were not addressed in others. Compliance was evaluated only in one trial; study methods cannot be relied on in some cases because of possible bias in design.

More rigidly controlled human clinical trials are needed before ginseng and its extracts can be recommended for improving cognitive and psychomotor functions.

Bold italic type indicates that reaction may be life-threatening.

Dosage

Dosages vary with the disease state; usually, 0.5 to 2 g of dry ginseng root P.O. daily or 200 to 600 mg of ginseng extract P.O. daily in one or two equal doses.

For improved well-being in debilitated elderly patients, 0.4 to 0.8 g of root daily P.O. on a continual basis.

Adverse reactions

CNS: headache, insomnia, nervousness.
CV: chest pain, hypertension, palpitations.
EENT: epistaxis.
GI: diarrhea, nausea, vomiting.
GU: impotence, mastalgia, vaginal bleeding.
Skin: pruritus, rash (with ginseng abuse).

Interactions

Antidiabetic agents, insulin: Increased hypoglycemic effect. Use together cautiously.

MAO inhibitors (hypericin, parnate, phenelzine, selegiline, tranylcypromine): Adverse reactions include headache, mania, and tremor. Avoid administration with ginseng.

Contraindications and precautions

Avoid using ginseng in pregnant or breast-feeding women; effects are unknown. Use cautiously in patients with CV disease, diabetes, hypertension, or hypotension and in those who are also receiving steroid therapy.

Special considerations

● Monitor the patient for signs and symptoms of ginseng abuse syndrome. This syndrome occurs when large doses of the herb are taken concomitantly with other psychomotor stimulants, such as tea and coffee. Symptoms include depression, diarrhea, edema, euphoria, hypertension, insomnia, loss of appetite, rash, and restlessness. The existence of this syndrome is debatable.

● Monitor the diabetic patient for signs and symptoms of hypoglycemia. Advise him to monitor his blood glucose level closely until effects are known.

● Advise the patient not to take ginseng for a prolonged period.

● Instruct the patient with preexisting medical conditions to check with his health care provider before taking ginseng.

● Urge the patient to watch for unusual symptoms (diarrhea, insomnia, nervousness, palpitations) because of the risk of ginseng toxicity.

● Advise the pregnant or breast-feeding patient to consult a health care provider before taking ginseng because safety has not been established.

Points of interest

● Ginseng has been given a positive evaluation from the German Commission E.

• It is estimated that 6 million people in the United States use ginseng regularly. In oriental cultures, it has been used for its medicinal properties for more than 2,000 years.

• Although it was abundant in eastern North America, American ginseng is now considered threatened because of aggressive harvesting for commercial sales.

Commentary

Public interest in ginseng has been increasing. Although the herb appears to have promising uses, additional human efficacy, toxicity, and interactions data are needed. Ginseng has an interesting and unique pharmacologic profile, but ingestion of the plant is not without risk, despite its use for centuries.

References

D'Angelo, L., et al. "A Double-Blind, Placebo-controlled Clinical Study on the Effect of a Standardized Ginseng Extract on Psychomotor Performance in Healthy Volunteers," *J Ethnopharmacol* 16:15-22, 1986.

Sorensen, H., and Sonne, J. "A Double-masked Study of the Effects of Ginseng on Cognitive Functions," *Curr Ther Res* 57:959-68, 1996.

Sotaniemi, E., et al. "Ginseng Therapy in Non-Insulin-Dependent Diabetic Patients," *Diabetes Care* 18:1373-75, 1995.

Suzuki, Y., and Hikino, H. "Mechanisms of Hypoglycemic Activity of Pnaxans A and B, Glycans of *Panax ginseng* Roots: Effects on the Key Enzymes of Glucose Metabolism in the Liver of Mice," *Phytotherapy Res* 3:15-19, 1989.

Wesnes, K.A., et al. "The Cognitive, Subjective, and Physical Effects of a Ginkgo Biloba/*Panax Ginseng* Combination in Healthy Volunteers with Neurasthenic Complaints," *Psychopharmacol Bull* 33:677-83, 1997.

Yun, T.K., and Choi, S. "A Case-Control Study of Ginseng Intake and Cancer," *Int J Epidemiol* 19:871-76, 1990.

GINSENG, SIBERIAN

ACANTHOPANAX SENTICOSUS, DEVIL'S SHRUB, ELEUTHEROCOCCUS SENTICOSUS, HEDERA SENTICOSA, SHIGOKA, TOUCH-ME-NOT

Taxonomic class

Araliaceae

Common trade names

Multi-ingredient preparations: Activex 40 Plus, Elton, Gincosan (with gingko biloba), Ginkovit, Ginseng Complex, Leuzea, Leveton, Minadex Mix Ginseng, Panax Complex, Siberian Ginseng, Taiga Wurzel, Vigoran

Common forms

Available as capsules, oils, powders, tablets, teas, and tinctures.

Source

The drug is extracted from the root and root bark of *Eleutherococcus senticosus,* which belongs to the same family as panax or chinese ginseng.

Chemical components

Constituents of the root include saponins (termed eleutherosides), which appear to be the active drug and are found in equal concentrations in above-ground parts and roots. The eleutherosides are subgrouped A to G. Other components include essential oil, resin, starch, and vitamin A.

Actions

The saponin portion of Siberian ginseng appears to have affinity for progestin, mineralocorticoid, and glucocorticoid receptors, although not to the extent of panax ginseng. Unlike panax ginseng, Siberian ginseng binds to estrogen receptors.

When the extract was injected into the peritoneal cavity of mice, a marked hypoglycemic effect was observed (Hikino et al., 1986). Orally administered *Eleutherococcus* was found to decrease blood glucose levels in rats but had no effect on plasma lactic acid, glucagon, insulin, or liver glycogen levels (Martinez et al., 1984). It is not known if this effect occurs in humans.

Despite the claim that Siberian ginseng enhances the ability to tolerate stress, ingestion of *Eleutherococcus* was not found to significantly affect the survival of mice under major environmental stress, but a more aggressive behavior was noted (Lewis et al., 1983).

Reported uses

Siberian ginseng is described as a pungent, bittersweet, warming herb with the purported ability to stimulate the immune and circulatory systems, regulate blood pressure, reduce inflammation, treat insomnia caused by prolonged anxiety, and increase stamina and the ability to cope with stress. Preliminary Russian studies have attempted to verify adaptogenic effects of ginseng in studies of both healthy and nonhealthy patients. These trial results are at best inconsistent but suggest some favorable effects in certain parameters associated with the patients' ability to withstand stressful conditions. An abstract of a trial published in a Russian journal describes a trial that supposedly documented an increase in working capacity and rehabilitation of trained athletes after a 20-day ingestion of new dosage formulations of *Eleutherococcus* (Azizov, 1997). Also, the apparent increase in blood coagulability seen with highly trained athletes was in part abrogated by the *Eleutherococcus* treatments. Another trial out of Poland concluded that an *Eleutherococcus* preparation, when given to 10 healthy men for 30 days, revealed a higher oxygen plateau, as measured by ergospirometry, and demonstrated beneficial effects on the lipid profile compared with echinacea (Szolomicki et al., 2000). Some questions exist in regard to the study's design.

Studies with animals have indicated no effect on stamina or stress tolerance. In a study involving highly trained distance runners, the herb had no effect on improving exercise tolerance (Dowling et al., 1996). As with other ginseng plants, Siberian ginseng claims to have immunomodulatory actions; it is thought to stimulate macrophages, promote antibody formation, activate complement, and increase T-lymphocyte proliferation. An increase in the T-lymphocyte count and in the activation state of T cells were shown in human patients (Bohn et al., 1987); neither the extent of the proliferation nor the duration of these effects can be determined from this study alone.

Extensive human studies are needed to verify claims of radioprotective or chemotherapeutic effects of Siberian ginseng.

Dosage
No guidelines exist. The most common regimen is 500 to 2,000 mg/day P.O. Use cautiously because of the lack of uniform content of capsules and the substitution of less expensive plants.

Adverse reactions
CNS: agitation, decreased concentration, dizziness, euphoria, insomnia, nervousness.
CV: hypertension.
GI: diarrhea.
GU: estrogenic effects, vaginal bleeding.
Hematologic: reduced coagulation potential (unknown mechanism).
Skin: rash.

Interactions
Digoxin: Elevated serum digoxin levels. Monitor digoxin use closely.
Hexobarbital: Inhibited hexobarbital metabolism. Avoid administration with Siberian ginseng.
Vitamins B$_1$, B$_2$, and C: Siberian ginseng may increase excretion of these vitamins. Avoid administration with Siberian ginseng.

Contraindications and precautions
Siberian ginseng use is contraindicated in children and in patients who are hypersensitive to ginseng, Siberian ginseng, or ingredients in the preparation.

Special considerations
• Advise the patient not to use Siberian ginseng for longer than 3 weeks.
• Siberian ginseng is not uniform in content when packaged, and less expensive plant products are commonly substituted for this herb.
• Siberian ginseng may be sold as a combination product with panax ginseng. Monitor for adverse reactions also associated with panax or Chinese ginseng.
• Urge the patient to report agitation, diarrhea, euphoria, insomnia, menstrual irregularities, nervousness, and rash.
• Caution the diabetic patient to closely monitor blood glucose levels and to watch for increased effects of antidiabetic drugs because of the herb's hypoglycemic effect in animals.

Commentary
The most prevalent claim for Siberian ginseng is its ability to improve energy, exercise performance, and stamina. This claim has proved to be

---

Bold italic type indicates that reaction may be life-threatening.

untrue. Also, the adaptogenic response, which claims increased resistance to stress, has also been found to be false.

The immunomodulating and radioprotective effects have been studied mostly in animal and foreign trials. Although the data thus far appear promising, particularly for a radioprotective action, larger controlled studies are needed in humans to determine whether the herb not only increases the T-lymphocyte count and response but also clinically prevents or hastens recovery from infections.

There are no data to substantiate other claims for Siberian ginseng. There are also no long-term studies, and thus its effects over time are not known. Consequently, the use of Siberian ginseng beyond 3 weeks is not recommended.

References

Azizov, A.P. "Effects of *Eleutherococcus,* Elton, Leuzea, and Leveton on the Blood Coagulation System During Training in Athletes," *Eksp Klin Farmakol* 60(5):58-60, 1997.

Bohn, B., et al. "Flow-Cytometric Studies with *Eleutherococcus senticosus* Extract as an Immunomodulatory Agent," *Arzneimittelforschung* 37:1193-96, 1987.

Dowling, E.A.., et al. "Effect of *Eleutherococcus senticosus* on Submaximal and Maximal Exercise Performance," *Med Sci Sports Exerc* 28:482-89, 1996.

Hikino, H., et al. "Isolation and Hypoglycemic Activity of Eleutherans A, B, C, D, E, F, and G: Glycans of *Eleutherococcus senticosus* Roots," *J Natl Prod* 49:293-97, 1986.

Lewis, W.H., et al. "No Adaptogenic Response of Mice to Ginseng and *Eleutherococcus* Infusions," *J Ethnopharmacol* 8:209-14, 1983.

Martinez, B., et al. "The Physiological Effects of Aralia, Panax *and Eleutherococcus senticosus* on Exercised Rats," *Jpn J Pharmacol* 35:79-85, 1984.

Szolomicki, J., et al. "The Influence of Active Components of *Eleutherococcus senticosus* on Cellular Defence and Physical Fitness in Man," *Phytother Res* 14(1):30-35, 2000.

GLUCOMANNAN

KONJAC, KONJAC MANNAN

Taxonomic class
Araceae

Common trade names
Glucomannan

Common forms
Available as capsules, powder, and tablets (600 mg).

Source
The tubers of the plant *Amorphophallus konjac* are typically harvested to yield a chemical called konjac mannan.

Chemical components
Konjac mannan, or glucomannan, is a polysaccharide composed of linked molecules of glucose and mannose. It is purified from konjac

flour by chemical treatment with cupric hydroxide and repeated ethanol washings or by dialysis against water.

Actions

Polysaccharide agents (guar gum, methylcellulose, tragacanth, bran, and pectin) such as glucomannan have been shown to delay the absorption of glucose from the bowel (Jenkins et al., 1978). Glucomannan ingestion changes intestinal microbial flora in rodents, but human microbial natural flora may be changed less dramatically (Fujiwara et al., 1991).

Other studies using rodents suggest that the water-soluble form of glucomannan can lower cholesterol levels, depending on the purity of the herb. A water-insoluble form (referred to as *konnyaku* in Japan) was unable to reduce rat plasma cholesterol levels (Kiriyama et al., 1969), but it appeared to lower the prevalence of murine lung cancers (Luo, 1992).

Reported uses

Bulk-forming agents such as guar gum (galactomannan, galactose, and mannose), methylcellulose, tragacanth, bran fiber, and pectin are known for their ability to draw water into the lumen of the bowel, promoting hydration of stool and facilitating relief of constipation. Anecdotal reports claim that glucomannan is an effective laxative because of these properties.

Hydrophilic agents have been included as part of weight-loss regimens because of the agents' supposed ability to produce early satiety and fullness. Glucomannan is becoming a popular component of weight-loss programs. Clinical trial data supporting the use of glucomannan as a weight-reducing agent are scarce and conflicting at best. Additional studies are needed in this area.

Studies in healthy human subjects have demonstrated the herb's ability to lower serum cholesterol and blood glucose levels. (See *Glucomannan as a cholesterol- and glucose-lowering agent.*)

Children with severe brain damage are known to have serious problems with chronic constipation because of their neurologic deficits. Stoiano and others (2000) evaluated the efficacy of glucomannan as a treatment for such children. A double-blind study of 20 patients randomized 10 subjects to glucomannan and 10 to placebo for 12 weeks. Konjac-mannan (glucomannan) significantly increased ($P<.01$) stool frequency, whereas findings in the placebo group were not significant. The use of glucomannan decreased the use of suppositories and laxatives. Glucomannan was also shown to significantly decrease the number of episodes of painful defecation. Neither glucomannan nor placebo had any measurable effect on colonic activity.

Dosage

For lowering blood glucose levels, 3.6 to 7.2 g of glucomannan P.O. daily was given to diabetic patients for 90 days.

For lowering cholesterol levels, one study used 3.9 g of glucomannan P.O. daily for 4 weeks, stopped for 2 weeks, and then resumed treatment for another 4 weeks. Another study used 100 ml of a 1% solution of glucomannan P.O. daily.

Bold italic type indicates that reaction may be life-threatening.

RESEARCH FINDINGS

Glucomannan as a cholesterol- and glucose-lowering agent

Glucomannan has been studied for its ability to lower serum cholesterol and blood glucose levels. The following trials have focused on the herb's ability to improve the lipid profile or lower blood glucose levels.

In one study, glucomannan was given to 13 diabetic patients for 90 days (Doi et al., 1979). After 20 days, serum cholesterol levels dropped by 11.2%, and at 30 days, blood glucose levels fell about 29% ($P<.025$) compared with baseline. Most patients were able to reduce their doses of oral antidiabetic drugs or insulin. Glucomannan was thought to reduce absorption of oral glucose, evidenced by lower peak blood glucose levels at 30 minutes after ingestion.

Additional evidence comes from a larger study of 72 patients with type 2 diabetes. A refined konjac food was given in various forms (powder, noodle, or toast) with normal foods consumed during meals. The diet and activity of the patients remained constant. After 65 days, fasting blood glucose and 2-hour postprandial glucose values were significantly lower than baseline ($P<.05$ for both), and patients lost an average of 2 kg of body weight. Glycosylated hemoglobin levels fell about 15% during this study ($P<.05$). Although LDL and total cholesterol levels fell slightly, only serum triglyceride levels were significantly reduced. HDL levels remained unchanged. The researchers concluded that konjac mannan food helped prevent and treat hyperglycemia (Huang et al., 1990).

In a controlled study, glucomannan improved metabolic control in high-risk patients with type 2 diabetes. Glycemia, lipidemia, and blood pressure were used as measuring tools in one controlled study. Compared with placebo, konjac mannan significantly reduced the metabolic control primary endpoints of decreased fructosamine, decreased HDL-cholesterol ratio, and decreased systolic blood pressure (Vuksan et al., 1999).

Another study supplemented a high-cholesterol diet with fiber from konjac mannan, to evaluate its effect on metabolic control in 278 patients ages 45 to 65 with insulin resistance syndrome. After an 8-week baseline, subjects were randomly assigned to take konjac mannan biscuits or wheat bran fiber biscuits for two 3-week periods followed by a 2-week washout. Serum cholesterol and fructosamine levels and apolipoprotein (apo) B–apo B/A-1 ratio decreased more in the konjac mannan group than in the wheat bran group. The conclusion was that a diet rich in high-viscosity konjac mannan improves glycemic control and lipid profiles (Vuksan et al., 2000).

For reducing body weight, an American study used 1.5 g of glucomannan b.i.d. for 8 weeks.

Because of the lack of consistency in trials, no specific dose can be recommended.

Adverse reactions

GI: changes in intestinal flora, diarrhea, esophageal and lower GI obstruction, esophageal perforation, flatulence, loose stools.
Metabolic: hypoglycemia.

Interactions

Cholesterol-lowering drugs: May increase the cholesterol-reducing effects of these drugs. Monitor the patient.
Insulin, oral antidiabetic drugs: May require dosage adjustment during herbal treatment. Monitor the patient.

Contraindications and precautions

Avoid using glucomannan in pregnant or breast-feeding women; effects are unknown. Use cautiously in patients who are prone to hypoglycemia or GI dysfunction or obstruction.

Special considerations

• Monitor patients who are prone to gastric obstruction as well as diabetic patients because insulin or oral antidiabetic drug doses may need to be reduced. Large doses are likely to produce laxative effects because of glucomannan's osmotically active properties in the bowel. GI effects may limit tolerance of the herb.
• Stagger administration of other drugs by a few hours; concomitant use may alter drug absorption.
• Monitor the patient for signs of GI or esophageal obstruction (abdominal pain, constipation, distended or tense abdomen, loss of appetite, nausea).
• **ALERT** Esophageal perforation as a complication of GI obstruction has occurred. Several of these cases required mechanical removal under general anesthesia.
• Monitor the patient for significant changes in bowel habit and periodically check serum electrolyte levels because of the glucomannan's potential to alter gut flora and act as a laxative.
• Urge the diabetic patient to closely monitor blood glucose levels and consider dosage reductions in insulin or oral antidiabetic drugs, if necessary
• Encourage the patient to report loss of efficacy of other drugs he is taking.
• Inform the patient that long-term effects of glucomannan are not well known.
• Advise the pregnant or breast-feeding patient to avoid using glucomannan.

Bold italic type indicates that reaction may be life-threatening.

Points of interest
• Adverse reactions have led to discontinuation of the tablet form of glucomannan in Australia since the mid-1980s.

Commentary
Both animal and human studies seem to support the efficacy of glucomannan as a cholesterol-lowering agent. The greater efficacy of modern pharmaceutical agents, such as the statins, forces glucomannan to take a back seat in the hyperlipidemia treatment program. Glucomannan may prove to be a valuable adjunct to lipid-lowering therapy, but larger trials are warranted to adequately describe its adverse reaction profile.

Glucomannan's substantial ability to lower blood glucose levels makes it an attractive choice for patients with coexisting hypercholesterolemia and diabetes.

Existing information on its use as a diet aid is conflicting and difficult to interpret.

References
Doi, K., et al. "Treatment of Diabetes with Glucomannan (Konjac Mannan)," *Lancet* 1:987-88, 1979.

Fujiwara, S., et al. "Effect of Konjac Mannan on Intestinal Microbial Metabolism in Mice Bearing Human Flora and in Conventional F344 Rats," *Food Chem Toxicol* 29:601, 1991.

Huang, C.Y., et al. "Effect of Konjac Food on Blood Glucose Level in Patients With Diabetes," *Biomed Environ Sci* 3:123-31, 1990.

Jenkins, D.J., et al. "Dietary Fibres, Fibre Analogues and Glucose Tolerance: Importance of Viscosity," *Br Med J* 1:1392, 1978.

Kiriyama, S., et al. "Hypocholesterolemic Effect of Polysaccharides and Polysaccharide-Rich Foodstuffs in Cholesterol-Fed Rats," *J Nutr* 97:382, 1969.

Luo, D.Y. "Inhibitory Effect of Refined *Amorphophallus konjac* on MNNG-Induced Lung Cancers in Mice," *Chung Hua Chung Chiu Tsa Chih* 14:48, 1992.

Stoiano, A., et al. "Effect of Dietary Fiber Glucomannan on Chronic Constipation in Neurologically Impaired Children," *J. Pediatrics* 136(1): 41-45, 2000.

Vuksan, V., et al. "Konjac-Mannan (Glucomannan) Improves Glycemia and Other Associated Risk Factors for Coronary Heart Disease in Type II Diabetes. A Randomized Controlled Metabolic Trial," *Diabetes Care* 22(6):913-19, 1999.

Vuksan, V., et al. "Beneficial Effects of Viscous Dietary Fiber from Konjac-Mannan in Subjects with the Insulin-Resistance Syndrome," *Diabetes Care* (1):9-14, 2000.

GLUCOSAMINE

CHITOSAMINE, GLUCOSAMINE SULFATE, GS

Common trade names
Multi-ingredient preparations: Arth-X Plus, Bioflex, Enhanced Glucosamine Sulfate, Flexi-Factors, Glucosamine Complex, Glucosamine Mega, Joint Factors, Nutri-Joint, Ultra Maximum Strength Glucosamine Sulfate

Common forms

Various molecular forms of glucosamine are available, including chlorhydrate, D-glucosamine, hydrochloride, N-acetyl, sulfate, and with potassium chloride added. The preferred form appears to be glucosamine sulfate.

Capsules: 250 mg, 375 mg, 500 mg, 600 mg, 1,000 mg
Tablets: 63 mg, 87 mg, 375 mg, 500 mg, 600 mg, 750 mg

Source

Glucosamine is a natural substance found in mucopolysaccharides, mucoproteins, and chitin. Glucosamine sulfate is synthetically manufactured.

Chemical components

Glucosamine sulfate is the sulfate salt of 2-amino-2-deoxy-D-chitin glucopyranose.

Actions

Glucosamine is believed to stimulate production of cartilage components and allow rebuilding of damaged cartilage (Anon., 1996). Early in vitro studies found that culture-derived fibroblast increased mucopolysaccharide and collagen synthesis when glucosamine was added (McCarty, 1994).

In vivo and in vitro studies conducted in rats demonstrated that glucosamine can severely impair insulin secretion and beta-cell secretory dysfunction similar to that observed in patients with type 2 diabetes mellitus (Balkan and Dunning, 1994).

Reported uses

Glucosamine is thought to be useful as an antarthritic in patients with osteoarthritis or other joint disorders. (See *Glucosamine and osteoarthritis.*)

Dosage

The dose used in several clinical trials was 500 mg P.O. t.i.d. Other dosages were based on patient weight: If weight is below 120 lb (54 kg), 1,000 mg of glucosamine plus 800 mg of chondroitin sulfates; between 120 and 200 lb (91 kg), 1,500 mg of glucosamine plus 1,200 mg of chondroitin sulfates; and above 200 lb, 2,000 mg of glucosamine plus 1,600 mg of chondroitin sulfates.

Adverse reactions

CNS: drowsiness, headache.
GI: abdominal pain, constipation, diarrhea, epigastic discomfort, heartburn, nausea.
Skin: rash.
Other: *anaphylaxis* (Matheu et al., 1999).

Interactions

None reported.

Bold italic type indicates that reaction may be life-threatening.

RESEARCH FINDINGS
Glucosamine and osteoarthritis

The three largest randomized, controlled trials to date were carried out by Reichelt and coworkers (1994), Drovanti and colleagues (1980), and Vaz (1982), who evaluated 155, 80, and 40 patients with established osteoarthritis, respectively, for 8 weeks or less. Reichelt and colleagues found significant differences favoring glucosamine over placebo, with lower scores in the Lequesne Index; this improvement was still present 2 weeks after treatment was concluded. In the Drovanti study, symptom scores and joint mobility significantly favored glucosamine over placebo. Vaz reported that the onset of pain relief was more rapid with ibuprofen than with glucosamine, but at 8 weeks, the pain scores were statistically significantly lower with glucosamine than with ibuprofen.

Trials using glucosamine combined with chondroitin have also been done. A 16-week randomized, double-blind, placebo-controlled crossover trial evaluated glucosamine 1,500 mg/day, chondroitin sulfate 1,200 mg/day, and manganese ascorbate 228 mg/day for degenerative joint disease of the knees or lower back (Leffler et al., 1999). Thirty-four men answered questionnaires and underwent physical examinations and running tests. Summary disease scores favored the combination over placebo. Investigators concluded that the therapy appeared safe and effective for the short term but suggested that larger trials are still warranted.

Rindone (2000) reported on a 2-month, randomized, double-blind parallel trial in 98 patients aged 34 to 81 with osteoarthritis of the knee. No difference was found between the glucosamine group and the placebo group on the visual analog scale for pain intensity while at rest or walking at both 30 and 60 days. Likewise, an 8-week trial in Canada of patients with osteoarthritis of the knee failed to identify any statistically significant differences in measurements (standardized questionnaire) over those of placebo (Houpt et al., 1999).

A systematic analysis (McAlindon et al., 2000) concluded that glucosamine is probably mildly to moderately effective. But many trials were linked to a manufacturer of glucosamine, explaining the likely bias toward heightened benefits.

Study design flaws and limitations may have biased some outcome endpoints, despite these studies exhibiting some of the best evidence for glucosamine to date. Limitations include the use of short treatment periods, small sample sizes, concomitant drugs, nonstandardized measurements, subjective endpoints, undisclosed blinding techniques, and unknown criteria for selecting patients.

Contraindications and precautions

Avoid using glucosamine in patients who are hypersensitive to glucosamine or any of its components, in pregnant or breast-feeding women, and in children; effects are unknown.

Special considerations

- Monitor blood glucose levels in diabetic patients.
- Inform the patient that human clinical trials evaluating glucosamine are lacking.
- Suggest other accepted pharmacologic treatment before starting therapy with glucosamine.
- Explain that the long-term effect on beta-cell secretory function in humans is unknown and could be harmful, especially to patients with diabetes or impaired glucose tolerance.

Points of interest

- The Arthritis Foundation does not recommend glucosamine for osteoarthritis or any forms of arthritis because of the lack of efficacy data (Anon., 1996).
- The FDA has not reviewed any studies that confirm claims made for this herb.

Commentary

Several trials have demonstrated that glucosamine sulfate can improve symptoms of osteoarthritis. Many contain major study design flaws and critical problems with data analysis, placing their conclusions in jeopardy. Furthermore, all trials do not support the efficacy of glucosamine over placebo. There are few large, controlled clinical trials evaluating the use of glucosamine with chondroitin sulfates that identify positive benefits. Large-scale, long-term, adequately designed, rigorous, controlled studies are needed before glucosamine's role in the treatment of bone and joint disorders can be determined.

References

Anon. *Glucosamine Sulfate Treatment*. Public information memo #96-05. Atlanta: Arthritis Foundation, March 4, 1996.

Balkan, B., and Dunning, B.E. "Glucosamine Inhibits Glucokinase In Vitro and Produces a Glucose-Specific Impairment of In Vivo Insulin Secretion in Rats," *Diabetes* 43:1173-79, 1994.

Drovanti, A., et al. "Therapeutic Activity of Oral Glucosamine Sulfate in Osteoarthrosis: A Placebo-controlled Double-blind Investigation," *Clin Ther* 3:260-72, 1980.

Houpt, J.B., et al. "Effect of Glucosamine Hydrochloride in the Treatment of Pain of Osteoarthritis of the Knee," *J Rheumatol* 26(11):2294-97, 1999.

Leffler, C.T., et al. "Glucosamine, Chondroitin and Manganese Ascorbate for Degenerative Joint Disease of the Knee or Low Back: A Randomized, Double-blind, Placebo-controlled Pilot Study," *Mil Med* 164(2):85-91, 1999.

Matheu, V., et al. "Immediate Hypersensitivity Reaction to Glucosamine Sulfate," *Allergy* 54(6):643, 1999.

Bold italic type indicates that reaction may be life-threatening.

McAlindon, T.E., et al. "Glucosamine and Chondroitin for Treatment of Osteo-arthritis: A Systematic Quality Assessment and Meta-analysis," *JAMA* 283(11): 1469-75, 2000.

McCarty, M.F. "The Neglect of Glucosamine as Treatment for Osteoarthritis," *Med Hypotheses* 42:323-27, 1994.

Reichelt, A., et al. "Efficacy and Safety of Intramuscular Glucosamine Sulfate in Osteoarthritis of the Knee," *Arzneimittelforschung* 44:75-80, 1994.

Rindone, J.P. "Randomized, Controlled Trial of Glucosamine for Treating Osteoarthritis of the Knee," *West J Med* 172(2):95, 2000.

Vaz, A.L. "Double-blind Clinical Evaluation of the Relative Efficacy of Ibuprofen and Glucosamine Sulphate in the Management of Osteoarthrosis of the Knee in Outpatients," *Curr Med Res Opin* 8:145-49, 1982.

GOAT'S RUE

FRENCH HONEYSUCKLE, FRENCH LILAC

Taxonomic class
Fabaceae

Common trade names
Goat's Rue

Common forms
Available as dried leaves and a tincture.

Source
Goat's rue refers to the dried stalks, leaves, and flowers of *Galega officinalis*. It is a perennial herb that grows in damp meadows and along riverbanks from central Europe to Iran.

Chemical components
Goat's rue is composed primarily of tannins, bitters, and the alkaloids galegine and paragalegine.

Actions
Goat's rue is reported to have diuretic activity. The galegine alkaloid may reduce blood glucose levels when administered orally, but its efficacy as a hypoglycemic agent has not been substantiated in controlled human studies. In 1873, Gillet-Damitte addressed the French Academy and stated that goat's rue increased milk secretion in cows by 35% to 50%. The herb's activity as a lactogenic in animals has since been confirmed (Remington et al., 1918). Its effects on milk production have not been demonstrated in breast-feeding women.

Interesting information comes from a study in mice that suggests *G. officinalis* has weight-reducing properties (Palit et al., 1999). When *G. officinalis* (10% w/w in diet) was added to the diet of normal and genetically obese mice for 28 days, statistically significant weight reductions were seen in both normal and obese mice compared with control mice fed the same diet. This reduction in weight was largely independent of a reduction in food intake for the normal mice, whereas obese mice maintained a reduced food intake level throughout the 28-day trial period.

Reported uses

Goat's rue has been claimed to be useful to reduce blood glucose levels in patients with hyperglycemia and to increase the flow of milk in breast-feeding women. The herb has also been used in the management of fever, snakebites, and the plague. Controlled human trials are lacking. The current use of the herb stems from traditional and anecdotal information.

Dosage

Goat's rue fluidextract is prepared by mixing 1 cup of boiling water with 1 tsp of the dried leaves; the extract is taken after 10 to 15 minutes P.O. b.i.d.

Adverse reactions

CNS: headache, nervousness, weakness.

Interactions

None reported.

Contraindications and precautions

Avoid using goat's rue extract in infants, children, and pregnant or breast-feeding women, unless approved by a health care provider. No problems occurring in breast-fed infants have been reported, but the risk of adverse reactions exists.

Special considerations

• Advise the patient to discontinue goat's rue and contact a health care provider if adverse reactions occur.
• Inform the patient taking goat's rue that saliva may be colored yellowish green.
• Advise the breast-feeding patient to avoid using this herb.

Points of interest

• Goat's rue has been associated with lethal poisonings in sheep grazing on the herb. Signs of animal toxicity include frothy nasal discharge, labored breathing, muscle spasms leading to seizures, and neck edema. Although the mechanism of goat rue's toxicity has not been established, the galegine and paragalegine alkaloids have been implicated (Gresham and Booth, 1991).

Commentary

Clinical data do not support the use of goat's rue as a lactogenic or hypoglycemic agent. Although considered an oral treatment for diabetes before the development of sulfonylureas, the extract was not considered an alternative to insulin (Remington et al., 1918). Because of questionable antihyperglycemic efficacy, the herb is not recommended in diabetes. Similarly, the herb should not be used as a lactogenic in women be-

---

Bold italic type indicates that reaction may be life-threatening.

cause the effects on the breast-fed infant are unknown. Intriguing data in mice for weight loss warrant further study.

References

Gresham, A.C.J., and Booth, K. "Poisoning of Sheep by Goat's Rue," *Vet Rec* 129:197-98, 1991.

Palit, P., et al. "Novel Weight-reducing Activity of *Galega officinalis* in Mice," *J Pharm Pharmacol* 51(11):1313-19, 1999.

Remington, J.P., et al., eds. *The Dispensatory of the United States of America*, 20th ed. Philadelphia: Lippincott-Raven Pubs., 1918.

GOLDENROD

AARON'S ROD, BLUE MOUNTAIN TEA, SWEET GOLDENROD, WOUNDWORT

Taxonomic class
Asteraceae

Common trade names
None known.

Common forms
Available as an alcoholic or aqueous extract.

Source
The active medicinal ingredients are found in the flowers and leaves of *Solidago virgaurea*. Only one species of goldenrod grows wild in England, but more than 130 species are found in the United States. The roots as well are valued for their medicinal use.

Chemical components
Chemical compounds identified as having medicinal value include bioflavonoids, saponins, carotenoids, diterpenes, and tannins. The plant also may contain a high concentration of nitrates. The phenolic glycosideleiocarposide has also been identified. Three cytotoxic compounds have been isolated from the plant: alpha-tocopherol-quinone, trans-phytol, and erythrodiol-3-acetate.

Actions
The flavonoids and saponins are used for their diuretic action because they stimulate fluid elimination from the kidneys. The tannins in the leaves, stems, and roots are noted for their astringent properties. Anti-inflammatory activity has been studied by several investigators with *Populus tremula* and *Fraxinus excelsior* (combination known as Phytodolor N). Aqueous and alcoholic extracts were tested alone and in combination in models of induced arthritis or edema in the rat paw. Arthritic paw volume and paw edema were reduced by the combinations and by the agents used alone. Anti-inflammatory activity was demonstrated and compared with that of diclofenac (Ghazaly et al., 1992).

Reported uses

Goldenrod has been endorsed by the German Commission E for use as an anti-inflammatory, a mild antispasmodic, and a diuretic. The herb is widely used in Europe to treat urinary tract inflammation and to prevent the formation or facilitate the elimination of kidney stones (Tyler, 1994). In folklore, Native Americans used goldenrod for treating sore throat and pain. Other uses included chronic diarrhea, kidney and intestinal inflammation, and stones in the bladder. Goldenrod has been used to induce abortion, and an antiseptic lotion and powder have been prepared to treat wounds. Leaves from goldenrod harvested in the Appalachians have been used to prepare Blue Mountain tea, prescribed for exhaustion and fatigue. The uses for goldenrod are founded on centuries of folklore medicine. No human studies demonstrating the medicinal value of goldenrod have been conducted.

Dosage

A decoction is prepared by mixing 1 or 2 tsp (3 to 5 g) of the dried herb with 8 oz of water. The mixture is boiled, allowed to stand for 2 minutes, and then strained. Another method uses 30 g of the herb mixed with 300 ml water. One tablespoon of the infusion is ingested t.i.d. or q.i.d.

Adverse reactions

Respiratory: *asthma*, hay fever (from extraneous pollens carried by *Solidago*).

Interactions

None reported.

Contraindications and precautions

Goldenrod is contraindicated in pregnant women because of its abortive properties.

Special considerations

• Goldenrod is considered to contain high concentrations of nitrates.
🔺**ALERT** Emesis, rapid respiration, and death have occurred with ingestion of the dried plant.
🔺**ALERT** Signs of toxicity include abdominal distention, emaciation, enlarged spleen, GI bleeding, and leg edema related to parasites, fungus, and rust present in plant.
• Advise the patient with allergies to avoid using goldenrod.
• Urge women to immediately report suspected pregnancy.
• Advise the patient to use goldenrod cautiously as a diuretic or in treating high blood pressure or kidney stones because its efficacy has not been proven. Also, advise him to consider the consequences of a delay in seeking medical attention for high blood pressure or kidney pain.
• Advise the patient to use goldenrod with caution for intestinal inflammation or chronic diarrhea.

Bold italic type indicates that reaction may be life-threatening.

Points of interest
- In folklore, herbalists used goldenrod to mask the bitterness of other medicines.
- Goldenrod has been popular with herbalists for curing bladder stones from as early as the mid-13th century and was described as an admirable plant for healing wounds.
- Goldenrod occurs commonly in the United States and can cause an allergic reaction in some people. Allergic rhinitis that occurs early in the spring and in the fall may be attributed more to ragweed, which blooms at the same time, than to goldenrod (Wunderlin and Lockey, 1988).
- Paradoxically, goldenrod has been used to treat allergy.

Commentary
There are no human studies documenting the clinical effects of goldenrod. Studies evaluating its anti-inflammatory, cytotoxic, and diuretic effects have been few and performed in vitro or on murine or rat models; adverse reactions, contraindications, and toxicity have not been reported. Even though the German Commission E endorsed goldenrod as an anti-inflammatory, an antispasmodic, and a diuretic, scientific evidence of its efficacy in humans is lacking.

References
Ghazaly, M., et al. "Study of the Anti-inflammatory Activity of *Populus tremula, Solidago virgaurea* and *Fraxinus excelsior,*" *Arzneimittelforschung* 42:333-36, 1992.

Sung, J.H., et al. "Cytotoxic Constituents from *Solidago virga-aurea* var. *gigantea* MIQ," *Arch Pharm Res* 22(6):633-37, 1999.

Tyler, V. *Herbs of Choice: The Therapeutic Use of Phytomedicinals.* New York: Pharmaceutical Products Press, Haworth Press Inc., 1994.

Wunderlin, R.P., and Lockey, R.F. "Questions and Answers," *JAMA* 260:3064-65, 1988.

GOLDENSEAL

EYE BALM, EYE ROOT, GOLDSIEGEL, GROUND RASPBERRY, INDIAN DYE, INDIAN TURMERIC, JAUNDICE ROOT, YELLOW PAINT, YELLOW PUCCOON, YELLOW ROOT

Taxonomic class
Ranunculaceae

Common trade names
Alvita, Dandelion Goldenseal, Golden Seal Extract, Golden Seal Extract 4:1, Golden Seal Glycerin Extract, Golden Seal Power, Golden Seal Root, Nu Veg Golden Seal Herb, Nu Veg Golden Seal Root

Common forms
Capsules, tablets: 250 mg, 350 mg, 400 mg, 404 mg, 470 mg, 500 mg, 535 mg, 540 mg

Also available as dried ground root powder, ethanol and water extracts, teas, and tinctures.

Source

The rhizome (root stock) of *Hydrastis canadensis* is commonly used to manufacture the dosage forms. The main chemical components are the alkaloids hydrastine and berberine. Also present are hydrastinine, canadine, berberastine, candaline, canadaline, chlorogenic acid, carbohydrates, fatty acids, volatile oil, resin, and meconin.

Actions

Goldenseal is claimed to have antihemorrhagic, anti-inflammatory, astringent, laxative, and oxytocic properties. The pharmacologic properties are attributed to berberine and hydrastine, and scientific studies have usually focused on these alkaloids rather than on the herb itself.

An alkaloid component of goldenseal was reported to inhibit muscle contractions in rodent smooth muscle, whereas others have shown an oxytocic effect. Goldenseal extracts reduce hyperphagia and polydipsia associated with streptozocin-induced diabetes in mice (Swanston-Flatt et al., 1989).

Berberine was found to decrease the anticoagulant effect of heparin in laboratory tests of heparinated animal and human blood (Preininger, 1975) and to act as a cardiac stimulant (at lower doses), increase coronary perfusion, and inhibit cardiac activity (at higher doses) in animals. Antipyretic activity (greater than aspirin) and anthelmintic, antihistaminic, antimicrobial, antimuscarinic, antitumorigenic, and hypotensive effects have also been documented for berberine in animal and laboratory models.

Hydrastinine causes vasoconstriction and can produce significant changes in blood pressure.

Reported uses

Claims for goldenseal include use for anorexia, cancer, conjunctivitis, dysmenorrhea, eczema, gastritis, GI disorders, mouth ulcers, otorrhea, peptic ulcer disease, postpartum hemorrhage, pruritus, tinnitus, and tuberculosis and as an anti-inflammatory, a diuretic, a laxative, and a wound antiseptic. There are few, if any, clinical trial data available to support these claims.

Goldenseal was found to be less effective than ergot alkaloids when used for postpartum hemorrhage in humans. Berberine has been shown to shorten the duration of acute *Vibrio cholera* diarrhea and diarrhea caused by some species of *Giardia*, *Salmonella*, and *Shigella* and some Enterobactereciae. Clinical studies in patients with hepatic cirrhosis have shown that berberine may correct some laboratory abnormalities and improve biliary secretion and function.

Dosage

Dried rhizome: 0.5 to 1 g P.O. t.i.d.
Ethanol and water extract: 250 mg P.O. t.i.d.

Bold italic type indicates that reaction may be life-threatening.

Adverse reactions
CNS: CNS depression, paralysis (with high doses), paresthesias, *seizures*.
CV: *asystole, bradycardia, heart block.*
EENT: mouth ulcers.
GI: abdominal cramps and pain, diarrhea, nausea, vomiting.
Respiratory: *respiratory depression* (with high doses).
Skin: contact dermatitis.

Interactions
Anticoagulants: Beneficial effects of therapeutic anticoagulants may be offset. Avoid administration with goldenseal.
Antihypertensives: Goldenseal or its extracts may interfere with or increase hypotensive effects. Do not use together.
Beta blockers, calcium channel blockers, digoxin: May increase or interfere with cardiac effects of these drugs. Do not use together.
CNS depressants (alcohol, benzodiazepines): May increase sedative effects. Avoid administration with goldenseal.

Contraindications and precautions
Goldenseal is contraindicated in patients with CV disease, particularly arrhythmias, heart failure, or hypertension, and in pregnant patients.

Special considerations
🐈 **ALERT** Death can result from the ingestion of large alkaloid doses. Symptoms of overdose include depression, exaggerated reflexes, GI upset, nervousness, and seizures that progress to respiratory paralysis and CV collapse.
- Monitor for unusual symptoms.
- Monitor for signs of vitamin B deficiency (angular stomatitis, cheilosis, glossitis, infertility, megaloblastic anemia, peripheral neuropathy, seborrheic dermatitis, and seizures).
- Caution the patient to avoid hazardous activities until CNS effects of goldenseal are known.
- Instruct the patient not to consume goldenseal because of its potential to cause toxicity.

Points of interest
- Chronic use of goldenseal has been reported to decrease the absorption of vitamin B and thereby promote its deficiency.
- Tolerance to the herb's pharmacologic effects is thought to develop after only a few weeks of chronic use.
- Berberine is also a component of barberry (*Berberis vulgaris*).
- Goldenseal extracts have been a component in sterile eyewashes for many years without supporting evidence for their inclusion. Also, the extracts or their components have been listed in the national pharmacopoeias of several countries.
- Goldenseal has been inappropriately used to mask the appearance of illicit drugs on urine drug screens in humans and race horses. This

information is false and originates from a fictional literary work that depicts the plant to be useful for hiding opioid ingestion.

• Goldenseal has been used as a dye. The rhizome is bright yellow and popular for staining many fabrics and materials.

• According to a survey inside a New York City emergency department, goldenseal tea is among the three most commonly cited herbal preparations consumed by patients (Hung et al., 1997).

Commentary

The pharmacologic effects of goldenseal have not been adequately studied. Because the risk of toxicity appears excessive for this plant, even some advocacy texts do not support its use for any disorder. Goldenseal and its alkaloids possess some promising pharmacologic properties; additional comprehensive, controlled studies in animals are needed before progressing to human studies.

References

Hung, O.L., et al. "Herbal Preparation Use Among Urban Emergency Department Patients," *Acad Emerg Med* 4(3):209-13, 1997.

Preininger, V. "The Pharmacology and Toxicology of the Papaveraceae Alkaloids," in *The Alkaloids,* vol. 15. Edited by Maske, R.H.F., and Holmes, H.L. New York: Academic Press, 1975.

Swanston-Flatt, S.K., et al. "Evaluation of Traditional Plant Treatments for Diabetes: Studies in Streptozotocin Diabetic Mice," *Acta Diabetol Latina* 26:51-55, 1989.

GOSSYPOL

AMERICAN UPLAND COTTON, COMMON COTTON, COTTON, UPLAND COTTON, WILD COTTON

Taxonomic class
Malvaceae

Common trade names
None known.

Common forms
Available as extracts.

Source
Gossypol is found in the roots, seeds, and stems of the cotton plant, *Gossypium hirsutum*. These plants grow in Florida and are cultivated throughout the southern United States. The seeds of the *Gossypium* species vary widely in the quantity of gossypol content.

Chemical components
A polyphenolic binaphthyl dialdehyde (dextro- and levo-rotatory enantiomers), gossypol is the active constituent of cottonseed and other parts of the cotton plant. Cottonseed is also high in protein and low in fat.

Bold italic type indicates that reaction may be life-threatening.

Actions

In animal and human sperm cells, gossypol produces visible morphologic damage and reductions in motility, accounting for the compound's antifertility actions. Gossypol's effects are related to its ability to impair the enzyme lactate dehydrogenase X of sperm and sperm-generating cells (Wu, 1989).

Gossypol exerts numerous effects on DNA replication, synthesis, and structural integrity. Tumorigenic potential, common in agents with similar DNA activity, has been reported with gossypol in small studies. Observed disruptions in DNA function in sperm and other cells, combined with gossypol's known inhibition of oxidative phosphorylation, have led researchers to suggest antitumorigenic potential for gossypol. In vitro studies have demonstrated gossypol's inhibitory effect on the growth of malignant human cancer cells and of cultured human benign prostatic hyperplasia cells (Shidaifat et al., 1997). Derivatives of gossypol have shown antitumorigenic activity against breast tumor epithelial cell lines (Liang et al., 1995).

Laboratory studies suggest that gossypol and a derivative (gossylic iminolactone) have anti-HIV activity; this activity is not considered to be caused by inhibition of reverse transcriptase (Royer et al., 1995).

U.S. patent rights have been granted to investigate the acetic acid derivative of gossypol as a treatment for breast and prostate cancers. Early study results indicate a lower adverse effect profile for this derivative than for other drugs used for these cancers (Federal Register, 1996).

Reported uses

Gossypol is claimed to be useful for easing labor and delivery and for promoting normal menstruation; these uses have not been validated.

Studies have shown gossypol to be an effective oral male contraceptive. Questions regarding the reversibility of these effects have precluded commercial development of this agent. Sperm counts usually return to normal about 3 months after the herb is discontinued, but long-term follow-up of patients has indicated that spermatogenesis may not always return to normal (Wu, 1989). One clinical trial examined gossypol administration as a contraceptive pill for about 1 year in 151 men from various countries (Coutinho et al., 2000). Subjects received 15 mg/day of gossypol for 12 to 16 weeks initially. After spermatogenesis was suppressed, patients were randomized to a smaller dose of either 7.5 or 10 mg/day for 40 weeks. Slightly more than 50% of patients achieved and maintained suppression of spermatogenesis. Eight of 43 patients experienced insufficient return of sperm counts at 1 year after cessation of gossypol therapy. Serum potassium levels appeared to fluctuate within the normal range.

A clinical trial examining gossypol, 10 mg P.O. twice daily, in 27 patients with recurrent glial cell tumors suggested some potential of gossypol as an antineoplastic for gliomas (Bushunow et al., 1999). Although promising, this information should be interpreted as preliminary data.

Other topical formulations of gossypol have been tested as vaginal spermicides and found to be comparable to other, existing spermicidal products. Gossypol appears effective in the presence of cervical mucus at low concentrations with minimal apparent systemic toxicity (Ratsula et al., 1983).

Dosage
For antifertility, Chinese studies used 20 mg/day P.O. for 60 to 90 days until the sperm count was reduced to a threshold of 4 million sperm/ml; then, doses of about 50 mg weekly were maintained.

Adverse reactions
CNS: paralysis.
CV: circulatory problems, ***heart failure,*** peripheral edema.
GI: diarrhea, ***hepatotoxicity.***
GU: ***nephrotoxicity*** (with high doses).
Hematologic: ***thrombocytopenia.***
Metabolic: hypokalemia (either caused by renal tubular damage or inhibition of 11beta-hydroxysteroid dehydrogenase: remains to be proven conclusively), malnutrition.
Musculoskeletal: muscle weakness, rapid muscle fatigue.
Skin: hair discoloration.

Interactions
Nephrotoxic drugs (amphotericin B): Increased risk of nephrotoxicity. Avoid administration with gossypol.
Potassium-wasting drugs (diuretics): May lead to significant potassium depletion. Do not use together.

Contraindications and precautions
Avoid using gossypol in pregnant or breast-feeding patients; effects are unknown. Use cautiously in patients with renal dysfunction because renal damage can occur.

Special considerations
🖑 **ALERT** Cotton seeds are potentially toxic and can cause death. Domesticated animals have been poisoned from consuming feed that contained cotton seeds; postmortem examinations revealed hepatic and pulmonary edema and heart tissue degeneration. Ruminating animals (bovines) appear to be less sensitive than nonruminants to the herb's toxic effects.
• Monitor BUN and serum creatinine and potassium levels in patient using gossypol.
• Periodically test muscle strength of patient taking this herb.
• Inform the patient who wants to use gossypol for its contraceptive effects that other products are available.
• Caution the patient that permanent infertility can occur with long-term use.

Bold italic type indicates that reaction may be life-threatening.

Points of interest

• Gossypol was first identified as an antifertility agent in Chinese epidemiological studies conducted during the 1950s.

• There is considerable debate as to whether gossypol should be pursued further as an antifertility agent for men. The World Health Organization has recommended that research on this agent be discontinued because of its potential to induce permanent infertility and hypokalemia. Published editorials highlight this interesting controversy in depth (Waites et al., 1998; Yu and Chan, 1998).

• Commercial processing of cottonseed oil removes the gossypol content of the cotton seeds.

• Gossypol-free cottonseed flour has been suggested as an economic and abundant source of protein and has been used in baked goods, livestock feed, and snacks.

Commentary

Gossypol continues to show promise as an oral contraceptive for men. Its routine systemic use is daunted by the potential for irreversible sterility. Commentaries have suggested the adverse effect profile may be sufficient to disregard use of the product, but this remains controversial. Further study is needed to determine optimal dosing, route of administration, and incidence of adverse reactions. Its use as a topical vaginal spermicide may be valuable, but definitive evidence of safety and efficacy in larger human clinical trials is needed to establish a role for this agent in contraception.

References

Bushunow, P., et al. "Gossypol Treatment of Recurrent Adult Malignant Gliomas," *J Neurooncol* 43(1):79-86, 1999.

Coutinho, E.M., et al. "Gossypol Blood Levels and Inhibition of Spermatogenesis in Men Taking Gossypol as a Contraceptive. A Multi-center, International, Dose-finding Study," *Contraception* 61(1):61-67, 2000.

"Gossypol Acetic Acid for Cancer Treatments," *Federal Register,* June 18, 1996.

Liang, X.S., et al. "Developing Gossypol Derivatives with Enhanced Antitumor Activity," *Invest New Drugs* 13(3):181-86, 1995.

Ratsula, K., et al. "Vaginal Contraception with Gossypol; A Clinical Study," *Contraception* 27:571, 1983.

Royer, R.E., et al. "Comparison of the Antiviral Activities of 3-azido-3-deoxythymidine and Gossylic Iminolactone Against Clinical Isolates of HIV-1," *Pharmacol Res* 31:49-52, 1995.

Shidaifat, F., et al. "Gossypol Arrests Human Benign Prostatic Hyperplastic Cell Growth at G_0/G_1 Phase of the Cell Cycle," *Anticancer Res* 17:1003-9, 1997.

Waites, G.M., et al. "Gossypol: Reasons for Its Failure to Be Accepted as a Safe, Reversible Male Antifertility Drug," *Int J Androl* 21(5):313, 1998.

Wu, D. "An Overview of the Clinical Pharmacology and Therapeutic Potential of Gossypol as a Male Contraceptive Agent and in Gynaecological Disease," *Drugs* 38:333-41, 1989.

Yu, Z.H., and Chan, H.C. "Gossypol as a Male Antifertility Agent—Why Studies Should Have Been Continued," *Int J Androl* 21(1):2-7, 1998.

GOTU KOLA
CENTELLA, HYDROCOTYLE, INDIAN PENNYWORT, INDIAN WATER NAVELWORT, TALEPETRAKO, TECA (TITRATED EXTRACT OF *CENTELLA ASIATICA*)

Taxonomic class
Apiaceae

Common trade names
Ginkgo/Gotu Kola Supreme, Gotu Kola Gold Extract, Gotu Kola Herb, Gotu Kola Herb Low Alcohol & Alcohol Free, Gotu Kola Leaf & Root

Common forms
Capsules: 221 mg, 250 mg, 435 mg, 439 mg, 441 mg
　　Also available as creams, extracts, and tinctures.

Source
Centella asiatica originated in Madagascar. It is also indigenous to India, Sri Lanka, and South Africa.

Chemical components
Gotu kola contains flavonoids (quercetin, kaempferol), various glycosides, terpenoids (asiaticoside, centelloside, madecasoside, brahmoside, brahminoside), madecassol, madecassic acid, asiatic acid, asiaticentoic acid, centellic acid, centoic acid, isothankuniside, fatty acids, amino acids, phytosterols, and tannin. The root region contains 14 polyacetylenes.

Actions
Most studies have been carried out in animals. Brahmoside and brahminoside showed CNS depressant effects (decreased motor activity, increased sleep time, and slightly decreased body temperature) in rats and mice in vivo. Asiaticoside has been shown to possess anti-HSV-1 and anti-HSV-2 activities in vitro (Yoosook et al., 2000).

Antifertility activity against human and rat sperm was demonstrated in vitro. Asiaticoside and brahminoside were believed to be the active constituents, but spermicidal or spermostatic action could not be shown. *Centella* extract was found to significantly reduce fertility in female mice. *C. asiatica* was shown to be effective in destroying cultured cancer tumor cells.

Topical formulations of *C. asiatica* extract have been studied in animal wounds and suggested to be of some value in promoting wound healing (Shukla et al., 1999a; Shukla et al., 1999b; Sunilkumar et al., 1998) and in reducing skin injury related to radiation (Chen et al., 1999). Asiaticoside, the purported active ingredient responsible for these beneficial effects, has demonstrated increases in tensile strength and collagen content and improved epithelialization, which appears to be most notable within the first 7 days after the injury.

Bold italic type indicates that reaction may be life-threatening.

Reported uses

Claims for gotu kola include uses as an anticancer agent, an antifertility agent, an antihypertensive, and an antipsoriatic; as an agent for wound healing; and as treatment for chronic hepatic disorders, mental fatigue, rheumatism, and varicose veins.

A cream formulation in which *C. asiatica* extract is an active ingredient may hold some value in reducing stretch marks related to pregnancy in women who are prone to stretch marks but appears to be of little value for the general population of pregnant women (Young and Jewell, 2000).

A cream formulation of hydrocotyle was shown to be effective in patients with psoriasis (Natarajan et al., 1973). In another study, a hydrocotyle extract was found to be useful for preventing and treating keloids and hypertrophic scars (Bosse et al., 1979); a cortisone-like effect has been proposed for the agent's action. Hydrocotyle has also been used in patients with chronic skin maladies, including cutaneous ulcers and gynecologic and surgical wounds.

Titrated extract of *C. asiatica* showed significant improvement of symptoms, including edema, in patients with venous insufficiency of the lower limbs (Pointel et al., 1987). Asiaticoside has been shown to improve the general ability and behavioral patterns of mentally retarded patients.

Dosage

Dosages vary with disease state and with the trial cited. Usual doses are 0.6 g of the dried leaf P.O. t.i.d. or 450 mg in capsule form once daily.

Adverse reactions

CNS: sedation (with large doses).
Metabolic: hypercholesterolemia, hyperglycemia.
Skin: burning sensation (with topical use), contact dermatitis, pruritus.

Interactions

Antidiabetic and cholesterol-lowering drugs: High doses of gotu kola may interfere with the actions of these drugs. Do not use together.

Contraindications and precautions

Gotu kola is contraindicated in pregnant or breast-feeding patients. Use cautiously in patients with a history of contact dermatitis.

Special considerations

• Two of the active ingredients of gotu kola have been reported to cause CNS depressant effects in animals; monitor the patient for these effects.
• Inform the patient that drowsiness and sedation may occur.
• Inform the patient that he may feel a burning sensation when the herb is applied topically.
• Advise the patient to use another contraceptive method if the herb is being used for this purpose.
• Urge women to report planned or suspected pregnancy.
• Instruct the patient not to use gotu kola continuously for longer than 6 weeks.

Points of interest
• After witnessing elephants chewing on the leaves of gotu kola, Sri Lankans propagated the myth that gotu kola promoted longevity.
• Do not confuse gotu kola with kola nuts, kola, or cola, an ingredient in Coca-Cola—all of which, unlike gotu kola, contain caffeine.

Commentary
Gotu kola appears to be an interesting herb with components that hold significant promise in the areas of wound healing and specific dermatologic disorders. More research in humans is needed to determine its long-term efficacy and safety profile.

References

Bosse, J-P., et al. "Clinical Study of a New Antikeloid Agent," *Ann Plast Surg* 3:13-21, 1979.

Chen,Y.J., et al. "The Effect of Tetrandrine and Extracts of *Centella asiatica* on Acute Radiation Dermatitis in Rats," *Biol Pharm Bull* 22(7):703-6, 1999.

Natarajan, S., et al. "Effect of Topical Hydrocotyle Asiatica in Psoriasis," *Indian J Dermatol* 18:82-85, 1973.

Pointel, J.P., et al. "Titrated Extract of *Centella asiatica* (TECA) in the Treatment of Venous Insufficiency of the Lower Limbs," *Angiology* 38:46-50, 1987.

Shukla, A., et al. "In Vitro and In Vivo Wound Healing Activity of Asiaticoside Isolated from *Centella asiatica*," *J Ethnopharmacol* 65(1):1-11, 1999a.

Shukla, A., et al. "Asiaticoside-induced Elevation of Antioxidant Levels in Healing Wounds," *Phytother Res* 13(1):50-54, 1999b.

Sunilkumar, J.S., et al. "Evaluation of Topical Formulations of Aqueous Extract of *Centella asiatica* on Open Wounds in Rats," *Indian J Exp Biol* 36(6):569-72, 1998.

Yoosook, C., et al. "Anti-Herpes Simplex Virus Activities of Crude Water Extracts of Thai Medicinal Plants," *Phytomedicine* 6(6):411-19, 2000.

Young, G.L., and Jewell, D. "Creams for Preventing Stretch Marks in Pregnancy," *Cochrane Database Syst Rev* 2:CD000066, 2000.

GRAPEFRUIT SEED EXTRACT
CITRUS PARADISI

Taxonomic class
Rutaceae

Common trade names
Citricidal, GSE, Traveler's Friend

Common forms
Liquid extract

Source
Grapefruit seed extract is synthesized from the pulp, seed, and inner rind of the fruit of *Citrus paradisi*.

Chemical components
The liquid concentrate contains 67% vegetable glycerin (derived from palm and coconut) and 33% Citricidal. Traveler's Friend is made up of 67% deionized water and 33% Citricidal.

Grapefruit juice contains naringin and naringenin, which inhibit the production of CYP3A4, leading to increased rates of absorption of certain drugs. Grapefruit seed extract contains about 0.1% of these compounds.

Actions
Grapefruit seed extract is part of the quaternary compound, and its structure is similar to that of benzylkonium chloride. The extract is reported to exhibit antibacterial, antifungal, and, potentially, antiviral activity. One study of the antimicrobial efficacy of six grapefruit seed extract products found that the preservative agents in the products, including benzethonium chloride, triclosan, and methyl parabens, were responsible for their activity (von Woedtke et al., 1999).

Reported uses
Grapefruit seed extract has been used topically as an antiseptic wound cleaner and to treat skin infections and internally as supportive treatment for various ailments, including *Candida* infections, GI upset, and sore throat. Grapefruit seed extract has also been used by campers and travelers to foreign countries to purify drinking water.

Dosage
One product reports a dosage of 10 to 15 gtt P.O. in water or juice b.i.d. or t.i.d.

Adverse reactions
GI: indigestion.

Interactions
Anticonvulsants, benzodiazepines, calcium channel blockers, certain antibiotics and antivirals, cyclosporine, nonsedating antihistamines, oral contraceptives, quinidine: Grapefruit extract may increase the bioavailability of these classes of drugs by inhibiting the cytochrome P-450 isoenzyme in the liver and gut wall (Dresser et al., 2000). Monitor the patient closely.

Contraindications and precautions
Avoid using grapefruit seed extract in pregnant or breast-feeding patients; effects are unknown. Do not use in the eyes. Do not use the extract with a mechanized toothbrush or tooth polisher because the acidic nature of the extract and abrasive actions of these instruments could cause tooth damage, including enamel erosion.

Special considerations
● Grapefruit seed extract concentrate has a pH of 2.2 and should be diluted before use.

• The extract is extremely bitter.
• Advise the patient to consult a health care provider before using herbal preparations because a treatment that has been clinically researched and proved effective may be available.

Points of interest
• The U.S. Department of Agriculture (USDA) confirmed that Citricidal was effective in inhibiting viral strains in cattle and hogs in the early 1980s and approved it for use in the USDA's Evian Influenza Eradication Program in 1984.

Commentary
Although grapefruit seed extract has been thought to be effective as an antimicrobial, limited studies have not supported this claim. Further investigation is needed into whether grapefruit seed extract alone possesses antimicrobial activity or if it lies with the product's preservative.

References
Dresser, G.K., et al. "Pharmacokinetic-Pharmacodynamic Consequences and Clinical Relevance of Cytochrome P450 3A4 Inhibition," *Clin Pharmacokinet* 38(1):41-57, 2000.
Von Woedtke, T., et al. "Aspects of the Antimicrobial Efficacy of Grapefruit Seed Extract and Its Relation to Preservative Substances Contained," *Pharmazie* 54(6):452-56, 1999.

GREEN TEA

MATSU-CHA, TEA

Taxonomic class
Theaceae

Common trade names
Ambootia Green Tea, Green Anti-Oxide, Green Chai Organic, Green Decaffin, Green Emerald, High Energy Chai Tea, Maitake Mai Green Tea, Tegreen 97 Capsules

Common forms
Available as capsules and teas.

Source
Green tea is prepared from the steamed and dried leaves of *Camellia sinensis*, a large shrub with evergreen leaves that is native to eastern Asia. Green tea is different from black tea in that it is produced from leaves that have been withered, rolled, fermented, and dried. Because of the curing process, the properties of green tea are similar to those of the fresh leaf.

Chemical components
Green tea contains polyphenols (catechins), tannins, flavonols, and methylxanthines (caffeine, theophylline, theobromine). Commercially prepared green tea extracts are standardized to contain 60% polyphe-

---

nols, and depending on the method of preparation, the tea may contain 1% to 4% caffeine.

Actions

The chemopreventive effect of green tea is attributed to the polyphenols (epigallocatechin and epigallocatechin-3-gallate); these agents are believed to inhibit cell proliferation and tumor promotion–related activities and have antioxidant actions. Animal models involving rodent lung, esophagus, stomach, intestine, skin, liver, and colon have shown the inhibitory activity of green tea against carcinogens. In vitro studies of green tea polyphenols induced programmed cell death (apoptosis) in human cancer cells (Hibasami et al., 1998; Ahmad et al., 1997). The mechanism of action of epigallocetechin gallate, the main green tea polyphenol, has been described (Fujiki et al., 1999).

The caffeine in green tea produces CNS stimulation, and the polyphenols inhibit ultraviolet-induced skin carcinogenesis (Zhao et al., 1999). Green tea has been suggested as an adjuvant to therapy for AIDS, to prevent drug-resistant mutants, because of its antimutagenic action (McCarty, 1997).

Green tea has been associated with cholesterol-lowering effects and decreased atherosclerosis (Yang and Koo, 1997, 2000). Antibacterial activity has been demonstrated against methicillin-resistant *Staphylococcus aureus* and *Yersinia enterocolitica* in vitro. The fluoride and tannins in green teas are believed to decrease the formation of dental caries (Rasheed and Haider, 1998).

Antithrombotic activities have been described in animal models, possibly because of green tea's antiplatelet effects (Kang et al., 1999).

Reported uses

The Chinese have used green tea leaf and its extracts for thousands of years. Therapeutic claims for this agent include the prevention of atherosclerosis, cancer, dental caries, and hypercholesterolemia. It has been promoted for its antibacterial, astringent, diuretic, radioprotective, and stimulant actions. Studies in animals and in in vitro human models have supported the chemopreventive effects and atherosclerosis claims.

Epidemiological studies in the Asian population have provided additional evidence. Although Japanese patients had a lower risk of cancer with green tea consumption, the difference was not significant (Imai et al., 1997).

In a clinical trial, single doses of green tea solids in doses of 0.6, 1.2, or 1.8 g dissolved in water inhibited prostaglandin E_2 levels in rectal mucosa. These preliminary data support further study of green tea as a colorectal chemoprotective agent (August et al., 1999).

Dosage

Epidemiological studies have suggested possible effects from drinking 6 to 10 cups daily; pharmacokinetic studies indicate that 3 capsules of green tea extract P.O. provide adequate plasma levels.

Adverse reactions
Other: *allergic reactions* (immunoglobulin E–mediated) in patients with green tea asthma.

Interactions
Doxorubicin: May increase antitumorigenic activity of doxorubicin. Monitor the patient.
Milk: May inhibit antioxidant effects of the polyphenol component. Avoid administration with green tea.
Warfarin: Green tea can be a significant source of vitamin K and thus antagonize the effects of warfarin (Taylor and Wilt, 1999). Monitor PT and INR.

Contraindications and precautions
No known contraindications. Avoid using green tea in patients with green tea asthma.

Special considerations
• Because of the risk of serious allergic reactions, green tea and other teas that contain epigallocatechin gallate should be avoided in people who are sensitive to tea.
• Inform the patient that green tea contains caffeine.
• Caution the patient not to self-treat symptoms of illness before seeking appropriate medical evaluation because this may delay diagnosis of a serious medical condition.

Points of interest
• Tea is grown in about 30 countries and, besides water, is the most commonly consumed beverage worldwide. It is considered one of the safest beverages because water is boiled in its preparation.
• Tea is generally recognized as safe in the United States.

Commentary
The potential uses of green tea as a preventive for atherosclerosis and cancer have been shown in many animals and suggested by various epidemiological evaluations and case-control and cohort studies in Asian populations. Although these reports and widespread usage over thousands of years suggest that green tea is relatively safe, further research is needed in other populations to clarify its impact on cancer risk. More mechanistic, dose-response studies and clinical trials are needed to verify and describe the effects of tea consumption on human carcinogenesis.

References
Ahmad, N., et al. "Green Tea Constituent Epigallocatechin-3-gallate and Induction of Apoptosis and Cell Cycle Arrest in Human Carcinoma Cells," *J Natl Cancer Inst* 89:1881-86, 1997.

August, D.A., et al. "Ingestion of Green Tea Rapidly Decreases Prostaglandin E_2 Levels in Rectal Mucosa in Humans," *Cancer Epidemiol Biomarkers Prev* 8(8):709-13, 1999.

Fujiki, H., et al., "Mechanistic Findings of Green Tea as Cancer Preventative for Humans," *Proc Soc Exp Biol Med* 220(4):225-28, 1999.

Bold italic type indicates that reaction may be life-threatening.

Hibasami, H., et al. "Induction of Apoptosis in Human Stomach Cancer Cells by Green Tea Catechins," *Oncol Res* 5:527-29, 1998.

Imai, K., et al. "Cancer-Preventative Effects of Drinking Green Tea Among a Japanese Population," *Prev Med* 26:769-75, 1997.

Kang, W.S., et al. "Antithrombotic Activities of Green Tea Catechins and (-)-Epigallocatechin gallate," *Thromb Res* 96(3):229-37, 1999.

McCarty, M.F. "Natural Antimutagenic Agents May Prolong Efficacy of Human Immunodeficiency Virus Drug Therapy," *Med Hypotheses* 48:215-20, 1997.

Rasheed, A., and Haider, M. "Antibacterial Activity of *Camellia sinensis* Extracts Against Dental Caries," *Arch Pharm Res* 21(3):348-52, 1998.

Taylor, J.R., and Wilt, V.M. "Probable Antagonism of Warfarin by Green Tea" *Ann Pharmacother* 33(4):426-28, 1999.

Yang, T.T., and Koo, M.W. "Hypocholesterolemic Effect of Chinese Tea," *Pharmacol Res* 35:505-12, 1997.

Yang, T.T., and Koo, M.W.. "Chinese Green Tea Lowers Cholesterol Level Through an Increase in Fecal Lipid Excretion," *Life Sci* 66(5):411-23, 2000.

Zhao, J.F., et al. "Green Tea Protects Against Psoralen Plus Ultraviolet A–Induced Photochemical Damage to Skin," *J Invest Dermatol* 113(6):1070-75, 1999.

GROUND IVY

ALEHOOF, CATSFOOT, CREEPING CHARLIES CAT'S PAW, GLECHOMA HEDERACEA, HAYMAIDS, HEDGEMAIDS

Taxonomic class
Lamiaceae

Common trade names
None known.

Common forms
Available as an infusion or tincture of leaves and flowers (aerial parts).

Source
Glechoma hederacea, with its kidney-shaped leaves and purple-blue flowers in whorls, is one of the most common plants growing wild in Great Britain.

Chemical components
Ground ivy contains sesquiterpenes, flavonoids, a volatile oil, a bitter principle (glechomine), saponin, resin, and tannins.

Actions
Ground ivy has not been well studied, and thus little is known about its action (Grieve, 1996). It appears to have astringent properties and is claimed to dry secretions and decrease inflammation. It has been used as a decongestant and a diuretic, but data to support these effects are unavailable.

Reported uses
Ground ivy has traditionally and anecdotally been recommended by herbalists to treat disorders of the ear, nose, throat, and digestive sys-

tem. Its astringent properties have been used to reduce phlegm in allergic rhinitis, bronchitis, hay fever, and sinusitis. Its binding nature has led to its use to treat diarrhea and to dry up watery and mucoid secretions. All the evidence of ground ivy's effectiveness comes from folklore and anecdotal reports; no animal or human trials have been reported.

Dosage
14 to 28 grains prepared as a fluidextract P.O. t.i.d.

Adverse reactions
None reported.

Interactions
None reported.

Contraindications and precautions
No known contraindications.

Special considerations
• Inform the patient that little information exists to support a therapeutic use of ground ivy.
• Suggest other, contemporary forms of therapy before starting therapy with this herb.
• Poisoning has occurred in horses that have ingested the plant. Symptoms include cyanosis, lung congestion, pupil dilation, salivation, and sweating.
• Although no known chemical interactions have been reported in clinical studies, consideration must be given to the pharmacologic properties of the herbal product and the potential for exacerbation of the intended therapeutic effect of conventional drugs.

Points of interest
• Ground ivy is known in parts of England as alehoof because it was used in medieval times to flavor and clarify ale.

Commentary
Ground ivy appears to be a well-tolerated herb often given to children to treat congestive conditions such as sinusitis. It may be safe at low doses, but animal toxicities have been reported at higher doses; thus, caution must be exercised. Because of the lack of controlled animal or human data, this product cannot be recommended.

References
Grieve, M. *A Modern Herbal.* New York: Barnes & Noble, Inc., 1996.

GUARANA
BRAZILIAN COCOA, GUARANA GUM, GUARANA PASTE, QUARANA, QUARANE, UABANO, UARANZEIRO, ZOOM

Taxonomic class
Sapindaceae

Common trade names
Guarana Plus, Guarana Rush, Happy Motion, Superguarana, Zoom

Common forms
Guarana is a source of caffeine and an ingredient in many soft drinks, including Dark Dog Lemon, Guts, and Josta. It is also available in alcoholic extracts, capsules, elixirs, tablets of varied strength, and teas and included as an ingredient in several aphrodisiacs, candies, chewing gum, energy drinks, vitamin supplements, and weight-loss supplements.

Source
Guarana is a dried paste made from the crushed seeds of *Paullinia cupana* (also known as *P. sorbilis)*, a woody vine or shrub that is native to Brazil and the Amazon basin. This plant is widely cultivated because of its market value as a caffeine source and an ingredient in soft drinks, nutritional supplements, and medicinal products worldwide. It is especially popular in South America, where it has long been used for various disorders.

Chemical components
Caffeine is the active ingredient in guarana. Roasted guarana seeds may have up to 6% caffeine, although one manufacturing process has resulted in soluble guarana that contains 10% caffeine. Guarana 800 mg has been reported to contain about 30 mg of caffeine. The plant may contain tannins (including catechutannic acid, d-catechin, tannic acid, and catechol) and saponins, including trace amounts of timbonine, similar to the timbo fish poisons used by Amazonian Indians.

Actions
The effects of guarana are attributed directly to its high caffeine content. The pharmacologic actions of caffeine include bronchial smooth-muscle relaxation; cardiac, CNS, and skeletal muscle stimulation; cerebrovascular vasoconstriction; coronary and peripheral vasodilation; diuresis; increased gastric acid secretion; and hyperglycemia. Although the effects of the saponins and tannins are not completely known, they may also participate in guarana's actions.

Guarana provides more CNS stimulation than tea or coffee, possibly because of the tannin action on caffeine or the effect of fats and saponin on caffeine's absorption (Bempong and Houghton, 1992; Henman, 1982). Antidiarrheal and astringent properties of guarana may also be attributed to the tannins. Catechutannic acid, catechol, and other astringents may relieve diarrhea but cause constipation in healthy people.

Studies in Brazil showed that guarana decreases thromboxane synthesis in platelets to reverse and inhibit platelet aggregation, effects that may be attributed to the plant's xanthine content.

Reported uses

Guarana has long been used as an aphrodisiac, an appetite suppressant, and a CNS stimulant; for treating diarrhea; and for protection against malaria and dysentery (Henman, 1982). It is included in many body-building, smoking cessation, and weight-loss products and in natural vitamin supplements to curb the appetite and provide a feeling of increased energy and mental alertness.

Guarana may be considered similar to coffee, colas, tea, and other caffeine products that are used to temporarily relieve drowsiness and enhance mental acuity. It may also be used in dermatologic preparations; claims have been made for tannins as protective agents, saponins as skin softeners, and xanthines as useful agents in reducing dermatitis.

Dosage

Dosage is highly variable and depends on the product and batch. Single doses usually contain 200 to 800 mg of guarana. Daily intake of guarana should not exceed 3 g P.O. of guarana powder or its equivalent.

A maximum daily caffeine intake of about 250 mg (3 to 5 g guarana) has been suggested for nonpregnant adults. Daily dosages of up to 1 g of caffeine have been used without apparent adverse effects, although withdrawal symptoms may occur after discontinuation.

Adverse reactions

Normal consumption
CNS: insomnia.
GU: diuresis.

Excessive consumption
CNS: agitation, anxiety, headache, irritability, ***seizures,*** tremor.
CV: premature ventricular contractions, tachycardia.
GI: diarrhea, nausea, vomiting.

Withdrawal after regular daily consumption
CNS: anxiety, headache, irritability.

Interactions

Adenosine: May decrease response. Monitor the patient.
Beta-adrenergic agonists: May enhance response. Monitor the patient.
Cimetidine, disulfiram, fluoroquinolones, oral contraceptives, phenylpropanolamine: May increase serum caffeine levels or prolong serum caffeine half-life. Monitor the patient.
Iron: Absorption may be decreased by coffee or tea if taken within 1 hour of a meal. Avoid administration with guarana.
Lithium: Caffeine may inhibit clearance of lithium. Monitor the patient.
Smoking: Increased elimination of caffeine and related xanthines. Avoid smoking.

Bold italic type indicates that reaction may be life-threatening.

Theophylline: May cause additive CNS and CV effects. Avoid administration with guarana and other sources of caffeine.

Contraindications and precautions

Guarana and other caffeine-containing products are contraindicated in patients with arrhythmias because high caffeine levels may worsen symptoms and arrhythmias and inhibit cardioversion with adenosine. Avoid or limit use of caffeine products in pregnant or breast-feeding patients because low birth weight is associated with caffeine consumption. Avoid or use cautiously in patients with anxiety disorders, CV disease, diabetes, gastric ulcer, or chronic headache and in those taking theophylline.

Special considerations

• The caffeine content of any particular guarana product cannot be accurately predicted.
• Caution the pregnant patient against using guarana because it contains caffeine.
🕭 **ALERT** Toxic symptoms (agitation, arrhythmias, irritability, seizures, tremor) can be produced in adults who consume more than 1 g of caffeine; an acute oral dose of 5 to 10 g of caffeine can be lethal.
• Counsel the patient to reduce guarana use if symptoms resulting from excessive caffeine use occur (headache, irritability, palpitations, tremor).
• Inform the patient that guarana may exacerbate gastroesophageal reflux disease, hiatal hernia, high blood pressure, and peptic ulcer disease.
• Caution the patient who is taking theophylline to avoid using guarana because of the risk of excessive CNS stimulation.
• Caution the patient that caffeine-containing products may increase muscle breakdown, especially if taken in high doses or in combination with other herbal products during periods of weight-training exercise.

Points of interest

• Guarana is listed as generally recognized as safe by the FDA for use as a food additive. (See *Uses of guarana,* page 376.)
• In 1989, the FDA prohibited the use of caffeine in OTC diet products because of increased agitation, hallucinations, restlessness, and tremor reported when caffeine was combined with phenylpropanolamine (DeSimone and Scott, 1995).
• In 1826, guaranine, the major alkaloid in guarana, was isolated and later shown to be nearly identical to caffeine; theophylline and theobromine were also isolated. Guaranine may still be used in labeling because some reports claim that it is a tetramethylxanthine, whereas caffeine is a trimethylxanthine.
• Small particles of the seed husk of guarana remain in the final product after processing, giving the herb a bitter, chocolate taste.
• Acute myoglobinuria has been reported after the first ingestion of a commercial mixture of guarana (500 mg), ginkgo biloba (200 mg), and kava (100 mg) extracts by a patient who had recently resumed low-

intensity weight training (Donadio et al., 2000). Methylxanthines can induce muscle contracture and rhabdomyolysis in high dosages (Wrenn and Oschner, 1989), and antidopaminergics, such as kava, may cause neuroleptic malignant syndrome, of which myoglobinuria may be a component.

Commentary

Guarana contains relatively high amounts of caffeine, although variations occur with product and preparation. The products are probably as safe as coffee, tea, and colas, but caffeine intake should be monitored. Many products contain guarana as an undisclosed ingredient (such as in body-building and weight-loss supplements), and the caffeine content is not always specified. Guarana elixirs contain alcohol and may contain higher amounts of caffeine than products that contain powdered guarana. Caffeine products should be avoided in pregnant or breast-feeding women because caffeine crosses the placenta and is excreted in breast milk.

References

Bempong, D.K., and Houghton, P.J. "Dissolution and Absorption of Caffeine from Guarana," *J Pharm Pharmacol* 44:769-71, 1992.

DeSimone, E.M., and Scott, D.M. "Nicotine and Caffeine Abuse," in *Applied Therapeutics: The Clinical Use of Drugs*, 6th ed. Edited by Young, L.Y., and Koda-Kimble, M.A. Vancouver, Wash.: Applied Therapeutics, 1995.

Donadio, V., et al. "Myoglobinuria After Ingestion of Extracts of Guarana, *Ginkgo biloba* and Kava," *Neurol Sci* 21:124, 2000.

Henman, A.R. "Guarana (*Paullinia cupana* var. *sorbilis*): Ecological and Social Perspectives on an Economic Plant of the Central Amazon Basin," *J Ethnopharmacol* 6:311-38, 1982.

Wrenn, K.D., and Oschner, I. "Rhabdomyolysis Induced by a Caffeine Overdose," *Ann Emerg Med* 18:94-97, 1989.

GUGGUL

GUGULIPID, GUM GUGGUL, GUM GUGGULU

Taxonomic class
Burseraceae

Common trade names
Guggulow, Guglip

Common forms
Available as powdered resin in capsules and as tablets (25 mg guggulsterone equivalent).

Source
Guggul is the oleoresin of the plant *Commiphora mukul* (gum guggul). The plant is indigenous to India, where it is well known as an ancient remedy in the Ayurvedic system of medicine (Indian plant medicine).

Chemical components
The gum resin exudate of *C. mukul* is composed primarily of ketonic steroid compounds, including E- and Z-guggulsterones, which are mainly responsible for its hypolipidemic activity. Gugulipid, the ethyl acetate extract of the gum, has been pursued commercially because it is thought to lack the toxic effects of the crude resin and petroleum ether extract.

Actions
Guggul has been shown to significantly lower serum lipid levels and change the lipoprotein profile in both animal and clinical studies, including decreases in serum cholesterol, triglyceride, LDL, and VLDL levels and an increase in HDL levels. This effect may be accounted for by guggul's ability to stimulate the thyroid gland. Conflicting evidence exists regarding an effect on the coagulation cascade. Data from both animal and human studies have shown an increase in PT and a tendency toward increased fibrinolytic activity and decreased platelet aggregation.

Reported uses
Guggul's therapeutic utility is based on emerging evidence that suggests an indication for treating dyslipidemia. One small, randomized, placebo-controlled trial showed significant reductions in serum cholesterol and triglyceride levels of 21.75% and 27.1%, respectively. The same study also showed an increase in serum HDL levels and a concomitant decrease in LDL and VLDL fractions after 16 weeks of therapy (Verma

and Bordia, 1988). A double-blind crossover trial compared lipid levels among patients who were randomized to receive either guggul or clofibrate, 500 mg, three times a day for 12 weeks. The results of this study showed a 12.6% and 14.7% decline in serum cholesterol levels with gugulipid and clofibrate therapy, respectively. Also, a lowering of serum triglyceride levels by 16.4% and 23.2% was noted with gugulipid and clofibrate, respectively. Among patients with hypercholesterolemia, response to gugulipid was better, whereas among patients with hyper-triglyceridemia, clofibrate produced a better response (Nityanand et al., 1989). Other reported uses stem from animal studies that have shown guggul to be beneficial in treating inflammation and in protecting cardiac enzymes and the cytochrome P-450 system against drug-induced myocardial necrosis.

Dosage

Commercially, guggul is marketed as the standardized ethyl acetate extract gugulipid, which provides a fixed amount of guggulsterones. Multicenter clinical trials showing hypolipidemic efficacy have tested gugulipid, 500 mg, given P.O. t.i.d. for 12 weeks. The authors of one small, double-blind, placebo-controlled trial recommended a typical daily dose of 100 mg of guggulsterones. A much smaller trial used 2,250 mg of crude gum guggul given P.O. b.i.d. in the morning and evening after meals.

Adverse reactions

Crude gum guggul (unpurified)
CNS: restlessness.
GI: diarrhea, hiccoughs.
GU: menstrual irregularities.
Skin: rash.

Gugulipid (ethyl acetate extract)
GI: epigastric fullness (only adverse event was documented in clinical trials with 400 mg three times a day for 4 weeks).

Interactions

None known.

Contraindications and precautions

Guggul is recognized as both an emmenogogue (enabling the onset of menstruation) and an abortifacient (inducing miscarriage) and, therefore, contraindicated in pregnant patients. Clinical data regarding the use of guggul in children and adolescents are not available. Use cautiously in patients taking antiplatelet drugs or anticoagulants because clinical data have shown increases in PT and variable effects on fibrinolytic activity and platelet aggregation.

Bold italic type indicates that reaction may be life-threatening.

Special considerations
• Advise the patient to report unusual bleeding or bruising.
• Inform the patient that the crude resin may be less well tolerated than the standardized extract, gugulipid.
• Urge the pregnant patient to avoid using guggul.
• Although no known chemical interactions have been reported in clinical studies, consideration must be given to the pharmacologic properties of the herbal product and the potential for exacerbation of the intended therapeutic effect of conventional drugs.

Points of interest
• An association between gum guggul and lipids was first described centuries ago in traditional Indian medicine. Two decades of animal and human research culminated in the approval of gugulipid for marketing as a potent hypolipidemic agent in 1987 by the prime minister of India. Double-blind, placebo-controlled trials have shown a lipid-lowering effect comparable to that of clofibrate.

Commentary
Clinical trials suggesting a role for guggul in the management of patients with dyslipidemia have mainly been conducted in India, where researchers have evaluated the use of the extract gugulipid. The most convincing evidence was obtained from a multicenter, double-blind, crossover trial that concluded that the drug caused reductions in serum cholesterol and triglyceride levels comparable to clofibrate, nicotinic acid, and cholestyramine. The study also reported significant increases in HDL levels and decreases in LDL levels. The results of these trials suggest that guggul may be characterized as a mild to moderate lipid-lowering agent. Further longer-term studies are needed to assess its exact role in the management of various lipid disorders. Such studies will also help to better illustrate the adverse effect profile because current studies suggest rather benign effects after treatment periods of less than 3 months. It would be interesting to know how gugulipid compares with the standard-of-care treatments of today, especially HMG-CoA reductase inhibitors.

References
Agarwal, R.C., et al. "Clinical Trial of Gugulipid a New Hypolipidemic Agent of Plant Origin in Primary Hyperlipidemia," *Indian J Med Res* 84:626-34, 1986.

Nityanand, S., et al. "Clinical Trials with Gugulipid a New Hypolipidaemic Agent," *J Assoc Phys India* 37:323-28, 1989.

Satyavati, G.V. "Gum Guggul (*Commiphora mukul*)—The Success Story of an Ancient Insight Leading to a Modern Discovery," *Indian J Med Res* 87:327-35, 1988.

Verma, S.K., and Bordia, A. "Effect of *Commiphora mukul* (Gum Guggulu) in Patients of Hyperlipidemia with Special Reference to HDL-Cholesterol," *Indian J Med Res* 87:356-60, 1988.

GUM ARABIC

ACACIA, ACACIA ARABICA GUM, ACACIA GUM, *ACACIA SENEGAL*, ACACIA VER, EGYPTIAN THORN, *GUMMAE MIMOSAE*, SENEGA

Taxonomic class
Fabaceae

Common trade names
Premium Granular Gum Acacia, Premium Granular Gum Arabic, Premium Powdered Gum Acacia, Premium Powdered Gum Arabic, Premium Spray Dried Gum Acacia, Premium Spray Dried Gum Arabic, Superwhite Spray Dried Gum Acacia

Common forms
Available as gum, a powder (20 g/package), and syrup (10% gum arabic).

Source
Gum arabic is extracted from the tree *Acacia senegal.* The quality of the gum varies according to the method of gum expression (beetle attack, extreme drought, or tapping) and the growing conditions.

Chemical components
Gum arabic is a complex mixture of calcium, magnesium, and potassium salts of arabic acid. It contains tannin, cyanogenic glycosides, oxidases, peroxidases, and pectinases. It is a heteropolysaccharide composed of D-galactopyranose, D-glucuronic acid, L-arabinose, and L-rhamnose. Acacia powder usually contains carbohydrate bases that contain fructose. The gum is soluble in water and insoluble in alcohol, ether, and oils.

Actions
Physiologic mechanisms are poorly described. Purified acacia gum may inhibit the growth and protease activity of suspected periodontal pathogens with marked differences in susceptibility (Clark et al., 1993). Tannins reportedly act as astringents with hemostatic and healing properties; cyanogenic glycosides, oxidases, peroxidases, and pectinases exhibit antimicrobial properties. Gum arabic may also be fermented in the colon, providing a substrate for bacterial nitrogen incorporation and growth. This action increases fecal nitrogen excretion and bacterial masses while lowering BUN levels.

Reported uses
In the early 1990s, two studies evaluated the efficacy of gum arabic in patients with hypercholesterolemia and found no beneficial effect (Haskell et al., 1992; Jensen et al., 1993). More recent studies show a conflicting picture. In one small study conducted by Mee and Gee (1997), an apple fiber and gum arabic supplement appeared to lower both total cholesterol and LDL levels in mildly hypercholesterolemic

---

Bold italic type indicates that reaction may be life-threatening.

men. In a larger trial by Davidson and colleagues (1998), a supplement containing a 4:1 ratio of gum arabic and pectin in apple juice was evaluated in 110 hypercholesterolemic men and women. Varying doses of the supplement were given for 12 weeks, with a 6-week apple juice–only washout period after the treatment phase. Mean serum total cholesterol and triglyceride levels actually rose 3.5% and 28.5%, respectively, during the treatment period ($P<.0001$). Total cholesterol levels increased an additional 2.4% ($P<.05$) during the washout phase, possibly implicating the apple juice as the cause of the elevated cholesterol levels. The gum arabic and pectin supplement failed to have a beneficial effect on cholesterol levels despite these subtle elevations.

Antiplaque and antibacterial effects were noted when gum arabic was used as a chewing gum; lower gingival and plaque scores were reported, implying inhibition of early deposition of plaque.

Gum arabic may also be useful in patients with chronic renal failure who are on a low-protein diet because it increases fecal nitrogen content and fecal bacterial mass and significantly decreases BUN levels (Bliss et al., 1996). Unsubstantiated claims include treatment of burns, colds, cough, diarrhea, dysentery, gonorrhea, inflammation, nodular leprosy, sore nipples, and sore throat.

Dosage
Dosages vary with the formulation.
For lowering cholesterol, 9.7 to 50 g daily P.O. of powdered gum arabic.
For reducing plaque, gum with an unknown quantity of the active ingredient is used.

Adverse reactions
GI: bloating, increased flatulence (dose-dependent effect), increased stool frequency, ***hepatotoxicity*** (with I.V. use).
GU: ***nephrotoxicity*** (with I.V. use).
Skin: contact dermatitis (after exposure to preservative).

Interactions
None reported.

Contraindications and precautions
Avoid using gum arabic in pregnant or breast-feeding patients; effects are unknown. Use cautiously in patients with a history of atopy or those who are prone to contact dermatitis.

Special considerations
• Gum arabic is considered a food supplement approved by the FDA and World Health Organization.
• Instruct the patient not to discontinue regular dental care in favor of this herb.
• Advise the patient to consult a health care provider before using herbal preparations because a treatment that has been clinically researched and proved effective may be available.

- Although no known chemical interactions have been reported in clinical studies, consideration must be given to the pharmacologic properties of the herbal product and the potential for exacerbation of the intended therapeutic effect of conventional drugs.

Points of interest

- In 1977, the United States imported more than 11,000 tons of gum arabic, primarily for the purpose of adding body and texture to processed food products.
- Gum arabic is used as an excipient in many OTC and prescription drugs to stabilize emulsions and act as a demulcent.

Commentary

Despite positive data from one small study, the overall clinical trial evidence in hypercholesterolemic patients seems to prove that gum arabic is not an effective agent for lowering cholesterol levels. Human study data do imply a role for gum arabic as an antiplaque agent in chewing gum; further studies are needed to define its dosage and use in treatment. There are no studies comparing gum arabic with standard-of-care drug therapies. Although allergic reactions have primarily been attributed to exposure to preservatives used along with gum arabic in various preparations, the potential for such reactions warrants discriminate use in atopic individuals.

References

Bliss, D.Z., et al. "Supplementation with Gum Arabic Fiber Increases Fecal Nitrogen Excretion and Lowers Serum Urea Nitrogen Concentration in Chronic Renal Failure Patients Consuming a Low-Protein Diet," *Am J Clin Nutr* 63:392-98, 1996.

Clark, D.T., et al. "The Effects of *Acacia arabica* Gum on the In Vitro Growth and Protease Activities of Periodontopathic Bacteria," *J Clin Periodontol* 20:238-43, 1993.

Davidson, M.H., et al. "A Low-viscosity Soluble-fiber Fruit Juice Supplement Fails to Lower Cholesterol in Hypercholesterolemic Men and Women," *J Nutr* 128(11):1927-32, 1998.

Haskell, W.L., et al. "Role of Water-soluble Dietary Fiber in the Management of Elevated Plasma Cholesterol in Healthy Subjects," *Am J Cardiol* 69:433-39, 1992.

Jensen, C.D., et al. "The Effect of Acacia Gum and a Water-soluble Dietary Fiber Mixture on Blood Lipids in Humans," *J Am Coll Nutr* 12:147-54, 1993.

Mee, K.A., and Gee, D.L. "Apple Fiber and Gum Arabic Lowers Total and Low-density Lipoprotein Cholesterol Levels in Men with Mild Hypercholesterolemia," *J Am Diet Assoc* 97(4):422-24, 1997.

HAWTHORN

CRATAEGUS EXTRACT, LI 132, MAY, MAYBUSH, WHITEHORN

Taxonomic class
Rosaceae

Common trade names
Alvita Teas Hawthorne Berry, Cardio Health Hawthorne Berry #6 Syrup, Cardiplant, Gaia Herbs Hawthorn Berry A/F, Gaia Herbs Hawthorn Berry Solid, Gaia Herbs Hawthorn Supreme, Gaia Herbs Hawthorn Supreme SFSE, Hawthorne Berry, Hawthorne Formula, Hawthorne Heart, Hawthorne Phytosome, Hawthorne Power, Heart Foods Company Hawthorne Plus, Heart Foods Company Power Caps Hot Cayenne with Hawthorne and Ginger, Herbalist and Alchemist Hawthorn-Cactus Extract, Herbalist and Alchemist Hawthorn-Fruit/Flower Extrac, Natrol Hawthorne Berry Capsules, Nature's Answer Hawthorne Berry Low Alcohol, Nature's Answer Hawthorne C+ Combo, Standardized Full Potency Hawthorne Berry Extract Vegicaps

Common forms
Available as biological extracts (4 mg/ml of vitexin-2-O-rhamnoside); capsules of berries (510 mg) or leaves (80 mg) standardized to 15 mg of oligomeric procyanidines; and extended-release capsules (300 mg of 1.8% vitexin-2-rhamnoside and hyperoside).

Source
Active ingredients are extracted from the berries, flowers, and leaves of *Crataegus* species, commonly *C. laevigata*, *C. monogyna*, or *C. folium*. More than 300 *Crataegus* species are found in the temperate regions of North America, Asia, and Europe.

Chemical components
Hawthorn is composed primarily of proanthocyanidins and flavonoids (quercetin, hyperoside, vitexin, vitexin-rhamnoside, rutin); other constituents include catechin and epicatechin.

Actions
Studies on animals and in vitro models have suggested CV actions that include ACE inhibition, beta-blocking activity, dilation of coronary arteries, hypotensive effects, and negative and positive inotropic effects. The high bioflavonoid content in some hawthorn species may show antioxidant activity and be cardioprotective in experimental ischemic animal models; the extracts decreased myocardial oxygen consumption and left ventricular work (Lianda et al., 1984). Prophylactic antiar-

rhythmic potential has also been shown in rabbits that received acon-itine. Mild CNS depressant effects have been documented for the haw-thorn flower extract.

Reported uses

Claims for hawthorn surround its use in arteriosclerosis, Buerger's disease, heart failure, hypertension, and paroxysmal tachycardia. It may be therapeutically useful in the treatment of New York Heart Association (NYHA) functional class II (mild to moderate) heart failure. Patients with this class of heart failure who received a daily dose of 600 mg of hawthorn extract showed significant clinical improvement over an 8-week period (Schmidt et al., 1994).

Hawthorn, either alone or with coenzyme Q10, was found to be beneficial and also compared favorably to captopril for patients with heart failure (Tauchert et al., 1994). Other studies have noted the herb's usefulness in patients with stable angina pectoris (Hanak and Bruckel, 1983).

Dosage

A dose of 160 to 900 mg of a standardized extract containing 2.2% flavonoids or 18.75% oligomeric procyanidins given P.O. b.i.d. or t.i.d. The amount of flavonoid (calculated as hyperoside) is 3.5 to 19.8 mg and that of procyanidins (as epicatechin) is 30 to 168.7 mg.

Adverse reactions

CNS: fatigue, sedation (with high doses).
CV: *arrhythmias* and hypotension (with high doses).
GI: nausea.
Respiratory: *respiratory failure* (in animals).
Skin: sweating.

Interactions

Antihypertensives, nitrates: Increased risk of hypotension. Monitor blood pressure closely.
Cardiac glycosides: Increased effects of these drugs. Use cautiously.
CNS depressants: May cause additive effects. Use cautiously.

Contraindications and precautions

Hawthorn is contraindicated in patients who are hypersensitive to other members of the Rosaceae family and in pregnant or breast-feeding patients.

Special considerations

• Monitor the patient for adverse CNS effects.
• Instruct the patient to use hawthorn only under medical supervision.
• Caution the patient to avoid hazardous activities until hawthorn's CNS effects are known.
• Inform the patient that other proven therapies for heart failure should be pursued before taking hawthorn.

Bold italic type indicates that reaction may be life-threatening.

• Urge the patient to seek emergency medical treatment if he becomes short of breath or if pain occurs in the heart region and spreads to the arm, lower jaw, or upper abdomen.
• Urge the patient who chooses to self-medicate to seek medical advice if symptoms continue for longer than 6 weeks.

Points of interest
• Germany's Federal Institute for Drugs and Medical Devices has approved the use of hawthorn leaf with flower extracts in the treatment of NYHA functional class II heart failure. The extract of berries has not been approved because efficacy has not been shown.
• Berry preparations are commonly advertised as a supplement to strengthen and invigorate the heart and circulatory system.

Commentary
Hawthorn has long been used for heart failure in Europe. Several foreign studies suggest that it may be effective in treating NYHA functional class II heart failure. Long-term studies using hawthorn that demonstrate prolonged survival are lacking. Future studies should focus on evaluating improvements in NYHA heart failure class, hospital admission rates, quality of life measurements, and whether hawthorn extracts have an effect on mortality.

References
Hanak, T.H., and Bruckel, M.H. "Behandlung Von Leichten Stabilen Formen der Angina Pectoris mit Crataegutt Novo," *Therapiewoche* 33:4331-33, 1983.

Lianda, L., et al. "Studies on Hawthorn and Its Active Principle. I. Effect on Myocardial Ischemia and Hemodynamics in Dogs," *J Tradit Chin Med* 4:283-88, 1984.

Schmidt, U., et al. "Efficacy of the Hawthorn *(Crataegus)* Preparation LI 132 in 78 Patients with Chronic Congestive Heart Failure Defined as NYHA Functional Class II," *Phytomedicine* 1:17-24, 1994.

Tauchert, M., et al. "Effectiveness of Hawthorn Extract LI 132 Compared with the ACE Inhibitor Captopril: Multicenter Double-Blind Study with 132 NYHA Stage II," *Munch Med* 136(Suppl):S27-33, 1994.

HELLEBORE, AMERICAN
FALSE HELLEBORE, GREEN HELLEBORE, INDIAN POKE, ITCHWEED, SWAMP HELLEBORE

Taxonomic class
Liliaceae

Common trade names
Cryptenamine

Common forms
Available as fluidextract, powder, root, and tincture.

Source

American or green hellebore is derived from the dried rhizome and roots of the perennial herb *Veratrum viride.* Related species include *V. album* (white hellebore), *V. californicum, V. japonicum,* and *V. officinale* (Cevadilla).

Chemical components

The main components of the root include several ester glycoalkaloids (pseudojervine, rubijervine, jervine, neogermitrine, cevadine, proto-veratrine, veratridine, and protoveratridine), starch, and resin. The alkaloids are chemically similar to steroids and are considered both medicinally active and toxic. All species contain varying amounts of alkaloids, which explains the varying degrees of action and toxicity.

Actions

The ester alkaloids are responsible for hellebore's physiologic effects, including lowering arterial pressure and heart and respiratory rates and stimulating blood flow to the kidneys, liver, and extremities. The CV response to *Veratrum* alkaloids depends on the agent and the dose administered. High doses have paradoxically elevated blood pressure (Arena and Drew, 1986).

   Veratrum alkaloids are known to have a depolarizing action on cardiac tissue, nerve membranes, and skeletal and visceral muscles. They are believed to increase nerve and muscle excitability, as noted by the adverse effects of increased muscle tone and paresthesia. These agents also produce nausea and emesis; large doses depress respiration and can cause respiratory failure.

Reported uses

Historically, hellebore has been used as an emetic and for neuralgias, peritonitis, pneumonia, and seizures. More recently, *Veratrum* alkaloids have been used to treat hypertension, acute hypertensive crises, hypertensive toxemia of pregnancy, and nephropathies (Arena and Drew, 1986). They have been given parenterally (with success) for managing pulmonary edema resulting from severe acute hypertensive crises. One *Veratrum* alkaloid, germine diacetate, has been used experimentally to treat myasthenia gravis (Anon., 1967).

   Hellebore and the *Veratrum* alkaloids are not currently used because of their narrow therapeutic index and highly toxic nature. Some herbalists may recommend American or green hellebore as a cardiac sedative.

Dosage

For cardiac sedation, 1 to 3 minims of fluidextract P.O. every 2 to 3 hours until pulse rate is reduced; or 1 to 2 grains of powder P.O.; or 10 to 30 minims of tincture P.O. I.V. doses are unknown.

Adverse reactions

CNS: paresthesia, ***seizures,*** syncope.
CV: ***arrhythmias, bradycardia,*** ECG changes, hypertension, hypotension.

Bold italic type indicates that reaction may be life-threatening.

EENT: dysgeusia, extraocular muscle paralysis, increased salivation, sneezing (inhalation).
GI: abdominal pain and distention, nausea, vomiting.
Musculoskeletal: increased muscle tone, muscle weakness.
Respiratory: dyspnea, respiratory depression.
Skin: pallor, sweating.

Interactions
None reported.

Contraindications and precautions
American hellebore is contraindicated in patients with aortic coarctation, digitalis intoxication, hypotension, increased intracranial pressure (unless caused by hypertensive crisis), or pheochromocytoma and in pregnant patients.

Special considerations
● American hellebore is considered highly toxic. It has a low therapeutic index that makes it unfavorable for medicinal purposes.
● **ALERT** Ingestion of any part of the plant can cause toxicity. Signs of overdose are abdominal pain, burning in throat, diarrhea, loss of consciousness, nausea, paralysis, shortness of breath, spasms, syncope, and vision changes. Most cases have not been fatal because of the rapid vomiting that occurs and the poor intestinal absorption of the *Veratrum* alkaloids.
● Although no known chemical interactions have been reported in clinical studies, consideration must be given to the pharmacologic properties of the herbal product and the potential for exacerbation of the intended therapeutic effect of conventional drugs.
● Advise the patient to consult a health care provider before using herbal preparations because a treatment that has been clinically researched and proved effective may be available.

Points of interest
● Veratrine, which once appeared in the USP (1898) and British Pharmacopoeia Codex, is derived from the plant *V. officinale* (Mexican hellebore) or sabadilla. It is used as a topical analgesic and a parasiticide. Veratrine contains many of the same alkaloids found in American hellebore in varying amounts.
● Ingestion of the plant *V. californicum,* related to American hellebore, has been associated with causing cyclopia and other related facial deformities in animals.
● Sneezing powders are known to have contained *Veratrum* alkaloids. The powders contained pulverized *V. album* root, which, when inhaled, caused many of the same adverse effects seen after ingestion, including bradycardia, hypotension, nausea, sweating, and vomiting (Fogh et al., 1983).
● Veracintine, an alkaloid isolated from *V. album,* and its derivatives have exhibited in vitro cytotoxic effects on leukemia cells.

Commentary

Despite its extensive use in the past for malignant hypertension, hellebore and *Veratrum* alkaloids are no longer preferred for these uses because of their narrow therapeutic index and the emergence of safer and more tolerable agents. The *Veratrum* alkaloids have clear pharmacologic activity, but their noxious and toxic adverse effects have limited their use. Because only small amounts of *Veratrum* alkaloid extracts are needed to cause toxic effects, their use is considered extremely dangerous. Hellebore is not recommended for medicinal use.

References

Anon. "Veratrum Alkaloids in the Therapy of Myasthenia Gravis," *Can Med Assoc J* 96:1534-35, 1967.

Arena, J.M., and Drew, R.H.,eds. *Poisoning: Toxicology, Symptoms, Treatments,* 5th ed. Springfield, Ill.: Charles C. Thomas Publisher, 1986.

Fogh, A., et al. "Veratrum Alkaloids in Sneezing-Powder: A Potential Danger," *J Toxical Clin Toxicol* 20:175-79, 1983.

HELLEBORE, BLACK

BLACK HELLEBORE, CHRISTE HERBE, CHRISTMAS ROSE, EASTER ROSE, MELAMPODE

Taxonomic class
Ranunculaceae

Common trade names
None known.

Common forms
Available as fluidextract, powdered root, seed, or a solid extract.

Source
The active components are extracted from the dried rhizome and root of the perennial plant *Helleborus niger.*

Chemical components
The extract may contain hellebrin, an aglycone, and two highly toxic crystalline glycosides—bufadienole helleborin and helleborcin. These glycosides may indicate contamination with other related species. Other components include saponosides, ranunculoside derivatives, resin, fat, and starch. The commercial hellebore roots consist mainly of *H. niger* and are mostly hellebrin-free. Other related species, especially *H. viridis,* tend to have higher levels of glycosides and aglycones.

Actions
The entire plant is considered poisonous. Extracts of black hellebore are claimed to promote menstrual flow and to have anthelmintic, narcotic, and purgative properties.

Protoanemonine is thought to cause abdominal pain, a burning sensation in the mouth and throat, dermatitis, eye irritation, and vomiting.

Bold italic type indicates that reaction may be life-threatening.

It combines with sulfhydryl groups, which results in subepidermal vesication. Topical application of the freshly bruised plant can cause serious irritation. Early in vitro studies using protoanemonine identified antifungal and cytotoxic properties (Erickson, 1948; Holden et al., 1947).

Reported uses

The plant has been used historically as a purgative and to treat amenorrhea, anxiety, heart failure, intestinal parasite infections, mental disorders, and skin ulcers. Other claims include its use as an anesthetic and a diuretic and to induce abortion.

In homeopathy, black hellebore tincture is said to be useful for eclampsia, encephalitis, epilepsy, meningitis, and psychoses. In Europe, black hellebore is used in homeopathy and as adjuvant therapy for cancer patients because of its claimed immunostimulatory properties. An in vitro study observed increased cytokine production in cells given an extract of black hellebore (Bussing and Schweizer, 1998). There have been no controlled, double-blind, randomized human trials involving black hellebore preparations.

Dosage

For laxative use, 1 to 10 gtt of fluidextract P.O., 1 to 2 grains of solid extract P.O., or 10 to 20 grains of powder P.O.

Adverse reactions

CV: *arrhythmias, bradycardia*, hypotension, irregular pulse (with contamination).
EENT: burning sensation in the mouth, conjunctival and nasal irritation, increased salivation, sneezing.
GI: abdominal pain, diarrhea, vomiting.
Respiratory: *respiratory failure* (with contamination), shortness of breath.
Skin: dermatitis.

Interactions

None reported.

Contraindications and precautions

Avoid using black hellebore in pregnant or breast-feeding patients; effects are unknown.

Special considerations

• Caution the patient that ingestion of the plant may result in abdominal pain, a burning sensation in the mouth and throat, diarrhea, increased salivation, and vomiting.
• Advise the patient that black hellebore is considered toxic and, therefore, should not be consumed.
• Advise the patient to consult a health care provider before using herbal preparations because a treatment that has been clinically researched and proved effective may be available.

- Although no known chemical interactions have been reported in clinical studies, consideration must be given to the pharmacologic properties of the herbal product and the potential for exacerbation of the intended therapeutic effect of conventional drugs.

Points of interest
- *H. niger* blossoms white flowers in the winter, from which it received its name Christmas rose.
- "Hellebore" is derived from the Greek *elein* (to injure) and *bora* (food), describing its toxic nature.

Commentary
Besides its use in homeopathy, black hellebore is used mainly as an ornamental garden plant. Although it is being used as a potential immunostimulant, controlled human trials to support this claim are lacking. Because of its recognized poisonous status and the lack of clinical data to support the medicinal use of black hellebore, products containing components of this plant should be avoided.

References
Bussing, A., and Schweizer, K. "Effects of Phytopreparation from *Helleborus niger* on Immunocompetent Cells In Vitro," *J Ethnopharmacol* 59:139-46, 1998.

Erickson, R.O. "Protoanemonin as a Mitotic Inhibitor," *Science* 108:533, 1948.

Holden, M., et al. "Range of Antibiotic Activity of Protoanemonin," *Proc Soc Exp Biol Med* 66:54, 1947.

HESPERIDIN

HESPERIDIN METHYLCHALCONE, HMC, METHYL HESPERIDIN

Common trade names
Multi-ingredient preparations: Alvenor, Ardium, Arventum 500, Capiven, Daflon 500, Detralex, Dios, Variton, Venitrol

Common forms
Available as effervescent granules for oral solution and as tablets (50 mg with diosmin 450 mg [flavone derivative]).

Source
The herb is extracted from *Aurantii fructus immaturi,* also known as unripe orange, and *Aurantii pericarpium,* or dried bitter-orange peel, both of which are derived from *Citrus aurantium*. It is also extracted from *Citri pericarpium*, known as dried lemon peel, which is derived from *Citrus limon.*

Chemical components
The agent is a crystalline flavonoid glycoside. Other chemical constituents include limonene (essential oil), pectin, coumarin derivatives, carotenoids, citric acid, and various other glycosidic flavonoids.

Bold italic type indicates that reaction may be life-threatening.

Actions

Reports describing the physiologic mechanisms of action have been largely based on the use of micronized purified flavonoid fraction (MPFF), composed of 90% diosmin and 10% hesperidin, as a phlebotropic agent. Clinical data have consistently shown a number of effects on venous hemodynamic parameters, including a reduction in venous emptying time, venous capacitance, venous distensibility, and increases in venous tone. Data from human trials also indicate that MPFF can exert effects on the microcirculation by modulating leukocyte-endothelial interactions and inhibiting proinflammatory mediators. One small clinical study demonstrated a reduction in surface expression of CD62L in neutrophils, monocytes, and the endothelial markers intercellular adhesion molecule-1 and vascular cell adhesion molecule-1, thus decreasing leukocyte chemotaxis and activation (Coleridge Smith et al., 1999). MPFF has also been shown to inhibit the release of prostaglandins and free radicals, resulting in decreased capillary permeability and increased capillary resistance.

Reported uses

Hesperidin is purported to be useful for treating chronic venous insufficiency (CVI). Numerous clinical studies have reported efficacy of the drug (as MPFF) in reducing the symptoms of CVI. The results of four randomized, double-blind, controlled trials showed significant reductions in subjective symptoms, including heaviness, nocturnal cramps, pain, and swelling and significant decreases in leg circumferences at the levels of the ankle and calf, after 2 to 3 months of therapy (Struckmann, 1999). Similar efficacy was noted after a 1-year period of administration. Hesperidin's ability to influence healing in patients with venous ulceration was assessed in a relatively small, double-blind, randomized, placebo-controlled trial, which reported that a significantly larger number of patients had complete ulcer healing at 2 months compared with placebo and a statistically shorter healing time. All patients were treated with a standard compression stocking, and it was among those patients with an ulcer size less than or equal to 10 cm that the results reached statistical significance. The ability of the drug to expedite ulcer healing is attributed to its effects on the microcirculation (Guilhou et al., 1997). One clinical study suggested that hesperidin may be valuable in patients with upper limb lymphedema secondary to breast cancer therapy, especially those with more severe lymphedema. Another role for this drug in the short-term treatment of hemorrhoids of pregnancy was suggested in an open study. Animal data from one source proposed a role for hesperidin in inhibiting neoplastic transformation in murine fibroblasts.

Dosage

Most trials that assessed the use of flavonoids for CVI and lymphedema secondary to breast cancer therapy tested Daflon 500. Patients received 2 tablets P.O. each day, equivalent to 1,000 mg.

Adverse reactions
CNS: anxiety, asthenia, dizziness, drowsiness, headache, insomnia, vertigo.
CV: hypotension, palpitations.
GI: abdominal cramps and pain, diarrhea, dyspepsia, epigastric discomfort, nausea, vomiting.
Skin: rash.

Interactions
None reported.

Contraindications and precautions
Use cautiously in patients taking anticoagulants. Adverse outcomes on human reproduction and lactation are unclear, but birth weight, fetal development, infant growth and feeding, and pregnancy were unaffected in an open study of 50 women with acute hemorrhoids. No teratogenic effects were observed among the offspring of rats treated with doses up to 8 g/kg/day. Photosensitization may occur because *C. aurantium* is known to contain furanocoumarins.

Special considerations
• Urge the patient to report unusual bleeding or bruising.
• Inform the patient that products containing hesperidin may cause photosensitization.
• Caution the patient not to self-treat symptoms of CVI before seeking appropriate medical evaluation because this may delay diagnosis of a serious medical condition.
• Although no known chemical interactions have been reported in clinical studies, consideration must be given to the pharmacologic properties of the herbal product and the potential for exacerbation of the intended therapeutic effect of conventional drugs.

Commentary
The preponderance of available clinical data comes from foreign studies evaluating MPFF (450 mg of diosmin and 50 mg of hesperidin). The most convincing human trial data suggest a role for hesperidin in managing CVI. Evidence indicates that this drug is efficacious in improving venous hemodynamic parameters and mitigating the microcirculatory changes underlying CVI, thereby ultimately reducing the symptoms of the disease and even accelerating complete healing of ulcers. Much of this evidence is based on double-blind, randomized, placebo-controlled trials, but sample size was consistently small and treatment duration was restricted to 1 year or less. Furthermore, these studies did not compare hesperidin with standard-of-care treatments. Although evidence seems to suggest that hesperidin is relatively benign with regard to adverse effects, it is important to note that available data are based on relatively small patient numbers. Overall, it seems that this agent could be considered a reasonable adjunct to current treatment modalities for CVI, including surgery, compression therapy, and pharmacotherapy.

Because it targets both the macrocirculation and the microcirculation, hesperidin may become a particularly beneficial therapy for venous ulceration, the most disabling and expensive stage of CVI. Further studies using larger study populations are needed to better define its place in therapy.

References

Coleridge Smith, P.D. "Neutrophil Activation and Mediators of Inflammation in Chronic Venous Insufficiency," *J Vasc Res* 36(suppl 1):24-36, 1999.

Guilhou, J., et al. "Efficacy of Daflon 500 mg in Venous Leg Ulcer Healing: A Double-blind, Randomized, Controlled Versus Placebo Trial in 107 Patients," *Angiology* 48:77-85, 1997.

Ibegbuna, V., et al. "Venous Elasticity After Treatment with Daflon 500 mg," *Angiology* 48:45-49, 1997.

Pecking, A., et al. "Efficacy of Daflon 500 mg in the Treatment of Lymphedema (Secondary to Conventional Therapy of Breast Cancer)," *Angiology* 48:93-98, 1997.

Struckmann, J.R. "Clinical Efficacy of Micronized Purified Flavonoid Fraction: An Overview," *J Vasc Res* 36(suppl 1):37-41, 1999.

HOPS

Taxonomic class
Cannabaceae

Common trade names
Multi-ingredient preparations: Alvita Teas Hops, Avena Sativa Compound in Species, HR 129 Serene, HR 133 Stress, Melatonin w/ Vitamin B_6, Nature's Answer Hops Low Alcohol, Nature's Herbs Hops-Valerian Combo, Nature's Way Hops Flowers, Sedative Tea, Snuz Plus, Stress Aid

Hops may also be sold as single-ingredient compounds under that name.

Common forms
Hops are usually taken in herbal tea preparations. However, both solid and liquid dosage forms are becoming popular. There are also anecdotal reports of dried hops being smoked.

Source
Humulus lupulus L., the hops plant, is a member of the Cannabaceae family (formerly classified within the Moraceae family; the only other genus of Cannabaceae is *Cannabis sativa/indica*). It is a perennial, dioecious vine that may grow 20' long. The leaves are trilobed, serrate, and, generally, opposite. The major source of active constituents is the strobile of the female plant. These fruits and flowers grow in conelike, leafy bracts and are usually 2" to 4" long.

Chemical components
The constituents of hops are well identified, with more than 330 distinct chemicals isolated. They are found in either a volatile oil fraction

(beta-myrcene, humulene, and linalool) or a resinous fraction (humulone, lupulone). Other active components of hops include estradiol, colupulone, avermectin, various alcohols such as 2-methyl-3-buten-2-ol, and prenylflavonoids and chalcones such as xanthohumol and 8-prenylnaringenin. Despite the fact that *Humulus* and *Cannabis* are members of the same family, hops does not contain delta-9-tetrahydrocannabinol as an active constituent.

Actions
Several distinct pharmacologic actions have been identified with the constituents of hops. In vitro studies indicate that the phytoestrogens exert direct estrogenic activity. 2-Methyl-3-buten-2-ol has demonstrated sedative-hypnotic effects in mice and humans as well as the ability to decrease vigilance and impair performance in humans. Colupulone and avermectin possess antibacterial activity as established both in vitro and in vivo. Humulone has been shown to decrease tumor formation and inflammation in mice. Colupulone induced hepatic microsomal enzymes, and xanthohumol inhibited the extramicrosomal hepatic enzyme DGAT in rats and mice. Xanthohumol also has been shown to inhibit human cytochrome P-450 enzymes in vitro (Henderson et al., 2000). Specifically, this activity was greatest in CYP1A1, CYP1B1, and CYP1A2 isozymes and relatively less in CYP2E3 and CYP3A4 isozymes. Conversely, the chalcones and flavonones have induced murine hepatic quinone reductase activity (Miranda et al., 2000). Certain constituents of hops, particularly 8-prenylnaringenin, possess estrogenic activity (Milligan et al., 1999). These phytoestrogens have demonstrated an ability to inhibit the growth of human breast cancer cells in vitro (Dixon-Shanies and Shaikh, 1999). Hops-derived flavonoids have also demonstrated in vitro antiproliferative and cytotoxic actions on colon and ovarian cancer cells (Miranda et al., 1999).

Reported uses
As with many herbal remedies, hops have a traditional reputation as a cure for many ailments. Historically, hops have been promoted as an anodyne, an antispasmodic, a nervine, a sedative, a soporific, a stomachic, and a vermifuge, among numerous other uses. The lay literature promotes the use of hops as an antidepressant and a sedative-hypnotic and for treating menopausal symptoms. The support of hops in this regard is primarily anecdotal. Based on more recent findings, hops is being proposed as a potential prevention and treatment for various cancers and as a symptomatic treatment for postmenopausal women (Humfrey, 1998).

Dosage
No dose specific for hops is available. Because hops are generally taken either in combination with other herbals or as a tea, the determination of a specific dose has not been accomplished. Based on combination products, the approximate dose of hops appears to be 2 to 4 mg of extract P.O.

Bold italic type indicates that reaction may be life-threatening.

Adverse reactions
CNS: decreased cognitive performance, sedation.
GI: indigestion, vomiting.
GU: menstrual irregularities.
Respiratory: bronchial irritation, bronchitis.
Skin: vesicular dermatitis.
Other: *allergic reactions, anaphylaxis.*

Interactions
Drugs metabolized by the cytochrome P-450 system: Subtherapeutic levels of these drugs because of the hepatic microsomal effects of hops. Monitor the patient closely.
Other CNS depressants (antihistaminics, anticholinergics, anxiolytics, antidepressants, antipsychotics, and alcohol): Additive effects. Patients taking these drugs should use caution when considering the use of hops.
Phenothiazine-type antipsychotics: Increased risk of hyperthermia. Patients taking these drugs should not use hops.

Contraindications and precautions
Given their estrogenic effects, hops are contraindicated in patients with estrogen-dependent tumors, such as breast, uterine, and cervical cancers. Use extreme caution in patients taking antipsychotics because of the risk of hyperthermia. Also use hops cautiously in patients who are taking CNS depressants.

Special considerations
• Advise the patient to consult a health care provider before using herbal preparations because a treatment that has been clinically researched and proved effective may be available.
• Hops loses their original activity when stored (only 15% remains after 9 months).
• Caution the patient to avoid hazardous activities until the CNS effects of hops are known.

Points of interest
• Hops are used in the commercial preparation of beer because of their bitter taste and preservative action.

Commentary
Other than their use in beers, hops have a long history of use as a sedative-hypnotic. This particular use has occurred over the centuries, and assuming no preexisting conditions or drug therapy that would contravene their use, they are probably safe when taken infrequently for occasional insomnia. Two studies indicated alterations in EEG results of human patients (Vonderheid-Guth et al., 2000) consistent with the sedative-calmative actions and efficacy of benzodiazepines (Schmitz and Jackel, 1998). In both of these studies, hops were given in combination with valerian. Therefore, the results cannot be positively correlated with hops alone. Despite their estrogenic activity, their touted use in menopause is less well founded. Given the complex scheme of

hormonal and physiologic changes that occur during this life phase, their use should probably be discouraged. Their traditional use as a vermifuge has been verified by the isolation of avermectin (a veterinary anthelmintic used in small animals). Surprisingly, herbalists have not emphasized this or the antibacterial, anti-inflammatory, or antitumorigenic effects of hops, even though laboratory data support these uses. As with many herbal preparations, the lack of specific dose and adverse effect–toxicity profiles is alarming. Hops may provide a source for many new pharmacologically active agents, but in-depth research is needed to isolate, quantify, and characterize the specific, potentially beneficial effects of hops.

References

Chappel, C.I., et al. "Subchronic Toxicity Study of Tetrahydroisohumulone and Hexahydroisohumulone in the Beagle Dog," *Food Chem Toxicol* 36(11):915-22, 1998.

Dixon-Shanies, D. and Shaikh, N. "Growth Inhibition of Human Breast Cancer Cells by Herbs and Phytoestrogens," *Oncol Rep* 6(6):1383-87, 1999.

Duncan, K.L., et al. "Malignant Hyperthermia-like Reaction Secondary to Ingestion of Hops in Five Dogs," *J Am Vet Med Assoc* 210(1):51-54, 1997.

Gerhard, U., et al. "Vigilance-decreasing Effects of 2 Plant-derived Sedatives," *Schweiz Rundsch Med Prax* 85(15):473-81, 1996.

Godnic-Cvar, J., et al. "Respiratory and Immunological Findings in Brewery Workers," *Am J Ind Med* 35(1):68-75, 1999.

Henderson, M.C., et al. "*In Vitro* Inhibition of Human P450 Enzymes by Prenylated Flavonoids from Hops, *Humulus lupulus*," *Xenobiotic* 30(3):235-51, 2000.

Humfrey, C.D. "Phytoestrogens and Human Health Effects: Weighing up the Current Evidence," *Natl Toxins* 6(2):51-59, 1998.

Mannering, G.J., and Shoeman, J.A. "Murine Cytochrome P4503A Is Induced by 2-Methyl-3-buten-2-ol, 3 Methyl-1-pentyn-3-ol(meparfynol), and Tert-amyl Alcohol," *Xenobiotica* 26(5):487-93, 1996.

Meznar, B., and Kajba, S. "Bronchial Responsiveness in Hops Processing Workers," *Plucne Bolesti* 42(1-2):27-29, 1990.

Milligan, S.R., et al. "Identification of a Potent Phytoestrogen in Hops (*Humulus lupulus* L.) and Beer," *J Clin Endocrinol Metab* 84(6):2249-52, 1999.

Miranda, C.L., et al. "Antiproliferative and Cytotoxic Effects of Prenylated Flavonoids from Hops (*Humulus lupulus*) in Human Cancer Cell Lines," *Food Chem Toxicol* 37(4):271-85, 1999.

Miranda, C.L., et al. "Prenylated Chalcones and Flavanones as Inducers of Quinone Reductase in Mouse Hepa 1c1c7 Cells," *Cancer Lett* 149(1-2):21-29, 2000.

Schmitz, M., and Jackel, M. "Comparative Study for Assessing Quality of Life of Patients with Exogenous Sleep Disorders (Temporary Sleep Onset and Sleep Interruption Disorders) Treated with a Hops-Valerian Preparation and a Benzodiazepine Drug," *Wien Med Wochenschr* 148(13):291-98, 1998.

Stevens, J.F., et al. "Prenylflavonoid Variation in *Humulus lupulus*: Distribution and Taxonomic Significance of Xanthogalenol and 4'-*O*-Methylxanthohumol," *Phytochemistry* 53(7):759-75, 2000.

Stricker, W.E., et al. "Food Skin Testing in Patients with Idiopathic Anaphylaxis," *J Allergy Clin Immunol* 77(3):516-19, 1986.

Tyler, V.E., et al. "Herbs and Health Foods," in *Pharmacognosy,* 8th ed. Philadelphia: Lea & Febiger, 1981.

Vonderheid-Guth, B., et al. "Pharmacodynamic Effects of Valerian and Hops Extract Combination (Ze 91019) on the Quantitative-Topographical EEG in Healthy Volunteers," *Eur J Med Res* 5(4):139-44, 2000.

Wohlfart, R., et al. "The Sedative-Hypnotic Action of Hops: Part 4. Pharmacology of the Hop Substance 2-Methyl-3-buten-2-ol," *Planta Med* 48(2):120-23, 1983.

Yasukawa, K., et al. "Humulon, a Bitter in the Hop, Inhibits Tumor Promotion by 12-*O*-Tetradecanoylphorbol-13-acetate in Two-stage Carcinogenesis in Mouse Skin," *Oncology* 52(2):156-58, 1995.

Zava, D.T., et al. "Estrogen and Progestin Bioactivity of Foods, Herbs, and Spices," *Proc Soc Exp Biol Med* 217(3):369-78, 1998.

HOREHOUND

COMMON HOREHOUND, HOARHOUND, MARRUBIUM, MARVEL, WHITE HOREHOUND

Taxonomic class
Lamiaceae

Common trade names
Alvita Teas Horehound Herb, Herbs for Kids Horehound Blend, Horehound Herb, Hore Hound Tea, Nature's Answer Horehound Herb Low Alcohol

Common forms
Available as capsules of fluidextract (300 mg), confectionaries, lozenges, powder, syrup, and tea.

Source
The extracts are derived mostly from fresh or dried leaves and the flowering tops of *Marrubium vulgare*. This plant, although native to Europe and Asia, has been naturalized to the United States and parts of North America.

Chemical components
The volatile oil marrubiin (a diterpene lactone) is the main bitter component of *M. vulgare;* extracted concentrations range from 0.3% to 1%. Horehound also contains diterpene alcohols, betonicine, tannins, volatile oils, beta-sitosterol (sterol), several flavonoids, waxes, ursolic acid, bitter glycosides, and various sesquiterpene moieties, mucilaginous and resinous substances, and marrubina.

Actions
Horehound is claimed to exert a laxative effect in large doses and a proarrhythmic effect when given in very large doses. In vitro studies with aqueous extracts of horehound have suggested that this herbal extract may antagonize the effects of serotonin (Cahen, 1970). Rabbit studies suggest that the extract can exert a hypoglycemic effect (Roman et al., 1992). Derivatives of marrubiin, but not marrubiin itself, may have minor transient effects on bile secretion.

Reported uses

Anecdotal reports and testimonials claim that horehound is useful as a diaphoretic, a digestive aid, a diuretic, and an expectorant and for intestinal parasites. Despite its bitter flavor, the herb occurs in several different candies and cough lozenges. The throat-soothing and expectorant properties of horehound have long been popularized by herbalists. No human, controlled clinical trials confirm these therapeutic claims.

Dosage

For coughs and throat ailments, 10 to 40 gtt of extract P.O. in warm water up to t.i.d.; 1 to 2 g of powder or by infusion P.O. t.i.d.; or lozenges P.O. as needed.

Adverse reactions

CV: *arrhythmias.*
GI: diarrhea.
Metabolic: hypoglycemia.
Other: spontaneous abortion.

Interactions

Drugs that enhance or antagonize serotonin release, such as antiarrhythmics, some antidepressants, antiemetics (granisetron, ondansetron), antimigraine drugs (ergot alkaloids, sumatriptan): May enhance serotonergic effects. Avoid administration with horehound.
Drugs used to lower blood glucose levels (oral antidiabetic drugs, insulin): May increase hypoglycemic effect of these drugs. Avoid administration with horehound.

Contraindications and precautions

Horehound is contraindicated in pregnant or breast-feeding patients and in those with diabetes mellitus or arrhythmias.

Special considerations

• Monitor blood glucose levels of diabetic patients.
• Monitor cardiac rate and rhythm.
• Inquire about the patient's use of horehound, and inform him that little information exists regarding its safety and efficacy.
• Urge women to report planned or suspected pregnancy.
• Inform the diabetic patient that the use of horehound may necessitate dose reductions in insulin or oral antidiabetic drugs.

Points of interest

• Although white horehound is listed by the Council of Europe as a natural source of food flavoring, its category (N2) permits only small quantities to be added to foodstuffs such as liqueurs, candy, and cough drops.
• Sometimes black horehound (*Ballota nigra*) can be found in compounds that reportedly contain only white horehound (*M. vulgare*).

Bold italic type indicates that reaction may be life-threatening.

Commentary

Although horehound has a long history of use as a cough remedy and a flavoring agent, evidence to promote its use for any other indication is lacking. Large doses of horehound should be avoided because it can adversely affect cardiac rhythms and blood glucose levels.

References

Cahen, R. "Pharmacological Spectrum of *Marrubium vulgare*," *CR Soc Biol* 164:1467, 1970.
Roman, R.R., et al. "Hypoglycemic Effect of Plants Used in Mexico as Antidiabetics," *Arch Med Res* 23:59, 1992.

HORSE CHESTNUT

AESCIN, CHESTNUT, ESCINE

Taxonomic class
Hippocastanaceae

Common trade names
Horse Chestnut Extract, Horse Chestnut Power, Horse Chestnut SFSE, Venostasin Retard, Venostat

Common forms
Capsules: 250 mg, 300 mg
   Also available as extract using aescin to standardize concentration.

Source
The seeds from *Aesculus hippocastanum* are used to formulate horse chestnut extract—sometimes known as *Hippocastani semen*. The bark of young branches should be used; the older bark is poisonous.

Chemical components
Horse chestnut is composed primarily of triterpene glycosides and flavonoids (quercetin, kaempferol, astragalin, isoquercetin, rutin), coumarins (aesculetin, fraxin, scopolin), allantoin, amino acids, choline, citric acid, and phytosterol. Products are adjusted to contain triterpene glycosides calculated as aescin (escin).

Actions
Anti-inflammatory actions have been documented for the saponins (aescin). Aescin reduces transcapillary filtration of water and protein and increases venous tone related to increased prostaglandin F_2 alpha (vasoconstrictor). Murine studies have demonstrated a reduction in vascular permeability from artificial insults (that is, acetic acid or histamine) after pretreatment with components of horse chestnut (escins, desaacylescins) (Matsuda et al., 1997). Aescin stabilizes cholesterol-containing membranes of lysosomes and limits the release of the enzymes. Usually, the release of the enzymes is increased in chronic pathological conditions of the vein. These enzymes normally break down the mucopolysaccharides in the cell membranes in the capillary walls,

but this action is inhibited by aescin (Bombardelli et al., 1996). Aescin has shown notable antiviral activity in vitro toward a strain of influenza virus.

Reported uses

Horse chestnut therapy has been claimed to be effective for treating diarrhea, fever, hemorrhoids, phlebitis, and enlargement of the prostate gland. Some data exist to support a role in venous insufficiency. (See *Horse chestnut and venous insufficiency.*)

Data also suggest a role for horse chestnut in treating varicose veins. Certain enzymes responsible for the metabolism of substances that regulate capillary rigidity and pore size were found to be reduced in patients with varicose veins treated with 900 mg of horse chestnut extract. Concentrations of these enzymes have been found to be elevated in patients with varicose veins and may play a role in this disorder (Kreysel et al., 1983).

Dosage

Dosages of 100 to 150 mg/day P.O. of the aescin component, given as a single dose or in divided doses b.i.d., have been clinically tested in humans.

Adverse reactions

CV: shock.
GI: *hepatotoxicity,* nausea (with oral use), vomiting.
GU: nephropathy.
Hematologic: severe bleeding and bruising (caused by antithrombotic activity of aesculin).
Musculoskeletal: muscle spasm.
Skin: hypersensitivity reactions, pruritus, urticaria.

Interactions

Anticoagulants, aspirin: Increased risk of bleeding because of aesculin, a hydroxycoumarin. Monitor the patient.

Contraindications and precautions

Horse chestnut is contraindicated in pregnant or breast-feeding patients; effects are unknown. Use cautiously in patients who are hypersensitive to other members of the horse chestnut family and in those with bleeding disorders.

Special considerations

• The fruit, leaves, and older bark of horse chestnut are poisonous.
• Monitor liver function test results.
• Inform the patient and health care staff that horse chestnut may color urine red.
• Instruct the patient to report fatigue, fever, unusual bleeding or bruising, and yellowing of skin or eyes.
• Advise the patient to only use products derived from the seeds or bark of young branches.

Bold italic type indicates that reaction may be life-threatening.

RESEARCH FINDINGS
Horse chestnut and venous insufficiency

Animal studies have suggested that some components (escins, desacylescins) of horse chestnut prevent vascular permeability from artificially induced causes (such as histamine or acetic acid) in murine models. This information has led to experiments in humans with chronic venous insufficiency. In one such trial, aescin, 50 mg twice daily, was shown to be equivalent to compression stocking therapy in reducing lower-leg edema in a 12-week, partially blind, placebo-controlled, parallel study of 240 patients (Diehm et al., 1996). A second study evaluated 51 postmenopausal women who received 100 mg of aescin daily compared with 1,000 mg of oxerutin daily for 4 weeks (51 patients) and then 500 mg daily for 12 weeks (35 patients). Both groups demonstrated a mean leg volume reduction of about 100 ml, similar to that reported with compression therapy (Rehn et al., 1996). A smaller study of 20 patients given placebo or 150 mg of aescin daily for 6 weeks found that leg volume was significantly reduced in the treatment group and then increased when the drug was withdrawn. Subjective symptoms of heaviness, leg fatigue, paresthesia, and tenseness improved (Diehm et al., 1992).

Most placebo-controlled trial data suggest that horse chestnut or some of its valuable components should be considered potential options for treating chronic venous insufficiency (Pittler and Ernst, 1998). The use of horse chestnut extract has been associated with significant reductions in lower-leg volume and leg circumference, leg pain and pruritus, and leg fatigue and tenseness.

• Advise the patient to report changes in effectiveness of other drug therapies.
• Urge the patient to check with his health care provider before taking other prescription or OTC drugs that may contain aspirin.

Points of interest
• Germany's Federal Institute for Drugs and Medical Devices recognizes horse chestnut extract as effective in treating chronic venous insufficiency.
• Do not confuse horse chestnut with buckeye, also called horse chestnut.
• Horse chestnut has been used I.V. in Europe for postoperative edema, presumably for its diuretic activity.

Commentary
Compression stocking therapy has been the primary treatment option for chronic venous insufficiency, although patient compliance is generally poor. No allopathic drugs are indicated for treating this disorder.

Standardized horse chestnut extracts or certain components (escins) have intriguing properties and may be useful in patients with symptoms associated with this disorder. Future studies should pursue this potential application. Of note, some data from previous controlled trials have examined parameters that might be considered subjective, such as fatigue, leg pain, pruritus, and tenseness. Additional large, randomized, double-blind, placebo-controlled trials that examine both efficacy and safety in a more objective manner are needed before horse chestnut or any of its components are given a definitive role in therapy.

References

Bombardelli, E., et al. "Review: *Aesculus hippocastanum* L," *Fitoterapia* 67:483-511, 1996.

Diehm, C., et al. "Medical Edema Protection—Clinical Benefits in Patients with Deep Vein Incompetence. A Placebo-controlled, Double-blind Study," *Vasa* 21:188-92, 1992.

Diehm, C., et al. "Comparison of Leg Compression Stocking and Oral Horse Chestnut Seed Extract in Patients with Chronic Venous Insufficiency," *Lancet* 347:292-94, 1996.

Kreysel, H.W., et al. "A Possible Role of Lysosomal Enzymes in the Pathogenesis of Varicosis and the Reduction in Their Serum Activity by Venostatin," *Vasa* 12:377-82, 1983.

Matsuda, H., et al. "Effects of Escins Ia, Ib, IIa and IIb from Horsechestnut, the Seeds of *Aesculus hippocastanum* L., on Acute Inflammation in Animals," *Biol Pharm Bull* 20(10):1092-95, 1997.

Pittler, M.H., and Ernst, E. "Horse-chestnut Seed Extract for Chronic Venous Insufficiency. A Criteria-based Systematic Review," *Arch Dermatol* 134(11):1356-60, 1998.

Rehn, D., et al. "Comparative Clinical Efficacy and Tolerability of Oxerutins and Horse Chestnut Extract in Patients with Chronic Venous Insufficiency," *Arzneimittelforschung* 5:483-87, 1996.

HORSERADISH

PEPPERROT

Taxonomic class
Brassicaceae

Common trade names
None known.

Common forms
Available as fresh root, powder, or semisolid paste for use as a condiment or spice.

Source
The root of *Armoracia rusticana,* a large, leafy perennial, is used to make commercial condiments.

Chemical components
Horseradish contains coumarins (aesculetin, scopoletin, caffeic and hydroxycinnamic acids), ascorbic acid, asparagin, peroxidase enzymes, resin, starch, and sugars. The leaf contains quercetin and kaempferol. The volatile oil contains glucosinolates (mustard oil glycosides), gluconasturtiin, and sinigrin. Isothiocyanate and other compounds are found in the root.

Actions
Horseradish has been used to relieve pain and expel afterbirth and as an anthelmintic and a diuretic; other claims include antiseptic, circulatory, and digestive stimulant properties. I.V. horseradish peroxidase has caused hypotension in cats (Sjaastad et al., 1984), and the extract has shown anticholinesterase activity (Leiner, 1980).

Reported uses
Horseradish is claimed to be useful for edematous states, certain infections, and inflamed joints.

Dosage
For all uses, 2 to 4 g of fresh root P.O. before meals.

Adverse reactions
GI: bloody diarrhea, vomiting (with large quantities).
Other: *hypersensitivity reactions*, severe mucous membrane irritation.

Interactions
Anticholinergics (atropine): May antagonize effects of the herb. Atropine may be useful in cases of excessive horseradish ingestion.
Cholinergic agents (bethanecol, neostigmine, pyridostigmine): May increase parasympathetic effects of these drugs. Monitor the patient.

Contraindications and precautions
The volatile oil of horseradish is contraindicated for any use. Avoid using horseradish in pregnant or breast-feeding patients; effects are unknown. Use cautiously in patients with thyroid disease.

Special considerations
• Inform the patient that this plant is poisonous; symptoms in animals include gastritis, excitation progressing to collapse, and hyperstimulation.
• Caution the patient not to grow wild horseradish because it can be confused with pokeweed root, which is considered toxic.
• Monitor the patient for adverse reactions.
• Urge the patient not to self-treat symptoms of edema, infection, or inflammation before seeking appropriate medical evaluation because this may delay diagnosis of a serious medical condition.

Points of interest
• The FDA considers horseradish to be generally safe. It is typically used in small quantities as a food flavoring.

- Horseradish is a common source of peroxidase enzymes.
- Allylisothiocyanate and butylthiocyanate combine with other compounds within the plant when it is destroyed or crushed to produce the characteristic pungent odor.
- Horseradish perioxidase has been used in some chemical tests for blood glucose (Jamnicky et al., 1988) and as a molecular probe in joint disorders (Shiozawa et al., 1983).
- The herb has been used as a taste repellent by mixing it with toxic substances to prevent accidental poisoning of domesticated animals.

Commentary
There is little clinical evidence to support the use of horseradish for any medicinal purposes. Consumption should be limited to quantities normally found in food and food flavorings until more is known about its action and adverse reactions.

References
Jamnicky, B., et al. "Application of Horseradish Peroxidase to Glucose Determination in Body Fluids," *Acta Pharm Jugo* 38:53, 1988.

Leiner, I.E. *Toxic Constituents of Plant Foodstuffs.* New York: Academic Press, 1980.

Shiozawa, S., et al. "Presence of HLA-DR Antigen on Synovial Type A and B Cells: An Immunoelectron Microscopic Study in Rheumatoid Arthritis, Osteoarthritis and Normal Traumatic Joints," *Immunology* 50:587, 1983.

Sjaastad, O.V., et al. "Hypotensive Effects in Cats Caused by Horseradish Peroxidase Mediated by Metabolites of Arachidonic Acid," *J Histochem Cytochem* 32:1328-30, 1984.

HORSETAIL

BOTTLE-BRUSH, DUTCH RUSHES, PADDOCK-PIPES, PEWTER-WORT, SCOURING RUSH, SHAVE GRASS

Taxonomic class
Equisetaceae

Common trade names
Goldenrod-Horsetail Compound (blend of liquid extracts containing 22.5% goldenrod flowering tips, 22.5% corn silk, 22.5% horsetail, 22.5% pipsissewa leaf, and 10% juniper berry), Horsetail Grass, Horsetail Grass Low Alcohol and Alcohol Free

Common forms
Capsules: 354 mg, 440 mg
   Also available as a liquid extract.

Source
Horsetail is obtained from the aerial stems of *Equisetum arvense* and other *Equisetum* species.

Chemical components

Horsetail contains silica and silicic acids, equisetonin (a saponin), flavone glycosides (isoquercitrin, equisetrin, and galuteolin), sterols (beta-sitosterol, campestrol, isofucosterol and cholesterol), trace amounts of alkaloids (nicotine, palustrine and palustrinine), thiaminase, aconitic acid, and dimethylsulfone.

Actions

The plant has a weak diuretic activity, probably because of equisetonin and the flavone glycosides. *E. hyemale* is a more potent diuretic. The herb may act similarly to hydrochlorothiazide; both increase sodium and potassium excretion and increase urinary pH (Hamon and Awang, 1992). Because *Equisetum* species contain monosilicic acid, which may be a ready source of silicon, horsetail may be useful in strengthening broken bones, connective tissue, and nails.

Reported uses

Horsetail has been used to treat several cancers, edema, fever, gonorrhea, gout, and rheumatism. It has also been used as a diuretic, a styptic, a tissue-strengthening agent in tuberculosis, and a urinary tonic. Horsetail ash has been used for dyspepsia. It is also used as a silicon supplement for healing broken bones and strengthening connective tissue, teeth, hair, and nails.

Dosage

For acute use, 20 to 40 gtt in water P.O. three to five times daily.
For chronic use, 20 to 40 gtt in water P.O. b.i.d. or t.i.d.

Adverse reactions

CNS: ataxia, fever.
CV: *arrhythmias.*
Metabolic: weight loss.
Musculoskeletal: muscle weakness.
Skin: seborrheic dermatitis.
Other: *hypersensitivity reactions.*

Interactions

CNS stimulants: Additive effect caused by nicotine content of herb. Use cautiously in patients using nicotine replacement aids for smoking cessation.
Diuretics: Potentiated effect. Avoid administration with horsetail.

Contraindications and precautions

Avoid using horsetail in pregnant or breast-feeding women; effects are unknown. Also avoid using large amounts of horsetail because nicotine toxicity can occur (abnormal heart rate, ataxia, cold extremities, fever, muscle weakness, weight loss).

Special considerations
• Urge the patient not to self-treat symptoms of illness before seeking appropriate medical evaluation because this may delay diagnosis of a serious medical condition.
• Inform the patient that horsetail contains nicotine.
• Advise the patient to keep horsetail out of the reach of children and pets.
• Advise pregnant or breast-feeding patients to avoid using horsetail.

Points of interest
• The FDA has classified horsetail as an herb of undefined safety.
• Cases have been reported of children being poisoned by using the stems as whistles or blowguns.
• Horsetail contains the toxin thiaminase, which inactivates thiamine and causes thiamine deficiency. Irreversible CNS damage can occur in severe thiamine deficiency. In Canada, manufacturers have to prove that their horsetail products are thiaminase-free.

Commentary
Horsetail exerts a weak diuretic activity. Because of its potential toxicity and the availability of safer and more effective diuretics, the use of horsetail as a diuretic should be avoided. Horsetail is also marketed as a urinary tonic and a silicon supplement to strengthen hair, bone, nails, and connective tissue, but no clinical data support these claims.

References
Hamon, N.W., and Awang, D.V.C. "Horsetail," *Can Pharm J* 125:399-401, 1992.

HYSSOP

Taxonomic class
Lamiaceae

Common trade names
Hyssop Herb, Hyssop Low Alcohol and Alcohol Free, Hyssop Organic, ViBlend (Echinacea/Hyssop for Kids) Liquid

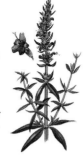

Common forms
Available as fluidextracts, oils, and tinctures. Fresh or dried flowering tops are used to prepare compresses or tea. Narcissus oil is used in fragrances. Narcissus pseudonarcissus lectin (also called narcissus pseudonarcissus agglutinin) is used in biochemistry.

Source
The plant belongs to *Hyssopus officinalis* of the Lamiaceae family.

Chemical components

Hyssop contains terpenoids (including marrubiin, oleanolic, and ursolic acids), a volatile oil (camphor, pinocamphone, thujone, isopinocamphone, with alpha- and beta-pinene, camphene, alpha-terpinene, linalool, bornylacetate, and others), flavonoids (including diosmin and hesperidiin), hyssopin (a glucoside), tannins, and resin.

Actions

Hyssop is reported to have anti-inflammatory, antiflatulent, antiseptic, antispasmodic, diaphoretic, expectorant, hepatic, sedative, and stimulant activities. It has been claimed to promote menstrual flow and to serve as a muscle relaxant. Crude extracts have been shown to inhibit HIV replication in vitro (Kaplan et al., 1990). A previously unidentified polysaccharide (MAR-10) isolated from aqueous extracts of *H. officinalis* has been shown to inhibit HIV-1 replication in vitro with no significant direct toxicity on lymphocyte functions or T-cell counts (Gollapudi et al., 1995).

Reported uses

Hyssop tea has been used for absence seizures, anxiety, asthma, bronchitis, colds, coughs, flatulence, hysteria, and indigestion. Hyssop preparations, especially the volatile oils, have been used externally for burns, cold sores, genital herpes sores, skin irritations, and wounds. Hyssop has been used with white horehound and colt's foot for bronchitis and coughs; with boneset, elder flower, and peppermint for colds; and with sage as a gargle for sore throats.

Dosage

Tea: Infuse 1 to 2 tsp of dried hyssop in 1 cup of boiling water for 10 to 15 minutes. Drink t.i.d. for cough; gargle t.i.d. for sore throat.
Tincture: 1 to 4 ml P.O. t.i.d.

Adverse reactions

CNS: *seizures* (hyssop's essential oil is known to possess strong convulsant chemicals; Burkhard et al., 1999).
GI: diarrhea, indigestion.

Interactions

None reported.

Contraindications and precautions

Hyssop is contraindicated in pregnant patients and in patients with seizure disorders until effects are known. Use low-strength preparations in elderly patients and in children aged 2 to 12. Avoid use in children under age 2.

Special considerations

• Do not confuse hyssop with giant hyssop, hedge hyssop, prairie hyssop, or wild hyssop.

• Instruct the patient to keep hyssop out of the reach of children and pets.
• Urge women to report planned or suspected pregnancy.
• Advise patients with seizure disorders to reconsider using hyssop because it may adversely affect seizure control.
• Advise the patient to use hyssop under medical supervision if he is taking it longer than 3 consecutive days.

Points of interest
• The volatile oil is an ingredient in many French liqueurs, specifically Chartreuse and Benedictine. Essential oil is also used in perfume.
• Commercial hyssop is not identical to the hyssop mentioned in the Bible; the latter is more commonly identified as *Marjoram* species or the caper plant, *Capparis spinosa*.

Commentary
Little clinical trial information exists for this herb. Hyssop might be generally recognized as safe, but medical supervision is suggested when using it longer than 3 consecutive days. There is no documented evidence that hyssop is effective in its external use in treating burns, wounds, and other infections. Even though hyssop extracts have been shown to inhibit HIV in vitro, there is no evidence for the usefulness of hyssop in treating patients with AIDS.

References
Burkhard, P.R., et al. "Plant-induced Seizures: Reappearance of an Old Problem," *J Neurol* 246(8):667-70, 1999.

Gollapudi, S., et al. "Isolation of a Previously Unidentified Polysaccharide (MAR-10) from *Hyssopus officinalis* That Exhibits Strong Activity Against Human Immunodeficiency Virus Type 1," *Biochem Biophys Res Commun* 210:145-51, 1995.

Kaplan, K.W., et al. "Inhibition of HIV Replication by *Hyssop officinalis* Extracts," *Antiviral Res* 14:323-37, 1990.

IBOGAINE
IBOGA, *TABERNANTHE IBOGA*

Taxonomic class
Apocynaceae

Common trade names
Endabuse

Common forms
Seeds

Source
This product is extracted from the root of the West African shrub *Tabernanthe iboga*.

Chemical components
Indole alkaloids constitute up to 6% of the dried root. The main alkaloid is ibogaine. Many other alkaloids exist in the root, including ibogamine, tabernanthine, ibagamine, iboluteine, desmethoxyiboluteine, hydroxyindoleninibogamine, hydroxyindoleninibogaine, ibochine, iboxygaine, kimvuline, kisantine, gabonine, and voacangine. Tannin has also been reported.

Actions
Ibogaine, the primary indole alkaloid in the root and a cholinesterase inhibitor, is a strong CNS stimulant, increases appetite and digestion, and causes hypotension. Ibogaine is a highly lipid-soluble chemical. Significant investigation into the complex pharmacology of ibogaine and its active metabolite, noribogaine, has shown activity as kappa agonists, N-methyl-D-aspartate antagonists, nicotinic antagonists, serotonin uptake inhibitors, and sigma-2 agonists in rats (Glick and Maisonneuve, 1998).

Reported uses
Historically, ibogaine has been used to reduce cocaine-induced locomotor stimulation in mice, prevent hunger and fatigue, and act as an aphrodisiac and a tonic. Chewing *T. iboga* roots may produce drunkenness, excitement, mental confusion, and, possibly, hallucinations. The product is in development as therapy for drug dependence, including alcohol, amphetamines, cocaine, and opioids. Anecdotally, a single oral dose of 6 to 19 mg/kg of ibogaine interrupts drug-seeking behavior in addicts for up to 6 months (Alburges and Hanson, 1999).

Dosage
No consensus exists.

Adverse reactions
CNS: anxiety, apprehension, drunkenness, hallucinations, mental confusion, ***dose- and species-dependent neurotoxicity.***
CV: hypotension, ***bradycardia.***

Interactions
Anticholinergics: May interfere with activity of these drugs. Monitor the patient.
Cholinergics, cholinesterase inhibitors: Potential for synergic effects of these drugs. Monitor the patient closely.
Reserpine: Documented antagonism of reserpine. Do not use together.

Contraindications and precautions
Avoid using ibogaine in pregnant or breast-feeding patients; safety of this herb has not been established.

Special considerations
• Of the hundreds of hallucinogenic plant species identified, only two plants are classified as DEA Schedule I controlled substances: *Cannabis sativa* and *T. iboga.*
• A number of toxicologists have deemed *T. iboga* dangerous (Duke, 1987).
• Toxic doses may result in paralysis, respiratory arrest, seizures, and death.
• Structurally, ibogaine resembles lysergic acid diethylamide.

Points of interest
• *T. iboga* root bark is ingested in ceremonies by the Bwiti people in Gabon to reconnect participants with their ancestors in the land of the dead beyond the sea.
• During the 1960s, ibogaine was used in underground cultures in the United States as a psychedelic.

Commentary
Considerable information is available regarding the activity of ibogaine in animals. Its use is legally prohibited in the United States because of its health dangers and potential for abuse. The use of ibogaine cannot be recommended.

References
Alburges, M.E., and Hanson, G.R. "Differential Responses by Neurotensin Systems in Extrapyramidal and Limbic Structures to Ibogaine and Cocaine," *Brain Research* 818:96-104, 1999.
Duke, J.A. *CRC Handbook of Medicinal Herbs.* Boca Raton, Fla.: CRC Press, 1987.
Glick, S.D., and Maisonneuve, I.M. "Mechanisms of Antiaddictive Actions of Ibogaine," *Ann NY Acad Sci* 844:214-26, 1998.

Bold italic type indicates that reaction may be life-threatening.

ICELAND MOSS

CETRARIA, CONSUMPTION MOSS, ICELAND LICHEN, *LICHEN ISLANDICUS*

Taxonomic class
Parmeliaceae

Common trade names
Iceland Moss, Juvinol Cell and Tissue Formula

Common forms
Available as capsules, creams, and throat lozenges.

Source
Cetraria islandica, a lichen that grows in the Northern hemisphere, is common in the mountains and heathlands of Iceland. The single-cell green algae are enclosed in a web of fungal hyphae (root filaments). The lichen may be gathered throughout the year, but it seems to be most abundant between May and September. It should be freed from attached impurities and dried in the sun or shade. The entire plant, or lichen, is used for extraction.

Chemical components
C. islandica is bitter and mucilaginous. Constituents include about 50% water-soluble polysaccharides, including lichenin, a linear cellulose-like polymer of beta-D-glucose, and isolichenin, a linear starchlike polymer of alpha-D-glucose. Iceland moss also comprises galactomannans; an acidic, branched polysaccharide containing D-glucose and D-glucuronic acid units; and trace amounts of iron and calcium salts. Other constituents are bitter-tasting lichen acids, including the depsidones fumarprotocetraric acid and protolichesterinic acid (ESCOP, 1997). Iceland moss has a high fiber content.

Actions
Protolichesterinic acid from Iceland moss was found to have antibacterial properties against *Mycobacterium tuberculosis, Streptococcus pyogenes,* and *Staphylococcus aureus.* It has also exhibited antitumorigenic activity against solid-type carcinoma in mice and been potent in vitro in inhibiting activity against the DNA polymerase activity of HIV type 1 reverse transcriptase (Ingolfsdottir et al., 1997). Protolichesterinic acid was shown to be antiproliferative and cytotoxic to T-47D and ZR-75-1 cell lines cultured from breast carcinomas and to K-562 from erythroleukemia. Significant inhibition of 5-lipoxygenase may stimulate these activities and contribute to protolichesterinic acid's reported anti-inflammatory actions (Ogmundsdottir et al., 1998).

Because of their antibacterial properties, the extracts have been studied for use in pharmaceutical and cosmetic products. The lichen extracts appear to be safe for use as preservatives without interfering with proprietary ingredients (Ingolfsdottir et al., 1985).

Extracts of Iceland moss were found to suppress the growth of *Helicobacter pylori*, the organism thought to contribute to the cause of gastritis and gastric and duodenal ulcers (Ingolfsdottir et al., 1997).

Reported uses

C. islandica has been used in European medicine to treat asthma, GI disorders such as gastritis, minor ailments (such as throat irritation and cough), and tuberculosis. Cough drops for sore throats and laxative and tonic formulations are available in European pharmacies. In a randomized trial, Iceland moss was found to prevent dryness and inflammation of the oral cavity in patients who had undergone surgery of the nasal septum and were subjected to prolonged mouth breathing after surgery. Emollient effects were noticeable with daily use of 0.48 mg of Iceland moss lozenges (Kempe et al., 1997).

The polysaccharides are thought to form a soothing, protective, mucilaginous layer on upper respiratory tract mucosa. In an open clinical trial, 100 patients with bronchial ailments, laryngitis, or pharyngitis were treated with lozenges containing 160 mg of an aqueous extract of Iceland moss. The results were determined to be positive in 86 cases, with good gastric tolerance and lack of adverse effects (ESCOP, 1997).

In Iceland, the plant has also been used for symptomatic relief of gastric and duodenal ulcers (Ingolfsdottir et al., 1997). Studies of the antitumorigenic and immunostimulating properties of the polysaccharides found comparable carbon clearance assay results as those for the fungal polysaccharide lentinan, which is used clinically in adjuvant cancer therapy in Japan (Ingolfsdottir et al., 1994).

Dosage

A decoction can be made by mixing 1 tsp of shredded moss in 1 cup of cold water, which should then be boiled for 3 minutes and taken P.O. b.i.d. Alternatively, 1 to 2 ml of the tincture can be taken P.O. t.i.d.

Of significance, powdered material must be soaked in lye for 24 hours or filtered through ash to properly extricate lichen acids. Studies demonstrate that poorly prepared Iceland moss may contain toxic levels of lead (Airaksinen et al., 1986).

Cough drops and laxative and tonic formulations are also available.

Adverse reactions

GI (with large doses or prolonged use): ***hepatotoxicity,*** indigestion, nausea.

Interactions

None reported.

Contraindications and precautions

Avoid using Iceland moss in pregnant or breast-feeding patients; effects are unknown. The bitterness of *Cetraria* is detectable in breast milk.

Bold italic type indicates that reaction may be life-threatening.

Special considerations
● Inform the patient that Iceland moss cannot be recommended for any use because of insufficient data.
● Advise the patient to watch for signs of toxicity (abdominal pain; bleeding; change in color of urine, stool, or skin; diarrhea; nausea; vomiting).
● Advise the patient to consult a health care provider before using herbal preparations because a treatment that has been clinically researched and proved effective may be available.

Points of interest
● Iceland moss has been exported from Iceland and is used abroad to manufacture herbal medicines (particularly in Germany). Because Iceland is regarded as one of the least polluted countries in the world, the purity of the plants growing in Iceland is desirable. The wild plants are grown organically; fertilizers are not used in the highlands, where many of these plants are found.
● Lichens lack roots and derive their energy and nutrients from their surroundings. They are susceptible to contamination by radioactivity and heavy metals. After the Chernobyl accident, the fallout contaminated the lichen in most of Europe, but in Iceland the radioactivity level was almost negligible.

Commentary
Iceland moss derivatives show promise as immunomodulating and antitumorigenic agents, and someday they may find a role in the treatment of *H. pylori* infections. Further research in human subjects is needed before any conclusions can be drawn. Definitive applications and clinical efficacy are not known. Although the lichen extracts appear to be relatively safe in small amounts, therapeutic application cannot be recommended.

References
Airaksinen, M.M., et al. "Toxicity of Iceland Lichen and Reindeer Lichen," *Arch Toxicol Suppl* 9:406-9, 1986.

ESCOP. "Lichen islandicus." *Monographs on the Medicinal Uses of Plant Drugs.* Exeter, U.K.: European Scientific Cooperative on Phytotherapy, 1997.

Ingolfsdottir, K., et al. "In Vitro Evaluation of the Antimicrobial Activity of Lichen Metabolites as Potential Preservatives," *Antimicrob Agents Chemother* 28:289-92, 1985.

Ingolfsdottir K., et al. "Immunologically Active Polysaccharide from *Cetraria islandica*," *Planta Med* 60:527-31, 1994.

Ingolfsdottir, K., et al. "In Vitro Susceptibility of *Helicobacter pylori* to Protolichesterinic Acid from the Lichen *Cetraria islandica*," *Antimicrob Agents Chemother* 41:215-17, 1997.

Kempe, C., et al. ("Icelandic Moss Lozenges in the Prevention or Treatment of Oral Mucosa Irritation and Dried Out Throat Mucosa [in German]"), *Laryngorhinootologie* 76(3):186-88, 1997.

McGuffin, M., et al. American Herbal Product Association's *Botanical Safety Handbook.* Boca Raton, Fla.: CRC Press, 1997.

Ogmundsdottir, H., et al. "Antiproliferative Effects of Lichen-derived Inhibitors of 5-Lipoxygenase on Malignant Cell-lines and Mitogen-stimulated Lymphocytes," *J Pharm Pharmacol* 50(1):107-15, 1998.

INDIGO

COMMON INDIGO, INDIAN INDIGO, QINGDAI

Taxonomic class
Fabaceae

Common trade names
None known.

Common forms
Available as a blue powder and as tablets.

Source
Indigo comes from the leaves and branches of a genus of plants called *Indigofera*. There are many *Indigofera* species worldwide, but only a few exist in the United States (such as *I. tinctoria* and *I. suffruticosa*). *I. tinctoria* is the source of natural blue indigo dye, which has been used for hundreds of years.

Chemical components
Leaf fermentation produces blue indigo dye. The dye comes from a glucoside component of several *Indigofera* species called indican, which is synthesized with different ingredients to produce various coloring agents.

Actions
Studies suggest that *I. tinctoria* may protect against hepatic damage induced by carbon tetrachloride, whereas other species may have a hepatotoxic effect. Aqueous decoctions of *I. arrecta* have decreased blood glucose levels in both animals and humans. Studies with *I. arrecta* in mice have demonstrated an increase in plasma insulin levels, and the herb is believed to cause insulin release by stimulating pancreatic beta cells.

Indirubin, a minor component of *I. tinctoria*, has been useful in treating chronic myelocytic leukemia and animal tumors. *I. tinctoria* has been found to significantly increase the survival of rats with cancer (Han, 1994). *I. aspalathoides*, similar to *I. tinctoria*, is believed to have anti-inflammatory activity.

Reported uses
I. arrecta has been reported to treat diabetes; the leaves and plant juice of *I. tinctoria* have been used to treat some cancers (gastric and ovarian). The Chinese have used *Indigofera* as an analgesic, an antipyretic, and an anti-inflammatory, and for purifying the liver. Natural indigo is also used to treat hemorrhoids and scorpion bites and as an emetic. Indigo is used with other plants to treat boils, carbuncles, hemorrhagic

disease, infantile febrile seizures, and mumps. No controlled therapeutic trials support these claims; indigo's use is based on anecdotal reports and traditional folklore.

Dosage
No consensus exists.

Adverse reactions
EENT: eye irritation.
Skin: dermatitis (with dyes).

Interactions
None reported.

Contraindications and precautions
No known contraindications.

Special considerations
• Caution the patient to keep indigo away from the eyes. Instruct him to flush eyes with water if contact occurs.
• Urge women to report planned or suspected pregnancy.
🔔 **ALERT** Indospicine, a component of *I. spicata*, has teratogenic and hepatotoxic properties and has caused cleft palate and embryo death in animals.

Points of interest
• All commercially available natural indigo is prepared synthetically. *I. tinctoria* is believed to be the active ingredient in a well-known, traditional Chinese medicine used for chronic myelocytic leukemia.

Commentary
The many species of the *Indigofera* plant are the common sources of natural blue dye. There is no clinical evidence to substantiate the therapeutic effects of natural indigo, alone or in combination with other ingredients. Because of the lack of clinical trials, this product cannot be recommended.

References
Han, R. "Highlight on the Studies of Anticancer Drugs Derived from Plants in China," *Stem Cells* 12:53-63, 1994.

INOSINE

Common trade names
None known.

Common forms
Available as dietary supplements in capsules and tablets.

Source
Inosine is found in organ meats and brewer's yeast.

Chemical components
A naturally occurring nucleoside, inosine is one of the basic compounds that make up cells.

Actions
Inosine, a precursor to adenosine, is involved in insulin release and protein synthesis and facilitates the use of carbohydrates by the heart.

Reported uses
Inosine has been reported to be ergogenic (energy boosting) by Eastern European athletes and is used to enhance athletic performance. Results of controlled clinical trials have not supported this use and have actually shown that inosine impairs performance (McNaughton et al., 1999; Starling et al., 1996).

Dosage
5,000 to 10,000 mg/day P.O.

Adverse reactions
Metabolic: hyperuricemia (with prolonged use or excessive ingestion).
Musculoskeletal: gout (with prolonged use or excessive ingestion).

Interactions
None reported.

Contraindications and precautions
Avoid using inosine in pregnant or breast-feeding patients; effects are unknown.

Special considerations
• No adverse reactions have been reported when inosine is used for only 2 to 5 days.
• Inform the patient that ingestion of an excessive amount of inosine may lead to gout.
• Advise the patient to consult a health care provider before using herbal preparations because a treatment that has been clinically researched and proved effective may be available.
• Although no known chemical interactions have been reported in clinical studies, consideration must be given to the pharmacologic properties of the herbal product and the potential for exacerbation of the intended therapeutic effect of conventional drugs.

Commentary
Controlled clinical trials do not support the use of inosine as an ergogenic agent but have shown that inosine increases uric acid levels, which can lead to long-term problems, such as gout. Therefore, the use of inosine is not recommended.

References
McNaughton, et al. "Inosine Supplementation Has No Effect on Aerobic or Anaerobic Cycling Performance," *Int J Sport Nutr* 9(4):333-44, 1999.

Bold italic type indicates that reaction may be life-threatening.

Starling, R.D., et al. "Effect of Inosine Supplementation on Cycling Performance,"
   Med Sci Sports Exerc 28(9):1193-98, 1996.

IRISH MOSS

CARRAGEEN, CARRAGEENAN, CHONDRUS, CHONDRUS
EXTRACT, IRISH MOSS EXTRACT

Taxonomic class
Gigartinaceae

Common trade names
Irish moss

Common forms
Used extensively in small quantities as a binder, an emulsifier, or a stabilizer in creams, hand lotions, tablets, and toothpastes. Also found in
some teas.

Source
The name Irish moss usually refers to a seaweed, *Chondrus crispus*, or is
applied to a mixture of *C. crispus* and *Mastocarpus stellatus*. It can be
collected at low tide on the rocky Atlantic coastlines of northwestern
Europe and Canada. Carrageenan, a seaweed gum, is processed from *C.
crispus* to commercial status through several procedures that can involve cleaning, extraction with sodium hydroxide, filtration and drum
rolling, or precipitation with alcohol. Carrageenan gels rapidly degrade
in an acidic environment or when exposed to heat. Degraded carra-
geenans lack the "gelling" or viscous properties.

Chemical components
Irish moss contains a large percentage of mucilage, carrageenan, iodine,
bromine, iron, and vitamins A and B. Carrageenan is a variable mixture
of potassium, sodium, calcium, magnesium, and ammonium sulfate esters of galactose and 3-6 anhydrogalactose copolymers. The major types
of hydrocolloid copolymers are kappa-carrageenan, iota-carrageenan,
and lambda carrageenan. Carrageenan readily dissolves in water to
form various types of gels with a wide range of characteristics, depending on the type of algae used, the manufacturing process, and the desired function.

Actions
Irish moss is reported to have demulcent and emollient properties.
Carrageenan extracted from the seaweed is used in the pharmaceutical
industry as an emulsifying, suspending, and gelling agent. The gelling
fractions are kappa-carrageenan and iota-carrageenan; lambda-
carrageenan does not gel. These hydrocolloid properties also make this
plant useful to the food industry for various types of jellies.
   Carrageenan has exhibited numerous pharmacologic effects in vitro
and in animals, including lowering cholesterol levels, limiting food ab-

sorption, decreasing gastric secretions (osmotically active), and producing cathartic effects and hypotension, as well as anticoagulant and immunosuppressive activities. Carrageenan has demonstrated antiproteolytic activity against pepsin and papain in vitro. Interestingly, carrageenan has been reported to cause GI ulceration in various animals (Anderson and Soman, 1965). (See *Carageenan and Ebimar*.)

When carrageenan is injected into a rodent's paw, it produces a consistent inflammatory response. The carrageenan-induced rat paw edema model is a popular and reliable model for testing potential anti-inflammatory compounds.

Reported uses

The herb's actions as a smooth binder have led to its use as a demulcent in treating ulcers and gastritis. Irish moss has also been reported to be valuable for bronchitis, colds, and other respiratory disorders, such as tuberculosis. There are no human data to verify these claims. It is used by the pharmaceutical industry as an emulsifying agent for such products as liquid petrolatum and cod liver oil.

Carrageenan has also been studied as a carrier for the GI delivery of various drugs. Absorption was enhanced with a carrageenan formulation of doxycycline (Grahnen et al., 1994).

Dosage

No dosages have been established based on controlled clinical trials. Irish moss is available in some countries in tablet form but usually is taken as a decoction.

To prepare the decoction, 1 oz of dried plant is added to 1 to 1½ pt of boiling water, simmered gently, and strained. It may be sweetened with lemon, cinnamon, or honey and taken b.i.d. or t.i.d. in 1-cup doses.

Adverse reactions

CV: hypotension.
GI: abdominal cramps, diarrhea, GI ulceration (in animals).
GU: renal disease (I.V. carrageenan–induced renal lesions in animals).
Hematologic: *bleeding.*
Other: infection.

Interactions

Anticoagulants: Increased risk of bleeding. Avoid administration with Irish moss.
Antihypertensives: May enhance hypotensive effects. Monitor the patient.
Other oral drugs: May impair absorption of these drugs. Avoid concomitant use of significant quantities of carrageenan.

Contraindications and precautions

Irish moss is contraindicated in patients with active peptic ulcer disease or in those with a history of peptic ulcer disease. Avoid using this herb in pregnant or breast-feeding patients; effects are unknown.

RESEARCH FINDINGS
Carageenan and Ebimar

Carageenan is a sulphated polysaccharide that can be extracted from a seaweed, *Chondrus crispus*, also known as Irish moss. Ebimar (Evans et al., 1965) is a pharmaceutical product derived from carageenan, but it has a slightly smaller molecular structure than carageenan. Ebimar's reduced viscosity allows it to be administered to patients more easily than carageenan.

Early studies have suggested that sulphated polysaccharides have antiulcerative effects. These data led to a comparative trial evaluating Ebimar with aluminum hydroxide gel (antacid) tablets in 35 patients with radiologically proven gastric or duodenal ulcers. The patients were randomly treated with either 1,000 mg P.O. three times a day (chewed and swallowed with meals) and 3,000 mg at bedtime of Ebimar, or 700 mg P.O. three times a day (chewed and swallowed with meals) and 2,100 mg at bedtime of aluminum hydroxide gel for the first 3 months, and then crossed over to the alternative treatment every 3 months thereafter. The patients were encouraged to eat dyspepsia-provoking meals and were frequently assessed for pain and discomfort and radiologic evidence of ulcer healing.

Neither treatment was found to be better than the other. Although at 5 months, aluminum hydroxide significantly reduced ulcers ($P<.05$), this effect was not maintained to the trial's end. Complete ulcer healing between the groups was similar. The investigators concluded that either treatment was beneficial but that Ebimar may cause less constipation. Some patients preferred Ebimar over aluminum hydroxide gel therapy because they claimed that the antacid particles accumulated beneath their dentures, making them uncomfortable.

Special considerations
• Monitor blood pressure.
• Monitor for signs of bleeding.
• Instruct the patient to avoid dizziness by rising slowly from a sitting or lying position.
• Urge the patient with a history of peptic ulcer disease to avoid using Irish moss until its safety and efficacy have been established.
• Instruct the patient to watch for signs of bleeding (bleeding gums, easy bruising, epistaxis, tarry stools).
• Inform the patient that carrageenan is considered safe only in small quantities in various foodstuffs and commercial creams and lotions. Consumption of larger quantities has not been adequately evaluated.

Points of interest
• Degraded carrageenan is used in preparations for treating peptic ulcers in France.
• Food-grade carrageenan (molecular weight over 50,000 daltons) is thought to be nontoxic because it is not absorbed.
• Carrageenan is used in milk products (chocolate milk, ice cream, sherbets, cottage cheese, evaporated milk, puddings, yogurts, and infant formulas) and to thicken sauces, gravies, jams, and jellies.
• Carrageenan is included in various herbal drinks, weight-loss products, fruit juices, and aloe vera lotions.

Commentary
Although carrageenan (main derivative of Irish moss) is widely used in the pharmaceutical and food industries, therapeutic claims have not been confirmed in controlled clinical human trials. Further study is warranted before Irish moss or its constituents can be recommended for any medical conditions.

References
Anderson, W., and Soman, P.D. "Degraded Carrageenan and Duodenal Ulceration in the Guinea Pig," *Nature* 3:101-2, 1965.

Evans, P.R.C., et al. "Blind Trial of a Degraded Carrageenan and Aluminum Hydroxide Gel in the Treatment of Peptic Ulceration," *Postgrad Med J* 41:48-52, 1965.

Grahnen, A., et al. "Doxycycline Carrageenate—An Improved Formulation Providing More Reliable Absorption and Plasma Concentrations at High Gastric pH than Doxycycline Monohydrate," *Eur J Clin Pharmacol* 46:143-46, 1994.

JABORANDI TREE

**ARRUDA BRAVA, ARRUDA DO MATO, INDIAN HEMP,
JABORANDI, JAMGUARANDI, JUARANDI, PERNAMBUCO
JABORANDI, *PILOCARPUS JABORANDI***

Taxonomic class
Rutaceae

Common trade names
Multi-ingredient preparations: Jaborandi, Origin Hair and Scalp Therapy, Wonder Gel, X-Tablets

Common forms
The leaves from the jaborandi tree are available as essential oil, fluidextract, a powder, and tincture. Combination products are found as gels and tablets. Pilocarpine, the main active ingredient, is available in many prescription products:
Ocular insert: 20 mcg, 40 mcg
Ophthalmic gel: 4%
Ophthalmic solution: 0.25%, 0.5%, 1%, 2%, 3%, 4%, 5%, 6%, 8%, 10%
Tablets: 5 mg

Source
Pilocarpus, or jaborandi, consists of the leaves of *Pilocarpus jaborandi (Pernambuco jaborandi), Pilocarpus microphyllus* (Maranham jaborandi), or *Pilocarpus pinnatifolius* (Paraguay jaborandi). The plant is native to the northern and northeastern parts of Brazil.

Chemical components
Three alkaloids are found in jaborandi: pilocarpine, pilocarpidine, and isopilocarpine. Also reported are jaborine, pilosine, volatile oils (including dipentene), and jaboric, pilocarpic, and tannic acids.

Actions
When applied topically to the eye, pilocarpine stimulates muscarinic receptors; this causes the pupil to constrict and the ciliary body to contract, thus improving the outflow of aqueous humor. Muscarinic alkaloids, when administered orally, stimulate the smooth muscles of the GI tract, increasing motility and tone. The tone and motility of other organs or organ systems (such as the ureter, bladder, gallbladder, and biliary ducts) may also be increased. Pilocarpine causes increased sweating and salivation in humans. It acts on the CV and respiratory systems as well (decreases blood pressure, heart rate, and vital capacity). In cats, pilocarpine has caused cortical stimulation (Brown and Taylor, 1996).

Jaborine, a component found in the leaves, may actually be antagonistic to pilocarpine. Tannic acid has local astringent properties that act on the GI mucosa and has shown antiulcerative and antisecretory effects within the GI tract.

Reported uses
Although jaborandi has several reported uses, pilocarpine is usually extracted and used to stimulate saliva secretion or as a diaphoretic or myotic (Claus, 1956). Pilocarpine is primarily used to treat glaucoma or xerostomia. Other reported uses of the jaborandi plant include treatment of Bright's disease, deafness, diabetes, edema, intestinal atony, jaundice, nausea, nephritis, pleurisy, psoriasis, rheumatism, syphilis, and tonsillitis. A decoction of the leaf applied locally has been used as a treatment for baldness.

Dosage
For glaucoma, 1 or 2 gtt applied t.i.d. or q.i.d. Refer to package insert for pilocarpine for specific dosing information.
For xerostomia, 15 to 30 mg P.O. daily; a dose of 100 mg P.O. is considered fatal.

The following daily doses have been suggested: powdered leaves, 5 to 60 grains (0.324 to 3.9 g); fluidextract, 10 to 30 gtt; tincture, ½ to 1 dram (1.75 to 3 ml).

Adverse reactions
CNS: headache.
CV: *bradycardia.*
EENT: increased salivation, lacrimation, visual changes.
GI: nausea, vomiting.
Skin: sweating.

Interactions
Anticholinergics (atropine, ipratropium, scopolamine, other belladonna-type alkaloids): May decrease effects of these drugs. Avoid administration with jaborandi.
Beta blockers: May cause conduction problems. Monitor the patient.
Glycosides, iron-containing compounds, other alkaloids: Tannic acid may interact with these drugs. Do not use together.
Other prescription products containing pilocarpine, other muscarinic agonists (arecoline, methacholine, muscarine), cholinesterase inhibitors (donepezil, edrophonium, physostigmine): May have additive effect when used concomitantly. Use cautiously to avoid toxicity.

Contraindications and precautions
Jaborandi is contraindicated in patients who are hypersensitive to pilocarpine and in those with uncontrolled asthma, acute iritis, and angle-closure glaucoma. Avoid use in pregnant or breast-feeding patients. Avoid large doses of jaborandi because hepatic injury can occur, especially in patients with preexisting hepatic disease. Use cautiously in pa-

---

Bold italic type indicates that reaction may be life-threatening.

tients with significant CV disease, biliary tract or urogenital abnormalities (cholelithiasis, nephrolithiasis), and preexisting cognitive or psychiatric disorders.

Special considerations
• Monitor intraocular pressure in patients at risk for glaucoma.
• Monitor liver transaminase levels; if they increase, the product should be discontinued immediately.
• Inform the patient that excessive sweating may lead to dehydration if fluids are not replenished.
🕭 **ALERT** Signs of pilocarpine toxicity include exaggerated muscarinic effects. Extreme cases may lead to severe bronchospasm, hypotension, pulmonary edema, and shock. Treatment consists of atropine administration and general support of the CV and respiratory systems to counteract the effects from pulmonary edema (Brown and Taylor, 1996).
• Urge the patient to immediately report symptoms associated with pilocarpine toxicity (excessive sweating, lacrimation, increased salivation, nausea, vomiting, hypotension, and bradycardia) or hepatic dysfunction (fever, jaundice, and pain in right upper quadrant). Instruct him to discontinue use of the product if they occur.
• Caution the patient that pilocarpine may cause visual changes, especially at night, which may impair his ability to drive.
• Advise the pregnant or breast-feeding patient not to use jaborandi.

Commentary
The jaborandi tree is regarded as a source for pilocarpine. Much information exists about the use of pilocarpine for treating glaucoma and xerostomia. No human studies are available that support the use of jaborandi leaves for any medicinal purpose. Patients with glaucoma, xerostomia, or other potentially treatable conditions should seek medical advice because self-medication with jaborandi is not advised.

References
Brown, J.H., and Taylor, P. "Muscarinic Receptor Agonists and Antagonists," in *Goodman and Gilman's The Pharmacological Basis of Therapeutics,* 9th ed. Edited by Hardman, J.G., and Limbird, L.E. New York: McGraw-Hill Book Co., 1996.
Claus, E.P. *Pharmacognosy,* 3rd ed. Philadelphia: Lea & Febiger, 1956.

JAMAICA DOGWOOD

FISHFUDDLE, FISH POISON TREE, WEST INDIAN DOGWOOD

Taxonomic class
Fabaceae

Common trade names
Jamaican Dogwood Rootbark, Willow-Meadowsweet Compound

Common forms

Available as dried preparations of root or bark, fluidextracts (30% to 60% alcohol), tinctures (45% alcohol), and unprocessed bark strips.

Source

Piscidia erythrina grows naturally in the West Indies and northern parts of South America; it has been transplanted to Mexico, Texas, and Florida.

Chemical components

Jamaica dogwood contains isoflavones (erythbigenin, piscidone, pis-cerythrone, ichthynone, listetin), rotenoids (rotenone, millettone, isomillettone, dehydromillettone, sumatrol), tartaric acid derivatives (piscidic fukiic, 3'*O*-methylfukiic acids), organic acids, beta-sitosterol, and tannins.

Actions

Isoflavone components, derived as fluidextracts from *P. erythrina* and other plant sources, showed spasmolytic activity in mice (Della-Loggia et al., 1988) and anxiolytic to sedative responses, depending on the dose of extract used (Della-Loggia et al., 1981). Anti-inflammatory, anti-pyretic, and antitussive activities have also been seen in animals.

Reported uses

Jamaica dogwood has been claimed to be a calming agent. It has been claimed to be an analgesic for toothache, an antispasmodic for asthma, and a hypnotic for insomnia and to treat migraines, neuralgias, renal or intestinal colic, and whooping cough. The herb also has been used in dysmenorrhea and to help with labor pains. No human trials attesting to the therapeutic benefits of Jamaica dogwood can be found.

Dosage

Doses vary among researchers.

Dried product: 2 to 4 g P.O. daily in divided doses, or 1 tsp in 1 cup of water, simmered for 10 minutes and then taken as a tonic.

Extract: 1 or 2 drams P.O. as a daily dose, starting with 5 to 20 gtt and increased cautiously.

Tincture: 5 to 15 ml P.O. as a daily dose, usually taken 2 to 3 ml at a time.

Doses for analgesic or antispasmodic effect are given three to five times daily; hypnotic doses are given at bedtime.

Adverse reactions

CNS: sedation.

GI: indigestion, nausea.

Interactions

CNS depressants (alcohol, benzodiazepines, narcotic analgesics): Jamaica dogwood may potentiate the effects of these drugs. Avoid concomitant use.

Bold italic type indicates that reaction may be life-threatening.

Contraindications and precautions

Jamaica dogwood is contraindicated in pregnant or breast-feeding patients. Avoid use in patients with CV disease because hypotension and mild myocardial depression may occur.

Special considerations

• Caution the patient who is at risk for hypotension or who has CV disease to avoid using Jamaica dogwood.
• Inform the patient that few, if any, studies have been conducted in humans and that no evidence exists to confirm a therapeutic benefit.
• Symptoms of overdose include increased salivation, sweating, and tremor. I.V. administration has resulted in toxicity in animals; oral administration appears to have a lower potential for toxicity.
• Caution the patient to avoid hazardous activity until CNS effects of the herb are known.
• Inform the patient that some constituents of the plant have shown carcinogenic activity.

Points of interest

• Central and South American fisherman use rotene and ichthynone to stun fish, but these components do not seem to have this effect in mammals.
• Jamaica dogwood is unrelated to the eastern U.S. plant, the common dogwood, *Cornus florida*.
• The European Council has found Jamaica dogwood unsuitable for use as a natural food flavoring.

Commentary

Information on Jamaica dogwood is scarce. Consumption of this plant should be avoided until data regarding its safety are available.

References

Della-Loggia, R. et al. "Evaluation of the Activity on the Mouse CNS of Several Plant Extracts and a Combination of Them," *Riv Neurol* 51:297-310, 1981.
Della-Loggia, R., et al. "Isoflavones as Spasmolytic Principles of *Piscidia erythrina*," *Prog Clin Bio Res* 280:365-68, 1988.

JAMBUL

BLACK PLUM, *EUGENIA CYANOCARPA*, *EUGENIA JAMBOLANA*, JAMBA, JAMBOLAN, JAMBOLÃO, JAMBOOL, JAMBU, JAMBULA, JAMBULON PLUM, JAVA PLUM, *SYZYGIUM JAMBOLANUM*

Taxonomic class

Myrtaceae

Common trade names

Jambul Seed

Common forms
Available as decoctions or a tea made from the seeds or dried leaves.

Source
The drug is extracted from the fruits, seeds, and leaves of *Syzygium cuminii,* a 50' to 80' tree with edible berries that is native to India and Sri Lanka.

Chemical components
The seeds of *S. cuminii* contain gallic acid, ellagic acid, corilagin, 3,6-hexahydroxydiphenoyl-glucose, 3-galloyl glucose, and quercetin.

Actions
Jambul seeds have been claimed to have antihyperglycemic, antihypertensive, and anti-inflammatory effects. In some South American countries, tea made from the leaves is used by diabetics for its antihyperglycemic effects (Teixeria et al., 1990). One study found no effect of jambul seed tea on postprandial blood glucose levels when compared with water in normal rats and rats with streptozotocin-induced diabetes mellitus (Teixeria et al., 1997).

The anti-inflammatory effects of jambul seed extract have been evaluated. Jambul seed extract was found to significantly reduce paw edema, although less effectively than phenylbutazone (Chaudhuri et al., 1990). An extract of jambul seeds was found to have neuropsychopharmacologic effects in mice; the animals became quieter and less active, with less spontaneous mobility. Loss of motor coordination and tone, decreased body temperature, and antagonism of amphetamine toxicity were also noted (Chakraborty et al., 1986).

Reported uses
Jambul seeds and extracts are thought to be useful in treating diarrhea and dysentery and in lowering blood glucose levels. Although the seeds have some anti-inflammatory and antipyretic properties, the extent of these properties has yet to be defined. Evidence for the therapeutic properties of jambul is anecdotal.

Teixeria and colleagues (2000) studied the effects of jambolan tea prepared from *S. cumini* in 30 nondiabetic patients after completing the original work in rats (Teixeria et al., 1997). In accordance with the results or the lack thereof found in rats, these investigators failed to find any hypoglycemic effect in humans after a glucose tolerance test and concluded that jambolan cannot be recommended as an antihyperglycemic agent.

Dosage
No consensus exists. In most cases, tea is prepared from the seeds or leaves of the tree.

Adverse reactions
None reported.

Bold italic type indicates that reaction may be life-threatening.

Interactions
CNS depressants: May cause altered behavior. Avoid administration with jambul.

Contraindications and precautions
No specific contraindications. Avoid using jambul in patients who are hypersensitive to this plant or related species and in pregnant or breast-feeding patients.

Special considerations
• Advise the patient to consult a health care provider before using herbal preparations because a treatment that has been clinically re-searched and proved effective may be available.
• Monitor the patient for changes in blood pressure or blood glucose levels.
• Urge the patient to report changes in behavior or coordination.
• Advise pregnant or breast-feeding patients to avoid using jambul.

Points of interest
• In Porto Alegre, a southern city of Brazil, a related species, *Syzygium jambos*, has also been used for treating diabetes. *S. jambos*, like *S. cumini*, is usually consumed in the form of a tea.

Commentary
Although jambul has been claimed to be effective for several medical conditions (diabetes, diarrhea, dysentery), there is little clinical evidence of its efficacy. In fact, animal and human clinical trials have failed to identify any significant hypoglycemic properties. Some studies have found extracts of jambul seeds and leaves to have anti-inflammatory, antipyretic, and neuropsychopharmacologic effects in animals. Further study on the active constituents of the seeds and leaves is warranted to determine the true pharmacologic properties of this plant.

References
Chakraborty, D., et al. "A Neuropsychopharmacologic Study of *Syzygium cuminii*," *Planta Med* 2:139-43, 1986.

Chaudhuri, A.K., et al. "Anti-inflammatory and Related Actions of *Syzygium cuminii* Seed Extract," *Phytotherapy Res* 4:5-10, 1990.

Teixeria, C.C., et al. "Effect of Tea Prepared from the Leaves of *Syzygium jambos* on Glucose Tolerance in Nondiabetic Patients," *Diabetes Care* 13:907-8, 1990.

Teixeria, C.C., et al. "The Effect of *Syzygium cumini* (L.) Seeds on Post-prandial Blood Glucose Levels in Nondiabetic Rats and Rats with Streptozotocin-induced Diabetes Mellitus," *J Ethnopharmacol* 56:209-13, 1997.

Teixeria, C.C., et al. "Absence of Antihyperglycemic Effect of Jambolan in Experimental and Clinical Models," *J Ethnopharmacol* 71(1-2):343-47, 2000.

JIMSONWEED

ANGEL'S TRUMPET, ANGEL TULIP, DEVIL'S APPLE, DEVIL'S
TRUMPET, DEVIL WEED, ESTRAMONIO, GREEN DRAGON,
GYPSYWEED, INFERNO, JAMESTOWN WEED, LOCO SEEDS,
LOCOWEED, MAD APPLE, MOON WEED, PERU APPLE,
STECHAPFEL, STINKWEED, STRAMOINE, THORN-APPLE,
TOLGUACHA, TRUMPET LILY, ZOMBIE'S CUCUMBER

Taxonomic class
Solanaceae

Common trade names
None known.

Common forms
Available in an oral and a rectal form. It is
also smoked in cigarettes or burned in powders
and the fumes inhaled.

Source
All parts of *Datura stramonium,* especially the seeds, are toxic. Parts that
are used include the leaves, flowering tops, roots, and, sometimes, seeds.
The plant is found in fields and roadside ditches and at refuse sites.

Chemical components
The leaves and seeds contain tropane alkaloids that consist of atropine,
hyoscyamine, hyoscine, and scopolamine. The seeds also contain fatty
acids (including oleic, linoleic, palmitic, stearic, and lignoceric) and un-
saponifiable matter (sitosterol and malic acid proteins). Other plant
constituents include flavonoids with anolides, coumarins, and tannins.
Although all plant parts are toxic, the constituents with the most anticholinergic effects occur in the seeds. Other isolated compounds include datugen, datugenin, total ash, potassium nitrate, and acid-insoluble ash.

Actions
Toxicity is caused by the pharmacologic activity of the tropane alkaloids, which are similar to those found in deadly nightshade (*Atropa
belladonna*). These alkaloids are potent central and peripheral anticholinergics. Symptoms usually occur within 30 to 60 minutes after ingestion and can continue for 48 hours or longer because of delayed GI
motility (Ellenhorn, 1997). Ingestion of *D. stramonium* manifests as
classic atropine toxicity.

Reported uses
There have been more reports of jimsonweed poisoning in humans
than in animals. Case reports in the literature abound of anticholinergic
syndrome secondary to seeds being intentionally ingested for the hallucinogenic effect. Fifty to 100 seeds can cause severe intoxication or

---

Bold italic type indicates that reaction may be life-threatening.

death. Jimsonweed has been used to treat several disorders, including asthma, muscle spasms, parkinsonism, and whooping cough. Because it acts similarly to belladonna and atropine, it potentially could be used as an antispasmodic or a mydriatic (Clause, 1961). It also relaxes the muscles of the GI, bronchial, and urinary tracts and reduces digestive and mucous secretions.

Dosage
The dose was formerly listed as 75 mg P.O. (Clause, 1961). The estimated lethal doses of atropine and scopolamine in adults are about 10 mg and more than 4 mg, respectively (Ellenhorn, 1997).

Adverse reactions
CNS: ataxia, difficulty speaking, extrapyramidal reactions, lack of coordination, mental status changes (confusion, disorientation, hallucinations, loss of short-term memory, psychosis), psychomotor agitation.
CV: hypertension, hypotension, sinus tachycardia.
EENT: blurred vision, mydriasis, photophobia.
GI: decreased bowel sounds, dysphagia, thirst.
GU: urine retention.
Metabolic: elevated body temperature (related to the inability to sweat).
Skin: dry, hot, flushed skin; dry mucous membranes.

Interactions
Other anticholinergics: May have additive effects. Avoid administration with jimsonweed.
Amantadine, antihistamines, disopyramide, levodopa, phenothiazines, procainamide, quinidine, thiazides, tricyclic antidepressants, other drugs that interact with atropine and hyoscyamine: May have adverse effects on CV system functioning. Avoid administration with jimsonweed.

Contraindications and precautions
Jimsonweed is contraindicated in pregnant or breast-feeding women and in patients with angle-closure glaucoma, myasthenia gravis, obstructive disease of the GI tract, obstructive uropathy, tachycardia, or thyrotoxicosis,

Special considerations
• Advise the patient to consult a health care provider before using herbal preparations because a treatment that has been clinically researched and proved effective may be available.
🕭 **ALERT** Jimsonweed poisoning resembles atropine toxicity. Signs and symptoms can occur 15 to 30 minutes after ingestion and include agitation, blurred vision, dizziness, dry mouth, euphoria, flushed skin, hallucinations, hyperthermia, nausea, palpitations, restlessness, symmetric dilation of pupils, and tachycardia. In cases of mild toxicity, treatment with activated charcoal and gastric lavage may suffice. For severe cases, some sources recommend treatment with physostigmine (Koevoets and van Harten, 1997; Chang et al., 1999).

• Monitor the patient for signs of anticholinergic toxicity, such as hyperthermia, lack of coordination, mental status changes, and tachycardia.

◆ ALERT Coma, CV collapse, respiratory failure, seizures, and death can occur with ingestion of the plant.

• Caution the patient to avoid consuming this herb.

Points of interest

• Jimsonweed is a popular recreational abuse herbal because of its hallucinogenic effects. Case reports of adverse reactions and poisonings from ingestion of jimsonweed are increasing (Thabet et al., 1999; Tiongson and Salen, 1998; Dewitt et al., 1997).

• Overdose and treatment of anticholinergic syndrome involve symptomatic and supportive care. Monitoring parameters include blood pressure, electrocardiograph tracings, heart and respiratory rates, and mental status. Gastric lavage, administration of activated charcoal, and induction of emesis may be helpful. Physostigmine is a potentially helpful but controversial treatment.

• *D. stramonium* is toxic at more than small doses and is subject to legal restrictions in most countries. It is an illegal drug for nonprescription use in the United States.

Commentary

D. stramonium has a narrow therapeutic window and has not shown promise over current treatments for antispasmodic, mydriatic, or respiratory purposes. Jimsonweed's use should be discouraged because of the lack of clinical data and the numerous reports of toxicity. It is also considered an illegal drug for nonprescription use.

References

Chang, S.S., et al. "Poisoning by *Datura* Leaves Used as Edible Wild Vegetables," *Vet Hum Toxicol* 41(4):242-45, 1999.

Clause, E.P. *Pharmacognosy,* 4th ed. Philadelphia: Lea & Febiger, 1961.

Dewitt, M.S., et al. "The Dangers of Jimsonweed and Its Abuse by Teenagers in the Kanawha Valley of West Virginia," *WV Med J* 93(4):182-85, 1997.

Ellenhorn, M.J. *Ellenhorn's Medical Toxicology—Diagnosis and Treatment of Human Poisoning,* 2nd ed. Baltimore: Williams & Wilkins Co., 1997.

Koevoets, P.F., and van Harten, P.N. "Thorn Apple Poisoning," *Ned Tijdschr Geneeskd* 141(29):1446-47, 1997.

Thabet, H., et al. "*Datura stramonium* Poisonings in Humans," *Vet Human Toxicol* 41(5):320-21, 1999.

Tiongson, J., and Salen, P. "Mass Ingestion of Jimson Weed by Eleven Teenagers," *Del Med J* 70(11):471-46, 1998.

JOJOBA

DEERNUT, GOATNUT, PIGNUT

Taxonomic class
Simmondsiaceae

Common trade names
Clearly Natural Soap Bar—Jojoba Oil, Derma-E Skin Care Jojoba and E Skin Oil, Desert Essence Jojoba 100 Percent Pure Oil, Queen Helene Beauty Jojoba Hot Oil Treatment

Common forms
Available as crude wax (jojoba oil), hydrogenated jojoba wax, jojoba butter, and wax beads. Jojoba is an ingredient in cosmetics and hair treatments.

Source
Jojoba oil is obtained from *Simmondsia chinensis* and *S. californica* seeds by expression or solvent extraction.

Chemical components
The highly stable jojoba oil (also referred to as liquid wax) contains long-chain polycarbon esters of fatty acids and alcohols (eicosenoic, docosenoic, oleic and palmitoleic acids, eicosenol, docosenol); simmondsin; small quantities of campesterol, stigmasterol, and sitosterol; vitamin E; B vitamins; silicon; chromium; copper; zinc; and iodine.

Actions
Jojoba oil is considered to have emollient properties that soothe chapped skin, psoriasis, and sunburn; relieve dry scalp; remove embedded sebum to help such scalp disorders as dandruff and hair loss; and reduce the acidity of the scalp. An atherogenic diet containing 2% jojoba oil lowered cholesterol levels in rabbits (Clarke and Yermanos, 1981). Antioxidant activity is probably related to the alpha-tocopherol content in jojoba (Mallet et al., 1994).

Interest in jojoba has centered around its application as a dietary supplement for animal and poultry feed (Hawthorne and Butterwick, 1998; Vermaut et al., 1999). Supplementation of the diet of broiler breeder hens with jojoba was found to promote smaller-sized eggs at a reduced rate of production. It was suggested that jojoba interfered with follicle growth, yolk deposition, progesterone production, and follicular maturation in the chickens (Vermaut et al., 1999).

Reported uses
Jojoba has been claimed to be effective in promoting hair growth and relieving skin problems. Its primary applications are to treat chapped and dry skin, dandruff, dry scalp, and psoriasis. Jojoba wax beads are used as an exfoliating agent in facial scrubs, skin conditioners, and soaps. Jojoba is also used as a replacement for petrolatum in creams, ointments, lotions, and lipsticks. Other claims include treatment of acne vulgaris, athlete's foot, cuts, eczema, hair loss, mouth sores, pimples, seborrhea, skin abrasions, warts, and wrinkles. Although little clinical evidence is available to support these claims, most applications appear to be based on theory and a long history of anecdotal use.

Dosage
No consensus on dosage exists.

Adverse reactions
Skin: contact dermatitis (with topical use).

Interactions
None reported.

Contraindications and precautions
Avoid systemic ingestion of large quantities of jojoba in pregnancy because of unknown and, possibly, detrimental effects.

Special considerations
• Advise the patient to consult a health care provider before using herbal preparations because a treatment that has been clinically researched and proved effective may be available.
• Inform the patient that jojoba oil is for topical use only.
◆ **ALERT** Ingestion of *S. chinensis* seeds has led to toxicity.
• Although no known chemical interactions have been reported in clinical studies, consideration must be given to the pharmacologic properties of the herbal product and the potential for exacerbation of the intended therapeutic effect of conventional drugs.

Points of interest
• Apache and American Southwest Indians and immigrants from Israel have been using jojoba oil to treat superficial conditions for many years.
• It has been suggested that jojoba would function well as an industrial lubricant because of its ability to maintain stability at high temperatures.

Commentary
Jojoba has been used for many years by Native Americans to promote hair growth and relieve skin problems. Numerous claims have been made regarding its efficacy in treating skin and scalp disorders, but no studies have been conducted to prove these claims. A long history of anecdotal use suggests that the oil is relatively safe if used topically.

References
Clarke, J.A., and Yermanos, D.M. "Effects of Ingestion of Jojoba Oil on Blood Cholesterol and Lipoprotein Patterns in New Zealand White Rabbits," *Biochem Biophys Res Commun* 102(4):1409, 1981.

Hawthorne, A.J., and Butterwick, R.F. "The Satiating Effect of a Diet Containing Jojoba Meal *(Simmondsia chinensis)* in dogs," *J Nutr* 128(12-Suppl):2669S-70S, 1998.

Mallet, J.F., et al. "Antioxidant Activity of Plant Leaves in Relation to Their Alpha-tocopherol Content," *Food Chem Toxicol* 49(1):61, 1994.

Vermaut, S., et al. "Evaluation of Jojoba Meal as a Potential Supplement in the Diet of Broiler Breeder Females During Laying," *Br Poult Sci* 40(2):284-91, 1999.

Bold italic type indicates that reaction may be life-threatening.

JUNIPER
A'RA'R A'DI, ARDIC, BACCAL JUNIPER, COMMON JUNIPER,
DWARF, GEMENER, GENIEVRE, GROUND JUNIPER,
HACKMATACK, HARVEST, HORSE SAVIN, JUNIPER
MISTLETOE, *JUNIPERI FRUCTUS*, YOSHU-NEZU, ZIMBRO

Taxonomic class
Cupressaceae

Common trade names
Multi-ingredient preparations: Cold-Plus, Cornsilk Buchu Formula,
Formula 600 Plus for Men, Juniper Berry, Naturalvite, PMS Aid,
Regeneration Softgels, SKB

Common forms
Available as capsules, essential oil, liquid, and tablets.

Source
The dried ripe fruit of the plant *Juniperus communis*, also known as female cones or berries, is used for medicinal purposes. The heartwood
and tops are used to a lesser extent.

Chemical components
This plant contains volatile oil, juniperin, resin, proteins, and formic
and malic acids. The volatile oils or essential oils constitute 0.8% to 3%
of the cones and consist of piene, sabinene, mycrene, and sesquiterpenes. The active constituent responsible for the diuretic action, ter-
pinen-4-ol, varies in concentration. Composition of the volatile oils depends on the season when the plant is harvested.

J. communis also contains isocupressic acid, which has been identified as an abortifacient.

Actions
The plant's berries have shown significant hypoglycemic effect when
given to normoglycemic and diabetic animals (Swanston-Flatt et al.,
1990); other observations included weight gain, increased peripheral
glucose consumption, and potentiation of glucose-induced insulin release (Sanchez de Medina et al., 1994).

Moderate anti-inflammatory activity was shown in vitro by *J. communis* (Tunon et al., 1995). *Juniper* species also appear to have mild antimicrobial activity. Extracts from bark, sapwood, and leaves have antimicrobial activity similar to that of streptomycin (Clark et al., 1990).
Ash from branches and needles is a good source of dietary calcium and
iron and a moderate source of magnesium.

Reported uses

J. communis has traditionally been used to treat kidney infections; a decoction of the branch with berries is used in some parts of the world (Ritch-Krc et al., 1996). This plant was considered an adjuvant to diuretic therapy in relieving dropsy caused by tubular kidney obstruction. A preparation of fresh berry juice diluted with water has been recommended as an effective diuretic for children. Although this plant is listed under the therapeutic category of diuretics, no studies confirm this property. Native Americans used bruised inner bark of juniper to relieve the odor of putrid-smelling wounds. Because of its antiflatulent properties, the oil has been used for flatulence and colic.

An herbal extract mixture of *J. communis* (juniper), *Urtica dioca* (nettle), and *Achillaea milefolium* (yarrow) was studied in vitro on the acid production of *Streptococcus mutans*. At doses of 6.3 mg/ml, the extract was found to have no inhibitory effects on this organism. A randomized, controlled trial was also conducted in 45 volunteers who had moderate gingival inflammation. Efficacy parameters included plaque index, modified gingival index, and angulated bleeding index. Participants were instructed to rinse with 10 ml of mouthwash composed of juniper, nettle, and yarrow twice a day for 3 months. Results showed that this mixture had no effect on plaque growth and gingival health (Van der Weijden et al., 1998).

Dosage

Dosages vary among researchers.
For anti-inflammatory activity, in vitro studies used 0.2 mg/ml.
For antimicrobial activity, in vitro studies used 20 mg/ml.
For colic and flatulence, 0.05 to 0.2 ml of juniper oil.
For hypoglycemic activity, in vivo doses ranged from 250 to 500 mg/kg every 24 hours.

Adverse reactions

GI: diarrhea (with large amounts).
GU: irritation of the urinary tract, especially the kidneys.
Skin: burning, erythema, possibly vesicles (with topical use).

Interactions

None reported.

Contraindications and precautions

Juniper is contraindicated in pregnant patients and in those with renal disease. Use cautiously in elderly patients and in those with contact dermatitis or diabetes or who are prone to hypersensitivity reactions. Do not apply to open wounds or skin abrasions.

Special considerations

🔊 **ALERT** *J. sabina,* a closely related species, has been used as an abortifacient, but this use is poorly substantiated. Daily doses of 190 and 245 mg of isocupressic acid in pregnant cattle (250 days' gestation) have

---

Bold italic type indicates that reaction may be life-threatening.

resulted in abortion after 3 to 4 days' administration. This plant and others in the *Juniperus* species are considered poisonous, causing mostly diarrhea and urinary tract irritation.

• Urge the patient to report significant diarrhea and urinary burning.
• Inform the patient that more potent preparations can cause irritation or blistering of skin or mucus membranes if applied topically.
• Inform the patient that juniper should not be used as a replacement for available diuretics.

Points of interest
• Juniper is used among the Carrier people of British Columbia. *J. communis* is always used fresh because of its abundant availability.

Commentary
Most clinical data are from in vitro animal studies. The traditional use of this plant as an antimicrobial and a diuretic for kidney infections has not been clinically documented. Although evidence suggests activity similar to that of streptomycin, studies in humans are needed. The hypoglycemic effect of the plant appears promising, but controlled studies in humans are needed before it can be recommended as an oral antidiabetic agent. Further studies regarding clinical use and dosage are needed to determine its therapeutic use.

References
Clark, A.M., et al. "Antimicrobial Properties of Heartwood, Bark/Sapwood and Leaves of *Juniperus* Species," *Phytother Res* 4:15-19, 1990.

Gardner, D.R., et al. "Abortifacient Effects on Lodgepole Pine (*Pinus contorta*) and Common Juniper *(Juniperus communis)* on Cattle," *Vet Hum Toxicol* 40(5):260-63, 1998.

Ritch-Krc, E.M., et al. "Carrier Herbal Medicine: Traditional and Contemporary Plant Use," *J Ethnopharmacol* 52:85-94, 1996.

Sanchez de Medina, F., et al. "Hypoglycemic Activity of Juniper Berries," *Planta Med* 60:197-200, 1994.

Swanston-Flatt, S., et al. "Traditional Plant Treatments for Diabetes. Studies in Normal and Streptozotocin Diabetic Mice," *Diabetologia* 33:462-64, 1990.

Tunon, N.H., et al. "Evaluation of Anti-inflammatory Activity of Some Swedish Medicinal Plants. Inhibition of Prostaglandin Biosynthesis and PAF-induced Exocytosis," *J Ethnopharmacol* 48:61-76, 1995.

Van der Weijden, G.G., et al. "The Effect of Herbal Extracts in an Experimental Mouthrinse on Established Plaque and Gingivitis," *J Clin Periodontol* 25(5):399-403, 1998.

KARAYA GUM

BASSORA TRAGACANTH, **I**NDIAN TRAGACANTH, KADAYA, KADIRA, KARAYA GUM, KATILA, KULLO, MUCARA, **S**TERCULIA, STERCULIA GUM

Taxonomic class
Sterculiaceae

Common trade names
Powdered Gum Karaya

Common forms
Karaya gum powder is used to form gels and pastes for bases in cosmetics, food, and pharmaceuticals.

Source
Karaya gum is the dried exudate of *Sterculia urens* and other *Sterculia* species. Native to India and Pakistan, this softwood tree grows to a height of about 30'. All parts of the tree exude a soft gum when injured. The gum is obtained by defacing the trunk, allowing the gum to seep out and be collected, washed, and dried.

Chemical components
Karaya gum is a high-molecular-weight complex polysaccharide composed of residues that contain galacturonic acid, beta-D-galactose, glucuronic acid, and L-rhamnose. Because the gum is partially acetylated, it may release acetic acid on degradation. Trimethylamine has also been identified in hydrolysis products.

Karaya gum contains 12% to 14% moisture and less than 1% acid-insoluble ash. The quality of karaya gum depends on how carefully impurities have been removed. Food-grade gum is usually a white to pinkish gray powder with a slight vinegar odor, whereas pharmaceutical grades may be almost translucent.

Actions
Karaya gum is essentially inert and not associated with significant pharmacologic activity. It is not digested or absorbed systemically. After contact with water, coarse particles in the gum swell, forming a discontinuous type of mucilage that exerts a laxative effect in the bowel. Although preliminary studies suggest that other gums of this type may normalize blood glucose and plasma lipid levels, karaya has not been investigated in this regard.

Reported uses

Karaya gum is used primarily in the pharmaceutical industry as a bulk laxative and in the food industry as an emulsifier, a binder, and a stabilizer in such products as bread and doughnut mixes, cheese spreads, frozen desserts, meringue powders, and whipped cream (Anderson, 1989).

The demulcent properties of karaya gum make it useful as an ingredient in lozenges to relieve sore throat. The bark has long been used as an astringent. A protective coating of karaya gum applied to dentures has been shown to reduce bacterial adhesion by 98%. Also, karaya gum is used as a denture adhesive in which the finely powdered gum is dusted onto the dental plate and swells when it touches the moist surface of the gums, providing a comfortable, tight fit for the plate. Karaya gum was also used in a clinical study of a new delivery system for administering salicylic acid in a skin patch to treat verruca vulgaris (warts). The patch achieved a cure rate of 69% compared with 35% for placebo controls. This treatment was considered safe, effective, and nonirritating (Bart, 1989).

Dosage

Dosage is expressed as a percentage of the karaya gum incorporated into the final product.

Adverse reactions

GI: abdominal pain, diarrhea, gastroesophageal or esophageal obstruction.

Interactions

None reported.

Contraindications and precautions

Avoid using karaya gum in pregnant or breast-feeding patients; effects are unknown. Use cautiously and in modest amounts in patients who are prone to gastric outlet obstruction.

Special considerations

• Advise the patient with diabetes to watch for signs and symptoms of hypoglycemia because large quantities of karaya gum may lower blood glucose levels.
• Instruct the patient to take other drugs at least 2 hours before or after ingesting karaya gum.
• Advise women to avoid using karaya gum products during pregnancy or when breast-feeding.
• Karaya gum is generally recognized as safe for internal consumption. Widespread experience with the product throughout the United States and Europe has not been associated with any significant adverse experiences.

Points of interest
• The use of karaya gum became widespread during the early 1900s, when it began to supplant tragacanth gum for many uses.

Commentary
Karaya gum has long been used as a bulk ingredient and emulsifying agent in the food and pharmaceutical industries. The gum appears to lack significant pharmacologic activity or toxicity. Clinical use as a bulk laxative appears safe and may be effective, but large, controlled clinical studies are unavailable.

References
Anderson, D.M. "Evidence for the Safety of Gum Karaya (*Sterculia* spp.) as a Food Additive," *Food Addit Contam* 6:189, 1989.
Bart, B.J. "Salicylic Acid in Karaya Gum Patch as a Treatment for Verruca Vulgaris," *J Am Acad Dermatol* 20:74-76, 1989.

KAVA

AVA, AWA, KAVA-KAVA, KAWA, KEW, SAKAU, TONGA, YAGONA

Taxonomic class
Piperaceae

Common trade names
Aigin, Antares, Ardeydystin, Cefkava, Kava Kava Liquid, Kava Kava Root, Kavarouse, Kavasedon, Kavasporal, Kava Stress, Kavatino, Kavatrol, Laitan, Mosaro, Nervonocton N, Potter's Antigian Tablets, Super 5HT with Kava, Viocava

Common forms
Prepared as capsules, a drink from pulverized roots, an extract, or tablets.

Source
Kava comes from the dried rhizome and root of *Piper methysticum,* a member of the black pepper family (Piperaceae). Kava, a large shrub with broad, heart-shaped leaves, is native to many South Pacific islands.

Chemical components
Pharmacologic activity is attributed to the kavapyrones that occur in the root. Biologically active components are obtained from chemical substitution of the basic pyrone structure. Alpha-pyrone components include yangonin, desmethoxyyangonin, 5,6-dehydromethysticin, 11-methoxyyangonin, and 11-methoxy-nor-yangonin. Methysticin, kawain, dihydromethysticin, and dihydrokawain are active components from the 5,6-dyhydro-alpha-pyrone structure. Pipermethystine is an alkaloid isolated from the plant leaves of kava.

Actions

More than one mode of action is involved. An unquantified synergism exists among kava components. Components of the root may produce local anesthetic activity similar to that of cocaine but lasting longer than that of benzocaine. Kava induced mephenesin-like muscle relaxation in animals but was found to lack curare-like activity. The limbic system is inhibited by kavapyrones, an effect associated with suppression of emotional excitability and mood enhancement. Kava also inhibited haloperidol-induced catalepsy in rats (Noldner and Chatterjee, 1999).

In human studies, kava produced mild euphoria with no effects on thought and memory. The neuropharmacologic effects of kava include analgesia, hyporeflexia, and sedation. Kava can impair gait and cause pupil dilation. Some pyrones show fungistatic properties against several fungi, including some that are pathogenic to humans.

Reported uses

Kava has been useful in attenuating spinal seizures and has antipsychotic properties. Therapeutic trials have shown a degree of seizure control in epileptic patients, suggesting involvement of gamma-aminobutyric acid receptors.

Kava extract has also been studied for treating anxiety disorders. In one study, 101 patients with anxiety of nonpsychotic origin showed improved scores on the Hamilton Anxiety Scale after being given a lipophilic extract of kava standardized to 70 mg of kavalactones three times a day (Volz et al., 1997). Both placebo and kava showed benefit as per the scale after 8 weeks, but kava fared significantly better than placebo at 16 weeks ($P<.0001$). No improvement was seen as measured on the Clinical Global Impression Scale. A meta-analysis of seven double-blind, randomized, placebo-controlled trials found some superiority of kava over placebo for treating anxiety in all trials but statistically significant superiority in only three trials (Pittler and Ernst, 2000).

Other claims for kava include treatment of asthma, depression, insomnia, muscle spasms, pain, rheumatism, and sexually transmitted disease and promotion of wound healing.

Dosage

Dosage is usually based on the kavapyrone content, which varies with preparation. Most studies in humans used 70 to 240 mg of kavapyrone P.O. daily. One study used 90 to 110 mg of dried kava extract P.O. t.i.d. for the treatment of anxiety (Volz et al., 1997). Doses of freshly prepared kava beverages average 400 to 900 g P.O. weekly.

Adverse reactions

CNS: changes in motor reflexes and judgment, headache, dizziness.
EENT: vision changes.

Long-term, heavy use
CV: hypertension.
GI: diarrhea.

Hematologic: decreased platelet and lymphocyte counts.
Metabolic: reduced plasma protein, urea, and bilirubin levels; weight loss.
Musculoskeletal: increased patellar reflexes.
Respiratory: shortness of breath.
Skin: hypersensitivity reaction (Schmidt et al., 2000).
Other: dopamine antagonism (potential for galactorrhea and breast engorgement), reddened eyes (may be related to cholesterol metabolism; Norton et al., 1994), and dry, flaking, discolored skin.

Interactions

Alcohol: Increased kava toxicity. Avoid administration with kava.
Alprazolam: May cause coma (Almeida et al., 1996). Avoid administration with kava.
Benzodiazepines, other CNS depressants: Additive sedative effects. Avoid administration with kava.
Levodopa: Increased parkinsonian symptoms. Avoid administration with kava.
Pentobarbital: May have additive effects. Avoid administration with kava.

Contraindications and precautions

Avoid using kava in pregnant or breast-feeding patients and in children under age 12; effects are unknown. Use cautiously in patients with neutropenia, renal disease, or thrombocytopenia. Avoid administration with psychotropic drugs.

Special considerations

• Inform the patient that significant adverse reactions may occur with long-term use of kava.
• Caution the patient to avoid alcohol and other CNS depressants because they enhance kava's sedative and toxic effects.
• Inform the patient that absorption of kava may be enhanced if it is taken with food.
• Advise women to avoid taking kava during pregnancy or when breast-feeding.

Points of interest

• Kava, although a depressant, is nonfermented, nonalcoholic, nonopioid, and nonhallucinogenic and does not appear to cause physiologic dependence, but the risk of psychological dependence exists.
• Kava is commonly used in the South Pacific as a ceremonial beverage. (See *Social significance of kava drinking.*)

Commentary

Kava has been used or studied most commonly for the treatment of anxiety, restlessness, and stress. These uses are supported by limited evidence from a few small clinical trials. In studies of kava as an anxiolytic, adverse reactions were minimal, but significant adverse reactions are reported with chronic, heavy use. Other therapeutic claims are poorly

---

Bold italic type indicates that reaction may be life-threatening.

documented. Additional trials are needed to establish dosing regimens,
drug interactions, therapeutic benefits, and adverse effects.

References
Almeida, J.C., et al. "Coma from the Health Food Store: Interaction Between Kava and Alprazolam," *Ann Intern Med* 125:940, 1996.

Dobelis, I.N. *Magic and Medicine of Plants.* Pleasantville, N.Y: Reader's Digest Association, Inc., 1986.

Noldner, M., and Chatterjee, S. "Inhibition of Haloperidol-induced Catalepsy in Rats by Root Extracts from *Piper methysticum F,*" *Phytomedicine* 6(4):285-86, 1999.

Norton, S.A., et al. "Kava Dermopathy," *J Am Acad Dermatol* 31:89-97, 1994.

Pittler, M.H., and Ernst, E. "Efficacy of Kava Extract for Treating Anxiety: Systematic Review and Meta-analysis," *J Clin Psychopharmacol* 20(1):84-89, 2000.

Schmidt, P., et al. "Delayed-type Hypersensitivity Reaction to Kava-kava Extract," *Contact Dermatitis* 42(6):363-64, 2000.

Volz, H.P., et al. "Kava-kava Extract WS-1490 versus Placebo in Anxiety Disorders —A Randomized Placebo-Controlled 25-Week Outpatient Trial," *Pharmacopsychiatry* 30:1-5, 1997.

KELP

BROWN ALGAE, HORSETAIL, *LAMINARIA*, SEA GIRDLES, SEAWEED, SUGAR WRACK, TANGLEWEED

Taxonomic class
Laminariaceae

Common trade names
Atlantic Kelp, Dr. Christopher Kelp-T #32 (Healthy Thyroid) V Caps, Kelp, Kelp Norwegian, Nature's Herbs Kelp-Norwegian Caps

Common forms
Capsules: 100 mg, 380 mg, 500 mg, 660 mg,
Tablets: 150 mcg, 225 mcg
   Also available as an aqueous extract, granules, powder, and sea spice kelp blends.

Source
Active components are derived from the fronds of the marine brown algae (*Laminaria digitata, L. japonica, L. saccharina,* and *Macrocystis pyrifera*) that grow along the northern Atlantic and Pacific coasts.

Chemical components
Kelp contains fucoidans, 1-3 beta glucans, algin, laminarin (a polysaccharide found in both soluble and insoluble forms in the plants), laminine, and histamine. Fucoidans have significant anticoagulant activity and may function in the same way as heparin as far as having an effect on heparin cofactor II (Mauray et al., 1998). Algin is a high-molecular-weight polysaccharide. Kelp is rich in vitamins, minerals, and iodine.

Actions
Kelp may have some antitumorigenic effects. It was found to protect female mice from the tumorigenic effects of a known carcinogen, and a kelp extract reduced DNA changes induced by several known carcinogens in *Salmonella typhimurium* bacteria (Okai et al., 1993). There is no conclusive evidence that kelp protects against carcinogenic substances. Sulfated laminarin has demonstrated anticoagulant, antilipemic, and antiviral properties (Kathan, 1965).

Reported uses
Kelp is claimed to have abortifacient, anticoagulant, antihypertensive, antiobesity, antirheumatic, and antitumorigenic actions. It was used in Japanese folk medicine for its alleged hypotensive attributes. The rate of breast cancer was found to be low in Japanese patients who had a high dietary intake of kelp (Teas, 1983). Kelp is also a high-quality source of natural iodine.

Dosage
Dosage is 1 tablet or capsule P.O. daily, providing 500 to 650 mg of ground kelp. This quantity of kelp will provide about 250 mcg of elemental iodine (about 150% of the RDA).

Adverse reactions
CV: hypotension.
Hematologic: abnormal erythropoiesis, *__autoimmune thrombocytopenia__*, *__bleeding__*.
Metabolic: thyroid dysfunction (transient hyperthyroidism caused by iodine component in kelp; Eliason, 1998; Kim and Kim, 2000).
Skin: acneiform lesions.

Bold italic type indicates that reaction may be life-threatening.

Interactions
Anticoagulants: Increased risk of bleeding complications in patients with coagulation or platelet defects or in those taking aspirin or warfarin concurrently. Avoid administration with kelp or monitor coagulation parameters intensively.

Antihypertensives: May have hypotensive effects; syncope or dizziness may occur. Avoid administration with kelp.

Antithyroid drugs, thyroid replacement: Iodine in kelp supplements may interfere with therapy for thyroid disease. Avoid administration with kelp.

Contraindications and precautions
Use kelp cautiously in pregnant patients because of cervical and placental effects associated with topical administration. *Laminaria* "tents," used as natural stents to dilate the cervix during delivery, have been associated with intrauterine fetal death (Agress and Benedetti, 1981).

Special considerations
• Patients who consume large quantities of kelp products on a daily basis should be evaluated for heavy metal poisoning. Edible marine algae has been found to be commonly contaminated with significant concentrations of various heavy metals and toxins (for example, arsenic, mercury, lead) as well as radioactive compounds (cesium-137, radium-226).

• Advise the patient who is prone to heart failure or hypotension, such as a patient taking an antihypertensive, not to use kelp because of its potential to produce hypotensive effects.

• Advise women to avoid using kelp products during pregnancy or when breast-feeding.

• Urge the patient on anticoagulant therapy to notify his health care provider if signs and symptoms of bleeding occur (bruises, bleeding gums, or blood in the stool).

Points of interest
• Natural stents or kelp "tents" have been used to maintain cervical dilation, but contamination of these tents has led to infectious complications and curtailed their use.

• Arsenic and other heavy metal poisonings have occurred with contaminated kelp (Walkin and Douglas, 1975). Foreign sources of kelp may contain some of the highest concentrations of these contaminants (Van Netten et al., 2000).

Commentary
Based on existing data, kelp cannot be recommended as a cancer preventive. Patients receiving anticoagulants or thyroid drugs should be made aware of kelp's potential to interact with their drug therapy. Prolonged consumption of large quantities of kelp products may increase the risk of heavy metal poisoning.

References

Agress, R.L., and Benedetti, T.J. "Intrauterine Fetal Death During Cervical Ripening with *Laminaria*," *Am J Obstet Gynecol* 141:587, 1981.

Eliason, B.C. "Transient Hyperthyroidism in a Patient Taking Dietary Supplements Containing Kelp," *J Am Board Fam Pract* 11(6):478-80, 1998.

Kathan, R.H. "Kelp Extracts as Antiviral Substances," *Ann N Y Acad Sci* 130:390-97, 1965.

Kim, J.Y., and Kim, K.R. "Dietary Iodine Intake and Urinary Iodine Excretion in Patients with Thyroid Diseases," *Yonsei Med J* 41(1):22-28, 2000.

Mauray, S., et al. "Comparative Anticoagulant Activity and Influence on Thrombin Generation of Dextran Derivatives and of a Fucoidan Fraction," *J Biomater Sci Polym Ed* 9(4):373-87, 1998.

Okai, Y., et al. "Identification of Heterogenous Antimutagenic Activities in the Extract of Edible Brown Seaweeds, *Laminaria japonica* (Makonbu) and *Undaria pinnatifida* (Wakame) by the Umu Gene Expression System in *Salmonella typhimurium*," *Mutat Res* 303:63-70, 1993.

Teas, J. "The Dietary Intake of *Laminaria*, a Brown Seaweed, and Breast Cancer Prevention," *Nutr Cancer* 4: 217-22, 1983.

Van Netten, C., et al. "Elemental and Radioprotective Analysis of Commercially Available Seaweed," *Sci Total Environ* 255(1-3):169-75, 2000.

Walkin, O., and Douglas, D.E. "Health Food Supplements Prepared from Kelp—A Source of Elevated Urinary Arsenic," *Clin Toxicol* 8:325-31, 1975.

KELPWARE

BLACK-TANG, BLADDER FUCUS, BLADDERWRACK, BLASEN-TANG, QUERCUS MARINA, SEA-OAK, SEAWRACK, SEETANG

Taxonomic class
Fucaceae

Common trade names
Bladderwrack, Kelp, Kelp Combination Tabs, Kelp/Lecithin/B6, Kelp Natural Iodine, Pacific Kelp

Common forms
Available as a dried plant, liquid extract, soft extract prepared with 45% alcohol, soft gel formulation with lecithin and vitamin B_6, and tablets.

Source
Fucus vesiculosus is a brown-green seaweed that grows in rocky areas along the northern coasts of the Atlantic and Pacific.

Chemical components
The plant is dried with periodic turning to avoid fungal growth and the development of a putrid odor. The active constituents are prepared from the dried thallus of the plant, which contains algin, iodine, bromine, mannite, and varying amounts of cadmium and lead. The plant also contains fucoidan, a sulfated polysaccharide.

Actions

F. vesiculosus has been studied mainly in vitro. The anticoagulant effects of fucoidan were found to prolong the activated partial thromboplastin time up to twofold (Dhrig et al., 1997). Kelpware also showed increased expression of platelet membrane activation markers that may play a role in thromboembolic events in patients with cancer and those undergoing percutaneous transluminal coronary angioplasty.

Kelpware has demonstrated antibacterial action against *Escherichia coli* and *Neisseria meningitidis* in vitro and antifungal action against *Candida guilliermondii* and *C. krusei* (Criado and Ferreiros, 1983, 1984).

Reported uses

The early literature reports the use of kelpware for obesity. It has been used in humans to reduce dietary fat content in patients with morbid obesity. The seaweed was also used to treat exophthalmic and simple goiter because of its iodine content and reported to be beneficial in patients under age 30. Kelpware has also been claimed to be useful in treating desquamative nephritis, fatty degeneration of the heart, inflammatory disease of the bladder, and menstrual irregularities such as menorrhagia.

Dosage

Alcoholic liquid extract: 4 to 8 ml P.O. before meals.
Alcoholic soft extract: 200 to 600 mg P.O.
Tablets: 3 tablets (3.75 grains) taken initially P.O. daily and then increased gradually up to 24 tablets P.O. daily.
For obesity, mix 16 g of bruised plant with 1 pt of water and then administer 2 fl oz P.O. t.i.d.

Adverse reactions

GU: elevated serum creatinine level, polydipsia, polyuria.
Metabolic: hyperglycemia.

Interactions

Anticoagulants, aspirin: May have additive effects. Monitor the patient.

Contraindications and precautions

Kelpware is contraindicated in pregnant or breast-feeding patients; effects are unknown. It is also contraindicated in patients with cancer, diabetes, heart failure, severe hepatic disease, recent myocardial infarction, or renal dysfunction; in elderly patients; and in those taking nephrotoxic drugs. (See *Kelpware and nephrotoxicity,* page 446.) Use cautiously in patients receiving amiodarone, anticoagulants, lithium, or thyroid hormone replacement therapy.

Special considerations

• Monitor laboratory results, including serum creatinine and blood glucose levels, PTT, PT, and INR.
• Advise women to avoid using kelpware during pregnancy or when breast-feeding.

RESEARCH FINDINGS

Kelpware and nephrotoxicity

Fucus vesiculosus was once thought to be harmless. However, a report of questionable nephrotoxicity has appeared in the literature. An 18-year-old female taking 1,200 mg P.O. three times a day of a product containing *F. vesiculosus* for weight loss presented with polyuria, polydipsia, and faintness.

Laboratory values revealed a significantly elevated serum creatinine level, and urinalysis revealed glucosuria (500 mg/dl), proteinuria, and leukocyturia. Renal biopsy showed moderate interstitial fibrosis, widespread tubular degeneration, and diffuse lymphomonocytic infiltrate. The glomeruli showed scarce and focal mesangial proliferation. Tested samples of the tablets contained 21.3 mg/kg of arsenic, 0.3 ppm of cadmium, 0.06 ppm of mercury, and 4 ppm of chromium. The arsenic content was believed to have contributed to the nephrotoxicity. The patient experienced a complete recovery 1 year after the onset of symptoms (Conz et al., 1998).

- Advise parents to avoid using kelpware in children because effects are unknown.
- Urge the diabetic patient not to use kelpware.
- Caution the patient that kelpware use may result in toxicity from cadmium, lead, arsenic, or bromide.
- Urge the patient to report signs of bleeding, increased thirst, and changes in urinary frequency or volume.
- Inform the patient that kelpware may contain iodine.

Points of interest

- *F. vesiculosus* has been reported to accumulate cadmium and lead in various plant parts, probably from the heavy metal content of seawater.
- Several *Fucus* species that are found along the French coastline are used to make kelpware tablets. The amount of iodine present in kelpware depends on the plant's origin; *F. digitatus* contains seven to eight times more iodine than *F. vesiculosus*.

Commentary

Although *F. vesiculosus* appears to possess anticoagulant activity, it cannot be recommended because of the lack of in vivo studies. Most experience with this plant's use is in Europe. The use of kelpware for obesity has received criticism and is generally excluded for morbid obesity.

References

Conz, P.A., et al. "*Fucus vesiculosus:* A Nephrotoxic Alga?" *Nephrol Dial Transplant* 13:526-27, 1998.

Bold italic type indicates that reaction may be life-threatening.

Criado, M.T., and Ferreiros, C.M. "Selective Interaction of *Fucus vesiculosus* Lectin-like Mucopolysaccharide with Several *Candida* Species," *Annales de Microbiologie* 134:149-54, 1983. Abstract.

Criado, M.T., and Ferreiros, C.M. "Toxicity of an Algal Mucopolysaccharide for *Escherichia coli* and *Neisseria meningitidis* Strains," *Rev Esp Fisiol* 40:227-30, 1984. Abstract.

Dhrig, J., et al. "Anticoagulant Fucoidan Fractions from *Fucus vesiculosus* Induce Platelet Activation in Vitro," *Thromb Res* 85:479-91, 1997.

KHAT

CAT, CHAT, GAD, KAHT, KAT, MIRAA, TSCHUT

Taxonomic class
Celastraceae

Common trade names
None known.

Common forms
Available as raw leaves.

Source
The raw leaves and tender twigs of *Catha edulis* are harvested for khat. The tree, a member of the staff tree family, grows to 80' and is native to East Africa and the highlands of the Arabian peninsula.

Chemical components
Leaves of khat contain the alkaloids cathinone and cathine. Cathinone is structurally related to amphetamine, and although it is a more powerful stimulant than cathine, it degrades rapidly in the presence of oxygen. Cathine has been identified as norpseudoephedrine. Other similar alkaloids (cathinine, cathidine, eduline, ephedrine), phenylpropyl, phenylpentenylamines, and tannins have also been identified. Fresh leaves contain the most cathinone.

Actions
Cathinone is a sympathomimetic agent with potent CNS-stimulating properties. Based on data obtained from animal and human studies, cathinone is considered a naturally occurring amphetamine analogue. Khat chewing causes anorexia, mydriasis, and vasoconstriction; elevates blood pressure; increases heart rate; and produces other amphetamine-like effects. CNS effects range from mild stimulation to euphoria to mania. Psychic dependence, tolerance, and addiction have also occurred.

Blood glucose levels were reduced in animals but not in humans (Elmi, 1983). An anti-inflammatory effect has been demonstrated in rats for a khat flavonoid. Cathinone suppresses serum testosterone levels, decreases sperm count and motility, and promotes degeneration of testicular tissue in animals (Islam et al., 1990).

Reported uses
Khat is claimed to be beneficial for treating depression, obesity, and ulcers. It is used in East Africa and the Arabian peninsula as an anorexiant and as a stimulant to offset fatigue.

Dosage
Usually, 100 to 200 g of raw leaf are chewed at a time. The leaves have a sweet taste and cause dryness of the mouth and oropharynx, typically leading to the consumption of large amounts of fluid.

Adverse reactions
CNS: aggressiveness, *cerebral hemorrhage,* euphoria, hallucinations (with overdose), hyperactivity, hyperthermia, mania, migraine headache, reduced performance on perceptual-visual memory and decision speed tests (with chronic use), psychoses.
CV: *arrhythmias*, hypertension, *cardiac arrest,* tachycardia.
EENT: decreased intraocular pressure, mydriasis, bilateral optic atrophy (possibly idiosyncratic reaction), oral cancers, periodontal disease.
GI: anorexia, constipation, esophagitis, gastritis, *hepatotoxicity,* stomatitis.
GU: decreased libido (in men), low sperm count, reduced sperm motility (animal and human studies).
Respiratory: *pulmonary edema.*
Skin: sweating.

Interactions
Antiarrhythmics, antihypertensives, beta blockers, decongestants, MAO inhibitors, other sympathomimetics: May cause similar interactions as with amphetamines. Avoid administration with khat.

Contraindications and precautions
Khat is contraindicated in patients with CV or renal disease or hypertension. Also avoid its use in pregnant or breast-feeding patients because cathinone is a suspected teratogen.

Special considerations
• Monitor the patient for psychological dependence to khat. Depression and sedation may be symptoms of khat withdrawal. Physical dependence and addiction appear unlikely.
• Caution the patient against chewing khat leaves or products because of the herb's deleterious effects on nutrition and GI function and its association with oral cancer.
• Inform the elderly patient that adverse reactions are likely to occur.
• Advise women to avoid using khat during pregnancy or when breast-feeding.

Points of interest
• At least one case of leukoencephalopathy has been linked with khat misuse (Morrish et al., 1999).

Bold italic type indicates that reaction may be life-threatening.

- Khat is consumed in daily social gatherings and deeply rooted in cultural tradition, especially among Yemen men. Khat chewing is also deeply rooted in religious beliefs; Muslims use it to gain a good level of concentration for prayer.
- Khat chewing has become a popular form of drug abuse in East Africa. The "red" type of khat is thought to be superior to the "white" type, which contains less cathinone.
- The sympathetic effects of khat may be described as greater than those of caffeine but less than those of amphetamine.

Commentary

Khat is chewed in Africa and Arabia for appetite suppression, euphoria, and stimulation. Many reports of adverse consequences of overuse and abuse exist in the literature. Symptoms of addiction, tolerance, and psychological dependence are less strong with khat than with amphetamines. Khat and its active ingredient, cathinone, have few, if any, appropriate medical uses.

References

Elmi, A.S. "The Chewing of Khat in Somalia," *J Ethnopharmacol* 8:163-76, 1983.

Islam, M.W., et al. "An Evaluation of the Male Reproductive Toxicity of Cathinone," *Toxicology* 603:223-34, 1990.

Morrish, P.K, et al. "Leukoencephalopathy Associated with Khat Misuse," *J Neurol Neurosurg Psychiatry* 67(4):556, 1999.

KHELLA

AMMI, BISHOP'S WEED, KHELLIN, VISNAGA, VISNAGIN

Taxonomic class
Apiaceae

Common trade names
Herb Pharm Khella, Khella, Quantam Herbal Products Khella

Common forms
Available as capsules, essential oil, extract, injectables, tablets, and teas.

Source
Active components are obtained from the fruit and seeds of *Ammi visnaga*, a member of the carrot family that is native to Egypt and other Middle Eastern areas.

Chemical components
Khella contains furanochromones, khellin, visnagin, khellol, and pyranocoumarins. Other compounds include flavonoids (quercetin, kaemperol, isorhamnetin), essential oils (camphor, terpineol, terpinen, linalool oxides), fixed oils, psoralens (methoxypsoralen), and protein.

Actions

Khellin and visnagin act as spasmolytic and vasodilatory agents on the muscles of the bronchi, GI tract, biliary tract, urogenital system, and coronary arteries, similar in action to calcium channel blockers.

When linked with an oxygen atom, khella forms a new compound called cromolyn sodium, formulations of which are used in the preventive treatment of asthma in children as well as for allergic reactions, bronchospasm, and hay fever.

The photobiological activity of khellin and visnagin against yeasts, bacteria, viruses, and fungi is being studied. In ultraviolet light, these compounds appear to affect cell division and alter DNA. Although still preliminary, research has shown antimutagenicity and antimicrobial activity in plant populations (Jansen et al., 1995; Borges et al., 1998). Furochromones from khella have shown anticonvulsant activity equivalent or superior to that of phenobarbital (Ragab et al., 1997).

Reported uses

Khella is claimed to be effective in treating biliary tract colic, spasmotic conditions of the GI tract, and dysmenorrhea. Traditionally, it has been used with hawthorn extracts to treat anginal symptoms. Early research appeared to yield impressive results in relieving anginal symptoms (Osher et al., 1951), but later studies have indicated that higher dosages of khella produce intolerable adverse reactions.

Khella may help to prevent asthma attacks but does not relieve an ongoing episode. It has been used to prevent bronchial asthma attacks and allergic reactions and has been used I.V. to treat anaphylaxis (Lowe et al., 1994). Extracts of khella have been used to treat psoriasis, and topical khellin with ultraviolet light irradiation has shown efficacy in treating vitiligo (Jansen et al., 1995). Topically applied khellin increases the carcinogenic effects of both ultraviolet light and sunlight (Borges et al., 1998).

Some components of khella may act favorably on total cholesterol levels, protein levels, and atherosclerotic changes in blood vessels, as evidenced by a study in which oral khella increased HDL levels without affecting total cholesterol or triglyceride levels (Harvengt and Desanger, 1983).

Dosage

Average daily doses of 20 mg of khellin P.O. have been recommended. *For treatment of angina,* 30 to 300 mg P.O. has been used. Sources are typically standardized to a 12% khellin content.

Adverse reactions

Skin: *allergic reactions* (itching), weak phototoxic activity, ***skin cancers*** (with topical use in patients predisposed to skin cancer).

With prolonged use or overdose
CNS: headache, insomnia, vertigo.
GI: anorexia, constipation, elevated liver function test results, nausea, vomiting.

Bold italic type indicates that reaction may be life-threatening.

Interactions
Antiarrhythmics: Khella may interfere with antiarrhythmic therapy. Avoid administration with khella.
Anticoagulants: May have additive effect. Avoid administration with khella.
Calcium channel blockers, other antihypertensives: May potentiate hypotensive effects. Avoid administration with khella.

Contraindications and precautions
Avoid using khella in pregnant or breast-feeding patients; effects are unknown. Use cautiously in patients with hepatic disease.

Special considerations
• Periodically monitor liver function test results.
• Recommend that the patient pursue a physician-supervised cardiac workup if khella is being taken as an antianginal.
• Inform the patient that concurrent use of khella may dramatically enhance hypotensive effects of antihypertensives.
• Urge the patient on anticoagulant therapy to report signs of bleeding (bruises, bleeding gums, or blood in the stool) to his health care provider.
• Advise women to avoid using khella during pregnancy or when breast-feeding.

Commentary
Khella appears to be a strong vasodilator, exerting activity similar to that of calcium channel blockers. It may be valuable in preventing bronchial and allergic reactions and is being studied for other disorders. Until adequate human clinical trials are conducted, khella should not be used without the supervision of a health care provider.

References
Borges, M.L., et al. "Photophysical Properties and Photobiological Activity of the Furanochromes Visnagin and Khellin," *Photochem Photobiol* 67:184-91, 1998.

Harvengt, C., and Desanger, J.P. "HDL Cholesterol Increase in Normolipaemic Subjects on Khellin: A Pilot Study," *Int J Clin Pharmacol Res* 3:363, 1983.

Jansen, T., et al. "Provocation of Porphyria Cutanea Tarda by KUVA-Therapy of Vitiligo," *Acta Derm Venereol* 75:232-33, 1995.

Lowe, W., et al. "A Khellin-like 7,7'Glycerol-bridged Bischromone with Anti-Anaphylactic Activity," *Arch Pharm (Weinheim)* 327:255-59, 1994.

Osher, H.L., et al. "Khellin in the Treatment of Angina Pectoris," *N Engl J Med* 244:315-21, 1951.

Ragab, F.A., et al. "Synthesis and Anticonvulsant Activity of New Thiazolidinone and Thioxoimidazolidinone Derivatives Derived from Furochromones." *Pharmazie (Cairo University, Egypt)* 52:926-29, 1997.

KUDZU

Dolichos lobatus, Pueraria lobata, Pueraria mirifica, Pueraria thomsonii, Pueraria thunbergiana, Pueraria tuberosa

Taxonomic class
Fabaceae

Common trade names
Fenge, Fen Ke, ge gen, Japanese arrowroot, Kudzu-Power, kudzu vine

Common forms
Capsules: 150 mg, 500 mg
Root powder: 250 g

Source
Kudzu is a rapidly growing bean vine that is native to China and Japan. It was introduced to the southeastern United States in 1876 and was first used as an ornamental shade plant. It was later used as groundcover for erosion control and soil fertility and is now considered by some to be a nuisance. The plant has three broad leaflets with large purple flowers and beans in flat pods.

Chemical components
Kudzu roots and flowers contain flavonoids, isoflavonoids, and isoflavones, such as daidzin and daidzein. Robinin has also been identified in the kudzu leaf. Other constituents of kudzu include formononetin, biochanin A, puerarin, and plant sterols.

Actions
Kudzu and its pharmacologically active components possibly inhibit the enzymes that metabolize alcohol or accelerate its clearance from blood.

Numerous studies in rats or Syrian golden hamsters have examined the use of *Pueraria lobata* and its major compounds—puerarin, daidzin, and daidzein—in the treatment of alcoholism. There are conflicting data on how *P. lobata* actually works. It was proposed that daidzein inhibited alcohol dehydrogenase and, therefore, interfered with alcohol metabolism. Later results hypothesize that daidzin and daidzein might accelerate alcohol clearance from blood or counter alcohol intoxication by suppressing the blood alcohol concentration through delayed stomach emptying (Xie et al., 1994; Overstreet et al., 1996). More studies are needed to determine kudzu's actual mechanism of action.

Reported uses
Historically, kudzu has been used to treat angina pectoris, arrhythmias, dysentery, gastritis, heart disease, hypertension, influenza, ischemia, migraine headache, and muscle aches and pain. There has been documen-

---

Bold italic type indicates that reaction may be life-threatening.

tation of kudzu's possessing antioxidant activity. Most notably, kudzu has been studied in the treatment of alcoholism.

Dosage
Typically, people take one or two 150-mg capsules containing kudzu root extract P.O. t.i.d.

Adverse reactions
None reported.

Interactions
None reported.

Contraindications and precautions
When taken appropriately, kudzu is considered safe. Because there is insufficient information about the use of kudzu in pregnant or breast-feeding women, it should be avoided.

Special considerations
• Patients using kudzu for treatment of alcoholism should be evaluated by a health care provider so that the herb is used appropriately.
• Advise pregnant and breast-feeding patients to avoid using kudzu.
• Advise the patient to consult a health care provider before using herbal preparations because a treatment that has been clinically researched and proved effective may be available.
• Although no known chemical interactions have been reported in clinical studies, consideration must be given to the pharmacologic properties of the herbal product and the potential for exacerbation of the intended therapeutic effect of conventional drugs.

Points of interest
• Apparently, under optimal growing conditions, kudzu can grow as fast as 12" per day and as much as 100' in a season.

Commentary
Human studies have not been conducted to examine the potential use of kudzu in treating alcoholism. There does not appear to be any toxic effects with this herb when used appropriately. More studies are needed to evaluate its use in humans.

References
Lin, R.C., and Li, T. "Effects of Isoflavones on Alcohol Pharmacokinetics and Alcohol-drinking Behavior in Rats," *Am J Clin Nutr* 68(suppl):1512S-5S, 1998.

Overstreet, D.H., et al. "Suppression of Alcohol Intake After Administration of Chinese Herbal Medicine, NPI-028, and Its Derivatives," *Alcohol Clin Exp Res* 20:221-27, 1996.

Xie, C-I., et al. "Daidzin, an Antioxidant Isoflavonoid, Decreases Blood Alcohol Levels and Shortens Sleep Time Induced by Ethanol Intoxication," *Alcohol Clin Exp Res* 18:1443-47, 1994.

LADY'S MANTLE

ALCHEMILLA, BEAR'S FOOT, DEWCUP, LEONTOPODIUM,
LION'S FOOT, NINE HOOKS, STELLARIA

Taxonomic class
Rosaceae

Common trade names
Lady's Mantle

Common forms
Available as compounded extracts, gelatin
capsules, teas, and tinctures.

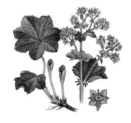

Source
The drug is extracted from the roots, leaves, and flowers of *Alchemilla mollis, Alchemilla vulgaris,* and others. The plant is native to Europe but naturalized to the northeastern United States and to Canada.

Chemical components
The major active ingredients are elligitannins and quercetin, a flavonoid. A glycoside and salicylic acid have also been isolated.

Actions
A water extract of *Alchemilla xantochlora* showed antioxidative activity, whereas an ethanol extract did not (Filipek, 1992). Flavonoid extracts of *A. vulgaris* inhibited the action of several proteolytic enzymes (elastase, trypsin, and alpha-chymotrypsin), suggesting that they may protect conjunctive and elastic tissues that are detrimentally affected by proteolytic enzymes (Jonadet et al., 1986). *A. vulgaris* did not affect the blood glucose and serum insulin levels in normal and streptozotocin diabetic mice (Swanson-Flatt et al., 1990).

Reported uses
Lady's mantle is claimed to be useful as an astringent and an aid to blood clotting. It has been applied topically to wounds to stop bleeding and to promote healing. Lady's mantle is used in women to reduce menstrual bleeding, alleviate menstrual cramps, and regulate menses. It has also been suggested to be effective in treating diarrhea because of its tannin content. No controlled trials in humans verify these claims.

Dosage
Various doses are used for the reported indications. An infusion or tea can be prepared from steeping 2 tsp of the dried herb in 1 cup of boiling water. The tea and tincture (2 to 4 ml) are taken P.O. t.i.d.

Adverse reactions

Hepatic: hepatic dysfunction (related to tannin component).

Interactions

None reported.

Contraindications and precautions

Lady's mantle is contraindicated during pregnancy because it may stimulate uterine muscle. Also avoid use in breast-feeding patients because effects are unknown.

Special considerations

• Periodically monitor liver function test results.
• Advise women to avoid using lady's mantle during pregnancy or when breast-feeding.
• Inform the patient that little is known about this herb.
• Urge the patient to report fatigue, jaundice, and weakness.

Points of interest

• The genus name, *Alchemilla*, is derived from the word alchemy because this herb was believed to bring about miraculous cures. The plant has also been associated with the Virgin Mary because the lobes of the leaves resemble the scalloped edges of a mantle.
• Lady's mantle is used as an ingredient in cleansing creams and other cosmetics.

Commentary

No clinical data support therapeutic claims for lady's mantle. Data from one animal study suggest that lady's mantle does not affect blood glucose or serum insulin levels, but it may have antioxidative properties and inhibit some proteolytic enzymes. Human clinical trials are needed to determine the safety and efficacy profiles of this herb.

References

Filipek, J. "Effect of *Alchemilla xantochlora* Water Extract on Lipid Peroxidation and Superoxide Anion Scavenging Activity," *Pharmazie* 47:717-18, 1992.

Jonadet, M., et al. "Flavonoids Extracted from *Ribes nigrum* L. and *Alchemilla vulgaris* L.: Part 1. In Vitro Inhibitory Activities on Elastase, Trypsin and Chymotrypsin. Part 2. Angioprotective Activities Compared In Vivo," *J Pharmacol* 17:21-27, 1986.

Swanson-Flatt, S.K., et al. "Traditional Plant Treatments for Diabetes. Studies in Normal and Streptozotocin Diabetic Mice," *Diabetologia* 33:462-64, 1990.

LADY'S SLIPPER, YELLOW

AMERICAN VALERIAN, MOCCASIN FLOWER, NERVE ROOT, NOAH'S ARK, WHIPPOORWILL'S SHOE, YELLOW INDIAN SHOE

Taxonomic class

Orchidaceae

Bold italic type indicates that reaction may be life-threatening.

Common trade names
None known.

Common forms
Available as dried rhizome, liquid extract, powdered root, teas, and tinctures. Commonly used in combination products with other herbal ingredients, such as valerian root.

Source
Active compounds are derived from the rhizome and root of the orchid, *Cypripedium pubescens,* or *C. calceolus.* Other species include *C. parviflorum* and are generally sparsely located in the forests of North America and Europe.

Chemical components
The rhizome of *Cypripedium* contains cypripedin, a complex resinoid. Other components include glycosides, resins, quinones, and tannic and gallic acids.

Actions
None reported.

Reported uses
Lady's slipper tea has been used for headaches and nervousness. The powdered root mixed in sugar water has been used as an antispasmodic, a mild hypnotic, and a sedative. Other claims include treatment of epilepsy, hysteria, low-grade fever, nervous depression associated with GI disorders, and neuralgia.

Dosage
Dried rhizome and root: 2 to 4 g P.O. t.i.d.
Liquid extract (1:1 water and 45% alcohol): 2 to 4 ml P.O. t.i.d.

Adverse reactions
CNS: excitement leading to hallucinations, giddiness, headache, restlessness.
Skin: contact dermatitis (quinone components).

Interactions
Dopamine agonists, similar drugs: May increase hallucinogenic effect. Avoid administration with lady's slipper.

Contraindications and precautions
Lady's slipper is contraindicated in patients with a history of plant allergies because quinone components may cause contact dermatitis. It is also contraindicated in patients who are susceptible to headaches or mental illness unless under medical supervision. Avoid its use in pregnant or breast-feeding patients; effects are unknown.

Bold italic type indicates that reaction may be life-threatening.

Special considerations
• Monitor the patient for psychotic behavior or headaches.
• Inform the patient that there are few clinical data to support therapeutic uses of this herb.
• Urge the patient not to perform hazardous activities until CNS effects of the herb are known.
• Advise women to avoid using lady's slipper during pregnancy or when breast-feeding.

Points of interest
• Native American healers used the root of *C. acaule* mixed into a solution for use in various illnesses, including influenza and hysteria (Sanchez et al., 1996).
• Lady's slipper may be found in combination products with valerian root *(Valerian officinalis)*, used for sedative and calming effects.

Commentary
Lady's slipper has not been adequately studied in animal or human models. Pending extensive testing for pharmacologic action, it cannot be recommended for any therapeutic use.

References
Sanchez, T.R., et al. "The Delivery of Culturally Sensitive Health Care to Native Americans," *J Holistic Nurs* 14:295-307, 1996.

LAVENDER

ASPIC, ECHTER LAVENDEL, ENGLISH LAVENDER *(LAVANDULA ANGUSTIFOLIA)*, ESPLIEG, FRENCH LAVENDER, GARDEN LAVENDER, LAVANDA, LAVANDE COMMUN, LAVANDIN, NARDO, SPANISH LAVENDER *(LAVANDULA STOECHAS)*, SPIGO, SPIKE LAVENDER, TRUE LAVENDER

Taxonomic class
Lamiaceae

Common trade names
Essent Oil Lavandin, Essent Oil Lavender, Lavender, Lavender Flowers, Massage Oil Lavender

Common forms
Available as flowers, leaves, and oils. Also included in cosmetic preparations, such as body mist, shower gel, conditioner, and deodorant.

Source
The flowering tops and stalks of *Lavandula officinalis* and other *Lavandula* species *(L. latifolia, L. angustifolia, L. stoechas)* are widely used for their active components. Native to the Mediterranean, lavenders are widely cultivated in American gardens for their color and fragrance. (Lavandin is a hybrid of spike lavender and true lavender.)

Chemical components

Lavender consists of essential oils, mainly monoterpenes. More than 100 compounds are identified in the oil, principally linaloyl acetate, linalool, and tannins; other compounds include ocimene, cineola, camphor, coumarins, flavonoids, phytosterols, pinene, limonene, caproic acid, and perillyl alcohol. Lavender oil, spike lavender oil, and lavadin oil are volatile oils that contain varying amounts of similar compounds.

Actions

Lavender was found to cause CNS depressant effects, anticonvulsant activity, and potentiation of sedative effects of chloral hydrate in rats. Spike lavender oil has been reported to exert a spasmolytic effect on animal smooth muscle, and *L. stoechas* caused hypoglycemia in normoglycemic rats.

Lavender oil fed to rats was found to cause regression of mammary tumors. The active ingredient has been suggested to be perillyl alcohol. The National Cancer Institute is examining this agent in phase II clinical trials in patients with advanced cancers of the breast, ovary, and prostate (Ziegler, 1996).

In vitro studies report promising results of topical lavender use to eradicate methicillin-resistant *Staphylococcus aureus* and vancomycin-resistant *Enterococcus faecium* (Nelson, 1997). No clinical trials are available to confirm these results.

Reported uses

Lavender is regarded by herbalists as a sedative to treat insomnia and restlessness. Other claims include its use in upper abdominal discomfort associated with nervousness, as an appetite stimulant, and to treat migraine headaches and neuralgia. Lavender has also been used as an astringent to treat minor cuts, bruises, and burns and for pain associated with strained muscles. It has been used as an indoor scent to induce a calming effect.

Dosage

Astringent (external): 20 to 100 g of lavender added to 7.7 gal (20 L) of water to avoid too strong a scent.
Lavender tea: 1 to 2 tsp in 150 ml of hot water; steep for about 10 minutes.
Oil (internal): 1 to 4 gtt of oil on a sugar cube.

Adverse reactions

With ingestion of large doses
CNS: CNS depression, confusion, drowsiness, euphoria, mental dullness, headache.
EENT: miosis.
GI: constipation, nausea, vomiting.
Respiratory: *respiratory depression.*
Skin: contact dermatitis.

Bold italic type indicates that reaction may be life-threatening.

Interactions
CNS sedatives (alcohol, benzodiazepines, narcotics): May potentiate sedative effects. Avoid administration with lavender.

Contraindications and precautions
Lavender is contraindicated in pregnant or breast-feeding patients and in those taking sedatives.

Special considerations
🔊 **ALERT** Lavender oil should be considered potentially poisonous. No more than 2 drops of the volatile oil should be consumed. Large doses are reported to exert narcotic-like effects.
• Monitor the patient using lavender and other sedatives for excessive sedation.
• Inform the patient suffering from insomnia that sedatives and hypnotic drugs with known risks and benefits are available. Also suggest techniques other than drug therapy (such as behavior modification, light therapy, and regular bedtime) to combat insomnia.
• Advise women to avoid using lavender during pregnancy or when breast-feeding.

Points of interest
• Lavender has been used in small concentrations to flavor food, but it is cultivated mainly for use as a perfume or potpourri and in decorations.
• France is a major producer of lavender products.

Commentary
Lavender has been used in traditional medicine for centuries, but clinical evidence of its efficacy for any disease or condition is inadequate. Controlled studies are needed before its use can be recommended.

References
Nelson, R.R.S. "In-Vitro Activities of Five Plant Essential Oils Against Methacillin-resistant *Staphylococcus aureus* and Vancomycin-resistant *Enterococcus faecium*," *J Antimicrob Chemother* 40:305-6, 1997.
Ziegler, J. "Raloxifene, Retinoids, and Lavender: 'Me Too' Tamoxifen Alternatives," *J Natl Cancer Inst* 88:1100-02, 1996.

LEMON BALM

BALM MINT, BEE BALM, BLUE BALM, CURE-ALL, DROPSY PLANT, GARDEN BALM, SWEET BALM,

Taxonomic class
Lamiaceae

Common trade names
Biodynamic Lemon Balm Liquid Herbal Extract.

Common forms

Lemon balm *(Melissa officinalis* L.) is usually taken as a tea made from either dried or fresh leaves. Liquid extracts are available. Preparation of a poultice has also been reported in the lay literature and a formulated cream has been used in some clinical trials.

Source

M. officinalis is a member of the mint family. Active chemical constituents can be found in the leaves and stems. The leaves are opposite, ovate, bluntly serrate, and acuminate. The flowers are bilabiate and range in color from white to light blue.

Chemical components

Numerous compounds have been isolated from lemon balm, including caffeic acid, citral, citronellal, eugenol, geraniol, choline, and an unidentified glycoside.

Actions

The efficacy of eugenol in dental analgesia is well established, and it is probably this component that accounts for the usefulness of lemon balm in toothache. Aqueous methanolic extracts have demonstrated a concentration-dependent inhibition of lipid peroxidation (Hohmann et al., 1999). Early scientific data reported possible antibacterial and antiviral properties of lemon balm. These reports have been supported by data that indicates potent activity against HIV-1 by aqueous extracts (Yamasaki et al., 1998). In vitro studies have also demonstrated antiprotozoal activity against *Trypanosoma brucei* specifically (Mikus et al., 2000). Additional research has indicated that certain constituents of the plant (caffeic acid and an unidentified glycoside) inhibit protein synthesis by direct interference with elongation factor 2. Numerous studies by various laboratories have supported these data. This may account for the antiviral activity of the herb. Ethanolic extracts have demonstrated an affinity for cholinergic receptors in human cerebral cortical tissue. This affinity was predominantly for nicotinic receptors with less but significant affinity for muscarinic receptors (Wake et al., 2000). Clinical trials of lemon balm cream for local treatment of herpes labialis demonstrated significant improvement in time to heal, spread of lesions, and attenuation of symptoms relative to placebo control (Koychev et al., 1999). No animal or human studies exist to establish the toxicity of lemon balm.

Reported uses

Nonmedical uses of lemon balm include its use in potpourri, herb pillows, and cosmetics and as a garnish or herb in cooking. The lay literature touts numerous therapeutic benefits for lemon balm, including its use as an antiflatulent, an antipyretic, an antispasmodic, a carminative, an emmenagogue, a sedative, a stomachic, and a sudorific. It has also been used by herbalists as a treatment for asthma, chronic bronchial catarrh, headache and vertigo in pregnancy, hysteria, melancholy, migraine headache, and toothache. Other uses purported for lemon balm

---

Bold italic type indicates that reaction may be life-threatening.

are as a poultice for local treatment of wounds, tumors, and insect bites; to relieve menstrual cramps; and in the treatment of herpes simplex lesions. Proposed cholinergic activity has led to lemon balm's being suggested as an alternative therapy for various derangements of memory, including Alzheimer's disease (Perry et al., 1999). No data exist that establish the extent of use of lemon balm by the public.

Dosage
Lemon balm is most often taken as a tea, prepared from either fresh or dried leaves. The tea is prepared by steeping a bag of leaves (1 tsp) for about 5 minutes in hot water. Sometimes a stronger tea is made by placing 1½ tbsp of the leaves in 1 pt of boiling water, covering it, and steeping it for 15 minutes before straining. Dosage for the liquid extract is recommended to be 2 to 4 ml P.O. t.i.d.

Adverse reactions
Skin: local irritation.
Other: *hypersensitivity reactions.*

Interactions
None reported.

Contraindications and precautions
No contraindications or precautions have been reported for lemon balm. One study that examined the ability of different antiviral compounds used in the treatment of herpes simplex to evoke a sensitivity reaction reported that an extract of lemon balm induced a weak response (less than the antiviral tromantadine) in guinea pigs. People who have a propensity to develop allergic reactions should use the herb cautiously. A second study examined the mutagenic properties of several medicinal plants, using an *Aspergillus nidulans* plate incorporation assay as the model. No mutagenic or genotoxic effects were noted for either aqueous or alcoholic extracts of lemon balm. No other studies using more stringent models of mutagenicity, teratogenicity, or genotoxicity exist. Given the ability of caffeic acid and the glycoside to inhibit protein synthesis, the use of lemon balm in pregnancy should be strongly discouraged, despite its purported efficacy in treating gravidal headache and dizziness.

Special considerations
• Caution the patient who is prone to allergic reactions to avoid using lemon balm.
• Advise pregnant patients to avoid using lemon balm.
• Advise the patient to consult a health care provider before using herbal preparations because a treatment that has been clinically researched and proved effective may be available.
• Although no known chemical interactions have been reported in clinical studies, consideration must be given to the pharmacologic properties of the herbal product and the potential for exacerbation of the intended therapeutic effect of conventional drugs.

Commentary

Potential benefit may be possible when lemon balm is used as recommended. A few scientific studies do support the possible efficacy of certain constituents as an anti-inflammatory and a memory aid. No clinical studies support these uses nor has the toxicological profile of these actions been determined.

The widespread use of lemon balm in cooking implies that it is probably safe when ingested in small amounts. Most information concerning its medical uses comes from the lay literature and does not constitute a valid recommendation for its use. Extensive scientific research is needed to provide a basis for the use of caffeic acid, the glycoside, or some derivative of these chemicals as an antiviral. Also, controlled scientific and clinical studies are needed to establish safe therapeutic doses and adverse effect and toxicity profiles of lemon balm.

References

Chabicz, J., and Galasinski, W. "The Components *of Melissa officinalis* L. That Influence Protein Biosynthesis *In Vitro*," *J Pharm Pharmacol* 38(11):791-94, 1986.

Galasinski, W., et al. "The Substances of Plant Origin That Inhibit Protein Biosynthesis," *Acta Pol Pharm* 53(5):311-18, 1996.

Hausen, B.M., and Schulze, R. "Comparative Studies of the Sensitizing Capacity of Drugs Used in Herpes Simplex," *Derm Beruf Umwelt* 34(6):163-70, 1986.

Hohmann, J., et al. "Protective Effects of the Aerial Parts of *Salvia officinalis, Melissa officinalis*, and *Lavandula angustifolia* and Their Constituents Against Enzyme-dependent and Enzyme-independent Lipid Peroxidation," *Planta Med* 65(6):576-78, 1999.

Koychev, R., et al. "Balm Mint Extract (Lo-701) for Topical Treatment of Recurring Herpes Labialis," *Phytomedicine* 6(4):225-30, 1999.

Kucera, L.S., et al. "Antiviral Activities of Extracts of the Lemon Balm Plant," *Ann NY Acad Sci* 130(1):474-82, 1965.

Mikus, J., et al. "*In Vitro* Effect of Essential Oils and Isolated Mono- and Sesquiterpenes on *Leishmania major* and *Trypanosoma brucei*," *J Planta Med* (66)4:366-68, 2000.

Perry, E.K., et al. "Medicinal Plants and Alzheimer's Disease: From Ethnobotany to Phytotherapy," *J Pharm Pharmacol* 51(5):527-34, 1999.

Ramos Ruiz, A., et al. "Screening of Medicinal Plants for Induction of Somatic Segregation Activity in *Aspergillus nidulans*," *J Ethnopharmacol* 52(3):123-27, 1996.

Robbers, J.E., et al. "Terpenoids," in *Pharmacognosy and Pharmacobiotechnology*. Baltimore: Williams & Wilkins, 1996.

Wake, G., et al. "CNS Acetylcholine Receptor Activity in European Medicinal Plants Traditionally Used to Improve Failing Memory," *J Ethnopharmacol* 69(2):105-14, 2000.

Yamasaki, K., et al. "Anti-HIV-1 Activity of Herbs in Labiatae," *Biol Pharm Bull* 21(8):829-33, 1998.

LICORICE

CHINESE LICORICE, LICORICE ROOT, PERSIAN LICORICE, RUSSIAN LICORICE, SPANISH LICORICE, SWEET ROOT

Taxonomic class
Fabaceae

Common trade names
Multi-ingredient preparations: Alvita Teas Licorice Root, Alvita Teas Licorice Sticks, Full Potency Licorice Root Vegicaps, Gaia Herbs Licorice Root A/F, Gaia Herbs Licorice Root SFSE, Licorice ATC Concentrate, Licorice and Garlic, Licorice Root Extract, Licorice Root Tea, Natrol Licorice Root Capsules, Natural Arthro-Rx, Nature's Answer Licorice Root Low Alcohol and Alcohol Free, Nature's Herbs Licorice Phytosome Capsules, Nature's Herbs Licorice Power-Certified Potency Capsules, Solaray Licorice Root, Tea with Mint, Tubi's Organic Licorice Licorice Bars and Chews, Tummy Soother

Common forms
Capsules: 100 to 520 mg licorice root
Liquid extracts: licorice extract, deglycyrrhizinized licorice extract
Tablets: 7 mg of licorice root and 333 mg of pure concentrated garlic
   Also available in candy, chewing gum, herbal teas, throat lozenges, and tobacco products.

Source
Most medicinal products use the roots and dried rhizomes of *Glycyrrhiza glabra,* a perennial herb or low-growing shrub. Spanish licorice, the most common variety, is derived from *G. glabra* var. *typica.* Licorice plants are native to the Mediterranean but widely cultivated in the United States, Russia, Spain, Turkey, Greece, India, Italy, Iran, and Iraq.

Chemical components
The rhizomes and roots contain 5% to 9% glycyrrhizin (glycyrrhizic acid), a glycoside that is 50 times sweeter than sugar. Hydrolysis of glycyrrhizin yields glycyrrhetic acid, which is not sweet. Other compounds include ammonia, oleane triterpenoids, glucose, mannose, and sucrose. Aqueous extracts of licorice contain 10% to 20% glycyrrhizin.

Actions
Glycyrrhizin is hydrolyzed by intestinal flora to the pharmacologically active form, glycyrrhetic acid. The main effect of licorice is to potentiate, rather than mimic, endogenous steroids (Davis and Morris, 1991).
   Studies in animals suggest that glycyrrhizin and glycyrrhetic acid have mild anti-inflammatory effects. Glycyrrhizin may stimulate gastric mucous synthesis through effects on prostaglandins, which may explain

RESEARCH FINDINGS
Licorice-derived products for peptic ulcer disease

Studies from Europe in the 1940s and 1950s suggested that licorice derivatives could be used to treat peptic ulcer disease. Adverse reactions ranged from headaches and edema to heart failure.

Interest in these agents was revived in the 1960s with the advent of carbenoxolone, a semisynthetic ester of glycyrrhetic acid. This was the first agent derived from traditional medicine to show efficacy against peptic ulcer disease. Ulcer healing was demonstrated in 50% to 70% of patients (Marks, 1980). Other studies failed to show that carbenoxolone or deglycyrrhizinized licorice was superior to cimetidine (Bardhan et al., 1978; LaBrooy et al., 1979; Maxton et al., 1990).

its ulcer-healing properties. (See *Licorice-derived products for peptic ulcer disease.*)

Anecdotally, licorice has effective demulcent (soothing) and expectorant properties and mild laxative and antispasmodic effects. A Chinese licorice preparation called Zhigancao has been found to have antiarrhythmic effects, including prolonged PR and QT intervals. Glycyrrhizin may also lower cholesterol and triglyceride levels and exert antianemic, antihepatotoxic, and immunosuppressive effects.

Reported uses
Because of its anecdotal use for gastric irritation, licorice derivatives have been studied for antipeptic action. Licorice was also evaluated as a treatment for Addison's disease and was found to enhance mineralocorticoid activity but could not mimic it when adrenal activity was absent.

Glycyrrhizic acid has been used as a shampoo to reduce sebum secretion from the scalp and for cold sores, eczema, and mouth ulcers.

In the United States, glycyrrhizin is used mainly as a flavoring and sweetening agent for bitter drugs, and in beverages, candies, chewing gum, tobacco products, and toothpastes. It is also added to some cough and cold preparations for its expectorant and demulcent effects.

Dosage
For peptic ulcer, 200 to 600 mg P.O. of glycyrrhizin daily for no longer than 6 weeks, according to the German Commission E.

The following tea is believed to provide glycyrrhizin in the middle of this dosage range: 1 tsp (2 to 4 g) of crude licorice to ½ cup (120 ml) of boiling water, simmered for 5 minutes. Cool, strain, and take P.O. t.i.d. after food.

Adverse reactions
CNS: *hypertensive encephalopathy* (Russo et al., 2000).
CV: *heart failure and cardiac arrest* (with overdose), *ventricular tachycardia* (Eriksson et al., 1999).
EENT: transient visual loss and disturbances after ingestion of ¼ to 2 lb of licorice candy (Dobbins and Saul, 2000).
Endocrine: growth retardation (Doeker and Andler, 1999), reduced serum testosterone levels (Armanini et al., 1999).
GU: renal tubular damage (Ishikawa et al., 1999).
Metabolic: hypokalemia (Ishikawa et al., 1999), pseudoprimary hyperaldosteronism (Heilmann et al., 1999).
Musculoskeletal: muscle weakness (with hypokalemia), myopathies, rhabdomyolysis.
Respiratory: *pulmonary edema* (Chamberlain and Abolnik, 1997).

Interactions
Antihypertensives, diuretics: May increase hypokalemic effects of some diuretics. Avoid administration with licorice.
Corticosteroids (including topicals): May increase effects. Use together cautiously.
Digoxin: May induce hypokalemia; risk of digitalis toxicity. Avoid administration with licorice.
Loratadine, procainamide, quinidine, other drugs that may prolong QT interval: May have additive effects. Use together cautiously.
Spironolactone: May block ulcer-healing and aldosterone-like effects of licorice. Avoid administration with licorice.

Contraindications and precautions
Licorice is contraindicated in patients with arrhythmias; CV, renal, or hepatic disease; or hypertension. Avoid using it in pregnant or breast-feeding patients; effects are unknown. Use cautiously under medical supervision in elderly patients.

Special considerations
• Monitor for hypokalemia in the patient receiving diuretics.
• A single large dose of licorice is less likely to cause toxicity than prolonged intake of smaller amounts.
🞂 **ALERT** Licorice poisoning may be insidious. Monitor for pseudoprimary hyperaldosteronism causing mineralocorticoid-like effects (headache, lethargy, sodium and water retention, hypokalemia, hypertension, and heart failure). Monitor for electrolyte (potassium, calcium, and sodium) imbalances, alkalosis, electrocardiographic abnormalities, and hypertension.
• Caution the patient about the dangers of excessive and chronic licorice intake, including fluid retention and electrolyte imbalances.
• Inform the patient of potential drug interactions.

Points of interest
• Licorice has been used medicinally since Roman times and is popular in Chinese herbal medicine.
• Most "licorice candy" sold in the United States is flavored with anise oil and does not actually contain licorice.

Commentary
Although licorice derivatives have been studied for use against peptic ulcer disease, such products have not performed better than H_2 antagonists and may be less well tolerated. Glycyrrhetic acid may play a role in increasing the topical action of low-potency steroids while minimizing systemic effects, but this research is still preliminary. Glycyrrhetic acid is the chief cause of licorice-induced pseudo-hyperaldosteronism syndrome seen with licorice ingestion, because of its inhibitory effect on the enzyme 11beta-hydroxysteroid dehydrogenase. Surprisingly, licorice in any form, even as candy, should be considered cautiously because chronic ingestion of low doses as well as high doses can be toxic, exemplified by a multitude of serious adverse events documented in the literature.

References

Armanini, D., et al. "Reduction of Serum Testosterone in Men by Licorice," *N Engl J Med* 341(15):1158, 1999. Letter.

Bardhan, K.D., et al. "Clinical Trial of Deglycyrrhizinised Licorice in Gastric Ulcer," *Gut* 19:779-82, 1978.

Chamberlain, J.J., and Abolnik, I.Z. "Pulmonary Edema Following a Licorice Binge," *West J Med* 167(3):184-85, 1997.

Davis, E.A., and Morris, D.J. "Medicinal Uses of Licorice Through the Millennia: The Good and Plenty of It," *Mol Cell Endocrinol* 78:1-6, 1991.

Dobbins, K.R., and Saul, R.F. "Transient Visual Loss After Licorice Ingestion," *J Neuroophthalmol* 20(1):38-41, 2000.

Doeker, B.M., and Andler, W. "Liquorice, Growth Retardation and Addison's Disease," *Horm Res* 52(5):253-55, 1999.

Eriksson, J.W., et al. "Life-threatening Ventricular Tachycardia Due to Licorice-induced Hypokalemia," *J Intern Med* 245(3):307-10, 1999.

Heilmann, P., et al. "Administration of Glycyrrhetinic Acid: Significant Correlation Between Serum Levels and the Cortisol/Cortisone-Ratio in Serum and Urine," *Exp Clin Endocrinol Diabetes* 107(6):370-78, 1999.

Ishikawa, S., et al. "Licorice-induced Hypokalemic Myopathy and Hypokalemic Renal Tubular Damage in Anorexia Nervosa," *Int J Eat Disord* 26(1):111-14, 1999.

LaBrooy, S.J., et al. "Controlled Comparison of Cimetidine and Carbenoxolone Sodium in Gastric Ulcer," *BMJ* 1:1308-9, 1979.

Marks, I.N. "Current Therapy in Peptic Ulcer," *Drugs* 20:283-99, 1980.

Maxton, D.G., et al. "Controlled Trial of Pyrogastrone and Cimetidine in the Treatment of Reflux Oesophagitis," *Gut* 31:351-54, 1990.

Russo, S., et al. "Low Doses of Licorice Can Induce Hypertension Encephalopathy," *Am J Nephrol* 20(2):145-48, 2000.

LILY-OF-THE-VALLEY

CONVALLARIA, JACOB'S LADDER, LADDER TO HEAVEN, LILY
CONSTANCY, LILY CONVALLE, MALE LILY, MAY LILY,
MUGUET, OUR LADY'S TEARS

Taxonomic class
Liliaceae

Common trade names
None known.

Common forms
Available as extracts.

Source
Active components are derived from leaves, roots, and flowers of *Convallaria majalis,* a low-growing perennial herb that is native to Europe and naturalized throughout North America.

Chemical components
The entire plant contains cardiac glycosides (convallatoxol, convallotoxin, convallarin, convallamarin, locundjosid, and convallosid—which transforms into convallatoxin when dried), volatile oil, saponins, asparagin, resin, rutin, chelidonic acid, calcium oxalate, choline, carotene, and wax.

Actions
Tea made from this herb is claimed to have diuretic, emetic, pyrogenic, and sedative actions. Cardiac effects stem from plant glycosides thought to be less toxic than those of foxglove (digitalis; McGuigan, 1984). The plant was also believed to exert hypoglycemic effects, but studies in diabetic mice have shown this to be false (Swanston-Flatt et al., 1990).

Reported uses
The plant was traditionally used as an antidote to poison gas and as a cardiotonic agent for treating valvular heart disease. Russian herbalists have also reported its use as an antiepileptic. The roots have been used in an ointment to help heal burn wounds and prevent them from scarring. In Germany, the flowers are mixed with raisins and made into wine.

Dosage
No consensus exists.

Adverse reactions
CNS: coma, dizziness, hallucinations, headache, paralysis.
CV: *arrhythmias, heart failure.*
EENT: burning pain in the mouth and throat, mydriasis, increased salivation.
GI: abdominal cramps and pain, diarrhea, nausea, vomiting.
GU: urinary urgency.

Metabolic: hyperkalemia.
Skin: cold, clammy skin; dermatitis (contact with leaves).
Other: *death.*

Interactions
Beta blockers, calcium channel blockers: Increased risk of heart block or bradycardia. Avoid administration with lily-of-the-valley.
Digoxin: May have additive effects. Avoid administration with lily-of-the-valley.

Contraindications and precautions
All parts of the plant are contraindicated.

Special considerations
• Lily-of-the-valley has been used in folk medicine as a digitalis substitute. However, it should not be used for any cardiac condition because of its potential for toxicity and lack of accurate dosage information.
🔻 **ALERT** The entire plant is toxic, causing digitalis-like symptoms. The water in which the cut flowers have been placed can also be toxic. Treatment includes emesis and gastric lavage followed by administration of activated charcoal and sorbitol cathartic as well as supportive care. Perform cardiac monitoring and restore normal sinus rhythm, if necessary, with atropine. Additional effects of plant ingestion may include other rhythm disturbances and hyperkalemia. Treatment is similar to that for digitalis toxicity.
• Advise the patient to consult a health care provider before using herbal preparations because a treatment that has been clinically researched and proved effective may be available.
• Keep lily-of-the-valley out of the reach of children and pets.

Points of interest
• The FDA considers lily-of-the-valley an unsafe and poisonous plant.
• The essential oils of the highly aromatic flowers have been used in perfumes and cosmetics.

Commentary
Digoxin and digitalis preparations are available for treating heart failure and other cardiac conditions. There is little use for a highly toxic, insufficiently studied herbal product that might have a similar therapeutic action.

References
McGuigan, M.A. "Plants—Cardiac Glycosides," *Clin Toxic Rev* 6:1-2, 1984.
Swanston-Flatt, S.K., et al. "Traditional Plant Treatments for Diabetes: Studies in Normal and Streptozotocin Diabetic Mice," *Diabetologia* 33:462-64, 1990.

LOBELIA

ASTHMA WEED, BLADDERPOD, CARDINAL FLOWER,
EYEBRIGHT, GAGROOT, GREAT LOBELIA, INDIAN PINK,
INDIAN TOBACCO, PUKEWEED, RAPUNTIUM INFLATUM,
VOMITWORT

Taxonomic class
Campanulaceae

Common trade names
Bantron Tablets, Dr. Christopher Mullein and Lobelia Massage Oil, Dr.
Christopher Mullein and Lobelia #12 Ointment, Lobelia Capsules,
Lobelia Extract, Lobeline Lozenges, Lobidram Computabs, Nature's
Herbs Lobelia Herb

Common forms
Capsules: 395 mg
Lozenges: 1 mg
Tablets: 2 mg
   Also available as an extract, liquid, ointment, and powder.

Source
The crude drug is primarily extracted from the dried leaves and tops of
Lobelia inflata, which is native to moist woodlands in eastern North
America. Other species include *L. berlandieri, L. cardinalis, L. inflata,*
and *L. siphilitica.*

Chemical components
Lobelia species contain at least 14 piperidine alkaloids. The primary alkaloid occurring in most species is lobeline; *L. cardinalis* has lobinaline
as its primary alkaloid. The emetic alkaloids lobelanine and lobelani-
dine are also found. Lobeline is similar to nicotine, both structurally
and pharmacologically.

Actions
Lobeline is similar to but less potent than nicotine. It acts on nicotine
receptors in the body and readily crosses both the blood barrier and the
placenta. Depending on the receptor site, lobeline produces several
pharmacologic responses. It causes a release of epinephrine and norepinephrine, producing positive inotropic and chronotropic effects on the
myocardium, and increases both systolic and diastolic blood pressure.
   At low doses, lobeline stimulates respiration, and at large doses, it
produces a curare-like effect. When administered at toxic doses, lobeline depresses respiration by inhibiting the respiratory centers in the
brain stem and causing paralysis of the respiratory muscles (Damaj et
al., 1997).
   Lobeline increases gastric acid secretion and GI tone and motility. It
is well absorbed from mucous membranes of the mouth, the GI tract,
and the respiratory system. It is metabolized primarily by the liver, kid-

neys, and lungs and is rapidly eliminated by the kidneys (Westfall and Meldrum, 1986).

Reported uses
Lobelia is claimed to be useful as an antasthmatic, an emetic, and a spasmolytic. Early settlers smoked lobelia to treat asthma, bronchitis, and other respiratory ailments. Some data suggest that lobelia may be useful as a smoking deterrent because of its nicotine-like effects (Rapp and Olen, 1955).

Dosage
As a smoking deterrent, 0.5 to 2 mg P.O. has been used in tablets and lozenges. The usual dose is 2 mg P.O. after each meal with ½ glass of water for no longer than 6 weeks. Doses as high as 8 mg P.O. have been used but caused significant GI distress. Lobeline doses exceeding 20 mg P.O. daily are considered toxic.

Adverse reactions
CNS: dizziness, *seizures,* tremor.
CV: decreased heart rate, hypertension, palpitations.
GI: epigastric discomfort, severe heartburn, nausea, vomiting (high doses).
Metabolic: fluid retention.
Respiratory: cough, *respiratory depression* (high doses) or stimulation (low doses).
Skin: sweating.

Interactions
Nicotine therapy: May potentiate adverse effects of lobeline. Avoid administration with lobeline.

Contraindications and precautions
Lobeline is contraindicated in children and pregnant or breast-feeding patients. Use cautiously in patients with hepatic or renal dysfunction.

Special considerations
• Urge the patient to stop smoking if lobeline is being used to avoid additive effects of nicotine and increased risk of adverse reactions.
• Encourage the patient who smokes to use smoking cessation programs, counseling, behavior modification, nicotine replacement, and other pharmacotherapy to help quit smoking.
🔺 **ALERT** Although less potent than nicotine, all *Lobelia* species should be considered dangerous. Death has occurred from respiratory depression and paralysis of the respiratory muscles. Symptoms of lobeline overdose include coma, extrasystoles, hypotension, hypothermia, muscle spasms, partial bundle-branch block, seizures, sinus arrhythmia, profound sweating, and tachycardia.
• Advise women to avoid using lobeline during pregnancy or when breast-feeding.
• Monitor the patient closely for adverse reactions.

Bold italic type indicates that reaction may be life-threatening.

• Caution the patient to avoid using lobeline for more than 6 weeks because of the lack of data on chronic use.

Points of interest
• The FDA advisory review panel on OTC drugs has classified lobeline as having insufficient data regarding its efficacy as an OTC drug.

Commentary
Because of its similarity to nicotine, lobeline has been used as a smoking deterrent. Long-term data are not available and clinical trials have not been conclusive. Other, safe and effective smoking deterrents are recommended for patients who want to stop smoking. The risk of serious adverse reactions appears to be higher with lobeline than with other clinically proven treatments, and therefore, its use as an herbal smoking cessation treatment is not recommended.

References
Damaj, M.I., et al. "Pharmacology of Lobeline, a Nicotine Receptor Ligand," *J Pharmacol Exp Ther* 282:410-19, 1997.

Rapp, G.W., and Olen, A.A. "A Critical Evaluation of a Lobeline-Based Smoking Deterrent," *Am J Med Sci* 230:9-14, 1955.

Westfall, T.C., and Meldrum, M.J. "Ganglionic Blocking Agents," in *Modern Pharmacology,* 2nd ed. Edited by Craig, C.R., and Stizel, R.E. Boston: Little, Brown, 1986.

LOVAGE

Aetheroleum levistici, Angelica levisticum, Hipposelinum levisticum, MAGGI PLANT, SEA PARSLEY, SMELLAGE

Taxonomic class
Apiaceae

Common trade names
None known.

Common forms
Available as capsules, essential oil, and tea.

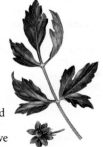

Source
Active components are obtained from the roots and seeds of *Levisticum officinale* and *Levisticum radix.* These plants are found in southern Europe and have been naturalized to the United States.

Chemical components
Lovage root contains essential oil that is primarily composed of phthalide lactones, giving it a characteristic aromatic, spicy odor (Gijbels et al., 1982). Other compounds include coumarins, terpenoids, and volatile acids.

Actions
When given parenterally in animals, lovage oils cause weak diuresis, presumably because of mild irritation of renal tubules. Lovage exerts sedative and spasmolytic effects in rodents and has been reported to stimulate salivation and gastric secretion.

Reported uses
Lovage has been used by herbalists mainly as a diuretic for patients with pedal edema. It is approved in Germany for irrigation therapy in urinary tract inflammation and to prevent renal calculus formation.

The herb is claimed to be useful for gastric discomfort (such as flatulence), as a spasmolytic and a sedative, to dissolve phlegm in the respiratory tract, and to induce menstruation.

Dosage
Tea: 1 cup (150 ml) of boiling water is poured into 1.5 to 3 g of finely cut root of *L. radix* and drained after 15 minutes. Dose is 4 to 8 g/day P.O.

Adverse reactions
Skin: photodermatosis (caused by furocoumarin compounds in leaves).

Interactions
Anticoagulants: May potentiate effects. Avoid administration with lovage.

Contraindications and precautions
Avoid using lovage in pregnant or breast-feeding patients; effects are unknown. Use cautiously in patients with a history of plant allergies.

Special considerations
• Monitor BUN and serum electrolyte and creatinine levels periodically during herbal therapy.
• Inform the patient taking lovage for its diuretic effect that pedal edema may indicate heart failure or other dangerous conditions. Advise him to undergo a complete physical examination to rule out the need for aggressive medical treatment.
• Inform the patient that other forms of proven diuretics are available.
• Lovage contains a compound known as sotolone (4,5-dimethyl-3-hydroxy-2[5H]-furanone), which has a characteristically sweet aroma. Sotolone has been identified in the urine of patients with maple syrup urine disease. An autosomal recessive inherited disorder of branched-chain amino acid metabolism, it is so named because of the sweet, syruplike odor that is present in body fluids of patients with the disease. Patients who ingest lovage may be mistaken for patients with this unique enzyme deficiency (Podebrad et al., 1999).

Points of interest
• Lovage oil is used as a fragrance in cosmetics, lotions, and soaps.

Commentary
There is some evidence of lovage's therapeutic use in animals, but human clinical trials and efficacy and safety data are lacking. Therefore, this herb cannot be recommended.

References
Gijbels, M.J.M., et al. "Phthalides in the Essential Oil from Roots of *Levisticum officinale*," *Planta Med* 44:207-11, 1982.

Podebrad, F., et al. "4-5,-Dimethyl-3-hydroxy-2[5H]-furanone (Sotolone)—The Odor of Maple Syrup Urine Disease," *J Inherit Metab Dis* 22(2):107-14, 1999.

LUNGMOSS

LOBARIA, LUNG LICHEN, LUNGWORT, LUNGWORT LICHEN, LUNGWORT MOSS, OAK LUNGS, TREE LUNGWORT

Taxonomic class
Pulmonaceae

Common trade names
Herbal trade names are unknown. Combination homeopathic preparations include Chestal, Cough & Cold Formula, HP7, Sinusitis PMD.

Common forms
Available as dried lichen powder, liquid extract, and tincture.

Source
Medicinal preparations are obtained from the dried thallus of the lichen *Lobaria pulmonaria* (syn. *Sticta pulmonaria, S. pulmonaceae*). This herb should not be confused with *Pulmonaria officinalis,* also known as lungwort.

Chemical components
Mucilage (arabitol), gyrophoric acid, stictinic acid, norstictinic acid, thelophoric acid, proteins, ergosterol and fugosterol, aliphatic hydrocarbons, and fatty acids (palmitic, oleic, and linoleic) have been isolated from this lichen.

Actions
The mucilage component of lungmoss imparts demulcent, expectorant, and mucolytic activity. Preparations of the lichen are also reported to exhibit anti-inflammatory, astringent, diaphoretic, orexigenic, and unexplained antibacterial effects. A polysaccharide of *L. pulmonaria* has been shown to possess radioprotective properties (Liu, 1991).

Reported uses
As its name suggests, lungmoss has traditionally been used to treat maladies of the respiratory tract, such as pertussis, pneumonia, and tuberculosis. It is used in herbal medicine to treat asthma, bronchitis, cough (especially in children), headache associated with hay fever and colds, muscle aches caused by influenza and upper respiratory tract infec-

tions, and pulmonary inflammation. A combination homeopathic remedy containing lungmoss was reported to be without adverse effects and, possibly, beneficial for treating sinusitis (Adler, 1999).

Dosage
Dried lichen (may be prepared as infusion): 1 to 2 g P.O. t.i.d.
Liquid extract (1:1 in 25% alcohol): 1 to 2 ml P.O. t.i.d.
Tincture (1:5 in 60% alcohol): 1 to 2 ml P.O. up to q.i.d.

Adverse reactions
None known.

Interactions
None reported.

Contraindications and precautions
Avoid using lungmoss in pregnant or breast-feeding patients; effects are unknown.

Special considerations
● Caution the patient not to self-treat symptoms of respiratory illness before seeking appropriate medical evaluation.
● Although no known chemical interactions have been reported in clinical studies, consideration must be given to the potential for adverse reactions with conventional drugs.
● Advise women to avoid using lungmoss during pregnancy or when breast-feeding.

Points of interest
● Lungmoss is found on old trees and on rocks throughout Europe and is used as an indicator of undisturbed ecosystems in Britain. Its traditional use arose from its physical resemblance to lung tissue; according to the Doctrine of Signatures, it was, therefore, prescribed for respiratory ailments. Lungmoss has a rich history of ethnobotanical use. In British Columbia, the Hesquiat people have used the lichen as a remedy for bloody sputum and arthritis. Hill men in India used lungmoss for curing eczema on the scalp, cleaning and strengthening the hair, and treating pulmonary disorders and hemorrhage. Lungmoss was used in Siberian monasteries for brewing bitter beer and has also been used as a dye and in making French perfume and tanning hides.

Commentary
Because of the lack of published clinical trial data for this product, its use for any therapeutic purpose cannot be recommended.

References
Adler, M. "Efficacy and Safety of a fixed-Combination Homeopathic Therapy for Sinusitis," *Adv Ther* 16:103-11, 1999.
Liu, S. "Radiosensitivity of Marrow Stromal Cells and the Effect of Some Radioprotective Agents," *Chung Kuo I Hsueh Ko Hsueh Yuan Hsueh Pao* 13:338-42, 1991. Abstract.

LUNGWORT

JERUSALEM COWSLIP, JERUSALEM SAGE, LUNG MOSS, LUNGS
OF OAK, SPOTTED COMFREY

Taxonomic class
Boraginaceae

Common trade names
Multi-ingredient preparations: Lungwort
Compound (formerly Bleeders Blend),
Lungwort Essence, Lungwort Herb

Common forms
Available as dried herb, extracts, and tablets.

Source
The drug is obtained from the leaves of *Pulmonaria officinalis*, a member of the borage family.

Chemical components
Lungwort leaves contain allantoin, flavonoids (quercetin and kaempferol), tannins, mucilage, ascorbic acid, saponins, potassium and iron salts, silicic acid, vitamin C, and an anticoagulant glycopeptide.

Actions
Lungwort is claimed to have anti-inflammatory, anti-irritant, antitussive, astringent, emollient, and expectorant actions. Its astringent and anti-inflammatory actions are probably attributed to tannins and flavonoids. When applied topically to wounds, tannins cause precipitation of proteins in the surrounding fluids to form a protective coating.

The nondialyzable fraction of the ammonia extract of lungwort contains a glycopeptide that possesses anticoagulant activity in animals (Byshevskii et al., 1990). Lungwort's antitussive activity may be attributed to its mucilage content. The emollient action may be produced by allantoin. The chemical basis for the plant's expectorant action has not been proved.

Reported uses
Lungwort has been used to treat such pulmonary disorders as bronchitis, coughs, hoarseness, and influenza. In race horses, lungwort is thought to have a strengthening effect on the animal's lungs to enhance performance; the same effect is thought to occur in humans with tuberculosis. These effects could be attributed to the plant's silica content, but there are no data to support these claims. Lungwort has also been claimed to be valuable as an astringent; in treating diarrhea, GI bleeding, hemorrhoids, and hypermenorrhea; and, topically, to promote wound healing.

Dosage
Infusion: 1 or 2 tsp of dried herb steeped in boiling water P.O. t.i.d.
Tincture: 1 to 4 ml P.O. t.i.d.

Adverse reactions
GI: GI irritation.
Hematologic: prolonged bleeding time.
Skin: contact dermatitis.

Interactions
Anticoagulants: May increase effects of warfarin. Avoid administration with lungwort.

Contraindications and precautions
Avoid using lungwort in pregnant or breast-feeding patients; effects are unknown. Also avoid its use in patients receiving anticoagulants. Use cautiously in patients with a history of GI bleeding, hypersensitivity reactions, or thrombocytopenia.

Special considerations
• Monitor PT and INR for increased bleeding time.
• Inform the patient that insufficient data exist to support a therapeutic use for lungwort.
• Encourage the patient with respiratory problems (such as asthma, bronchitis, or emphysema) to pursue conventional medical therapy.

Points of interest
• Historically, lungwort has been used to treat pulmonary ailments because the spotted leaves resemble the lung's surface.

Commentary
The chemical basis for lungwort's pulmonary effects is poorly understood. It may be effective as an astringent because of its tannin content. Because no human studies support the safety and efficacy of lungwort, its use cannot be recommended.

References
Byshevskii, A., et al. "Nature, Properties and the Mechanism of the Effect of Blood Coagulation of the Preparation Obtained from *Pulmonaria officinalis*," *Gematol Transfuziol* 35:6-9, 1990.

LUTEIN

VEGETABLE LUTEOL, VEGETABLE LUTIEN, XANTHOPHYLL

Taxonomic class
Asteraceae

Common trade names
Bo-Xan, Eyebright +, FloraGlo Lutein, and as the dipalmitate ester (helenien) in Adaptinol
Multi-ingredient preparations: Carotene-Power, Lutein Carotenoid Complex Vegicaps, Natural Lutein Lycopene Carotene Complex Softgels, Ocutone, Phytonutrient Carotenoid Complex

---

Common forms
Nondietary sources of lutein are available in solid dosage forms, primarily capsules.

Source
Lutein was first isolated from egg yolks. It may also be isolated from nettles or algae, but most commercial lutein is isolated from the leaves of the Aztec marigold (*Tagetes erecta*) or other marigolds (*Tagetes* spp. L.).

Chemical components
Lutein is a single-chemical entity (beta, epsilon-carotene-3,3'-diol). It is classified as a hydroxycarotenoid and is closely related chemically, botanically, and physiologically to the xanthophyll zeaxanthin.

Actions
The literature on lutein is quite extensive, encompassing both laboratory and clinical data. Physiologically, lutein may play a dietary role by serving as an antioxidant and a component of cellular membranes, contributing to membrane structure and function (Socaciu et al., 2000). Research using cell culture techniques and animal models has demonstrated anticarcinogenic and antimutagenic activity. Specifically, lutein has been shown to inhibit colon carcinogenesis in both mice and rats and mammary tumors in mice.

Although human data are less conclusive, an inverse relationship has been demonstrated between lutein and cancers of the breast, lung, liver (Kozuki et al., 2000), prostate (Cohen et al., 2000), and kidney (Yuan et al., 1998).

A similar inverse relationship has been found between lutein and the incidence of coronary heart disease (Martin et al., 2000), cerebrovascular accident (Suter, 2000), cholestatic hepatic disease (Floreani et al., 2000), neural tube defects (Shaw et al., 1999), diabetes mellitus (Ford et al., 1999), and cognitive impairment (Schmidt et al., 1998). The specific action thought to be responsible for these effects is the antioxidant activity exhibited by lutein, a feature common to most carotenoids.

Lutein is one of the primary pigments in the human retina. It is present in higher concentrations in people with dark eyes and decreases in retinal concentration as the eyes become lighter, with blue-eyed individuals having the lowest concentration. Antioxidant activity in the eye is thought to be responsible for the protection offered by lutein in response to short wavelength visible light. It has also been strongly supported in the literature that lutein decreases age-related macular degeneration and cataract formation (Brown et al., 1999; Chasan-Taber et al., 1999). A second mechanism that may contribute to the retinal protective effects of lutein is its ability to bind to retinal tubulin, thus increasing the retinal concentration of lutein. Other demonstrated actions of lutein include immunomodulatory activity (lymphocyte proliferation and antibody production in older animals; Kim et al., 2000) and enhanced gap junctional communication, both of which may contribute to its anticarcinogenic activity, as well as gastroprotective effects (decreases development of acid-induced mucosal lesions).

Reported uses

The majority of lay literature proposes the benefits of lutein in the prevention or slowing of age-related macular degeneration and its subsequent blindness. Although the evidence is strong for potential benefits in decreasing cancer risk, it is the ophthalmic activity that has historically been promoted. Raised public awareness of the potential protective effects with certain cancers is gaining acceptance and increasing the use of lutein-containing products.

Dosage

No RDA for lutein has been published. Studies that have used lutein have used doses ranging from 6 mg/week to 30 mg/day. Available products contain 7.5 mcg to 15 mg/dosage unit, with the recommended dose usually being 2 capsules P.O. up to t.i.d.

Adverse reactions

None reported.

Interactions

Smoking, ethanol: Decreased lutein concentration. The exact mechanism of these interactions is not known, but it may be related to the oxidation of lutein in response to the effects of either compound. Avoid smoking and alcohol consumption.

Contraindications and precautions

No specific contraindications or precautions have been published for lutein.

Special considerations

• Caution the patient not to self-treat symptoms of macular degeneration or cancer before seeking appropriate medical evaluation because this may delay diagnosis of a serious medical condition.
• Urge the patient to notify the prescriber and pharmacist of any herbal or dietary supplement he is taking when filling a new prescription.

Points of interest

• The bioavailability of lutein may be dependent on several dietary factors, including fat (increased bioavailability; Roodenburg et al., 2000), fiber (decreased bioavailability; Hoffmann et al., 1999), and food type (juices provide greater amount of lutein than fresh or cooked fruits and vegetables; Van Het Hof et al., 2000).

Commentary

The ability of lutein to slow macular degeneration and thus prevent its subsequent blindness is well documented. Also, the potential role of lutein in reducing the risk of certain forms of cancer is compelling. This underscores the importance of inclusion of lutein-rich foods (broccoli,

Brussels sprouts, collards, corn, kale, spinach, and tomatoes) in the diet. For those who want to use lutein as a true dietary supplement (especially those who smoke), common sense should prevail and a dose chosen that would provide additional benefit without undue risk. The literature indicates that lutein in small doses and in combination with other carotenoids provides greater antioxidant activity than any single carotenoid taken alone. Because lutein is a fat-soluble compound, it could bioaccumulate. The effects of vitamin A toxicity are well documented. However, lutein is not converted to vitamin A, and its toxicity profile could differ radically from that of vitamin A. Given the lack of literature on potential lutein toxicity, care should be taken to avoid potential oversupplementation. Regardless of the source (dietary or supplemental), adequate lutein intake probably improves eye and, possibly, overall health. Health care providers should encourage a healthy diet that includes adequate sources of lutein, thus decreasing the need for non-dietary sources. Because some studies indicated a dose-dependent pro-oxidant effect associated with an increased risk for cancer, the International Agency for Research on Cancer published a review stating that "pending further research, . . . lutein. . . should not be recommended for cancer prevention in the general population" (Vainio and Rautalahti, 1998). Reasonable supplementation, especially from dietary sources, should be safe and effective.

References

Bernstein, P.S., et al. "Retinal Tubulin Binds Macular Carotenoids," *Invest Ophthalmol Vis Sci* 8(1):167-75, 1997.

Brown, L., et al. "A Prospective Study of Carotenoid Intake and Risk of Cataract Extraction in U.S. Men," *Am J Clin Nutr* 70(4):517-24, 1999.

Budavari, S., ed. Abstract 9972, in *The Merck Index,* 11th ed. Rahway, N.J.: Merck & Co., 1989.

Chasan-Taber, L., et al. "A Prospective Study of Carotenoid and Vitamin A Intakes and Risk of Cataract Extraction in U.S. Women," *Am J Clin Nutr* 70(4):509-16, 1999.

Chew, B.P., et al. "Effects of Lutein from Marigold Extract on Immunity and Growth of Mammary Tumors in Mice," *Anticancer Res* 16(6B):3689-94, 1996.

Cohen, J.H., et al. "Fruit and Vegetable Intakes and Prostate Cancer Risk," *J Natl Cancer Inst* 92(1):61-68, 2000.

Comstock, G.W., et al. "The Risk of Developing Lung Cancer Associated with Antioxidants in the Blood: Ascorbic Acid, Carotenoids, Alpha-tocopherol, Selenium, and Total Peroxyl Radical Absorbing Capacity," *Cancer Epidemiol Biomarkers Prev* 6(11):907-16, 1997.

Floreani, A., et al. "Plasma Antioxidant Levels in Chronic Cholestatic Liver Disease," *Aliment Pharmacol Ther* 14(3):353-58, 2000.

Ford, E.S., et al. "Diabetes Mellitus and Serum Carotenoids: Findings from the Third National Health and Nutrition Examination Survey," *Am J Epidemiol* 149(2):168-76, 1999.

Hoffmann, J.J., et al. "Dietary Fiber Reduces the Antioxidant Effect of a Carotenoid and Alpha-tocopherol Mixture on LDL Oxidation Ex Vivo in Humans," *Eur J Nutr* 38(6):278-85, 1999.

Howard, A.N., et al. "Do Hydroxy-carotenoids Prevent Coronary Heart Disease? A Comparison Between Belfast and Toulouse," *Int J Vitam Nutr Res* 66(2):113-18, 1996.

Khachik, F., et al. "Identification of Lutein and Zeaxanthin Oxidation Products in Human and Monkey Retinas," *Invest Ophthalmol Vis Sci* 38(9):1802-11, 1997.

Kim, H.W., et al. "Dietary Lutein Stimulates Immune Response in the Canine," *Vet Immunol Immunopathol* 74(3-4):315-27, 2000.

Kim, H.W., et al. "Modulation of Humoral and Cell-mediated Immune Responses by Dietary Lutein in Cats," *Vet Immunol Immunopathol* 73(3-4):331-41, 2000.

Kozuki, Y., et al. "Inhibitory Effects of Carotenoids on the Invasion of Rat Ascites Hepatoma Cells in Culture," *Cancer Lett* 151(1):111-15, 2000.

Landrum, J.T., et al. "A One Year Study of the Macular Pigment: The Effect of 140 Days of a Lutein Supplement," *Exp Eye Res* 65(1):57-62, 1997.

Martin, K.R., et al. "The Effect of Carotenoids on the Expression of Cell Surface Adhesion Molecules and Binding of Monocytes to Human Aortic Endothelial Cells," *Atherosclerosis* 150(2):265-74, 2000.

Roodenburg, A.J., et al. "Amount of Fat in the Diet Affects Bioavailability of Lutein Esters But Not of Alpha-carotene, Beta-carotene, and Vitamin E in Humans," *Am J Clin Nutr* 71(5):1187-93, 2000.

Schmidt, R., et al. "Plasma Antioxidants and Cognitive Performance in Middle-aged and Older Adults: Results of the Austrian Stroke Prevention Study," *J Am Geriatr Soc* 46(11):1407-10, 1998.

Shaw, G.M., et al. "Periconceptional Nutrient Intake and Risk for Neural Tube Defect–Affected Pregnancies," *Epidemiology* 10(6):711-16, 1999.

Snodderly, D.M. "Evidence for Protection Against Age-related Macular Degeneration by Carotenoids and Antioxidant Vitamins," *Am J Clin Nutr* 62(6 Suppl.):1448S-61S, 1995.

Socaciu, C., et al. "Competitive Carotenoid and Cholesterol Incorporation into Liposomes: Effects on Membrane Phase Transition, Fluidity, Polarity, and Anisotropy," *Chem Phys Lipids* 106(1):79-88, 2000.

Stahl, W., et al. "Carotenoid Mixtures Protect Multilamellar Liposomes Against Oxidative Damage: Synergistic Effects of Lycopene and Lutein," *FEBS Lett* 427(2):305-9, 1998.

Suter, P.M. "Effect of Vitamin E, Vitamin C, and Beta-carotene on Stroke Risk," *Nutr Rev* 58(6):184-87, 2000.

Vainio, H., and Rautalahti, M. "An International Evaluation of the Cancer Preventive Potential of Carotenoids," *Cancer Epidemiol Biomarkers Prev* 7(8):725-28, 1998.

Van Het Hof, K.H., et al. "Dietary Factors That Affect the Bioavailability of Carotenoids," *J Nutr* 130(3):503-6, 2000.

Yuan, J.M., et al. "Cruciferous Vegetables in Relation to Renal Cell Carcinoma," *Int J Cancer* 77(2):211-16, 1998.

LYCOPENE

Common trade names

Lyc-O-Cycle, Lyco-O-Mato, Lyc-O-Pen, Lycopene, Lyco-Red, Lycosan, Power-Herbs-Tomato-Power, Radicopene, Tomato Lycopene, Tomato-O-Red

Multi-ingredient preparations: Cellimum, Lady'Mato, Lyco Plus, Nobilin Lyco

---

Bold italic type indicates that reaction may be life-threatening.

Common forms
Capsules and softgels: 5 mg, 6 mg, 10 mg, 15 mg

Source
Lycopene is commonly found in tomatoes and tomato-based foods, such as tomato sauce and spaghetti sauce. Ingestion of concentrated tomato puree provides significantly more lycopene to the body than eating cooked whole tomatoes. Lycopene from intact cells (cooked whole tomato) is less bioavailable than lycopene from processed tomato products (Holloway et al., 2000). An earlier study examining human buccal mucosal cellular content of lycopene seemed to favor supplementation with tomato oleoresin and lycopene beadlets over that with lycopen-rich tomato juice (each containing 70 to 75 mg of lycopene), as far as the agents' ability to increase cellular lycopene (Paetau et al., 1999). Watermelon and guava also contain significant quantities of lycopene.

Chemical components
Lycopene is a carotenoid and belongs to the same family of antioxidants as beta-carotene and vitamin A.

Actions
Lycopene possesses antioxidant properties (Rao and Agarwal, 1998). In vitro evidence suggests that lycopene may have free radical–trapping properties, be a scavenger of singlet oxygen and peroxyl radicals, or exert a combination of these effects. Notably, lycopene supplementation (15 mg/day) resulted in a decrease in the levels of the essential fatty acid linoleic acid in a study of 23 healthy subjects (Wright et al., 1999). Studies evaluating the bioavailability of lycopene in plasma after ingestion of tomato juice, tomato oleoresin, or lycopene beadlets found that plasma lycopene levels increased to a similar degree with all treatments in 15 healthy subjects. Elevations of plasma lycopene levels were about 0.23 to 0.24 micromol/L for all entities and were found to be statistically significant from placebo (Paetau et al., 1998).

Reported uses
Lycopene has been suggested to be a potential anticancer agent based on its antioxidant status. Some population studies have associated a decreased risk of cancer with dietary intake of tomatoes, a major source of lycopene (Rao and Agarwal, 1998). In a comprehensive review of the available evidence for lycopene or tomato-based foods, Giovannucci (1999) determined that about one-half of the epidemiological studies available (35 of 72) showed statistically significant benefits favoring diets high in lycopene or tomato-based foods. This evidence for a cancer-protective role was highest for cancers of the prostate, lungs, and stomach but also seemed to confer protection against cancers of the pancreas, colon, and rectum. The data from these studies are primarily observational and, therefore, do not necessarily prove a cause-effect relationship.

One trial examined lycopene's potential effects on lipoprotein oxidation (Agarwal and Rao, 1998). Dietary supplementation with tomato juice, tomato oleoresin, or spaghetti sauce had no effect on the lipid profile as far as LDL, HDL, or total cholesterol level. It was determined, however, that serum lipid peroxidation and LDL oxidation were significantly decreased (Agarwal and Rao, 1998).

Dosage
No consensus exists. Manufacturers of lycopene dietary supplements recommend anywhere from 5 to 15 mg/day of lycopene P.O.

Adverse reactions
None reported.

Interactions
Trace element (zinc 20 mg, selenium 100 mcg) supplementation: Serum lycopene levels were significantly decreased in a large population of institutionalized elderly subjects (Galan et al., 1997). Avoid administration with lycopene.

Contraindications and precautions
Avoid using lycopene in pregnant or breast-feeding patients; effects are unknown. Also avoid its use in patients who are allergic to tomatoes or tomato-based foods.

Special considerations
• Inform the patient that modern medicine cannot guarantee the prevention of certain cancers simply by ingestion of tomatoes or tomato-based foods or by lycopene supplementation. Such factors as the environment and genetics play a role in the incidence and development of cancer.
• Urge the patient to eat a balanced diet that includes foods that contain carotenoids (such as beta-carotene and lycopene). This is probably the best recommendation that can be made for general, overall good health and cancer prevention.
• Urge the patient to notify the prescriber and pharmacist of any herbal or dietary supplement he is taking when filling a new prescription.
• Avoid using lycopene in pregnant or breast-feeding patients.

Points of interest
• The tomato was once referred to as the "Apple of Paradise."
• A medium-sized California tomato contains about 40% of the RDA for vitamin C.

Commentary
Lycopene is an interesting antioxidant that is related to beta-carotene and other carotenoids. Its role in cancer protection has been suggested by in vitro investigations and epidemiological studies that link dietary intake of tomatoes with a reduced risk of cancer development. Data describing this relation (beneficial effect) come from observational, epidemiological studies and, therefore, must be interpreted with caution. Studies such as these do not prove a cause-effect relationship but mere-

ly suggest rationale for future prospective investigations. Many other chemicals present in tomatoes and tomato-based foods may be responsible for the cancer benefit rather than lycopene. Which source (lycopene supplementation versus tomato foodstuffs) provides the most "usable" lycopene remains a subject of debate. Long-term, prospective trials examining cancer rates and dietary supplements are needed before intake of oral dosage forms can be recommended routinely for cancer prevention.

References
Agarwal, A., and Rao, A.V. "Tomato Lycopene and Low Density Lipoprotein Oxidation: A Human Dietary Intervention Study," *Lipids* 33(10):981-84, 1998.

Galan, P., et al. "Effects of Trace Element and/or Vitamin Supplementation on Vitamin and Mineral Status, Free Radical Metabolism and Immunological Markers in Elderly Long-term Hospitalized Subjects," *Int J Vitam Nutr Res* 67(6):450-60, 1997.

Giovannucci, E. "Tomatoes, Tomato-based Products, Lycopene, and Cancer: Review of the Epidemiologic Literature," *J Natl Cancer Inst* 91(4):317-31, 1999.

Holloway, D.E., et al. "Isomerization of Dietary Lycopene During Assimilation and Transport in Plasma," *Free Radic Res* 32(1):93-102, 2000.

Paetau, I., et al. "Carotenoids in Human Buccal Mucosa Cells After 4 Weeks of Supplementation with Tomato Juice or Lycopene Supplements," *Am J Clin Nutr* 70(4):490-94, 1999.

Paetau, I., et al. "Chronic Ingestion of Lycopene-rich Tomato Juice or Lycopene Supplements Significantly Increases Plasma Concentrations of Lycopene and Related Tomato Carotenoids in Humans," *Am J Clin Nutr* 68(6):1187-95, 1998.

Rao, A.V., and Agarwal, S. "Bioavailability and In Vivo Antioxidant Properties of Lycopene from Tomato Products and Their Possible Role in Prevention of Cancer," *Nutr Cancer* 31(3):199-203, 1998.

Wright, A.J., et al. "Beta-carotene and Lycopene, But Not Lutein, Supplementation Changes the Plasma Fatty Acid Profile of Healthy Male Non-smokers," *J Lab Clin Med* 134(6):592-98, 1999.

LYSINE

L-LYSINE

Common trade names
Lysine Ascorbs, L-Lysine Capsules, Lysine Extra, L-Lysine Tablets

Common forms
Available as dietary supplements in the form of capsules and tablets.

Source
An essential amino acid that can be derived from such food sources as meat, poultry, fish, dairy products, wheat germ, and soy.

Chemical components
Lysine is a naturally occurring essential amino acid in the body.

Actions
Lysine may aid the body in absorbing and maintaining calcium (Civitelli et al., 1992). Together with other essential amino acids, lysine aids in maintaining growth, lean body mass, and nitrogen stores.

Reported uses
As an essential amino acid, lysine has been suggested to help in treating diarrhea, diverticulitis, heartburn, heart disease, hypertension, low immunity, indigestion, infertility, intermittent claudication, and prostate problems and as an aid in wound healing. Uncontrolled human studies have suggested that lysine is also effective in treating herpes simplex infections (Curry, 1980; Griffith et al., 1978).

Dosage
For herpes simplex infections, 1 to 6 g/day P.O. (Werbach and Murray, 1994).

Adverse reactions
None reported.

Interactions
None reported.

Contraindications and precautions
Avoid using lysine in pregnant or breast-feeding patients; effects are unknown.

Special considerations
• Although no known chemical interactions have been reported in clinical studies, consideration must be given to the pharmacologic properties of the herbal product and the potential for exacerbation of the intended therapeutic effect of conventional drugs.
• Advise the patient to consult a health care provider before using this herbal preparation as a treatment for herpes simplex .
• Urge the patient to notify the prescriber and pharmacist of any herbal or dietary supplement he is taking when filling a new prescription.
• Advise pregnant or breast-feeding patients to avoid using lysine.

Points of interest
• In animals, high doses have been reported to increase the risk of gallstone formation and elevate cholesterol levels (Lininger, 1998). A 1% solution of lysine added to chick amniotic fluid resulted in muscle spasticity and weakness in the chick legs, but the total dose of lysine is unknown (Bergstrom et al., 1970).

Commentary
Because no adequate clinical data support lysine's various therapeutic claims, it cannot be recommended for any use.

Bold italic type indicates that reaction may be life-threatening.

References

Bergstrom, R.M., et al. "Teratogenic Effects of Lysine in the Chicken," *Naturwissenschaften* 57:134, 1970.

Civitelli, R., et al. "Dietary L-lysine and Calcium Metabolism in Humans," *Nutrition* 8:400-4, 1992.

Curry, S.S. "Cutaneous Herpes Simplex Infections and Their Treatment," *Cutus* 26:41-58, 1980.

Griffith, R.S., et al. "A Multicentered Study of Lysine Therapy in Herpes Simplex Infection," *Dermatologica* 156:257-67, 1978.

Lininger, S., ed. *The Natural Pharmacy*. Rocklin, Calif.: Prima Health Publishing, 1998.

Werbach, M.R., and Murray, M.T. *Botanical Influences on Illness: A Sourcebook of Clinical Research.* Tarzana, Calif.: Third Line Press, 1994.

MADDER

DYER'S-MADDER, FARBERROTE, GARANCE, KRAPP,
MADDER ROOT, ROBBIA, *RUBIAE TINCTORUM RADIX*

Taxonomic class
Rubiaceae

Common trade names
Multi-ingredient preparations: Madder Whole Root,
Nephrubin, Rubia Teep, Rubicin, Uralyt

Common forms
Available as dried root, fluidextract, and root
powder.

Source
The crude drug is obtained from the dried roots of
Rubia tinctorum. The plant is native to parts of the Mediterranean,
Europe, and Asia and naturalized to areas of North America.

Chemical components
Madder root contains anthraquinone derivatives (ruberythric acid,
alizarin, and purpurin), glycosides (including alizarinprimeveroside
and lucidinprimeveroside, which is converted to lucidin), an iridoid
(asperuloside), resin, and calcium.

Actions
Madder is claimed to have antispasmodic, diuretic, and renal calculus–
inhibiting properties. *R. tinctorum* preparations have proved to be genotoxic in rats (Blomeke et al., 1992) and to form DNA adducts in murine
liver, kidney, duodenum, and colon tissue (Poginsky et al., 1991). No
acute or subacute toxicity was found when fresh madder root extract was
added to the diet of mice over a 3-month period (Ino et al., 1995); however, rats that for 2 years were fed a diet that contained madder root experienced dose-dependent increases in benign and malignant liver and kidney tumor formation (Westendorf et al., 1998). Purpurin has been reported to possess antimutagenic properties (Marczylo et al., 2000).

Reported uses
Madder was traditionally used to treat amenorrhea, jaundice, paralysis,
renal disorders, and sciatica. It is now used in herbal medicine to prevent or treat calcium-containing calculi in the kidneys and bladder.
Calcium oxalate crystallization and stone formation have reportedly
been inhibited in the kidneys of rats and rabbits by dietary intake of

fresh madder root. In a rabbit model, administration of anthraquinone derivatives from *R. tinctorum* was found to reduce the rate of calculus formation in the bladder (Berg et al., 1976).

Dosage
The German Commission E reports a dose of 30 mg of hydroxyanthracene derivatives P.O., calculated as ruberythric acid. Other sources suggest 20 gtt of fluidextract or 1 capsule (from dried root tincture) P.O. t.i.d. for up to 2 months.

Adverse reactions
Other: red color of bone, breast milk, perspiration, saliva, tears, or urine.

Interactions
None reported.

Contraindications and precautions
Madder is contraindicated in pregnant or breast-feeding patients because of mutagenic potential.

Special considerations
• Caution the patient about the dangers associated with madder use, especially if treatment is prolonged.

▲ **ALERT**   Madder has been shown to be carcinogenic, genotoxic, and mutagenic in rodents.

• Instruct women to report planned or suspected pregnancy.

• Advise women to avoid using madder during pregnancy or when breast-feeding.

• Inform the patient who wears contact lenses that madder consumption may stain the lenses.

Points of interest
• Madder was formerly cultivated for the red dye (alizarin) obtained from its roots. Cloth dyed with madder has been found on Egyptian mummies. Madder also was used to color the trousers of French soldiers and Turkish fezzes. The production of synthetic alizarin ceased the demand for the natural product.

• Alizarin colors bone red and was used as a histologic stain in the 1800s to trace bone development and bone cell function.

Commentary
Because of a lack of documented human safety and efficacy and the potential for carcinogenicity and genotoxicity, the use of madder is strongly discouraged.

References
Berg, W., et al. "Influence of Anthraquinones on the Formation of Urinary Calculi in Experimental Animals," *Urologe [A]* 15:188-91, 1976. Abstract, author's translation.

Blomeke, B., et al. "Formation of Genotoxic Metabolites from Anthraquinone Glycosides Present in *Rubia tinctorum* L.," *Mutat Res* 265:263-72, 1992.

Bold italic type indicates that reaction may be life-threatening.

Ino, N., et al. "Acute and Subacute Toxicity Tests of Madder Root, Natural Colorant Extracted from Madder (*Rubia tinctorum*), in (C57BL/6 X C3H)F1 Mice," *Toxicol Ind Health* 11:449-58, 1995.

Marczylo, T., et al. "Protection Against Trp-P-2 Mutagenicity by Purpurin: Mechanism of In Vitro Antimutagenesis," *Mutagenesis* 15:223-28, 2000. Abstract.

Poginsky, B., et al. "Evaluation of DNA-Binding Activity of Hydroxyanthraquinones Occurring in *Rubia tinctorum* L.," *Carcinogenesis* 12:1265-71, 1991.

Westendorf, J., et al. "Carcinogenicity and DNA Adduct Formation Observed in ACI Rats After Long-term Treatment with Madder Root, *Rubia tinctorum* L.," *Carcinogenesis* 19:2163-68, 1998.

MAGNOLIA

MAGNOLIA FLOWER BUD: FLOS MAGNOLIAE, *MAGNOLIA BIONDII*, *MAGNOLIA DENUDATA*, OTHER SPECIES OF *MAGNOLIA*. MAGNOLIA BARK: BEAVER TREE, HOLLY BAY, HOU PO, INDIAN BARK, *MAGNOLIA OBOVATA*, *MAGNOLIA GLAUCA*, RED OR WHITE BAY, SWAMP LAUREL, SWAMP SASSAFRAS, SWEET BAY, WHITE LAUREL

Taxonomic class
Magnoliaceae

Common trade names
None known.

Common forms
Available as liquid extract and powder.

Source
Indigenous to North America, magnolia's medicinal parts are derived from the bark of the stem and root. The main active components are obtained from the bark of several magnolia species; the flower bud is also used in Chinese medicine. Drying and age cause its volatile, aromatic properties to be lost.

Chemical components
The active components found in the bark are alkaloids (for example, magnocurarine and tubocurarine) and essential oils (for example, magnolol, tetrahydromagnolol, isomagnolol, machiolol, and honokiol).

Actions
Components of magnolia bark have been studied in vitro and in animals for antimicrobial activity in the treatment of periodontal disease (Chang et al., 1998), for antifungal activity (Bang et al., 2000), and as antitumorigenic promoters (Konoshima et al., 1991). The lignans isolated from the flower buds have been studied for their inhibitory effects on tumor necrosis factor–alpha production (Chae et al., 1998). Few, if any, data exist from human clinical trials. Magnolol, the active principle of the herb, has anti-inflammatory properties and has been shown to

---

reduce prostaglandin E_2 and leukotriene-B_4 levels in the pleural fluid of mice and to suppress thromboxane-B_2 formation (Huang, 1999).

Decoctions made from magnolia have been cited to cause uterine contractions.

Reported uses
Magnolia has been claimed to be useful as an antasthmatic, an anti-inflammatory, a muscle relaxant, and a stimulant. Its use has also been suggested for appetite stimulation, digestive disorders, dysentery, flatulence, nausea, and shortness of breath.

Dosage
No standard dosing is available.

Adverse reactions
Other: allergic reaction.

Interactions
None reported.

Contraindications and precautions
Magnolia is contraindicated in pregnancy because of empiric uterine-stimulating activity (flower buds).

Special considerations
• Although primary allergy to magnolia is seldom reported, caution the hypersensitive patient to be wary of allergic reactions to magnolia. One patient, described as having allergies to several sesquiterpene lactone-containing plants, experienced a severe case of chronic lichenfied dermatitis to *Magnolia grandiflora* (Guin, 1990).
• Advise the patient to consult a health care provider before using herbal preparations because a treatment that has been clinically researched and proved effective may be available.
• Advise the pregnant patient not to ingest magnolia.

Points of interest
• A report in an FDA bulletin suggests that a *M. stephania* preparation may lead to acute renal failure and, possibly, permanent renal dysfunction.
• The genus *Magnolia* is named after Pierre Magnol, a professor of medicine and botany at Montpellier in the early 18th century.

Commentary
Although magnolia is popular in Chinese medicine, scientific information from human trials to support its pharmacologic actions does not exist. Evidence to support claims is lacking. More research is needed before definitive recommendations can be made.

References
Bang, K.H., et al. "Anti-fungal Activity of Magnolol and Honokiol," *Arch Pharm Res* 23(1):46-49, 2000.

Chae, S.H., et al. "Isolation and Identification of Inhibitory Compounds on TNF-alpha Oroduction from *Magnolia fargesii*," *Arch Pharm Res* 21(1):67-69, 1998.

Chang, B., et al. "Anti-microbial Activity of Magnolol and Honokiol Against Perio-dontopathic Microorganisms," *Planta Med* 64(4):367-69, 1998. Letter.

Guin, J.D. "*Magnolia grandiflora* dermatitis," *Dermatol Clin* 8(1):81-84,1990.

Huang, K.C. *Hou Po: The Dried Bark of Magnolia officinalis. The Pharmacology of Chinese Herbs,* 2nd ed. Boca Raton, Fla.: CRC Press, 1999.

Konoshima, T., et al. "Studies on Inhibitors of Skin Tumor Promotion. Part 9. Neo-lignans from *Magnolia officinalis*," *J Natl Prod* 54(3):816-22, 1991.

MAIDENHAIR FERN

FIVE-FINGER FERN, HAIR OF VENUS, MAIDEN FERN, ROCK FERN, VENUS HAIR

Taxonomic class
Adiantoideae

Common trade names
None known.

Common forms
Available in decoctions, infusions, syrups, and teas.

Source
Maidenhair fern, *Adiantum capillis-veneris (A. pedatum),* is a member of the Adiantoideae family of ferns. It is native to eastern Asia and North America but has been naturalized throughout Europe as well. Related species may be found throughout the world. The fern typically grows about 1' high. The stems are darkly colored with 6" fronds composed of alternate, triangular, and oblong (or fan-shaped) notched pinnae. The aerial portions of the fern are used to make decoctions, infusions, syrups, and teas.

Chemical components
Maidenhair fern's numerous constituents, including volatile oils, sugars, tannins, mucilages, and bitters, have been poorly characterized. Triterpenoids, beta-sitosterol, stigmasterol, and capesterol have also been isolated from the fern (Berti et al., 1969; Marino et al., 1989).

Actions
There are no clinical or laboratory data describing known actions of maidenhair fern or its constituents. All purported actions are anecdotal.

Reported uses
Historically, maidenhair fern has been used to treat various pulmonary cattarhs (asthma, cough, pleurisy) and renal disorders (gravel) and as a hair-darkener and restorer. Modern recommendations for its use include alopecia, bronchitis, dysmenorrhea, and whooping cough and as an expectorant and a refrigerant drink for erysipelas and fever. Numerous

---

Bold italic type indicates that reaction may be life-threatening.

other uses are mentioned in the lay literature. There is no evidence to support its use in any disease state.

Dosage
Decoction and infusion: 1 to 4 fl oz P.O.
Syrup: 1 or 2 tbsp P.O.
Tea: 1.5 g in 150 ml of water P.O.

Adverse reactions
GI: vomiting.
Other: allergic reaction.

Interactions
None reported.

Contraindications and precautions
Maidenhair fern is contraindicated in pregnant patients.

Special considerations
• Caution the patient not to self-treat symptoms of respiratory illness before seeking appropriate medical evaluation because this may delay diagnosis of a serious medical condition.
• Although no known chemical interactions have been reported in clinical studies, consideration must be given to the pharmacologic properties of the herbal product and the potential for exacerbation of the intended therapeutic effect of conventional drugs.
• Urge the patient to notify the prescriber and pharmacist of any herbal or dietary supplement he is taking when filling a new prescription.

Points of interest
• About 9,500 species of ferns exist. The genus *Adiantum* has more than 200 species of ferns. The American Fern Society, which is more than 100 years old, provides information and specimens (spores) to those who are interested in cultivating ferns.

Commentary
The use of maidenhair fern is regulated in the United States, and it is permitted to be used only as a flavoring agent in alcoholic beverages (McGuffin et al., 1997). Some sources indicate that if maidenhair fern is taken in small quantities, there is no reason to expect adverse drug, herb, or food interactions (Jellin et al., 1999). Because laboratory and clinical data on potential mechanisms of action, pharmacodynamic effects, therapeutic benefits, toxicity profiles, and interactions are lacking, there is no basis for recommending maidenhair fern for any reason.

References
Berti, G., et al. "Structure and Stereochemistry of a Triterpenoid Epoxide from Adiantum capillus-veneris," *Tetrahedon* 25(15):2939-47, 1969

Grieve, M. *Maidenhair, True in A Modern Herbal.* Chatham, Kent: Jonathan Cape, Ltd., 1931, pp. 303-4.

Jellin, J.M., et al. "Maidenhair Fern," in *Pharmacist's Letter/Prescriber's Letter Natural Medicines Comprehensive Database.* Stockton, Calif.: Therapeutic Research Faculty, 1999, p. 611.

Kofler, H., et al. "Fern Allergy," *Allergy* 55(3):299-300, 2000.

Marino, A., et al. "Phytochemical Investigation of Adiantum capillus veneris," *Boll Soc Ital Biol Sper* 65(5):461-63, 1989.

McGuffin, M., et al. "*Adiantum pedatum* L.," in *American Herbal Products Association's Botanical Safety Handbook.* Boca Raton, Fla.: CRC Press, 1997, p 4.

MALE FERN

BEAR'S PAW ROOT, ERKEK EGRELTI, HELECHO MACHO, KNOTTY BRAKE, MALE SHIELD FERN, SWEET BRAKE, WURMFARN

Taxonomic class
Malvaceae

Common trade names
Aspidium Oleoresin, Bontanifuge, Extractum Filicis, Extractum Filicis Aethereum, Extractum Filicis Maris Tenue, Male Fern Oleoresin, Paraway Plus

Common forms
Extract: 1.5% to 22% filicin
Male fern extract draught: 4 g of male fern extract
   Also available as single-ingredient or combination-product capsules.

Source
The drug is prepared from the dried rhizomes (runners) and roots of *Dryopteris filix-mas,* a perennial fern that grows in Europe, Asia, North America, South America, and northern Africa. Fresh rhizomes are treated with ether to yield the active components. When stored, the rhizomes lose pharmacologic activity in about 6 months.

Chemical components
The active components consist of ether-soluble derivatives of phloroglucinol. Filicic and flavaspidic acids are mainly responsible for the plant's pharmacologic activity and are inactivated in an alkaline environment. Other compounds include volatile oils, tannin, albaspidin, and desaspidin. Filicin is the collective name given to the mixture of ether-soluble substances obtained in the drug assay and extract. An ethereal extract of European plant material contains about 25% filicin, whereas Indian plant material contains about 30% filicin.

Actions
Male fern is well known for its anthelmintic action. (See *Efficacy of male fern extracts against tapeworms.*) Several in vivo trials in humans have been conducted describing successful expulsion of *Taenia solium* (pork tapeworm), *T. saginata* (beef tapeworm), and *Diphyllobothrium latum* (fish tapeworm) after treatment with the plant extracts. In the 1950s

---

Bold italic type indicates that reaction may be life-threatening.

RESEARCH FINDINGS

Efficacy of male fern extracts against tapeworms

Two studies evaluated the efficacy of male fern extract in patients who didn't respond to other anthelmintics. The eradication cure rate of pork and beef tapeworm was studied in 100 patients ages 5 to 68; the appearance of scoleces (tapeworm heads and mouth parts) in feces after treatment signalled successful therapy. Adults received 6 to 7 g of male fern ethereal extract and children were given 0.25 to 0.50 g for each year of age; the maximum dose was 7 g. The drug was administered by duodenal intubation. Based on the appearance of scoleces, the cure rate achieved was 97%. Three patients in this study experienced adverse effects (nausea and vomiting), but no one experienced intolerance to the extract (Alterio, 1969).

In another study, the effect of male fern against fish tapeworm was tested against three prescribed agents (Laparin, Antiphen, and pumpkin seeds) for tapeworm infestations (Palva, 1963). Although clinical efficacy (expulsion of tapeworms) occurred in all treatment groups, the clinical cure rate (no microscopic evidence of ova in feces) for *Extractum filicis,* Laparin, Antiphen, and pumpkin seeds was 95%, 35%, 52%, and 0%, respectively. The author believed that reinfection couldn't be a cause of finding ova in stools during follow-up examination and attributed the poor results to inferior anthelmintic activity for these substances (except male fern).

Another study (Mello et al., 1978) examined the efficacy of male fern ethereal extract in 29 patients aged 12 to 60 who had not previously responded to other anthelmintic therapy. The patients received the extract orally, preceded by a hypertonic magnesium sulfate solution. Three cases revealed *Taenia solium* and 26 cases revealed *T. saginata.* The total cure rate was 86%; the cure rates from specific groups weren't provided.

and 1960s, mepacrine (quinacrine), dichlorophen, and niclosamide were commonly used to expel tapeworms. Male fern is thought to have fewer adverse effects than those drugs and to achieve a better cure rate when given by duodenal tube.

Dryopteris phlorophenone derivatives were studied in vitro and in vivo for antitumorigenic activity against the Epstein-Barr virus antigen. Among the 33 phlorophenone derivatives tested, aspidin and desaspidin were found to be most active in vitro and showed significant antitumorigenic activity in the mouse. The percentage of induced papillomas per mouse decreased by 50% after 10 to 20 weeks of topical therapy; papilloma production was also reduced (Kapadia et al., 1996).

Reported uses

Male fern is known as a remedy for intestinal tapeworms. The patient typically received a light diet (to starve the worm) and a laxative the evening before treatment. On arising and before eating, the patient was given male fern and another laxative.

Dosage

Adults (fasting state): 3 to 6 ml P.O.
Children over age 2: 0.25 to 0.5 ml P.O. per year of age; maximum, 4 ml P.O. in divided doses.
Children up to age 2: up to 2 ml P.O. in divided doses.

Male fern draught may be given by duodenal tube in a dose of 50 ml to limit GI intolerance. Treatment may need to be repeated. Seven to 10 days should elapse between treatments. Male fern may be given as capsules but is considered more effective as a draught.

Adverse reactions

CNS: headache.
GI: abdominal cramps (severe), diarrhea, nausea, vomiting.
GU: albuminuria.
Metabolic: hyperbilirubinemia (in animals and humans).
Respiratory: dyspnea.

Interactions

Antacids: Inactivate male fern. Avoid taking male fern within 1 to 2 hours of taking an antacid.
Fats, oils (such as castor oil): May increase absorption and risk of toxicity. Avoid administration with male fern.
Proton pump inhibitors (lansoprazole, omeprazole) and other alkaline agents: Inactivate male fern. Avoid administration with male fern.

Contraindications and precautions

Male fern is contraindicated in elderly or debilitated patients, during pregnancy, and in infants. It is also contraindicated in patients with anemia; cardiac, hepatic, or renal dysfunction; or GI ulceration. Use cautiously in patients receiving drugs that are known to affect bilirubin conjugation or increase liver enzymes, such as HMG CoA reductase inhibitors.

Special considerations

• Hepatocellular damage has occurred in animals with doses of 500 mg/kg of crude extractum filicis.
• Monitor liver function test results. Test abnormalities and pathologic changes were reversed within several days of receiving the initial dose (Valtonen and Takki, 1968).
🕭 **ALERT** Cardiac failure, coma, optic neuritis, respiratory failure, seizures, and death have occurred with severe poisoning. Treatment consists of administering a saline cathartic followed by demulcent fluids but avoiding fats and oils. Benzodiazepines and ventilatory assistance may be needed for seizures and respiratory failure, respectively.

Bold italic type indicates that reaction may be life-threatening.

- Advise the patient to take male fern on an empty stomach.
- Advise women to avoid using male fern during pregnancy or when breast-feeding.

Points of interest
- The Foods Standards Committee of London, England, has recommended that male fern not be used in foods as a flavoring agent.
- Male fern was used by the ancients and mentioned as an anthelmintic by Galen, Dioscorides, Theophrastus, and Pliny.

Commentary
Male fern has shown promise in treating human tapeworms, but clinical evidence is sparse. It is not clear whether the plant exerts sole action or is helped by adjuncts, such as a low-residue diet and laxatives. It would be interesting to compare this plant with praziquantel to determine equivalent efficacy, especially in patients who cannot tolerate praziquantel or niclosamide. The anthelmintics available today for tapeworms are much safer than male fern. Herbal therapy may be considered if current anthelmintic therapy fails, with thorough consideration of the contraindications and adverse reactions beforehand.

References

Alterio, D.L. "Treatment of Taeniasis with Ether Extract of Male Fern Administered by Duodenal Intubation," *Trop Dis Bull* 66:831, 1969.

Kapadia, G.J., et al. "Anti-Tumor Promoting Activity of *Dryopteris* Phlorophenone Derivatives," *Cancer Lett* 105:161-65, 1996.

Mello, E.B.F., et al. "Oral Treatment of Human Taeniasis by Ethereal Extract of Male Fern (Aspidium) Preceded by the Administration of Hypertonic Solution of Magnesium Sulfate," *Abl Bakt Hyg I* Orig A 248:384-87, 1978. Abstract.

Palva, I.P. "The Effectiveness of Certain Drugs in the Expulsion of Fish Tapeworm," *Ann Med Intern Fenn* 52:89-92, 1963.

Valtonen, E.J., and Takki, S. "Acute Hepatocellular Damage Caused by Oleoresin of the Male Fern in the Rat: An Electron Microscope Study," *Acta Pharmacol Toxicol (Copenh)* 26:169-76, 1968.

MALLOW

BLUE MALLOW, CHEESEFLOWER, CHEESEWEED, DWARF MALLOW, FIELD MALLOW, FLEURS DE MAUVE, HIGH MALLOW, *MALVAE FLOS* (MALLOW FLOWER), *MALVAE FOLIUM* (MALLOW LEAF), *MALVA PARVIFLORA*, MALVE, MAULS, ZIGBLI

Taxonomic class
Malvaceae

Common trade names
Malvedrin, Malveol

Common forms
Available as dried herb and fluidextract.

Source
The drug is obtained from the dried leaves and flowers of *Malva sylvestris,* a member of the mallow family, and is related to the cultivated hibiscus.

Chemical components
Mallow contains flavonol glycosides, mucilage (when hydrolyzed yields arabinose, glucose, rhamnose, galactose, and galacturonic acid), anthocyanins (about one-half is malvin), tannins, and leukocyanins.

Actions
The mucilage contained in the leaves and flowers is responsible for the herb's emollient and demulcent properties. This mucilage has been shown to inactivate complement, which is a host defense system component (Tomoda et al., 1989). The plant is also reported to have astringent and expectorant properties.

Reported uses
Mallow preparations are used to treat bladder complaints, bronchitis, hoarseness, irritations of the oral and pharyngeal mucosa, irritative cough, laryngitis, and tonsillitis and as a mild astringent. It is also used topically to reduce swelling and allergic cutaneous irritation, eliminate toxins, and relieve the pain of skin abrasions and insect stings. The leaves have been used as a laxative and for gut irritation. Sometimes mallow preparations have been given to children to ease teething pains. Mallow has been used with yarrow (*Achillea* species) as a douche for vaginal irritation.

Dosage
The suggested dose is 5 g/day P.O. of the chopped, dried herb or by infusion.

Adverse reactions
None reported in humans. Some *Malva* species have been linked to muscle spasms in cattle.

Interactions
None reported.

Contraindications and precautions
Avoid using mallow in pregnant or breast-feeding patients; effects are unknown.

Special considerations
• Do not confuse mallow with the similar-sounding marshmallow (*Althaea officinalis*) or country mallow (*Sida cordifolia*).
• Inform the patient that human clinical trial data are lacking.
• Although no known chemical interactions have been reported in clinical studies, consideration must be given to the pharmacologic properties of the herbal product and the potential for exacerbation of the intended therapeutic effect of conventional drugs.

Bold italic type indicates that reaction may be life-threatening.

• Advise women to avoid using mallow during pregnancy or when breast-feeding.

Points of interest
• Young mallow leaves and shoots have been eaten since the 8th century B.C. The traditional importance of the herb is captured in the Spanish adage, "A kitchen garden and mallow, sufficient medicines for a home."
• Mallow's mucilage and anthocyanin components have been analyzed for structural and molecular properties (Classen and Blaschek, 1998; Farina et al., 1995; Gonda et al., 1990).
• Mallow leaf is rich in vitamin C.
• Mallow flower is used as a food-coloring agent.

Commentary
Although this herb is approved by the German Commission E for treating bronchitis, cough, and inflammation of the mouth and pharynx, clinical data supporting the use of mallow for any indication are lacking. Because of its tannin component, mallow may reasonably be used as a topical astringent. Long-term or heavy use should be avoided.

References
Classen, B., and Blaschek, W. "High Molecular Weight Acidic Polysaccharides from *Malva Sylvestris* and *Alcea Rosea*," *Planta Med* 64:640-44, 1998. Abstract.

Farina, A., et al. "HPTLC and Reflectance Mode Densitometry of Anthocyanins in *Malva silvestris L.*: A Comparison with Gradient-Elution Reversed-Phase HPLC," *J Pharm Biomed Anal* 14:203-11, 1995. Abstract.

Gonda, R., et al. "Structure and Anticomplementary Activity of an Acidic Polysaccharide from the Leaves of *Malva sylvestris* var. *mauritiana*," *Carbohydr Res* 198:323-29, 1990. Abstract.

Tomoda, M., et al. "Plant Mucilages. Part 42. An Anticomplementary Mucilage from the Leaves of *Malva sylvestris* var. *mauritiana*," *Chem Pharm Bull (Tokyo)* 37:3029-32, 1989. Abstract.

MARIGOLD

CALENDULA, GARDEN MARIGOLD, POT MARIGOLD

Taxonomic class
Asteraceae

Common trade names
Aura Cacia Essential Oil Tagetes, Boiron Homeopathics Calendula Lotion, Hyland's Standard Homeopathics Calendula Spray

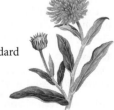

Common forms
Available as an ointment of 5% flower extract, infusion, and mouthwash.

Source
Components are extracted from the small, bright yellow-orange flower heads of *Calendula officinalis*. The shoots and leaves also have been investigated for potentially active compounds. *C. officinalis* is an annual herb that is native to southern Europe and the eastern Mediterranean and naturalized in many parts of the United States and Canada.

Chemical components
Compounds isolated from *C. officinalis* include triterpenoids, oleanic acid glycosides, lutein, carotenoid pigment, sterols, and fatty acids.

Actions
The anti-inflammatory activity of marigold has been demonstrated in mice (Akihisa et al., 1996; Zitterl-Eglseer et al., 1997), and the triterpenoids, primarily faradiol monoester, are thought to be the active components. The unesterfied faradiol equals indomethacin in activity.

Marigold extracts appeared to show antiviral activity against HIV type 1, rhinovirus, and vesicular stomatitis virus (De Tommasi et al., 1991; Kalvatchev et al., 1997).

The healing effect of an ointment containing 5% calendula extract was shown in a rat model. Surgically induced wounds treated with the ointment demonstrated marked physiologic regeneration and epithelialization (Klouchek-Popova et al., 1982).

Dietary lutein derived from marigold extract increased tumor latency, suppressed mammary tumor growth, and enhanced lymphocyte proliferation in mice given tumor cell infusions (Park et al., 1998; Chew et al., 1996). Observational evidence suggests that macular degeneration and cataracts are less likely to develop in people who eat foods that contain lutein, such as green vegetables (Mares-Perlman et al., 1995).

Reported uses
Therapeutic claims for marigold extract include antiseptic and skin-healing activities. Ointments have been suggested for leg ulcers, pressure ulcers, and varicose veins. Advocates recommend oral infusions to aid in digestion and promote bile production. Mouthwashes that contain marigold extract have been promoted for gum healing after tooth extraction.

Calendula oil has been used for skin treatments during aromatherapy. The herbal agent has also been promoted for soothing chapped lips, cracked nipples from breast-feeding, and skin inflammation.

Dosage
Ointment: apply topically as needed.
Tincture and tea: 1 to 4 ml P.O. t.i.d.

Adverse reactions
Other: allergic reaction (reported with other members of the Asteraceae family of plants).

Interactions
None reported.

Contraindications and precautions
Avoid using marigold in pregnant or breast-feeding patients; effects are unknown.

Special considerations
• Do not confuse *C. officinalis* with other ornamental marigolds, such as *Tagetes patula* (French marigold), *T. erecta* (African marigold), and *T. minuta* (Inca marigold). These plants are known for their ability to repel insects and soil nematodes and are commonly included in vegetable gardens.
• Inform the patient of the risk of allergic reactions.
• Advise women to avoid using marigold during pregnancy or when breast-feeding.

Points of interest
• The plant flowers continuously from May to October and was given the name calendula because it was always in bloom on the first day of the month.
• Calendula is believed to have originated in Egypt, where it was valued as a rejuvenating herb.
• During the American Civil War, field doctors are believed to have used marigold leaves on open wounds.

Commentary
Marigold has been used for centuries for its healing effects without documented problems. Animal models have supported its healing and anti-inflammatory effects, but human studies are lacking. Further research is needed to confirm other claims for the use of marigold.

References
Akihisa, T., et al. "Triterpene Alcohols from the Flowers of Compositae and Their Anti-Inflammatory Effects," *Phytochemistry* 43:1255-60, 1996.

Chew, B.P., et al. "Effects of Lutein from Marigold Extract on Immunity and Growth of Mammary Tumors in Mice," *Anticancer Res* 16:3689-94, 1996.

De Tommasi, N., et al. "Structure and In Vitro Antiviral Activity of Triterpenoid Saponins from Calendula arvensis," *Planta Med* 57:250-53, 1991.

Kalvatchev, Z., et al. "Different Effects of Phorbol Ester Derivatives on Human Immunodeficiency Virus 1 Replication in Lymphocytic and Monocytic Human Cells," *Acta Virol* 41:289-92, 1997.

Klouchek-Popova, E., et al. "Influence of the Physiological Regeneration and Epithelialization Using Fractions Isolated from Calendula officinalis," *Acta Physiol Pharmacol Bulg* 8:63-67, 1982.

Mares-Perlman J.A., et al. "Diet and Nuclear Lens Opacities," *Am J Epidemiol* 141:322-34, 1995.

Park J.S., et al. "Dietary lutein from marigold extract inhibits mammary tumor development in BALB/c mice," *J Nutr* 128(10):1650-56, 1998.

Zitterl-Eglseer, K., et al. "Anti-Oedematous Activities of the Main Triterpendiol Esters of Marigold (*Calendula officinalis* L.)," *J Ethnopharmacol* 57:139-44, 1997.

MARJORAM

COMMON MARJORAM, KNOTTED MARJORAM, OLEUM
MAJORANAE (OIL), OREGANO, SWEET MARJORAM, WILD
MARJORAM

Taxonomic class
Lamiaceae

Common trade names
Marjoram, Marjoram Essential Oil, Sweet
Marjoram Essential Oil

Common forms
Available as dried or powdered leaves and tea.

Source
Products identified as marjoram are generally composed of the dried leaves and flowering tops of
Origanum majorana L., a member of the mint family. The name wild
marjoram is generally a synonym for *O. vulgare*, one of the species
more commonly referred to as oregano. Essential oils identified as oil of
marjoram or wild marjoram oil have been obtained from thyme
(*Thymus mastichina*) and other species.

Chemical components
The essential oil of wild *O. majorana* plants contains the phenolic terpene isomers carvacrol and thymol. Other compounds include triacontane, sitosterol, oleanolic and ursolic acids, rosmarinic acid, flavonoids,
hydroquinone, tannins, and phenolic glycosides (arbutin and methylarbutin).

Actions
An aqueous extract of *O. compactum* inhibited responses to acetylcholine, histamine, serotonin, and nicotine, increasing calcium concentrations and electrical stimulation in smooth muscle from rat and guinea
pig ileum and duodenum. These effects were attributed to thymol and
carvacrol present in the plants (Van Den Broucke and Lemli, 1980).
Marjoram was found to exert some antiviral activity, possibly because
of tannins in the plants. Hydroquinone exerted dose-dependent cytotoxic activity on cultured rat hepatoma cells (Assaf et al., 1987). Thymol
has been shown to have bactericidal action against several oral bacteria;
it is included in some antiseptic mouthwashes and in Cervitec, a varnish used in dentistry. There are several reports of antibacterial, antifungal, and antiviral effects of thymol, carvacrol, and essential oils of
the Lamiaceae family.

Reported uses
The dried leaves and flowering tops of the marjoram plant are used
mainly in cooking. Marjoram is among the many plants that have been
labeled as oregano, but it generally has a milder flavor than the other

---

Bold italic type indicates that reaction may be life-threatening.

species. Medicinally, it has been used as an antidote for snakebite and for treating amenorrhea, bruises, certain cancers, conjunctivitis, cough, headache, infant colic, insomnia, menstrual pain, motion sickness, muscle and joint pain, and nausea. *O. majorana* and *O. vulgare* have been used to stimulate digestion and prevent flatulence (Van Den Broucke and Lemli, 1980).

Dosage
Tea: 1 or 2 tsp of dried leaves and flower tops steeped for 10 minutes in 1 cup of boiling water; no more than 3 cups should be taken P.O. daily. Alternatively, three doses of ½ to 1 tsp of the tincture P.O. daily.

Adverse reactions
None reported.

Interactions
None reported.

Contraindications and precautions
The use of marjoram in pregnant women should be limited to normal amounts used for cooking because of the slight risk of uterine contractions with herbal overdoses. Use cautiously in children and infants because marjoram's safety has not been evaluated for this age group.

Special considerations
ALERT Although no suspected cases of harm from marjoram consumption have been reported, several preparations of essential oil warn against internal use. Thymol and hydroquinone may be toxic.
• The content of thymol, carvacrol, hydroquinone, and other active components varies among plants (and thus in products), and the volatile oil content may decrease with age.
• Instruct the patient to reduce the dose or discontinue using marjoram if diarrhea, nausea, or vomiting occurs.
• Urge the patient to notify his health care provider of nausea or diarrhea that lasts longer than a few days because these symptoms may indicate serious disease or cause electrolyte imbalance if left untreated.
• Advise the patient to avoid using the volatile oil.
• Advise the patient not to exceed consumption of marjoram in an amount greater than that commonly found in foods.

Points of interest
• Early Greeks believed that marjoram was cultivated by Aphrodite, the goddess of love. The herb is still included in love potions and placed in hope chests or under women's pillows to ensure happy marriages.
• Marjoram is generally regarded as safe by the FDA.

Commentary
The antispasmodic effect of the extracts may account for its use to treat colic, menstrual pain, and nausea. Because marjoram is recognized as a safe food additive, moderate consumption in foods or teas is unlikely to

cause harm and may be beneficial for these conditions. Although antibacterial, antifungal, and antiviral effects of thymol and carvacrol have been shown in vitro, their concentration is variable; therefore, marjoram should not be relied on to treat or prevent infections. Its use as a toothache remedy may be related to the antimicrobial activity of thymol on oral bacteria. Suspected oral infections should be treated with conventional drugs.

There is little clinical evidence to support most of the therapeutic claims made for marjoram. Use of marjoram products should be restricted to oral intake or topical use on the skin if desired. Application of marjoram to open wounds or rashes and, especially, the eyes should be discouraged.

References

Assaf, M.H., et al. "Preliminary Study of Phenolic Glycosides from *Origanum majorana*; Quantitative Estimation of Arbutin; Cytotoxic Activity of Hydroquinone," *Planta Med* 53:343-45, 1987.

Van Den Broucke, C.O., and Lemli, J.A. "Antispasmodic Activity of *Origanum compactum*," *Planta Med* 38:317-31, 1980.

MARSHMALLOW

ALTHAEA ROOT, ALTHEA, MORTIFICATION ROOT, SWEET WEED

Taxonomic class
Malvaceae

Common trade names
Frontier Marshmallow Root Org Caps, Gaia Herbs Marshmallow Root, Nature's Answer Marshmallow Root Alcohol Free

Common forms
Available as capsules that contain powdered root and as dried leaves or flowers, extracts, and whole dried root.

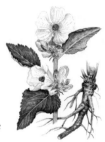

Source
The crude drug is obtained from the dried roots of *Althaea officinalis*, a perennial herb that is native to Europe and naturalized to the United States. Flowers and leaves may also be used.

Chemical components
Marshmallow root contains starch, mucilage, pectin, and sugar plus asparagine, flavonoids, phenolic acids, and calcium oxalate. The leaves and flowers also contain mucilage, a substance that swells in water and develops a gel-like consistency. Althea-mucilage O, a representative mucous polysaccharide isolated from marshmallow root, contains rhamnose, galactose, and glucuronic acid. Althea-mucilage OL is a similar acidic polysaccharide that occurs in the leaves. The root has also been

found to contain scopoletin, quercetin, kaempferol, chlorogenic acid, caffeic acid, and p-coumaric acids.

Actions
Althea-mucilage O and OL have been shown to exert a hypoglycemic effect in nondiabetic mice (Tomoda et al., 1987), but these effects have not been studied in humans. Antibacterial activity has also been shown in vitro (Recio et al., 1989).

Although polysaccharides from other plant sources, such as tragacanth, have been used as bulk-forming laxative products, the laxative effects of marshmallow mucilages have not been evaluated. Plant mucilages are commonly used as pharmaceutical vehicles, usually as suspending agents or viscosity-increasing agents.

Reported uses
Marshmallow has been used as a cough suppressant and to soothe irritated throats. It is also thought to be useful for intestinal conditions, such as constipation, gastritis, irritable bowel syndrome, and peptic ulcer disease. Applied topically, marshmallow purportedly soothes inflamed skin and helps to heal minor abrasions.

Dosage
Leaf: 5 g P.O. daily.
Root: 6 g P.O. daily in crude form or formulations.

Adverse reactions
None reported.

Interactions
Insulin, sulfonylureas: May increase hypoglycemic effects. Avoid administration with marshmallow.
Other drugs: Delayed absorption of other drugs when administered with marshmallow. Stagger administration.

Contraindications and precautions
Avoid using marshmallow in pregnant or breast-feeding patients; effects are unknown.

Special considerations
• Advise the patient to consult a health care provider before using herbal preparations because a treatment that has been clinically researched and proved effective may be available.
• Urge the patient to notify the prescriber and pharmacist of any herbal or dietary supplement he is taking when filling a new prescription.
• Monitor the diabetic patient for hypoglycemic effects.
• Advise women to avoid using marshmallow during pregnancy or when breast-feeding.

Commentary
Marshmallow cannot be recommended for any condition or disease because of the lack of data. Mucilaginous substances may be useful as

pharmaceutical agents, but this warrants additional investigation. Consumption of marshmallow in quantities other than that used in foods is not recommended.

References

Recio, M.C., et al. "Antimicrobial Activity of Selected Plants Employed in the Spanish Mediterranean Area, Part II," *Phytother Res* 3:77-80, 1989.

Tomoda, M., et al. "Hypoglycemic Activity of Twenty Plant Mucilages and Three Modified Products," *Planta Med* 53:8-12, 1987.

MAYAPPLE

DEVIL'S-APPLE, HOG APPLE, INDIAN APPLE, MANDRAKE, MAY APPLE, UMBRELLA PLANT, WILD LEMON

Taxonomic class
Berberidaceae

Common trade names
Condylox, Podocon-25, Podofilm, Warix, Wartec

Common forms
Available as dried rhizome, prescription-only resinous extract available as a solution or gel (0.5 % podophyllotoxin in alcohol), and concentrated tincture (5% to 25% solution in alcohol or compound benzoin tincture). A component of mayapple is available commercially in various synthetic anticancer drugs.

Source
Active components are derived from rhizome extracts; the USP powdered mixture of resins from *Podophyllum peltatum* is obtained by percolation of the plant with alcohol and precipitation with acidified water. Mayapple is a perennial herb that grows wild in the forests of North America and should not be confused with *Mandragora officinarum*, also known as mandrake, which is native to the Mediterranean and has different physiologic actions.

Chemical components
Mayapple contains a neutral crystalline substance, podophyllotoxins, amorphous resin, picropodophyllin, quercetin, starch, sugar, fat, and yellow coloring matter. The dried rhizomes and roots of *P. peltatum* yield some resin. The resin contains aryltetralin lignans calculated as podophyllotoxin. The "podophyllum" resin extract (incorrectly named podophyllin) contains at least 16 physiologically active compounds, including podophyllotoxin, picropodophyllin (the *cis* isomer of podophyllotoxin), alpha- and beta-pelotins, and quercetin.

Actions
A small quantity of the dried root powder produces a powerful cathartic effect. The resin is a potent spindle poison that blocks mitosis in metaphase, an effect it shares with the vinca alkaloids.

Bold italic type indicates that reaction may be life-threatening.

Reported uses
The fruits are the only edible portion of this plant and can be consumed in drinks, marmalades, and jellies. Mayapple is thought to be useful for treating hepatic congestion and as a counterirritant, an emetic, and a stimulant. It has also been used as a powerful cathartic. Antitumorigenic effects are well documented, and mayapple compounds have been incorporated into various synthetic anticancer drugs to treat acute myelogenous and lymphoblastic leukemia, lymphomas, small-cell lung cancers, and testicular and ovarian germ cell cancers.

Chinese mayapple (or bajiaolian) has been used for dysmenorrhea, hepatomas, lymphadenopathy, neck masses, postpartum recovery, snakebites, and weakness (Kao et al., 1992).

The concentrated tincture is claimed to be useful for treating warts. The resinous black extract is available by prescription only to topically treat anogenital and plantar warts. The Centers for Disease Control and Prevention recommends this treatment as an alternative to cryotherapy for external genital or perianal warts, vaginal warts, and urethral meatus warts.

Dosage
Powdered root: 10 to 30 grains P.O.

Resin: Apply to warts b.i.d. for 3 successive days; repeat at weekly intervals for up to 5 weeks. Treat a small number of warts at one time; don't wash off.

5% to 25% solution in alcohol or compound benzoin tincture: Apply to wart once weekly. Leave the solution on for 1 to 6 hours and then wash off. If application is unsuccessful after 4 weeks, consider an alternative therapy.

Tincture: 1 to 10 gtt P.O. once or twice daily.

Adverse reactions
CNS: acute psychotic reactions, ataxia, *coma,* confusion, dizziness, hallucinations, hypotonia, *seizures,* and stupor that may take 10 to 15 days to resolve (Dobb et al., 1984); EEG changes for several days; paresthesia.

CV: orthostatic hypotension, tachycardia.

EENT: irritation of eyes and mucous membranes (resin).

GI: abdominal pain, diarrhea, elevated liver function test results noted with bajiaolian (Kao et al., 1992), nausea, vomiting.

GU: *renal failure,* urine retention.

Hematologic: *leukopenia*, *thrombocytopenia.*

Hepatic: *hepatotoxicity.*

Musculoskeletal: decreased reflexes, muscle weakness.

Respiratory: *apnea.*

Skin: irritation.

Interactions
None reported.

Contraindications and precautions

Mayapple is contraindicated in pregnant or breast-feeding patients. It is also contraindicated in patients with diabetes, in those taking steroids, and in those who have poor circulation. Avoid applying resin to friable, bleeding, unusual warts with hair growing from them and to recently biopsied warts, moles, and birthmarks.

Use cautiously because extremely violent cathartic and CNS effects can occur.

Special considerations

• Monitor for adverse CNS effects.

▪ **ALERT** Except for the ripe fruits, the entire mayapple plant is toxic and should be used with extreme caution. Severe systemic toxicity can occur after ingestion or topical application. Neuropathy and death have resulted from applying large amounts of the resin to multiple and wide-spread skin lesions (Rate et al., 1979).

• Caution the patient to use only FDA-labeled pharmaceutical preparations of mayapple components. Resin and tincture are for external application only, and their use should be supervised by a primary health care provider. Commercial products are available only by prescription.

• Instruct the patient to keep the resin away from the eyes.

• Advise women to avoid using mayapple during pregnancy and when breast-feeding.

• Urge the patient to immediately report easy bruising, signs of infection, and unusual bleeding.

• Instruct the patient to keep these products out of the reach of children and pets.

Commentary

Mayapple compounds have many established uses because of documented antimitotic effects. These effects are valuable in treating tumors and genital warts, but they also contribute to the herb's toxicity. Other claims, including its efficacy as a liver tonic, lack documentation and need further investigation.

References

Dobb, G.J., et al. "Coma and Neuropathy After Ingestion of Herbal Laxative Containing Podophyllin," *Med J Aust* 140:495, 1984.

Kao, W.F., et al. "Podophyllotoxin Intoxication: Toxic Effect of Bajiaolian in Herbal Therapeutics," *Hum Exp Toxicol* 11(6):480-87, 1992.

Rate, R.G., et al. "Podophyllin Toxicity," *Ann Intern Med* 90:723, 1979.

MEADOWSWEET

BRIDEWORT, DOLLOFF, DROPWORT, *FILIPENDULA*, FLEUR
D'ULMAIRE, FLORES ULMARIAE, GRAVEL ROOT, LADY OF
THE MEADOW, MEADOW-WORT, MEADSWEET, QUEEN OF THE
MEADOW, SPIERSTAUDE, *SPIREAEA FLOS* (MEADOWSWEET
FLOWER), *SPIREAEA HERBA* (MEADOWSWEET HERB)

Taxonomic class
Rosaceae

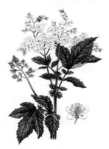

Common trade names
Multi-ingredient preparations: Arkocaps, Artival,
Neutracalm, Rheuma-Tee, Rheumex, Santane,
Spireadosa

Common forms
Available as fluidextract, infusion, powder, tablets
of dried herb (300 mg), and tincture.

Source
Active components are obtained from the dried flowers and aerial parts
of *Filipendula ulmaria*, a hardy perennial herb that is native to Europe
and northern Asia and naturalized to the United States as an ornamental plant. A member of the rose family, it is also known as *Spireaea ulmaria*.

Chemical components
Meadowsweet contains flavonoids (mainly glycosides of quercetin and
kaempherol, spiraeoside in the flowers, and avicularin and hyperoside in
the leaves), phenolic glycosides (spiraein in the flowers, monotropin in
the flowers and leaves, and the primaverosides of salicylaldehyde and
methyl salicylate polyphenols), and tannins. The volatile oil contains salicylates (salicylaldehyde, gaultherin, isosalicin, methyl salicylate, mono-
tropitin, salicin, salicylic acid, and spirein), phenylethyl alcohol, benzyl
alcohol, anisaldehyde, and methyl salicylate. Other compounds include
benzaldehyde, ethyl benzoate, heliotropin, phenylacetate, vanillin, citric
acid, mucilage, heparin, carbohydrates, and ascorbic acid.

Actions
Meadowsweet has traditionally been used for its antiemetic, antiflatulent,
anti-inflammatory, antimicrobial, antirheumatic, antiulcerative, astringent, diaphoretic, digestive aid, diuretic, laxative, sedative, and mild urinary antiseptic properties. In Russian animal studies, meadowsweet was
reported to lower motor activity and rectal temperature, relax the muscles, and potentiate the action of narcotics (Barnaulov et al., 1977); prolong life expectancy of mice (Barnaulov and Denisenko, 1980); lower vascular permeability and prevent stomach ulcers in mice and rats (Yanutsh
et al., 1982); increase bronchial tone in cats; potentiate histamine bronchospasm; increase the impact of histamine on ulcers; increase intestinal

tone in guinea pigs; and increase uterine tone in rabbits (Barnaulov et al., 1978). An ointment prepared from *F. ulmaria* showed positive effects in preventing induced cervical and vaginal cancer in mice (Peresun'ko et al., 1993). Meadowsweet extract has been shown to possess antibacterial properties (Rauha et al., 2000). Heparin isolated from *F. ulmaria* was found to be structurally and functionally similar to heparin of animal origin (Kudriashov et al., 1990; Kudriashov et al., 1991). Extracts from the flowers and seeds have shown in vitro and in vivo anticoagulant activity (Liapina and Koval'chuk, 1993). The tannins present in meadowsweet have an astringent action that may ease GI complaints.

Reported uses
Meadowsweet has been used in folk medicine for arthritis, cancer, chills, colds, cystitis, diarrhea, gastritis, heartburn, indigestion, irritable bowel syndrome (with other herbs), peptic ulcer disease, respiratory disorders, rheumatic joints and muscles, skin diseases, sprains, and tendinitis. The French use the herb as a diaphoretic and a diuretic and to treat headache and toothache pain. In Belgium, the herb is used for painful articular conditions. Although salicylates are present, they appear to cause less GI irritation than acetylsalicylic acid. In Europe, meadowsweet is used as a natural food flavoring. The FDA lists meadowsweet as an herb of undefined safety.

Dosage
For treatment of diarrhea, 1 cup decoction P.O. b.i.d. or t.i.d.
Dried flowers: 2.5 to 3.5 g P.O. up to t.i.d.
Dried herb: 2 to 6 g P.O. up to t.i.d.
Liquid extract (1:1 in 25% alcohol): 1.5 to 6 ml P.O. up to t.i.d.
Oral infusion: 100 ml P.O. every 2 hours.
Powder: ½ tsp P.O. with a small amount of water t.i.d.
Tincture (1:5 in 25% alcohol): 2 to 4 ml P.O. up to t.i.d.

Adverse reactions
GI: indigestion, nausea.
Respiratory: *bronchospasm.*
Skin: rash.

Interactions
Narcotics: May potentiate the effects of narcotics. Monitor the patient closely.
Other salicylate-containing herbs and drugs: May interact with these other herbs and drugs and cause interactions similar to those seen with salicylates. Use together cautiously.

Contraindications and precautions
Avoid using meadowsweet in pregnant or breast-feeding patients; effects are unknown. Also discourage its use in patients with asthma or salicylate or sulfite sensitivity and in children.

Bold italic type indicates that reaction may be life-threatening.

Special considerations
• Monitor for signs of bleeding.
• Caution asthmatic patients not to use meadowsweet.
• Advise women to avoid using meadowsweet during pregnancy or when breast-feeding. Although not substantiated, a link between salicin and birth defects has been reported.

Points of interest
• Meadowsweet was one of the most sacred herbs of the Druids; it is unknown whether it was used medicinally. It was used to flavor mead in the Middle Ages, thus the synonyms meadwort and meadsweet.
• Meadowsweet was used as a source of salicylates for aspirin in the late 1800s. Some sources report that aspirin derived its name from this herb (*S. ulmaria*).

Commentary
The German Commission E reports no known adverse effects or contraindications, except that of salicylate sensitivity, for meadowsweet and has approved its use for treating bronchitis, colds, and coughs. Its use cannot be recommended because of the scarcity of human clinical data, but further studies are warranted because of its potential therapeutic value and low reported toxicity.

References
Barnaulov, O.D., et al. "Chemical Composition and Primary Evaluation of the Properties of Preparations from *Filipendula ulmaria* (L) Flowers," *Rastit Resur* 13:661-69, 1977.

Barnaulov, O.D., et al. "Preliminary Evaluation of the Spasmolytic Properties of Some Natural Compounds and Galenic Preparations," *Rastit Resur* 14:573-79, 1978.

Barnaulov, O.D., and Denisenko, P.P. "Antiulcerogenic Action of the Decoction from Flowers of *Filipendula ulmaria*," *Pharmakol Toksikol* 43:700-05, 1980.

Kudriashov, B.A., et al. "The Content of a Heparin-like Anticoagulant in the Flowers of the Meadowsweet *(Filipendula ulmaria)*," *Farmakol Toksikol* 53:39-41, 1990. Abstract.

Kudraishov, B.A., et al. "Heparin from the Meadowsweet *(Filipendula ulmaria)* and Its Properties," *Izv Akad Nauk SSSR* [Biol] 6:939-43, 1991. Abstract.

Liapina, L.A., and Koval'chuk, G.A. "A Comparative Study of the Action on the Hemostatic System of Extracts from the Flowers and Seeds of the Meadowsweet *(Filipendula ulmaria)*," *Izv Akad Nauk Ser Biol* 4:625-28, 1993. Abstract.

Peresun'ko, A.P., et al. "Clinico-Experimental Study of Using Plant Preparations from the Flowers of *Filipendula ulmaria* (L.) Maxim for the Treatment of Precancerous Changes and Prevention of Uterine Cervical Cancer," *Vopr Onkol* 39:291-95, 1993. Abstract.

Rauha, J.P., et al. "Antimicrobial Effects of Finnish Plant Extracts Containing Flavonoids and Other Phenolic Compounds," *Int J Food Microbiol* 25:3-12, 2000.

Yanutsh, A.Y., et al. "A Study of the Antiulcerative Action of the Extracts from the Supernatant Part and Roots of *Filipendula ulmaria*," *Farm Zh* 37:53-56, 1982.

MELATONIN

MEL, N-ACETYL-5-METHOXYTRYPTAMINE

Common trade names
Multi-ingredient preparations: Bevitamel, Chronoset, Knockout, Mela-T
Melatonin, Melatonix, Rapi-Snooze, Super Melatonin, Tranzone

Common forms
Capsules: 1 mg, 3 mg, 5 mg
Capsules (extended-release): 2 mg, 3 mg
Liquid: 500 mcg/ml, 1 mg/ml
Lozenge: 3 mg
Tablets: 300 mcg, 500 mcg, 1 mg, 1.5 mg, 3 mg
Tablets (sustained-release): 1 mg, 3 mg
   Also available as cream and tea.

Source
Melatonin is a hormone produced by the pineal gland in response to
darkness. It is extracted from beef cattle pineal gland; it can also be synthesized chemically from 5-methoxyindole. The synthetic product may
be preferred to avoid viral contamination from a beef by-product. Exogenously administered hormone may be a concern in its potential for
negative feedback reduction of natural hormone production.

Chemical components
Melatonin has the chemical name of N-2-(5-methoxyindol-3-ethyl) ac-
etamide. Physiologically, melatonin is available when tryptophan is
converted to serotonin, which is then enzymatically converted to melatonin in the pineal gland. Commercial products may also contain the
inactive ingredients cellulose, lactose, cornstarch, magnesium stearate,
and isopropyl alcohol.

Actions
Melatonin release corresponds to sleeping periods. Serum levels of melatonin are very low during the day, with peak levels occurring between 2
and 4 a.m. This partly explains melatonin's role in sleep and circadian
rhythms. Prolonged intake can reset the sleep-wake cycle. Melatonin secretion declines with age but has not been proved responsible for sleep
disturbances. Serum prolactin levels, growth hormone release, and response to growth hormone–releasing hormone stimulation increase after acute doses of melatonin. Long-term use may also decrease serum
luteinizing hormone levels in women. Melatonin has been found to be a
free radical scavenger and may be more effective than mannitol, vitamin
E, or glutathione (Brzezinski, 1997). Its efficacy may be associated only
with patients whose endogenous melatonin levels are low.

Reported uses
Melatonin has been studied for many conditions. It has been widely
promoted for the prevention and treatment of jet lag, as a hypnotic, for

---

Bold italic type indicates that reaction may be life-threatening.

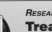

RESEARCH FINDINGS
Treating jet lag with melatonin

Prevention and treatment of jet lag appear to be the most popular indications for using melatonin. Several studies have evaluated melatonin's effect on sleep disturbance, recovery of energy, fatigue, mental alertness, and mood. In most studies, melatonin showed a modest improvement in these outcomes compared with placebo.

In one study, 20 subjects took either placebo or melatonin to prepare for a flight between England and New Zealand. The dosage regimen was 5 mg once daily for 3 days before the flight, during the flight, and for 3 days after arrival. The melatonin group required significantly less time to return to normal sleep patterns and energy levels than the placebo group. The study also found that jet lag symptoms were much worse on the return flight, suggesting that melatonin may play an important role during the return portion of a journey (Petrie et al., 1989).

In a subsequent study, the authors compared two dosage regimens and found that 5 g daily for 5 days after arrival was superior to 5 mg 2 days before departure through 5 days after arrival. The former group experienced significantly less jet lag and sleep disturbance, but there was no difference in recovery of energy and alertness. An interesting finding was that the melatonin group experienced worse jet lag than the placebo group (Petrie et al., 1993).

In contrast, another study found that melatonin wasn't statistically superior to placebo in improving sleep quality, morning sleepiness, or mood (Claustraut, 1992).

---

blind entrainment, for cancer protection, as an oral contraceptive, and as a treatment for tinnitus. Many of these claims lack scientific support. (See *Treating jet lag with melatonin*.) Melatonin is thought to induce sleep similarly to benzodiazepines rather than altering sleep cycles. A preliminary study suggests that melatonin supplementation can initiate and maintain sleep in elderly melatonin-deficient patients with insomnia (Haimov et al., 1995). Orphan drug status has been given to melatonin in the treatment of circadian rhythm disorders that can occur in blind people who lack light perception.

As an anticancer agent, melatonin may produce partial response in treating solid tumors and stabilization of disease (Lissoni et al., 1991). Larger clinical trials are needed to confirm these results. The use of melatonin has also led to significantly less weight loss in patients with cancer (Lissoni et al., 1996). It may also be a future contraceptive option because decreased levels of luteinizing hormone, progesterone, and estradiol have been noted.

Research has been conducted concerning melatonin's use as a sleep aid in patients with schizophrenia or major depression. It may be useful in treating subjective tinnitus in patients with high Tinnitus Handicap Inventory scores or difficulty sleeping (Rosenberg et al., 1998). There is growing evidence of melatonin's effect on the immune system through the release of cytokines by activated T cells and monocytes (Neri et al., 1998). Also, melatonin has been compared with midazolam for decreasing anxiety and increasing sedation before anesthesia induction (Naguib et al., 1999).

Dosage
For blind patients with sleep problems, 5 mg P.O. at bedtime.
For cancer (solid tumors) as single agent, 20 mg I.M. for 2 months and then 10 mg/day P.O.
For cancer (with interleukin-2 [IL-2]), 40 to 50 mg P.O. at bedtime starting 7 days before IL-2 and continued through cycle.
For chronic insomnia, 75 mg P.O. at bedtime.
For delayed sleep phase syndrome, 5 mg P.O. at bedtime (10 p.m.).
For elderly patients with insomnia, 1 to 2 mg P.O. sustained-release 2 hours before bedtime
For jet lag, 5 mg/day P.O. starting 3 days before departure and ending 3 days after departure. (Alternate regimen: 5 mg/day P.O. for 5 days after arrival.)
For normalization of nocturnal levels, 4 mcg/hour continuous I.V. for 5 hours.

Adverse reactions
CNS: altered sleep patterns, confusion, headache, hypothermia, sedation, **transient depression with doses higher than 8 mg.**
CV: tachycardia.
Skin: pruritus.

Interactions
Benzodiazepines: Increased anxiolytic action. Use cautiously.
Beta blockers: Decreased nocturnal production of melatonin. Monitor the patient.
DHEA: Altered cytokine production in murine studies. Monitor the patient.
Magnesium, zinc: Additive inhibitory effects on the N-methyl-D-aspartate receptor (animal studies). Avoid administration with melatonin.
Methamphetamine: Increased monoaminergic effects of methamphetamine; may exacerbate insomnia. Avoid administration with melatonin.
Succinylcholine: Potentiated blocking properties of succinylcholine. Avoid administration with melatonin.

Contraindications and precautions
Melatonin is contraindicated in patients with hepatic insufficiency, especially cirrhosis, because of reduced clearance of the drug. It is also contraindicated in patients who have a history of cerebrovascular dis-

---

ease, depression, or neurologic disorders. Use cautiously in patients with renal dysfunction.

Special considerations
• The content of commercial melatonin products may not be uniform.
• Comprehensive therapy for sleep disorders may include behavior modification, light therapy, pharmacology, and counseling.
• Monitor for adverse CNS effects.

Commentary
Melatonin is a popular alternative drug. The efficacy rates from clinical trials may lead to conservative recommendation for certain indications.

For jet lag, melatonin appears promising in mitigating symptoms. More controlled trials are needed to determine whether the dosing regimen should be changed to taking the first dose on the departure day rather than for days after. Melatonin is an orphan drug as an aid to blind patients with abnormal circadian rhythms.

Theoretically, melatonin may possess contraceptive characteristics. Trials evaluating whether melatonin can inhibit pregnancy are ongoing. Despite promise as a chemotherapeutic agent, larger studies are needed to define rigid controls in the use of melatonin as an adjunct or single agent for solid tumor treatment. Thus, this drug may be useful in treating sleep disorders and certain cancers and as a contraceptive. Recommendations for its use cannot be made until long-term studies are completed.

References
Brzezinski, A. "Melatonin in Humans," *N Engl J Med* 336:186-95, 1997.

Claustraut, B. "Melatonin and Jet Lag: Confirmatory Result Using a Simplified Protocol," *Biol Psychol* 32:705-11, 1992.

Haimov, I., et al. "Melatonin Replacement Therapy of Elderly Insomniacs," *Sleep* 18:598-603, 1995.

Lissoni, P., et al. "Clinical Results with the Pineal Hormone Melatonin in Advanced Cancer Resistant to Standard Antitumor Therapies," *Oncology* 48:448-50, 1991.

Lissoni, P., et al. "Is There a Role for Melatonin in the Treatment of Neoplastic Cachexia?" *Eur J Cancer* 32A:1340-43, 1996.

Naguib, M., et al. "Premedication with Melatonin: A Double-blind, Placebo-controlled Comparison with Midazolam," *Br J Anaesth* 82(6):875-80, 1999.

Neri, B., et al. "Melatonin as Biological Response Modifier in Cancer Patients," *Anticancer Res* 18(2B):1329-32, 1998.

Petrie, K., et al. "Effect of Melatonin on Jet Lag After Long Haul Flights," *BMJ* 298:705-7, 1989.

Petrie, K., et al. "A Double-Blind Trial of Melatonin as a Treatment for Jet Lag in International Cabin Crew," *Biol Psych* 33:526-30, 1993.

Rosenberg, S.I., et al. "Effect of Melatonin on Tinnitus," *Laryngoscope* 108(3):305-10, 1998.

METHYL-SUFONYL-METHANE
M-S-M

Common trade names
Mineral sulfur

Common forms
Methyl-sufonyl-methane is available in 100-mg capsules or tablets.

Source
Organic forms of sulfur are produced or derived from amino acids in laboratories.

Chemical components
Methyl-sufonyl-methane is primarily taken to supplement the intake of sulfur, which is the active component in methyl-sufonyl-methane.

Actions
The mineral sulfur is needed for the manufacture of many proteins in the body, including those that form hair, muscles, bone, teeth, and skin (the proteins in connective tissues; Richmond, 1986). Sulfur contributes to fat digestion and absorption because it is needed to make bile acids. No human or animal trials could be found that specifically used methyl-sufonyl-methane.

Reported uses
Claims have been made regarding methyl-sufonyl-methane in disorders ranging from arthritis to diabetes. No clinical trials have substantiated any of the reported uses. The use of methyl-sufonyl-methane in arthritis can be traced to an old study of low levels of cystine and, therefore, possibly sulfur (a component of cystine), in people with arthritis (Sullivan et al., 1935). This study, coupled with the fact that sulfur-containing proteins are present in bone, has led to the use of supplemental dietary sulfur, such as methyl-sufonyl-methane, in arthritis. The rationale for using methyl-sufonyl-methane in diabetes is that sulfur is a component of insulin, and therefore, supplementation could be beneficial. This association has never been proved.

Dosage
No recommended intake levels have been established, but the usual dose is 100 mg P.O. one to three times a day.

Adverse reactions
None reported.

Interactions
None reported.

Contraindications and precautions
Methyl-sufonyl-methane is contraindicated in patients who are allergic to sulfa.

Bold italic type indicates that reaction may be life-threatening.

Special considerations
● Most dietary sulfur is provided by protein-rich foods and is found in garlic and onions. Sulfur deficiency has not been documented.
● Advise the patient to consult a health care provider before using herbal preparations because a treatment that has been clinically researched and proved effective may be available.
● Although no known chemical interactions have been reported in clinical studies, consideration must be given to the pharmacologic properties of the herbal product and the potential for exacerbation of the intended therapeutic effect of conventional drugs.

Commentary
The supplementation of sulfur through a product such as methylsufonyl-methane has not been studied. Because sulfur deficiency has not been documented and the theoretical link between sulfur deficiency and any medical disorder has not been found, methyl-sufonyl-methane appears to serve no useful purpose and cannot be recommended.

References
Richmond, V.L. "Incorporation of Methylsulfonylmethane Sulfur into Guinea Pig Serum Proteins," *Life Sci* 39: 263-68, 1986.
Sullivan, M.X., et al. "The Cystine Content of the Finger Nails in Arthritis," *J Bone Joint Surg* 16:185-88, 1935.

MILK THISTLE
CARDUUS MARIANUS L., *CNICUS MARIANUS*, HOLY THISTLE, LADY'S THISTLE, MARIAN THISTLE, MARY THISTLE, ST. MARY THISTLE

Taxonomic class
Asteraceae

Common trade names
Beyond Milk Thistle, Milk Thistle Extract, Milk Thistle Phytosol, Milk Thistle Plus V-Caps, Milk Thistle Power, NU VEG Milk Thistle Power, Silymarin, Super Milk Thistle

Common forms
Capsules: 50 mg, 100 mg, 175 mg, 200 mg, 505 mg
Tablets: 85 mg (standardized to contain 80% silymarin with the flavonoid silibinin)
     Also available as an extract.

Source
The seeds from *Silybum marianum*, a member of the Asteraceae family (daisies and thistles), are used to formulate milk thistle preparations. The plant is indigenous to the Mediterranean area but also found in Europe, North America, South America, and Australia.

Chemical components
Milk thistle contains silymarin, which consists of three flavonolignan compounds (silibinin, silidyanin, and silychristin). Other flavonolignans include dehydrosilybin, siliandrin, silybinome, and silyhermin. Apigenin, silybonol, linoleic and oleic acids, myristic, stearic and palmitic acids, betaine, histamine, and triamine also are found.

Actions
Silymarin exerts antihepatotoxic and hepatoprotective actions against hepatotoxins, such as *Amanita phalloides* and other cyclopeptide-containing mushrooms (*Galerina* and *Lepiota* species). Silymarin alters the outer liver membrane cell structure so that toxins cannot enter the cell; it also stimulates RNA polymerase A, which enhances ribosome protein synthesis and leads to activation of the regenerative capacity of the liver through cell development. Other suggested protective mechanisms are the inhibition of lipid peroxidation through silymarin's free radical scavenging and inhibition of cytochrome P-450 enzymes responsible for the bioactivation of various hepatotoxins.

Reported uses
Milk thistle seeds or seed extracts are believed to be useful as liver "cleansing" agents. The extracts have been used as an antidote after the accidental ingestion of *A. phalloides* and other poisonous mushrooms. Successful outcomes were noted in two human trials using silymarin after hepatotoxic mushroom ingestion (Flora et al., 1998).

   In patients with psychotropic drug–induced hepatic dysfunction, silymarin improved liver function test results and blunted halothane hepatotoxicity. Data exist regarding the use of extracts in both acute and chronic hepatic disease. (See *Milk thistle and hepatic disease.*) There is anecdotal evidence about its use in hepatitis C and by liver transplant patients.

Dosage
The doses evaluated ranged from 420 to 800 mg/day P.O. as a single dose or in divided doses b.i.d. or t.i.d. The German Federal Institute for Drugs and Medical Devices recommends 200 to 400 mg of silymarin P.O. daily, calculated as the silibinin component. The bioavailability of silibinin in conventional milk thistle products is extremely low (about 2%). A new formulation, silipide (a complex of silibinin and phosphatidylcholine), drastically increases silibinin plasma levels.

Adverse reactions
GI: mild laxative effect (with standardized extracts).
GU: menstrual and uterine stimulation.

Interactions
CYP450-, CYP3A4-, and CYP2C9-mediated drug metabolism; enzymes responsible for conjugation with glucuronic acid (UGTs): May inhibit drug metabolism. Monitor the patient closely.

Bold italic type indicates that reaction may be life-threatening.

RESEARCH FINDINGS
Milk thistle and hepatic disease

Milk thistle extract has been studied in the treatment of acute and chronic hepatic disease. In patients with acute alcoholic hepatitis, the extract caused more patients than controls to normalize (as measured by hepatic transaminase levels) and significantly reduced the time to normalization (Fintelmann and Albert, 1980). In a double-blind study, compared with placebo, varying doses of silymarin improved liver function test results, reduced complications, hastened recovery, and shortened hospitalization in patients with acute viral hepatitis (Flora et al., 1998).

During a 6-month treatment period in patients with chronic alcoholic hepatitis, liver function test results normalized and liver histology improved compared with placebo (Feher et al., 1989; Salmi and Sarna, 1982). In a third trial of biopsy-confirmed cirrhotics, laboratory findings weren't statistically different, but mortality was significantly reduced in the treated group. The largest trial involved more than 2,500 patients with chronic hepatic disease and showed improvement in both objective and subjective parameters of hepatic function (Albrecht et al., 1992).

Most data supporting the use of silymarin in hepatic dysfunction are from foreign studies. These trials were flawed in design; inconsistent in measuring parameters of hepatic dysfunction and in including a control group; sometimes failed to control alcohol intake; included patients with varied etiology and severity of disease; sometimes used small study populations; and used inconsistent definitions of endpoints and variable dosing regimens. Moreover, adverse effects of milk thistle extract are largely undefined.

Despite these limitations, the future of silymarin appears promising in the treatment of hepatic disease.

Contraindications and precautions
Milk thistle is contraindicated in pregnant or breast-feeding patients. Use cautiously in patients with hypersensitivity to plants belonging to the Asteraceae family.

Special considerations
ALERT Milk thistle therapy is generally regarded as safe, but a report of an adverse reaction to the herb has been documented. In Australia, a 57-year-old woman presented with a 2-month history of various GI-related symptoms, including abdominal pain, nausea, and vomiting (Adverse Drug Reactions Advisory Committee, 1999). Other than signs of dehydration, all pertinent laboratory results were normal. On questioning, the patient admitted taking Microgenics Herbal Milk Thistle

Vegicaps for the past 2 months. At one point, she stopped taking the medication and her symptoms improved. Several weeks later, she resumed therapy and was, ultimately, admitted to the hospital. It is possible that the symptoms experienced by the woman could be linked to another ingredient in the herbal preparation.

• Monitor liver function test results during therapy with milk thistle.
• Advise the patient to consult a health care provider specialized in hepatic disease before pursuing this therapy.
• Advise women to report planned or suspected pregnancy.
• Urge the patient to report unusual symptoms immediately.

Points of interest
• The German Federal Institute for Drugs and Medical Devices approves the use of milk thistle for toxic liver and as supportive treatment in chronic inflammatory hepatic disease and hepatic cirrhosis.
• In vitro studies in human liver microsomes and cultured hepatocytes suggest that silymarin inhibits CYP450-mediated drug metabolism. Spurred by the hypothesis that one of milk thistle's hepatoprotective actions involves the inhibition of liver enzymes, work has focused on the possibility of herb-drug interactions that could occur as a result of this inhibition. A study using human liver microsomes reported that the possibility of CYP3A4- and CYP2C9-mediated inhibition by silibinin at normal concentrations could not be excluded. Another study that looked at CYP3A4 enzymes and enzymes responsible for conjugation with glucuronic acid in primary cultures of human hepatocytes showed a reduction in the metabolism of substrates of these enzymes when treated with silymarin (Venkataramanan et al., in press). Studies to establish whether this relation exists in humans are under way.

Commentary
Studies and the traditional use of milk thistle for hepatic diseases in Europe suggest that this agent may play a role in preventing acute toxin-induced hepatic dysfunction. Because no hepatoprotective or antihepatoxic allopathic alternatives are available, a trial use of milk thistle may be warranted in life-threatening situations. Clinicians should be cognitive of the potential for drug interactions in patients who consume milk thistle on a chronic basis.

References
Adverse Drug Reactions Advisory Committee. "An Adverse Reaction to the Herbal Medication Milk Thistle (Silybum marianum)," *Med J Aust* 170:170-71, 1999.

Albrecht, M., et al. "Therapy of Toxic Liver Pathologies with Legalon," *Z Klin Med* 47:87-92, 1992.

Feher, J., et al. "Hepatoprotective Activity of Silmarin (Legalon) Therapy in Patients with Chronic Liver Disease," *Orv Hetil* 130:2723-27, 1989.

Fintelmann, V., and Albert, A. "Nachweis der therapeutischen Wirksamkeit von Legalon bei Toxischen Lebererkrankungen im Doppelblindversuch," *Therapiewoche* 30:5589-94, 1980.

Flora, K., et al. "Milk Thistle (*Silybum marianum*) for the Therapy of Liver Disease," *Am J Gastroenterol* 93:139-43, 1998.

Bold italic type indicates that reaction may be life-threatening.

Morazzoni, P., et al. "Comparative Pharmacokinetics of Silipide and Silymarin in Rats," *Eur J Drug Metab Pharmacokinet* 18:289-97, 1993.

Salmi, A., and Sarna, S. "Effect of Silymarin on Chemical, Functional, and Morphological Alterations of the Liver," *Scand J Gastroenterol* 174:517-21, 1982.

Venkataramanan, R., et al. "Milk Thistle, a Herbal Supplement, Decreases the Activity of CYP3A4 and UGT in Human Hepatocyte Cultures," *Drug Metab Disp* (in press).

MINT

BALM MINT, BRANDY MINT, GREEN MINT, LAMB MINT, OUR LADY'S MINT, PEPPERMINT, SPEARMINT

Taxonomic class
Lamiaceae

Common trade names
Ben-Gay, Rhuli Gel, Robitussin Cough Drops, Vicks VapoRub

Common forms
Peppermint and spearmint are available as inhalant preparations, liquid extracts, oil, and tea. Peppermint oil is also available as enteric-coated capsules. Menthol is an active component of several topical analgesics, anesthetics, and antipruritics; it is also available as an antitussive ointment, lozenge, creams, lotions, and throat spray.

Source
The best known and most cultivated members of the fragrant mint family are peppermint and spearmint. Peppermint (*Mentha piperita*) is a hybrid between *M. spicata* (spearmint) and *M. aquatica* (water mint). The essential oils of peppermint and spearmint are extracted from the leaves and flowering tops of these plants. Both are members of the mint family. They are native to Europe and widely cultivated in the United States and in Canada.

Chemical components
Peppermint oil is a volatile oil composed primarily of menthol. Menthol stereoisomers include neomenthol, menthone, menthofuran, eucalyptol, and limonene. Other components are methyl acetate, piperitone, tannins, flavonoids, and tocopherols. The most popular types of peppermint are white peppermint (*M. piperita* var. *officinalis*) and black peppermint (*M. piperita* var. *vulgaris*). More than 100 other chemical components are found but vary with growth stage, cultivation method, and geographical location. Spearmint oil contains carvone, limonene, phellandrene, and pinene; menthol is absent. Fresh leaves are reported to contain as much vitamin C as oranges and more provitamin A than carrots.

Actions

Peppermint essential oil is reported to have in vitro antibacterial and antiviral activity. It also relaxes the sphincter of Oddi by reducing calcium influx and stimulates bile flow in animals by the choloretic action of its flavonoid components.

Most of peppermint's pharmacologic activity is caused by menthol, which, in concentrations of 0.1% to 1%, depresses sensory cutaneous receptors and alleviates itching and irritation. In higher concentrations, it acts as a counterirritant by stimulating the nerves that perceive cold while depressing the nerves that perceive pain and itching. When applied to the skin, menthol produces an initial feeling of coolness followed by a sensation of warmth. The cooling effect may result from direct desensitization of warmth receptors, and warming follows vasodilation of small blood vessels under the skin (Jacknowitz, 1996).

Menthol also has a direct spasmolytic effect on smooth muscles of the digestive tract. Its spasmolytic activity is reportedly mediated through a calcium antagonist effect. Azulene (cyclopentacycloheptane) occurs in small amounts in peppermint oil and exerts anti-inflammatory and anti-ulcerative effects in animals (Taylor et al., 1983; Hills and Aaronson, 1991).

The medicinal action of spearmint is not documented in the literature. It is reported to have antispasmodic and antiflatulent properties similar to those of peppermint, but its effects are weaker.

Reported uses

Peppermint is a popular medicinal and commercial mint with several uses. It is considered an anesthetic, an antiemetic, an antiflatulent, an antiseptic, an aromatic, a diaphoretic, a digestive aid, a flavoring agent, and a stimulant. The leaf is also a classic folk remedy for stomach cancer. Peppermint's antiflatulent and antispasmodic activities have been used for abdominal pain, colic, diarrhea, dyspepsia, flatulence, and indigestion. Peppermint oil has demonstrated effectiveness in reducing colonic spasms during barium enema and endoscopy (Jarvis et al., 1992; Leicester and Hunt, 1982; Sparks et al., 1995). Enteric-coated peppermint oil capsules have been reported to be effective for reducing symptoms of irritable bowel syndrome (Dew et al., 1984; Pittler and Ernst, 1998; Rees et al., 1979). Other studies have failed to demonstrate a significant symptomatic improvement favoring peppermint oil (Nash et al., 1986).

Menthol has been used traditionally to relieve the pain of headache, neuralgia, rheumatism, throat infections, and toothache by acting as an antipruritic, an antiseptic, a counterirritant, a disinfectant, a local anesthetic, and a vascular stimulant. It is used externally in liniments, rubs, and ointments to treat the itching, minor pain of sunburn and the musculoskeletal pain of arthritis, neuralgia, and rheumatism.

Menthol is also used in inhalant preparations to alleviate bronchitis, chest complaints, cold, cough, laryngitis, and nasal congestion. As a local anesthetic, menthol is used in sprays and lozenges for sore throat, and it is occasionally used to anesthetize gastric nerve endings in motion sickness and nausea.

Peppermint oil is widely used in cosmetics, flavoring, mouthwashes, pharmaceuticals, and toothpastes as well as in anesthetic, antipruritic, and local antiseptic preparations. It is gaining popularity in aromatherapy to increase concentration and stimulate the mind and body and has even been used topically for headaches.

Spearmint is mainly used as a flavoring agent, but it is also considered a milder antispasmodic and antiflatulent for colic and other digestive problems and is claimed to be useful in tumors and stomach cancer. Spearmint is thought to whiten teeth, cure mouth sores, alleviate nausea and vomiting, heal the bites of a rabid dog, relieve pain of wasp stings, and repel rodents. Because its effects are less powerful than those of peppermint, it is considered to cause fewer problems in children.

Dosage

The following dosages have been reported for peppermint, but consensus is lacking. Considerably less information on dosing exists for spearmint preparations.

Capsules (enteric-coated): 1 or 2 capsules (0.2 ml/capsule) P.O. t.i.d. between meals for irritable bowel syndrome. Enteric coating is claimed to minimize esophageal irritation.

Inhalation: 3 or 4 gtt of peppermint oil in hot water t.i.d., as needed.

Oil: 0.2 to 0.4 ml P.O. t.i.d. in dilute preparations. Average daily amount should be 6 to12 gtt.

Spirits (10% oil and 1% leaf extract): 1 ml (20 gtt) with water P.O. t.id., as needed.

Tea: 1 to 1.5 g (1 tbsp) leaves in 160 ml of boiling water P.O. b.i.d. or t.i.d.

Tincture (1:% preparation; 45% ethanol): 2 to 3 ml P.O. t.i.d.

Topicals (as external analgesic; menthol 1.26-16%): Apply to affected area t.i.d. or q.i.d.; for external use only.

The fatal dose of menthol in humans is estimated to be 1,000 mg/kg (Murray, 1995).

Adverse reactions

GI: abdominal pain, gastroesophageal reflux disease, worsening symptoms of heartburn, hiatal hernia, relaxation of lower esophageal sphincter and GI smooth muscle, perianal burning.

Respiratory: *asthma exacerbation, bronchial or laryngeal spasms* (in infants and young children; with menthol in teas).

Skin: contact dermatitis (with external use).

Other: *allergic reactions* (flushing, headache, heartburn, irritation of mucous membranes, muscle twitching, rash; with internal use).

Interactions

Calcium channel blockers: May increase effects on smooth muscle. Use cautiously with peppermint oil.

Drugs that block gastric acid secretion: Some references suggest that peppermint oil should be used cautiously with drugs that block gastric acid secretion.

Contraindications and precautions

Mint is contraindicated in patients with hypersensitivity or known allergy to peppermint, menthol, or other members of the mint family. It is also contraindicated in pregnant patients because peppermint oil may stimulate menstrual flow. Do not apply topically on or near mucous membranes (eyes, nares, lips, genitalia) or open or abraded skin or use in patients with biliary duct occlusion, gallbladder inflammation, gallstones, gastroesophageal reflux disease, hiatal hernia, or severe hepatic dysfunction. Avoid use in patients with achlorhydria and in young children. Peppermint leaf may cause choking.

Use with caution because menthol can also cause sensitization and allergic reactions in adults and children. Symptoms include erythema, urticaria, and other cutaneous lesions.

Special considerations

⬛ ALERT Peppermint oil has been shown to cause dose-related neurotoxicity and brain lesions in rats fed up to 100 mg/kg/day for 28 days (Olsen and Thorup, 1984).

⬛ ALERT Applying a mentholated ointment to an infant's nostrils for cold relief may cause a syncopal event.

• Caution the patient not to give peppermint or spearmint products to infants or young children.

• Caution the patient not to apply topical mentholated products to broken skin.

• Instruct the patient not to use topical menthol preparations with a heating pad because skin damage can occur.

• Caution the patient to avoid prolonged use of peppermint oil as an inhalant.

• Peppermint-flavored toothpaste has been reported to exacerbate asthma symptoms in a young adult (Jacknowitz, 1996).

• Advise the patient with gastroesophageal reflux disease to avoid taking mint products internally.

• Advise women to avoid using mint during pregnancy or when breast-feeding.

Points of interest

• The German Commission E monographs give approval for the use of peppermint oil and peppermint leaf in GI, gallbladder, and biliary spasms; internally for upper respiratory tract symptoms of colds or bronchitis; and externally for myalgias and neuralgias.

• Notably, peppermint oil was dropped from nonprescription drug status in 1990 by the FDA Advisory Review Panel on OTC Miscellaneous Internal Drug Products because it lacked safety and efficacy information for use internally as a digestive aid.

Commentary

Peppermint and spearmint are used extensively as flavoring agents in foods, pharmaceuticals, and cosmetics. The internal use of spearmint has not been widely studied and is not recommended. Peppermint has

---

Bold italic type indicates that reaction may be life-threatening.

been used internally for treating some GI disorders, including irritable bowel syndrome, and respiratory tract complaints. Efficacy data in these areas are inconclusive and do not include sufficient safety information, especially with regard to children. The external use of peppermint, or menthol, is generally recognized as safe as an antipruritic and a local analgesic or anesthetic if used appropriately.

References

Dew, M.J., et al. "Peppermint Oil for the Irritable Bowel Syndrome: A Multicentre Trial," *Br J Clin Pract* 38:394-98, 1984.

Hills, J.M., and Aaronson, P.I. "The Mechanism of Action of Peppermint Oil in Gastrointestinal Smooth Muscle," *Gastroenterology* 101:55-65, 1991.

Jacknowitz, A.I. "External Analgesic Products," in *Handbook of Nonprescription Drugs.* Edited by Covington, T.R., et al. Washington, D.C.: American Pharmaceutical Association, 1996.

Jarvis, L.J., et al. "Topical Peppermint Oil for the Relief of Colonic Spasms at Barium Enema," *Clin Radiol* 46:A435, 1992. Abstract.

Leicester, R., and Hunt, R. "Peppermint Oil to Reduce Colonic Spasm During Endoscopy," *Lancet* 2:989, 1982. Abstract.

Murray, M. *The Healing Power of Herbs.* Rocklin, Calif.: Prima Publishing, 1995.

Nash, P., et al. "Peppermint Oil Does Not Relieve the Pain of Irritable Bowel Syndrome," *Br J Clin Pract* 40:292-93, 1986.

Olsen, P., and Thorup, I. "Neurotoxicity in Rats with Peppermint Oil and Pulegone," *Arch Toxicol* (Suppl) 7:408-9, 1984.

Pittler, M.H., and Ernst, E. "Peppermint Oil for Irritable Bowel Syndrome: A Critical Review and Metaanalysis," *Am J Gastroenterol* 93:1131-35, 1998.

Rees, W., et al. "Treating Irritable Bowel Syndrome with Peppermint Oil," *Br Med J* 2:835-36, 1979.

Sparks, M., et al. "Does Peppermint Oil Relieve Spasms During Barium Enema?" *Br J Radiol* 68:841-43,1995.

Taylor, B.A., et al. "Inhibitory Effect of Peppermint on Gastrointestinal Smooth Muscle," *Gut* 24:A992, 1983. Abstract.

MISTLETOE

ALL-HEAL, BIRDLIME, DEVIL'S FUGE, EUROPEAN
MISTLETOE, GOLDEN BOUGH, *VISCUM*

Taxonomic class
Viscaceae

Common trade names
Helixor, Iscador (aqueous extract), Iscador Qu Spezial, Iscucin, Plenosol, Viscum Album Quercus Frischsaft

Common forms
Available as capsules, dried leaves, infusion, liquid extract, tablets, and tincture.

Source
Active components are commonly derived from the leaves, branches, and berries of European mistletoe, *Viscum album,* and related species,

V. abietis and *V. austriacum.* These plants live as parasites on tree branches and are native to England, Europe, and Asia. North American mistletoes, including *Phoradendron flavescens, P. serotinum,* and *P. tomentosum*, are primarily used as Christmas greens. They are also parasitic and commonly grow on fruit trees, poplars, and oaks.

Chemical components

Mistletoe plants contain amines, acetylcholine, choline, beta-phenylethylamine, histamine, tyramine, phoratoxins, viscotoxins, flavonoids, flavonol derivatives (quercetin), lectins, terpenoids, alkaloids, and acids. Other compounds include mucilage, polyols, sugars, starch, tannins, and syringin.

Actions

Mistletoe is claimed to have cardiac depressant, hypotensive, and sedative effects. In vitro studies with *V. album* showed antineoplastic activity. The phoratoxins, viscotoxins, and various lectins display cytotoxic activity to varying extents. The lectins' cytotoxic effect is reportedly inactivated by heat, but the cytotoxic effects of the alkaloid fractions and the viscotoxins are preserved despite heating for at least 60 minutes (Park et al., 1999). Lectins are also reported to increase the secretion of some cytokines (interleukins-I-beta, 2, 6, and 10) and tumor necrosis factor (TNF)-alpha (Hajto et al., 1990). Different preparations of *V. album* extracts produced varying results as far as their ability to induce the cytokines and TNF-alpha (Elsasser-Beile et al., 1998). Stoss and colleagues (1999) in Germany demonstrated an increase in CD3/25-positive lymphocyte counts in a small study of HIV-positive and HIV-negative individuals. Although a debate continues as to which components are responsible, *V. album* extracts have demonstrated the ability to stimulate the functional activity of granulocytes (Stein et al., 1999).

Other effects demonstrated by mistletoe include bradycardia, increased GI motility, dose-dependent hypotension and hypertension, and increased uterine activity.

Reported uses

Mistletoe has been claimed to be beneficial in treating arteriosclerosis, cancer, depression, epilepsy, hypertension, hypertensive headache, insomnia, nervousness, sterility, tachycardia, tension, ulcers, and urinary disorders.

Iscador, prepared from crude juice of the plant, caused a slight improvement in patients with colon cancer and appeared to prolong survival in a patient with small-cell carcinoma of the lung (Bradley et al., 1989). Because the extract has relatively weak antineoplastic activity, it may be useful as an adjuvant therapy with surgery or radiotherapy.

Based on seemingly beneficial changes in hematologic parameters of HIV-positive patients, some investigators have suggested a role for *V. album* extracts in HIV disease (Gorter et al., 1999). This work should be considered preliminary data.

Dosage
Dried leaves: 2 to 6 g P.O. t.i.d.
Liquid extract (1:1 solution in 25% alcohol): 1 to 3 ml P.O. t.i.d.
Tincture (1:5 solution in 45% alcohol): 0.5 ml P.O. t.i.d.

Adverse effects
CNS: *coma,* delirium, fever, hallucinations, *seizures.*
CV: *bradycardia*, *cardiac arrest,* hypertension, hypotension.
EENT: gingivitis, miosis, mydriasis.
GI: diarrhea, gastroenteritis, *hepatitis,* nausea, vomiting.
GU: elevated BUN and serum creatinine levels (Gorter et al., 1999).
Hematologic: neutrophilic and monocytic leukocytosis (Gorter et al., 1998), eosinophilia (Van Wely et al., 1999; Gorter et al., 1999).
Metabolic: dehydration, diminished protein stores (Gorter et al., 1999).
Other: injection site redness.

Interactions
Antihypertensives: May increase hypotensive effects of these drugs. Avoid administration with mistletoe.
CNS depressants: Increased sedative effects. Avoid administration with mistletoe.
Immunosuppressants: Cytotoxic and immunostimulant effects. Consider carefully before using in combination.

Contraindications and precautions
Avoid using mistletoe in pregnant or breast-feeding patients; two types of mistletoe have shown uterine stimulant activity in animals.

Special considerations
■ **ALERT** All plant parts of mistletoe are toxic. Institute supportive emergency treatment for symptomatic patients.
● Subcutaneous injections of aqueous extracts of *V. album* cause an inflammatory reaction at the injection site. This reaction is predominantly a result of dense leukocyte (lymphocyte and monocyte) infiltration of both the dermal and the subcutaneous areas surrounding the site (Gorter et al., 1998). Some investigators suggest that this local reaction, as long as it remains tolerable (less than 5 cm), is desirable and might be used as an indicator of response (Stoss et al., 1999).
● A study examining the tolerability of escalating subcutaneous doses of an Iscador product (Iscador Qu Spezial) reported that HIV-positive patients were more likely than healthy subjects to experience adverse effects related to the preparation. Adverse effects were thought to be mild and included flulike symptoms, gingivitis, fever, local erythema, and eosinophilia (Van Wely et al., 1999).
● Monitor the patient taking mistletoe for dehydration and electrolyte imbalances.
● Caution the patient about the potential cardiac, CNS, and GI toxicity of mistletoe.

• Advise the patient taking mistletoe to treat cancer that conventional treatments should be considered first.

◆ **ALERT** Advise the patient to keep mistletoe out of the reach of children.

Commentary

Despite its known toxic effects, mistletoe continues to be pursued as a natural remedy for various ailments in other countries, especially Germany, where the bulk of the investigational research seems to originate. Some components of mistletoe appear to exert unique effects on cytokines, TNF-alpha, and leukocytes and demonstrate some antineoplastic activity. Some preliminary study suggests that toxicity from parenteral administration is mild, yet clinical investigations have been too small and too short. Larger trials for longer periods are needed to assess the plant's true safety and efficacy profile.

Based on worldwide research directions, it appears unlikely that mistletoe will be pursued for its use as an antineoplastic agent in the near future, although clinical investigations of this rather interesting entity in the immunosuppressed population are anticipated.

References

Bradley, G.W., et al. "Apparent Response of Small Cell Lung Cancer to an Extract of Mistletoe and Homeopathic Treatment," *Thorax* 44:1047-48, 1989.

Elsasser-Beile U, et al. "Comparison of the Effects of Various Clinically Applied Mistletoe Preparations on Peripheral Blood Leukocytes," *Arzneimittelforschung* 48(12):1185-89, 1998.

Gorter, R.W., et al. "Subcutaneous Infiltrates Induced by Injection of Mistletoe Extracts (Iscador)," *Am J Ther* 5(3):181-87, 1998.

Gorter, R.W., et al. "Tolerability of an Extract of European Mistletoe Among Immunocompromised and Healthy Individuals," *Altern Ther Health Med* 5(6):37-44, 1999.

Hajto, T., et al. "Increased Secretion of Tumor Necrosis Factors Alpha, Interleukin 1, and Interleukin 6 by Human Mononuclear Cells Exposed to Beta-galactoside-specific Lectin from Clinically Applied Mistletoe Extract," *Cancer Res* 50:3322-26, 1990.

Park, J.H., et al. "Cytotoxic Effects of the Components in Heat-treated Mistletoe (Viscum album)," *Cancer Lett* 139(2):207-13, 1999.

Stein, G.M., et al. "Viscotoxin-free Extracts from European Mistletoe (Viscum album) Stimulate Activity of Human Granulocytes," *Anticancer Res* 19(4B):2925-28, 1999.

Stoss, M., et al. "Study on Local Inflammatory Reactions and Other Parameters During Subcutaneous Mistletoe Application in HIV-positive Patients and HIV-negative Subjects over a Period of 18 Weeks," *Arzneimittelforschung* 49(4):366-73, 1999.

Van Wely, M., et al. "Toxicity of a Standardized Mistletoe Extract in Immunocompromised and Healthy Individuals," *Am J Ther* 6(1):37-43, 1999.

Bold italic type indicates that reaction may be life-threatening.

MOTHERWORT

I-MU-TS'AO, LION'S EAR, LION'S TAIL, LION'S TART, THROW-
WORT

Taxonomic class
Lamiaceae

Common trade names
None known.

Common forms
Available as dried leaves, extract, and liquid.

Source
Extracts are obtained primarily from the seeds or nutlets contained in
the dry and spinose flowering heads of *Leonurus cardiaca.* Active components of *L. artemisia* are extracted from the dried leaves. These members of the mint family have been naturalized to the United States and
Canada from Europe. Other species that may be referred to as motherwort include *L. glaucescens, L. heterophyllus, L. quinquelobatus,* and *L.
sibiricus.*

Chemical components
Extracts of various *Leonurus* species have yielded active substances,
such as alkaloids, cardanolides, flavones, saponins, and phenylpropanoid glycosides (from *L. artemisia*). Furanoid derivatives have been purified from *L. cardiaca,* nitrate compounds have been isolated from *L.
quinquelobatus,* and guanidine derivatives have been isolated from *L.
sibiricus.*

Actions
Few data exist on the therapeutic action of *L. cardiaca.* The herb exerts
CV effects, including inhibiting pulsating myocardial cells in vitro and
improving coronary circulation and microcirculation in rats, and
platelet-aggregation inhibitory effects in rats (Xia, 1983). *L. quinquelobatus* may exert CNS effects in animals, including slowing the heart rate
and increasing the force of cardiac contractility. *L. artemisia* has shown
uterotonic effects in the rat uterus in vitro.

   Human studies performed with *L. heterophyllus* noted decreased
blood viscosity and fibrinogen volume, increased RBC flexibility, and
decreased platelet aggregation (Zou, 1989). It is possible that the anticoagulant effect may be attributed to prehispanolone, a motherwort component.

   Anti-inflammatory and antineoplastic activity has been noted in animal models. A Russian study reported possible antioxidant properties
in humans (Bol'shakova, 1997).

Reported uses
Motherwort has long been used as a remedy for such cardiac conditions
as palpitations, hence the name *cardiaca.* It has also been used as a pain

reliever for menstrual cramping and as a uterotonic to assist in childbirth. These claims have not been confirmed by human therapeutic trials.

Dosage
No consensus exists.

Adverse reactions
Hematologic: increased bleeding time.
Skin: photosensitivity (at high doses).

Interactions
Beta blockers, digoxin, other cardiac drugs: Decreased heart rate and increased contractility (in animals). Avoid administration with motherwort.
Heparin, warfarin: Risk of increased bleeding effects. Avoid administration with motherwort.

Contraindications and precautions
Motherwort is contraindicated during pregnancy because of its potential uterotonic and prostaglandin synthesis effects. It is also contraindicated in patients with thrombocytopenia.

Special considerations
• Caution the patient not to self-treat symptoms of cardiac disease before seeking appropriate medical evaluation because this may delay diagnosis of a serious medical condition.
• Advise the patient using this herb to avoid direct sunlight.
• Urge the patient to report signs of unusual bruising or bleeding.
• Instruct the patient to notify the prescriber and pharmacist of any herbal or dietary supplement he is taking when filling a new prescription.

Commentary
Some studies suggest that motherwort may have promising antineoplastic and antioxidant properties. Further investigation and clinical trials are needed to support any therapeutic claims.

References
Bol'shakova, I.V. "Antioxidant Properties of a Series of Extracts from Medicinal Plants," *Biofizika* 42:480-83, 1997.

Xia, Y.X. "The Inhibitory Effect of Motherwort Extract on Pulsating Myocardial Cells In Vitro," *J Tradit Chin Med* 3:185-88, 1983.

Zou, Q.Z. "Effect of Motherwort on Blood Viscosity," *Am J Chin Med* 17:65-70, 1989.

MUGWORT

AI YE, ARMOISE COMMUNE, *ARTEMESIA*, CARLINE THISTLE, FELON HERB, GEMEINER BEIFUSS, HIERBA DE SAN JUAN, SAILOR'S TOBACCO, ST. JOHN'S PLANT, *SUMMITATES ARTEMISIAE*, WILD WORMWOOD

Taxonomic class
Asteraceae

Common trade names
Phyto Surge

Common forms
Available as dried leaves and roots, fluidextract, infusion, and tincture.

Source
The dried herb is obtained from the leaves and roots of *Artemisia vulgaris,* a shrubby perennial and member of the daisy family that is native to northern Europe, Asia, and North America. The herb should not be confused with wormwood (*A. absinthium*).

Chemical components
The volatile oil contains camphor, thujone, linalool, 1,8-cineole, 4-terpineol, borneol, spathulenol, alpha-cadinol, and monoterpene. Other components include sesquiterpenes, sesquiterpene lactones (including the eudesmane derivative vulgarin, also known as tauremisin), psilostachyin, psilostachyin C, flavonol glycosides (including quercetin and rutin), coumarins (including aesuletin, aesculin, umbelliferone, scopoletin, coumarin, and 6-methoxy-7,8-methylene-dioxycoumarin), polyacetylenes, pentacyclic triterpenes, sitosterol, stigmasterol, and carotenoids.

Actions
Mugwort is reported to have abortifacient, analgesic, anthelmintic, antibacterial, antiflatulent, antifungal, antirheumatic, antiseptic, aphrodisiac, appetite stimulant, bile stimulant, CNS depressant, counterirritant, diaphoretic, digestive, diuretic, emetic, expectorant, hemostatic, laxative, sedative, uterine stimulant, and uterine vasodilator activities. An aqueous extract of the herb has been shown to possess antibacterial activity against *Streptococcus mutans* (Chen et al., 1989).

Reported uses
Mugwort was traditionally used similarly to wormwood (*A. absinthium*)—as an anthelmintic and for treating amenorrhea and dysmenorrhea. It is used in Chinese traditional medicine for *moxa* treatments (moxibustion), in which small cones of dried mugwort leaves are burned in cups on certain points of the body, many of which coincide with acupuncture points. Moxibustion is growing in popularity in the

United States. Its use in correction of breech presentation has been evaluated clinically with positive results (Cardini and Weixin, 1998).

Mugwort is also used to treat GI conditions, such as abdominal cramps, colic, constipation, diarrhea, and weak digestion, and for chills, circulatory problems, mild depression, epilepsy, fever, hysteria, menopausal and menstrual complaints, rheumatism, seizures in children, stress, and persistent vomiting.

The roots are claimed to be useful as a tonic and for treating anxiety, depression, hypochondria, insomnia, general irritability and restlessness, neurasthenia, neuroses, and psychoneuroses. Other uses include anorexia, asthma, dermatitis, dysentery, flatulence, gout, headache, hematemesis, hemoptysis, infertility, muscle spasm, neuralgia, nosebleed, opioid addiction, pinworms, roundworms, snakebite, threadworms, and whitlow. The essential oil is used for antibacterial and antifungal purposes.

Immunotherapy with *A. vulgaris* has successfully decreased cutaneous and bronchial sensitivity as well as serum-specific immunoglobulin E (IgE) antibodies in patients who are allergic to mugwort pollen (Olsen et al., 1995; Leng et al., 1990).

Dosage

As an appetite stimulant, 150 ml of boiling water poured over 1 or 2 tsp of the dried herb, allowed to steep for 5 to 10 minutes, and then strained. Two to three cups of the tea are taken before meals.

For heavy menstruation, infusion of 15 g of dried herb added to 500 ml of water P.O., or as tincture, up to 2.5 ml P.O. t.i.d.

For stress, 5 ml of root tincture P.O. 30 minutes before bedtime.

For other complaints, 1 to 4 ml of tincture (1:1 in 25% ethanol) P.O. t.i.d.

Adverse reactions

GI: *significant uterine stimulant effects.*
Skin: contact dermatitis.
Other: allergic reaction, *anaphylaxis.*

Interactions

Anticoagulants: May increase anticoagulant effects. Avoid administration with mugwort.

Contraindications and precautions

Mugwort is contraindicated in pregnant or breast-feeding patients and in those with bleeding abnormalities. Avoid its use in patients with previous sensitization. Use cautiously in patients with gastroesophageal reflux disease.

Special considerations

• Mugwort pollen is a known allergen that contributes to hay fever in some patients. It demonstrates IgE cross-reactivity with hazelnut (Caballero et al., 1997).

• Patients who are hypersensitive to mugwort pollen may be allergic to other foods in the Asteraceae family (Garcia Ortiz et al., 1996).

Bold italic type indicates that reaction may be life-threatening.

• Patients who are hypersensitive to tobacco, honey, or royal jelly may experience an allergic reaction to mugwort.
• Urge the patient who is taking anticoagulants to avoid using mugwort.
• Caution the pregnant or breast-feeding patient to avoid using mugwort.
• Inform the patient about the lack of clinical safety and efficacy data for this herb.

Commentary
Because of the lack of clinical data to support mugwort's safety and efficacy for its reported indications, its use cannot be recommended.

References
Caballero, T., et al. "IgE Cross-reactivity Between Mugwort Pollen (Artemisia vulgaris) and Hazelnut (Abellana nux) in Sera from Patients with Sensitivity to Both Extracts," *Clin Exp Allergy* 27:1203-11, 1997. Abstract.

Cardini, F., and Weixin, H. "Moxibustion for Correction of Breech Presentation: A Randomized Controlled Trial," *JAMA* 280:1580-84, 1998.

Chen, C.P., et al. "Screening of Taiwanese Crude Drugs for Antibacterial Activity Against Streptococcus mutans," *J Ethnopharmacol* 27:285-95, 1989. Abstract.

Garcia Ortiz, J.C., et al. "Allergy to Foods in Patients Monosensitized to Artemisia Pollen," *Allergy* 51:927-31, 1996.

Leng, X., et al. "A Double-blind Trial of Oral Immunotherapy for Artemesia Pollen Asthma with Evaulation of Bronchial Response to the Pollern Allergen and Serum-specific IgE Antibody," *Ann Allergy* 64:27-31, 1990.

Olsen, O.T., et al. "A Double-blind, Randomized Study Investigating the Efficacy and Specificity of Immunotherapy with Artemisia vulgaris or Phleum pratense/betula verrucosa," *Allergol Immunopathol (Madr)* 23:73-78, 1995. Abstract.

MULLEIN
AARON'S ROD, BUNNY'S EARS, CANDLEWICK PLANT, FLANNEL-LEAF, GREAT MULLEIN, JACOB'S STAFF

Taxonomic class
Scrophulariaceae

Common trade names
Mullein Flower Oil, Mullein Leaves, Verbascum Complex

Common forms
Capsules: 290 mg, 330 mg (leaf)
Flower oil: 1 oz, 2 oz
Liquid extract: 250 mg (2 oz)

Source
The crude drug is obtained from the dried leaves and flowers of *Verbascum thapsus,* a tall, biennial herb of the snapdragon family. The plant is native to Europe and Asia and naturalized to the United States. It is easily noted by its characteristic fuzzy leaves and yellow flower spikes.

Chemical components
Mullein contains saponins, an iridioid glycoside (verbascoside), and several carbohydrates. Bitter amorphous substances and mucilage are found in the leaves; the seeds contain hemolytic saponins but no alkaloids. Flavonoids have also been noted.

Actions
The pharmacology of verbascoside, an iridoid glycoside isolated from *V. thapsus,* is being studied. Preliminary studies suggest that it may have significant anti-inflammatory, antioxidant, and antitumorigenic effects. The presence of four phenolic hydroxyl groups in the structure of verbascoside may contribute to its antioxidant activity (Zheng et al., 1993).

Because verbascoside also inhibits 5-lipoxygenase, the enzyme that catalyzes formation of inflammatory leukotrienes, it may play a role in inflammatory and allergic diseases. Some glycosides of *V. thapsus* also have documented antitumorigenic effects. One in vitro study found that verbascoside has cytotoxic effects on rat hepatoma and sarcoma cells and cytostatic activity on human epithelial carcinoma cells (Saracoglu et al., 1995). Another in vitro trial found antiviral effects in an alcoholic extract of mullein (Zanon et al., 1999).

Reported uses
Touted therapeutic claims for mullein include its use as an antitussive, a demulcent, and an expectorant, but clinical trial data to document its efficacy are lacking. It is believed to tone the mucous membranes of the respiratory system, increasing fluid production and thus promoting a productive cough. It has been combined with white horehound, colt's foot, and lobelia for bronchitis; with elder and red clover for coughs; and with gumweed for asthma. An extract of mullein prepared with olive oil and applied externally is used for healing and soothing inflamed surfaces. This oil has also been used in the ear to stimulate secretion of cerumen and systemically to control painful urination in chronic cystitis, hyperuricemia, and urinary calculi.

Dosage
Traditional uses suggest the following dosages:
Capsules: Two 290-mg capsules P.O. with two meals daily or as needed.
Flower oil: 5 to 10 gtt P.O.
Leaves: 1 cup of boiling water mixed with 1 or 2 tsp of dried leaves and steeped for 10 to 15 minutes. Tea can be decanted and taken t.i.d.

Adverse reactions
CNS: sedation.
Skin: contact dermatitis.

Interactions
None reported.

Contraindications and precautions
Avoid using mullein in children and in pregnant or breast-feeding patients; effects are unknown. Mullein is also contraindicated in patients who are hypersensitive to the herb.

Special considerations
• Advise the patient to consult a health care provider before using herbal preparations because a treatment that has been clinically researched and proved effective may be available.
• Advise women to avoid using mullein during pregnancy or when breast-feeding.
• Inform the patient that clinical data about mullein products are lacking.
• Although no known chemical interactions have been reported in clinical studies, consideration must be given to the pharmacologic properties of the herbal product and the potential for exacerbation of the intended therapeutic effect of conventional drugs.

Points of interest
• During the 19th century, dried flowers and roots of mullein were smoked for treatment of respiratory diseases and asthma symptoms, a practice copied from the Mohegan and Penobscot Indians.

Commentary
Clinical data do not support the use of mullein for treating chronic respiratory conditions and for other therapeutic claims made. Although preliminary data suggest that glycosides might have therapeutic value, human studies have not confirmed initial results. Because information regarding treatment is lacking, mullein cannot be recommended for use.

References
Saracoglu, I., et al. "Studies on Components with Cytotoxic and Cytostatic Activity of Two Turkish Medicinal Plants," *Biol Pharm Bull* 18:1396-400, 1995.

Zanon, S., et al. "Search for Antiviral Activity of Certain Medicinal Plants from Cordoba, Argentina," *Rev Latinoam Microbiol* 41(2):59-62, 1999.

Zheng, R.L., et al. "Inhibition of the Autooxidation of Linoleic Acid by Phenylpropanoid Glycosides from Pedicularis in Micelles," *Chem Phys Lipids* 65:151-54, 1993.

MUSTARD

BLACK MUSTARD, BROWN MUSTARD, CALIFORNIA RAPE, CHARLOCK, CHINESE MUSTARD, INDIAN MUSTARD, WHITE MUSTARD, WILD MUSTARD

Taxonomic class
Brassicaceae

Common trade names
Multi-ingredient preparations: Act-On Rub, Musterole

Common forms
Available as ground mustard seeds (mustard flour), mustard oil, and a tea.

Source
The active component is the volatile oil, derived from the seeds by steam distillation or expression. Black and white mustard plants (*Brassica nigra* and *B. alba*) are native to the southern Mediterranean area. Other *Brassica* species occur in Eastern Europe, India, and the Middle East. White mustard is also referred to as *Sinapis alba*.

Chemical components
Components include sinigrin (potassium myronate), myrosin, sinapic acid, sinapine, fixed oils (erucic, eicosenoic, arachic, oleic, and palmitic acid glucosides), globulins, and mucilage. Most mustards contain allyl isothiocyanate and *p*-hydroxybenzyl isothiocyanate precursors in their volatile oils. Sinigrin releases allyl isothiocyanate when in contact with myrosin.

Actions
Potent local irritant effects allow mustard to serve as a rubefacient when applied topically. Irritation and copious tearing in the eyes can be attributed to allyl isothiocyanate. Isothiocyanate compounds have produced goiter in animals. The volatile mustard oil has strong antimicrobial properties. Sinigrin has been reported to have antilarvicidal properties against some insects.

Mustard oil has been reported to exhibit anticarcinogenic effects in animals with arsenic-induced chromosomal aberrations. This effect was greater than that seen with garlic extract (Choudhury et al., 1997).

Reported uses
Anecdotally, mustard has been used in footbaths for rheumatism and arthritis of the feet and topically to alleviate muscle aches and pains. The herb has also been used as an antiflatulent, a diuretic, an emetic, and a stimulant and both orally and applied topically to the chest to relieve pulmonary congestion.

Dosage
As a footbath, mix 1 tbsp of mustard seeds with 1 L of hot water as a soak.
As a topical rubefacient, prepare a paste with 120 g (4 oz) of ground black mustard seeds in warm water. The irritant effect can be eased by applying olive oil after the paste is removed.

Adverse reactions
Skin: severe contact irritation of skin and mucous membranes.

Contraindications and precautions
Mustard is contraindicated in pregnant or breast-feeding patients; effects are unknown. Use cautiously in patients with pulmonary disease because inhalation may aggravate airways.

Bold italic type indicates that reaction may be life-threatening.

Special considerations

🕭 ALERT Because of its toxic nature, volatile mustard oil should not be tasted or inhaled in undiluted form.

• Caution the patient to use care when preparing mustard herbal products and to wash hands after using products and avoid contact with eyes.

• Caution the patient not to apply mustard preparations to mucous membranes.

• Advise parents to keep mustard products out of the reach of children and pets.

Points of interest

• Mustard flour typically lacks the characteristic pungent aroma when dry, but the aroma is released on contact with water, which frees allyl isothiocyanate by hydrolysis.

• White mustard does not contain the toxic allyl isothiocyanate.

• The average maximum level of mustard oil in foods is about 0.02%.

• Topical application of white mustard seed as a poultice is approved in Germany for pulmonary congestion and joint and soft-tissue inflammation.

Commentary

The unique pungent properties of mustard entice people to use it as an herbal remedy. If not handled properly, mustard can damage the tissues. Although white mustard has been used in Germany, data regarding its use are not available.

References

Choudhury, A.R., et al. "Mustard Oil and Garlic Extract as Inhibitors of Sodium Arsenite-induced Chromosomal Breaks in Vivo," *Cancer Lett* 121:45-52, 1997.

MYRRH

AFRICAN MYRRH, ARABIAN MYRRH, BAL, BOL, BOLA, GUM MYRRH TREE, HEERABOL, SOMALI MYRRH, YEMEN MYRRH

Taxonomic class
Burseraceae

Common trade names
Astring-O-Sol, Myrrh Gum, Odara

Multi-ingredient preparations: Goldenseal with myrrh.

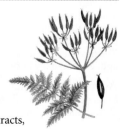

Common forms
Available in capsules (525 mg, 650 mg), fluidextracts, mouthwashes, salves, and tinctures.

Source
Myrrh is a mixture of volatile oil, gum, and resin (oleo-gum-resin) obtained from *Commiphora molmol* and other *Commiphora* species. These shrubs are native to Ethiopia, Somalia, and the Arabian Peninsula.

Chemical components
Myrrh is composed of volatile oils (dipentene, cadinene, heerabolene, limonene, pinene, eugenol, m-creosol, cinnamaldehyde, cuminaldehyde, cumic alcohol), resin (commiphoric acid), steroids (campesterol, cholesterol, beta-sitosterol), terpenoids (particularly alpha-amyrin), and gum.

Actions
Components of myrrh are reported to have antibacterial, antiflatulent, antifungal, antiseptic, astringent, expectorant, and local anesthetic properties (Dolara et al., 2000). Anti-inflammatory and antipyretic activity has been noted in rodent studies (Atta and Alkofahi, 1998). Myrrh extracts, alone and with other plants, have shown hypoglycemic activity, perhaps by involving increased target cell glucose use and decreased gluconeogenesis (Al-Awadi and Gumaa, 1987).

A lipid (guggulipid) from a related plant, *C. mukul,* appeared to reduce serum cholesterol levels and associated lipid parameters in some patients (Malhotra and Ahuja, 1971) and to affect thyroid metabolism in baby chicks (Tripathi et al., 1975).

Reported uses
Myrrh has been used for abrasions, aphthous ulcers, gingivitis, pharyngitis, pulmonary congestion, and wounds. It has also been incorporated into salves used externally for hemorrhoids, pressure ulcers, and wounds. Myrrh is primarily used today as a fragrance and flavoring agent.

Anecdotally, myrrh has been used with echinacea for infections and in mouthwash to treat ulcers. It has also been combined with witch hazel for external use. External preparations that contain myrrh, golden seal root powder, and marigold flowers have been claimed to be useful for their antimicrobial activity in patients with HIV infection or AIDS.

Dosage
Traditional uses suggest the following dosages:
Tea: 1 or 2 tsp of resin added to 1 cup of boiling water, allowed to steep for 10 to 15 minutes, and taken P.O. t.i.d.
Tincture: Resin is dissolved in alcohol; 1 to 4 ml of the tincture can be applied externally t.i.d.

Adverse reactions
Skin: dermatitis (conflicting reports).
Other: diarrhea, hiccups, and restlessness (reported with *C. mukul).*

Interactions
Insulin, sulfonylureas: Hypoglycemic effects may increase when administered with myrrh. Monitor blood glucose levels.

Bold italic type indicates that reaction may be life-threatening.

Contraindications and precautions

Avoid using myrrh in pregnant or breast-feeding patients; effects are unknown.

Special considerations

- Closely monitor the patient who is prone to hypoglycemia.
- Inform the patient that few clinical data exist on human use of myrrh.
- Urge the patient to immediately report signs and symptoms of hypoglycemia.

▲ ALERT Large doses of *C. myrrha* extract (injection) given to rats have decreased total protein and albumin levels; increased serum creatinine, bilirubin, cholesterol, and hepatocellular enzyme levels; and caused jaundice, macrocytic anemias, leukopenias, and death (Omer et al., 1999a). Similar toxic results were seen in goats who were given large doses (Omer and Adam, 1999b).

- Advise women to avoid using myrrh during pregnancy or when breast-feeding.

Points of interest

- The Federal Register recommends that myrrh tincture not be recognized as safe and effective. It should be considered misbranded if labeled for oral health care.

Commentary

Insufficient human data exist to support any therapeutic application of myrrh. In vitro studies suggest some interesting properties of myrrh and its components. Potential applications in HIV infection require thorough clinical investigation. *C. mukul* extracts appear to reduce serum lipid levels, but this use also needs further study. Animal studies suggest some potentially serious toxicities when given in substantial doses.

References

Al-Awadi, F.M., and Gumaa, K.A. "Studies on the Activity of Individual Plants of an Antidiabetic Plant Mixture," *Acta Diabetol Lat* 24:37-41, 1987.

Atta, A.H., and Alkofahi, A. "Anti-nociceptive and Anti-inflammatory Effects of Some Jordanian Medicinal Plant Extracts," *J Ethnopharmacol* 60(2):117-24, 1998.

Dolara, P., et al. "Local Anesthetic, Antibacterial and Antifungal Properties of Sesquiterpenes from Myrrh," *Planta Med* 66(4):356-58, 2000. Letter.

Malhotra, S.C., and Ahuja, M.M. "Comparative Hypolipidemic Effectiveness of Gum Guggulu (Commiphora mukul) Fraction, Alpha-ethyl-p-chlorophenoxy-isobutyrate, and Cica-13437-Su," *Indian J Med Res* 59:1621-32, 1971.

Omer, S.A., et al. "Effects of Commiphora myrrha Extract Given by Different Routes of Administration," *Vet Human Toxicol* 41(4):193-96, 1999a.

Omer, S.A., and Adam, S.E. "Toxicity of Commiphora myrrha to Goats," *Vet Human Toxicol* 41(5):299-301, 1999b.

Tripathi, S.N., et al. "Effect of a Keto-Steroid of Commiphora mukul on Hypercholesterolemia and Hyperlipidemia Induced by Neomercazole and Cholesterol Mixture in Chicks," *Indian J Exp Biol* 13:15-18, 1975.

MYRTLE

BRIDAL MYRTLE, COMMON MYRTLE, DUTCH MYRTLE,
JEW'S MYRTLE, MIRTIL, ROMAN MYRTLE

Taxonomic class
Myrtaceae

Common trade names
None known.

Common forms
Available as extracts.

Source
Active components are derived from the seeds and leaves of *Myrtus communis,* a plant that is native to the Mediterranean and the Middle East. This plant should not be confused with Madagascar myrtle (*Eugenia jambolana)* or common periwinkle (*Vinca minor).*

Chemical components
The volatile oil contains myrtol or gelomyrtol as well as eucalyptol, dextro-pinene, and camphor. Tannins and polyphenolic compounds have also been found in the leaves.

Actions
An alcoholic extract of myrtle demonstrated weak anti-inflammatory activity in animal models (Al-Hindawi et al., 1989). Myrtle extract showed unique hypoglycemic properties in mice (Elfellah et al., 1984). A leaf tincture may minimize antibiotic resistance to some pathogenic staphylococci (Pochinok et al., 1968).

Reported uses
Myrtle has been used as an astringent antiseptic for wounds, a pulmonary decongestant, and a tonic for digestive and urinary disorders. Although myrtle has been investigated as an antidiabetic agent, this effect has not been adequately documented in humans. Phytohemagglutinins from myrtle seeds have been used to reduce turbidity of lipemic sera, enabling spectrophotometric determination of blood glucose levels; serum bilirubin, uric acid, and hepatic transaminase levels; and other components of the sera (Ortega and Rodenas, 1979).

Dosage
The suggested dose is 1 to 2 ml of essential oil P.O. daily.

Adverse reactions
Metabolic: hypoglycemia.
Other: allergic reaction.

Bold italic type indicates that reaction may be life-threatening.

Interactions
Drugs undergoing significant detoxification through the cytochrome P-450 system of the liver: May increase hepatic microsomal enzyme function (in animals). Monitor response to drug therapy.
Insulin, oral sulfonylureas: May increase hypoglycemic effects. Use cautiously.

Contraindications and precautions
Avoid using myrtle in pregnant or breast-feeding patients; effects are unknown. Use cautiously in diabetic patients.

Special considerations
• Caution the patient not to take the essential oil internally except under the supervision of a health care provider.
• Advise women to avoid using myrtle during pregnancy or when breast-feeding.
• Monitor blood glucose levels and liver function test results.
• Caution the diabetic patient that myrtle may increase effects of antidiabetic drugs.
• Inform the patient that myrtle may affect the metabolism of other drugs.

Points of interest
• Myrtle is used as a dye in some regions of Greece.

Commentary
Although myrtle shows some promise as an antidiabetic agent in animals, human clinical data are lacking. Therefore, it cannot be recommended for any therapeutic use.

References
Al-Hindawi, M.K., et al. "Anti-inflammatory Activity of Some Iraqi Plants Using Intact Rats," *J Ethnopharmacol* 26:163-68, 1989.

Elfellah, M.S., et al. "Anti-hyperglycemic Effect of an Extract of *Myrtus communis* in Streptozotocin-induced Diabetes in Mice," *J Ethnopharmacol* 11:275-81, 1984.

Ortega, M., and Rodenas, S. "*Myrtus communis* L. Phytohemagglutinins as a Clarifying Agent for Lipemic Sera," *Clin Chim Acta* 92:135-39, 1979.

Pochinok, V., et al. "Possibility of Control of Resistance to Antibiotics of Pathogenic Staphylococci by the Tincture of *Myrtus communis* Leaves," *Farm Zh* 23:72-74, 1968. Abstract.

NETTLE

COMMON NETTLE, GREATER NETTLE, STINGING NETTLE

Taxonomic class
Urticaceae

Common trade names
Nettles Capsules, Nettles Liquid Extract

Common forms
Available as capsules (150 mg, 300 mg) and dried leaf and root extract or tincture.

Source
The active chemical components are found in the leaves, stems, and roots of *Urtica dioica*, a perennial herb of the nettle family. It is one of three species that are native to Europe and is naturalized throughout the United States and parts of Canada.

Chemical components
Nettle roots and flowers contain scopoletin, steryl derivatives, lignan glucosides, and flavonol glycosides. The roots contain phenylpropanes and lignans. The plant has B-group vitamins as well as vitamins C and K and steroid-related compounds such as sitosterol. The stinging, hair-like projections on the stems contain amines, such as histamine, serotonin, and choline, and formic acid. The lectin found in the roots is specific to this plant and may help to standardize preparations.

Actions
Nettle acts primarily as a diuretic by increasing urine volume and decreasing systolic blood pressure. It has been observed to stimulate uterine contractions in rabbits, but the mechanism is unknown.

Other compounds identified have known pharmacologic activity. The *U. dioica* agglutinin, a lectin protein, has immunostimulating activity. Scopoletin has anti-inflammatory activity. A 20% methanolic extract of stinging nettle roots inhibited benign prostatic hyperplasia (BPH) in mice (Lichius and Muth, 1997). The plant extract was effective in reducing urine flow, nocturia, and residual urine in human patients. Another study of stinging nettle extract reported it to have an antiproliferative effect on human prostatic cancer cells (Konrad et al., 2000).

Reported uses
Nettle has been used to treat rheumatism and is claimed to be helpful as an antispasmodic and an expectorant. The leaves have been smoked to

treat asthma. Nettle tea has been used to treat cough and tuberculosis. The juice has been applied to the scalp to stimulate hair growth. The plant's styptic or astringent action has been useful for treating nosebleeds and uterine bleeding. Other claims include treatment of cancer, diabetes, eczema, and gout and wound healing.

Nettle's diuretic properties have prompted its use in heart failure, hypertension, and urinary, bladder, and renal disorders. It was studied with other herbs as a bladder irrigant for treating prostatic adenoma in humans and was found to reduce postoperative blood loss, bacteriuria, and inflammation. The German Commission E recognizes this irrigant for treating urinary tract inflammation and for preventing and treating kidney gravel. Nettle is widely used in Germany for the early treatment of BPH and has been shown to be effective for treating allergic rhinitis (Mittman, 1990). However, there is stronger evidence for the use of saw palmetto, beta-sitosterols, and pygeum in the treatment of BPH than for nettle.

Dosage
For allergic rhinitis, 150 to 300 mg in capsule form P.O. t.i.d., as needed.
Root: 4 to 6 g P.O. daily.
Tea: 1 or 2 tsp of dried herb mixed in 1 cup of boiling water; up to 2 cups P.O. daily.
Tincture: ½ to 1 tsp P.O. up to b.i.d.

Adverse reactions
Skin: contact urticaria (leaves).
CV: edema (internal use).
GI: abdominal distress, diarrhea, indigestion (internal use).
GU: oliguria (internal use).

Interactions
Diuretics: May potentiate effects. Avoid administration with nettle.

Contraindications and precautions
Nettle is contraindicated in pregnant or breast-feeding women because of its diuretic and uterine stimulation properties. It is also contraindicated in children under age 2. Use cautiously and in reduced doses in older children and adults over age 65.

Special considerations
• Advise the patient to eat foods high in potassium, such as bananas and fresh vegetables, and to replenish electrolytes lost through diuresis.
• Caution the patient against self-medicating with nettle for BPH or to relieve fluid accumulation associated with heart failure without approval and supervision of a health care provider.
🕮 **ALERT** If rubbed against the skin, nettles can cause intense burning for 12 hours or longer. Instruct the patient to wash thoroughly with soap and water, use antihistamines and steroid creams, and wear heavy gloves if the plant is to be handled.

Bold italic type indicates that reaction may be life-threatening.

RESEARCH FINDINGS

Nettle for arthritic pain

A randomized, controlled, double-blind, crossover trial studied 27 patients, mean age 60 years, over 12 weeks. The perception of pain in the base of the thumb was measured after application of nettle leaf. Patients were instructed how to cut a leaf with the hand protected in a plastic bag and then to apply the underside of the leaf to the painful finger area. The treatment period lasted 1 week followed by a washout period of 5 weeks. Another treatment week with a further washout period of 5 weeks followed. Pain was measured by means of a patient diary, a visual analogue pain scale, and a verbal rating scale for pain. The investigators observed that after 1 week's treatment, pain scores were significantly reduced compared with placebo. Patients were permitted to continue taking analgesics or anti-inflammatories during the treatment periods, and it was noted that use of these drugs declined. The potential use of this treatment in osteoarthritic pain deserves further research (Randall et al., 2000).

Points of interest
- The FDA considers this herb to be of undefined safety.
- Nettle plants were used in weaving in the Bronze Age; archeologists have found burial shrouds made of nettle fabric.
- Nettle juice was an ingredient in hair-growth preparations in the 19th century.
- Native American women believed that nettle tea eased delivery and stopped uterine bleeding after childbirth.

Commentary
Despite its traditional use for several conditions, the only proven pharmacologic action of nettle is as a diuretic. It is considered relatively safe in the amounts recommended, and adverse effects from the oral form are rare. The herb has been studied in the treatment of allergic rhinitis, BPH, and osteoarthritis and as a component in postoperative bladder irrigation, but more studies are needed to determine its role for these uses. (See *Nettle for arthritic pain.*)

References
Konrad, L., et al. "Antiproliferative Effect on Human Prostate Cancer Cells by Stinging Nettle Root (Urtica dioica) Extract," *Planta Med* 66(1):44-47, 2000.

Lichius, J.J., and Muth, C. "The Inhibiting Effects of Urtica dioica Root Extracts on Experimentally Induced Prostatic Hyperplasia in the Mouse," *Planta Med* 63:307-10, 1997.

Mittman, P. "Randomized, Double-blind Study of Freeze-dried *Urtica dioica* in the Treatment of Allergic Rhinitis," *Planta Med* 56:44-47, 1990.

Randall, C., et al. "Randomized Controlled Trial of Nettle Sting for Treatment of Base-of-thumb Pain," *JR Soc Med* 93(6):305-9, 2000.

NIGHT-BLOOMING CEREUS

Cactus grandiflorus, *Cereus grandiflorus*, LARGE-FLOWERED CACTUS, QUEEN OF THE NIGHT, SWEET-SCENTED CACTUS, VANILLA CACTUS

Taxonomic class
Cactaceae

Common trade names
Multi-ingredient preparations: Cactus Grandiflorus, Cactus-Hawthorn Compound, Cereus Grandiflorus, Night-Blooming Cereus

Common forms
Available as liquid extract and tincture.

Source
Active components are derived from the stems and flowers of *Selenicereus grandiflorus*, which is native to tropical and subtropical America, including the West Indies.

Chemical components
The plant contains a digitalis-like glycoside, either cactine or hordenine (*N,N*-dimethyl-4-hydroxy-beta-phenethylamine). Other reported components include betacyanin, isorhamnetin-3-glucoside, narcissin, rutin, cacticine, kaempferitrin, grandiflorine, hyperoside, isorhamnetin-3-beta-galactosyl-rutinoside, and isorhamnetin-3-beta-xylosyl-rutinoside.

Actions
Night-blooming cereus is thought to elevate arteriolar tension by increasing the muscular energy of the heart and causing arteriolar contraction. This theory has not been confirmed by human data. Early research with commercial preparations of the active compound proved it to be physiologically inert. More recently, in studies with rats and dogs, hordenine showed a positive inotropic effect on the heart, with increased systolic and diastolic blood pressures and peripheral blood flow volume (Hapke, 1995). Flavonoids and their derivatives (rutin, rutinoside, and kaempferitrin) are thought to improve capillary function by decreasing abnormal leakage (Wadworth and Faulds, 1992).

Reported uses
In Europe, the liquid plant extract has been used to treat angina pectoris, irritable bladder, kidney congestion, nervous headache, palpitations, and prostatic diseases. The herb has been used as an antirheumatic and a cardiotonic in Cuba. Other indications for its use include cystitis, dyspnea, edema, endocarditis, and myocarditis. Anecdotal reports claim that the herb is valuable as a cardiac stimulant and a partial substitute for digitalis in heart disorders related to anemia, dyspepsia, Graves' disease, neurasthenia, and tobacco toxicity.

Dosage
Traditional uses suggest the following dosages:
Liquid extract: 0.7 ml (12 minims) P.O. every 4 hours.
Tincture: 1 to 1.8 ml (15 to 30 minims) P.O. every 4 hours.

Adverse reactions
EENT: burning sensation in the mouth.
GI: diarrhea, nausea, vomiting.

Interactions
ACE inhibitors, antiarrhythmics, beta blockers, calcium channel blockers, cardiac glycosides: May increase effects of these drugs. Avoid administration with night-blooming cereus.

Contraindications and precautions
Night-blooming cereus is contraindicated during the first trimester of pregnancy.

Special considerations
• Monitor the patient's heart rate and blood pressure if he is also taking prescription cardiac drugs.
• Encourage the patient with a CV disorder to be evaluated by a health care provider and, if necessary, receive prescribed cardiac drugs. Because the use of night-blooming cereus as a substitute for digitalis has not been confirmed by human clinical trials, it should not be used by itself for heart-related disorders.
• Urge the patient to immediately report heart-related adverse effects (blood pressure changes, increased heart rate, and palpitations) to his health care provider.
• Instruct women to report planned or suspected pregnancy.
• Advise women to avoid using night-blooming cereus during pregnancy or when breast-feeding.

Commentary
Although night-blooming cereus contains a digitalis-like glycoside, its use as a substitute for digitalis preparations (digoxin or digitoxin) or for treating heart-related disorders has not been evaluated in humans. Patients with such conditions should strongly be encouraged to seek professional medical advice. Also, patients who are taking prescription digitalis or other cardiac drugs should avoid concurrent use of this herb.

References
Hapke, H.J. "Pharmacological Effects of Hordenine," *Deutsche Tierarztliche Wochenschrift* 102:228-32, 1995. Abstract in English.
Wadworth, A.N., and Faulds, D. "Hydroxyethylrutosides: A Review of Pharmacology and Therapeutic Efficacy in Venous Insufficiency and Related Disorders," *Drugs* 44:1013-32, 1992.

Bold italic type indicates that reaction may be life-threatening.

NOTOGINSENG ROOT

PANAX NOTOGINSENG, PSEUDOGINSENG ROOT, SAN QI

Taxonomic class
Araliaceae

Common trade names
None known.

Common forms
Available as loose, dried roots and as tablets.

Source
The drug is extracted from the root of *Panax notoginseng* (also known as *Aralia quinquefolia* var. *notoginseng*), which belongs to the same family as panax or Chinese ginseng. The plant is native to the southern regions of China, and the root is cultivated before the plant flowers or after the fruit has ripened.

Chemical components
Active constituents of the root appear to be saponins. The plant root also contains heteroglycans composed of glucose, galactose, arabinose, mannose, and xylose.

Actions
The extract of the roots of *P. notoginseng* has exhibited antitumorigenic activity on mouse skin tumors (Konoshima et al., 1999). Studies have also demonstrated some calcium channel antagonism leading to antihypertensive and vasodilatory actions (Kwan, 1995; Feng et al., 1997). A study using dogs found that notoginseng had electrophysiologic effects similar to those of amiodarone (Wu et al., 1995). An in vitro study found that notoginseng extract improved sperm motility as well (Chen et al., 1999). Notoginseng also was shown to improve learning and decrease memory deficits in rats (Hsieh et al., 2000).

Reported uses
Notoginseng root is traditionally used in Chinese medicine to treat internal and external bleeding. It is taken internally to quell nosebleeds and blood in stool, urine, or lungs and for acute attacks of Crohn's disease. Applied externally, it is used to relieve pain and swelling from bruises, cuts, sprains, and other external wounds. None of these treatments has been supported by controlled clinical trials in humans.

Notoginseng has been promoted to treat angina and hypertension based on animal studies that showed effects on circulation and blood pressure. The lack of controlled human trials with notoginseng root limits its therapeutic usefulness.

Dosage
No standard guidelines exist because most consumption is as a tea mixture with other Chinese herbs.

Notoginseng root can be made into a liniment or compress for external use on wounds and bruises.

Adverse reactions
CNS: dizziness, headache.
CV: hypotension.
GI: constipation.
GU: *miscarriage.*

Interactions
Beta blockers: May have additive effects. Monitor the patient closely.

Contraindications and precautions
Notoginseng is contraindicated in pregnant or breast-feeding patients; it may cause a miscarriage.

Special considerations
• Inform the patient that clinical data supporting the use of notoginseng are lacking.
• Advise the patient to consult a health care provider before using herbal preparations because a treatment that has been clinically researched and proved effective may be available.
• Although no known chemical interactions have been reported in clinical studies, consideration must be given to the pharmacologic properties of the herb and the potential for exacerbation of the intended therapeutic effect of conventional drugs.

Commentary
Traditionally, notoginseng root has been used to treat bleeding disorders. There is no clear clinical evidence to support this use or any other, and thus, it cannot be recommended. Animal trials have found some potential use in CV disorders, but further human clinical trials are needed to determine the exact effect of notoginseng and the doses that are safe in humans.

References
Chen, J.C., et al. "Effect of *Panax notoginseng* Extracts on Inferior Sperm Motility In Vitro," *Am J Chin Med* 27(1):123-28, 1999.

Feng, P.F., et al. "Clinical and Experimental Study of Improving Left Ventricular Diastolic Function by Total Saponins of *Panax notoginseng*," *Chung Kuo Chung His I Chieh Ho Tsa Chih* 17(12):714-17, 1997.

Hsieh, M.T., et al. "The Ameliorating Effects of the Cognitive-enhancing Chinese Herbs on Scopolamine-induced Amnesia in Rats," *Phytother Res* 14(5):375-77, 2000.

Konoshima, T., et al. "Anti-carcinogenic Activity of the Roots of *Panax notoginseng*," *Biol Pharm Bull* 22(10):1150-52, 1999.

Kwan, C.Y. "Vascular Effects of Selected Antihypertensive Drugs Derived from Traditional Medicinal Herbs," *Clin Exp Pharmacol Physiol* 22(Suppl 1): S297-99, 1995.

Wu, W., et al. "Effects of *Panax notoginseng* Saponin RG1 on Cardiac Electrophysiological Properties and Ventricular Fibrillation Threshold in Dogs," *Chung Kuo Yao Li Hsueh Pao* 16(5):459-63, 1995.

Bold italic type indicates that reaction may be life-threatening.

NUTMEG

MACE, MACIS, MUSCADIER, MUSKATBAUM, MYRISTICA, NOZ
MOSCADA, NUEZ MOSCADA, NUX MOSCHATA

Taxonomic class
Myristicaceae

Common trade names
Multi-ingredient preparations: Agua del Carmen, Aluminum Free Indigestion, Incontinurina, Klosterfrau Magentonikum, Melisana, Nervospur, Vicks Vaporub

Common forms
Available as capsules (200 mg), essential oil, and powders.

Source
Nutmeg is the dried kernel of seeds of the nutmeg tree, *Myristica fragrans*. Inside the fruit lies a netlike substance, the aril, from which another spice (mace) is produced. The aril is wrapped around the brittle shells that contain the nutmeg kernel. Nutmeg trees grow in Sri Lanka, the West Indies, and the Molucca Islands.

Chemical components
Nutmeg seeds contain a fixed oil (nutmeg butter), consisting of myristic acid and glycerides of lauric, tridecanoic, stearic, and palmitic acids. Also present is an essential oil composed of *d*-camphene, dipentene, myristicin, elemicin, and small amounts of iso-elemicin, gerianiol, eugenol, isoeugenol, *d*-pinene, *l*-pinene, borneol, safrole, limonene, sabinene, cymene alpha-thujene, gamma-terpinene, lysergide, and monoterpene alcohols.

Actions
Nutmeg's components eugenol and isoeugenol may inhibit renal prostaglandin synthesis in rats (Misra et al., 1978). Nutmeg may have MAO inhibitor properties as well (Blumenthal et al., 1998). Many preliminary data surround nutmeg's claim as an antidiarrheal (Barrowman et al., 1975; Shafran and McCrone, 1975). Components of nutmeg have been shown to impair release of toxins from *Escherichia coli* bacteria. The herb may have value in veterinary medicine as an antidiarrheal in cattle.

Nutmeg may play a role in improving glucose and insulin metabolism, as shown in an in vitro study using a rat epididymal adipocyte assay (Broadhurst et al., 2000).

Total cholesterol levels were found to be significantly reduced and platelet aggregation inhibited in albino rabbits after receiving an ethanolic extract of nutmeg for 60 days (Ram et al., 1996). Nutmeg's potent hallucinogenic effect is thought to be attributed to lysergide, borneol, eugenol, geraniol, and safrol (Giannini et al., 1986); it is often sought by recreational drug users when stronger chemicals, such as LSD, cannot be obtained.

Reported uses

Commonly used as a cooking spice, nutmeg has also been used as an antiemetic and an aphrodisiac and for chronic CNS disorders, indigestion and other GI disorders, and renal disorders. The essential oil is claimed to be useful for bad breath, rheumatic pain, and toothaches. Although nutmeg is used for GI disorders in Germany, its use is controversial. Homeopathy supports the use of nutmeg for anxiety and depression. Nutmeg may possess antibacterial activity (Dorman and Deans, 2000).

Dosage

Some suggested doses are within the hazardous range.
For chronic diarrhea, indigestion, and nausea, 1 or 2 capsules of nutmeg "kernel" P.O. as a single dose, or 3 to 5 gtt of essential oil on a sugar lump or 1 tsp of honey P.O., or 4 to 6 tbsp of powder P.O. daily (for diarrhea).
For toothache, 1 or 2 gtt of essential oil applied to the gum around the aching tooth until the dental visit.

Adverse reactions

CNS: delusions (with excessive doses), euphoria, hallucinations.
With ingestion of nutmeg oil or doses over 5 g:
CNS: confusion, *seizures,* stupor.
CV: tachycardia.
EENT: dry mouth.
GI: constipation, nausea, vomiting.
GU: *miscarriage.*
Other: flushing, *death.*

Interactions

Antidiarrheals: May have additive effects. Monitor bowel function.
Neuroleptic drugs (clozapine, haloperidol, olanzapine, thiothixene): May cause loss of symptom control or interference with existing therapy for psychiatric illnesses. Avoid administration with nutmeg.

Contraindications and precautions

Nutmeg is contraindicated in pregnant or breast-feeding patients; it may cause a miscarriage. Use cautiously in patients with psychiatric illnesses.

Special considerations

• Inform the patient that nutmeg may be carcinogenic (Blumenthal et al., 1998).
• Monitor for CNS effects.
• Monitor the patient's bowel habits if nutmeg is being used as an antidiarrheal.
• Nutmeg has been abused and misused.
• Urge women to report planned or suspected pregnancy.
• Advise the patient to avoid hazardous activities until the herb's CNS effects are known.

Bold italic type indicates that reaction may be life-threatening.

• Caution the patient against consuming large amounts of nutmeg because of its toxic potential.

🔊 ALERT Symptoms of overdose include chest or abdominal pressure, confusion, extended periods of alternating bouts of delusions and somnolence, hypothermia, nausea, faint pulse, and vomiting. Anticholinergic hyperstimulation, palpitations, and psychosis can also occur. Treatment consists of gastric lavage and supportive therapy (Abernethy and Beckel, 1992).

• Caution the patient to keep nutmeg products out of the reach of children and pets.

• Inform the patient that nutmeg can precipitate symptoms associated with disease in a patient with psychiatric illness.

• Counsel the patient taking nutmeg for its antidiarrheal effects to consider less toxic agents, such as bulk laxatives, casanthrol with docusate sodium, and milk of magnesia.

Points of interest
• Nutmeg is most popular for its uses as a spice in foods and drinks and as a fragrance in cosmetics and soaps.

• Nutmeg is one of the active ingredients in Aromatic Ammonia Spirits NF, which causes reflex stimulation when inhaled.

Commentary
Despite nutmeg's interesting pharmacologic profile, its therapeutic use is limited because of the risk of toxicity and abuse or misuse. Death has resulted from ingestion of excessive quantities. Less toxic agents are available for treating diarrhea. Nutmeg cannot be recommended for any indication because of its risks.

References
Abernethy, M.K., and Beckel, L.B. "Acute Nutmeg Intoxication," *Am J Emerg Med* 10:429-30, 1992.

Barrowman, J.A., et al. "Diarrhea in Thyroid Medullary Carcinoma: Role of Prostaglandins and Therapeutic Effect of Nutmeg," *Br Med J* 3:11-12, 1975.

Blumenthal, M., et al. "Herb Guide by Pharmacological Action (Unapproved Herbs)," in *The Complete German Commission E Monographs: Therapeutic Guide to Herbal Medicines.* Austin, Tex.: American Botanical Council, 1998.

Broadhurst, C.L., et al. "Insulin-like Biological Activity of Culinary and Medicinal Plant Aqueous Extracts In Vitro," *J Agricultural Food Chem* 48(3):849-52, 2000.

Dorman, H.J., and Deans, S.G. "Antimicrobial Agents from Plants: Antibacterial Activity of Plant Volatile Oils," *J Appl Microbiol* 88(2):308-16, 2000.

Giannini, A.J., et al. "Contemporary Drugs of Abuse," *AFP* 33:208, 1986.

Misra, V., et al. "Role of Nutmeg in Inhibiting Prostaglandin Biosynthesis," *Indian J Med Res* 67:482, 1978.

Ram, A., et al. "Hypolipidaemic Effect of *Myristica fragrans* Fruit Extract in Rabbits," *J Ethnopharmacol* 55:49-53, 1996.

Shafran, I., and McCrone, D. "Nutmeg and Medullary Carcinoma of Thyroid," *N Engl J Med* 293:1266, 1975. Letter.

OAKS

BRITISH OAK, BROWN OAK, COMMON OAK, CORTEX
QUERCUS, ECORCE DE CHENE, EICHERINDE, EICHENLOHE,
ENCINA, ENGLISH OAK, GRAVELIER, NUTGALL, OAK
APPLES, OAK BARK, OAK GALLS, PENUNCULATE OAK,
STONE OAK, TANNER'S BARK

Taxonomic class
Fagaceae

Common trade names
Multi-ingredient preparations: Conchae Com-pound, Eichenrinden-
Extrakt, Entero-Sanol, Hamon No. 14, Kernosan Elixir, Menodoron,
Peerless Composition Essence, Pektan N, Silvapin, Tisanes de l'Abbe,
Tonsilgon-N, Traxaton, White Oak Bark, White Oak Inner Bark, Wild
Countryside White Oak

Common forms
Available as capsules, decoctions, extracts, unground or powdered oak
bark, oak galls, ointments, ooze (a tea of oak bark), and tincture. Oak
bark is included in some prepared herbal mixtures and several commercially prepared GI remedies, such as Entero-Sanol.

Source
Oak bark is obtained from the English oak, *Quercus robur*, and the dur-
mast oak, *Q. petraea,* members of the beech family. Oaks are slow-
growing deciduous trees that occur in Eurasia, North America, and
Australia. The bark is taken from young branches and twigs and can be
up to 4 mm thick; it is grayish brown on the outside and brownish red
on the inner surface.

   Oak galls are abnormal growths produced on oak stems and leaves,
primarily by insects and nematodes. Many galls are rich in tannins. The
leading gallmakers are tiny gall-wasps, which belong to the genus *Cynips*
(Cynipidae family). The insect pierces the shoots and young boughs of
the oak and deposits its egg in the wound. After hatching from the egg,
the larva secretes an enzyme-containing fluid that changes starch in ad-
jacent oak cells into sugar, which the larva consumes as a food source.
This sugar is also used by growing plant cells, which form a large, protective growth around the developing insect. When the insect reaches the
adult stage, it eats its way out of the gall.

Chemical components
Oak bark contains tannins, including quercitannic acid and varying
amounts of catechins, ellagitannins, and proanthocyanidins. The galls

contain tannic acid, gallic acid, resin, calcium oxalate, and starch. Acorns contain primarily tannic acid, gallic acid, and pyrogallol. The content of the tree components varies, depending on the time of harvesting and age of the branches, galls, or acorns. Other compounds found in the bark and galls include beta-sitosterol, friedelin, leucocyanidin, leucodelphinidin, levulin, pectin, quercetin, quercin, quercitol, and the glycoside quercitrin.

Actions

The active ingredients associated with oak bark and galls are the tannins. These highly astringent compounds act locally by precipitating proteins and decreasing cell membrane permeability. Tannic acid exerts astringent action on the mucous membranes of the GI tract; it can also be absorbed from damaged skin and mucous membranes. Although several properties have been reported for other components of oak, these chemicals exist in trace amounts and are unlikely to have clinical effects.

Quercitrin and quercetin have been reported to exert a vasodilating effect. However, studies have found that quercetin is extensively bound to cellular proteins and that it has no effect on CV or thrombogenic risk factors (Boulton et al., 1998; Conquer et al., 1998).

Reported uses

Traditionally, oak bark has been used as an anti-inflammatory, an antiseptic, and an astringent. Although oak galls may be used instead of the bark in small quantities, their use internally is not recommended. Astringent compresses were commonly applied to treat contact dermatitis and eczema in their early, weeping stage. Decoctions, such as vaginal douches, were used to treat leukorrhea; they were also used externally to treat anal fissures, small burns and other dermatologic conditions, foot odor, eye inflammation, hemorrhoids, and varicose veins. A decoction was also reportedly used as a gargle to treat bleeding gums, laryngitis, sore throat, and tonsillitis.

Powdered oak bark was used as a snuff to treat nasal polyps and sprinkled on weeping eczema to dry the affected area. The German Commission E recommends the external use of oak bark for inflammatory skin disorders and the internal use for the local treatment of acute diarrhea and mild inflammatory conditions of the oral cavity, pharyngeal region, and urogenital areas.

Tannic acid has been used in suppositories for hemorrhoids, locally for sore throat and stomatitis, and to harden nipples during breastfeeding. It has been shown to inhibit gastric enzyme activity in pigs, an effect attributed to its antisecretory and antiulcerative properties (Murakami et al., 1992).

Other claims advanced for tannic acid include its use as an antimutagenic, an antinephritic, an antioxidant, an antiviral, a bactericidal, a cancer preventive, a hepatoprotective, an immunosuppressant, a psychotropic, and a viricide.

Bold italic type indicates that reaction may be life-threatening.

Dosage
As an antidiarrheal, German Commission E recommends 3 g of the powdered oak bark or equivalent preparations P.O. daily. If diarrhea persists for longer than 4 days, the patient should consult a health care provider. Alternatively, 1 cup of tea P.O. t.i.d., made by adding 1 g of finely cut or coarsely powdered drug or 1 or 2 tsp of chopped bark to 500 ml of water, or 1 tsp of bark per 250 ml of water, boiled for 15 minutes, strained, cooled, and used undiluted.

Baths: 5 g of drug per 1 L of water. Several ready-to-use oak bark extracts are available; typically, 1 to 3 tsp are added to a partial bath.

Capsules: 2 capsules P.O. with meals t.i.d.

Compress, rinse, gargle: Prepare fresh decoction daily by boiling 20 g of drug per 1 L water for 10 to 15 minutes. Use strained liquid undiluted; apply compresses loosely to the affected area to enable free evaporation. External application should typically be needed for only a few days and should not exceed 3 weeks.

Tincture: 1 to 2 ml P.O. t.i.d.

Adverse reactions
GI: abdominal pain, constipation (with possible fecal impaction), gastroenteritis, ***hepatic necrosis*** (with more than 1 g of tannins), ***hepatotoxicity*** (with tannic acid enemas and prolonged skin application), indigestion, nausea, vomiting.

GU: nephritis (with tannic or gallic acid in animals).

Respiratory: ***respiratory failure*** (with tannic or gallic acid in animals).

Skin: rash around the anus followed by a generalized nonspecific rash and blisters on the roof of the mouth (reported after ingestion of White Oak Bark Tablets).

Other: ***death*** (with tannic acid enemas, prolonged skin application).

Interactions
Alkaloids, glycosides, heavy metal salts: Precipitation and reduced absorption of these drugs. Avoid administration with oak products internally.

Contraindications and precautions
Avoid using oak products in pregnant or breast-feeding patients; effects are unknown. External use is contraindicated if extensive skin surface damage is present. Full baths are contraindicated, according to the German Commission E, in patients with discharging, extensively large eczema and skin injuries; febrile and infectious diseases; New York Heart Association classes III and IV; and hypertonia state IV (World Health Organization).

Special considerations
• Caution the patient to avoid having oak come in contact with areas of extensive skin damage, large areas of the body, or the eyes. Instruct him to wash the exposed areas of skin with soap and water and to flush the eyes with tepid water for at least 15 minutes if contact occurs.

Bold italic type indicates that reaction may be life-threatening.

FOLKLORE
History of oaks

The genus name of the oak, *Quercus*, is thought to be derived from the Celtic *quer* (fine) and *cuez* (tree). The oak tree was sacred to the Druids in prehistoric Britain and to the ancient Greeks and Romans and has long been esteemed in European herbal medicine for its astringent bark, leaves, and acorns. The bark was used to tan leather and smoke fish, and an infusion of the bark or galls was used as a dye for wool or yarn. The acorns were made into a meal by Native Americans. A coffee substitute made from roasted acorns and mixed with cream and sugar was considered a remedy for a type of tuberculous adenitis (Dobelis, 1986).

• Advise women to avoid using oak during pregnancy or when breast-feeding.
• Caution the patient to avoid full-body baths with the herb.
• Advise the patient not to take the herb internally for longer than a few weeks.

Points of interest
• Oaks have a long history of medical use. (See *History of oaks*.)
• At one time, tannic acid was included in barium enemas. Because of reports of some deaths from hepatic necrosis, such use is no longer recommended.
• White oak bark (*Q. alba*) makes a yellowish tea with a slightly bitter, astringent taste.

Commentary
Limited external use of oak decoctions may provide some relief for certain forms of dermatitis, such as eczema and contact dermatitis, and minor burns. Although there are anecdotal reports of the herb's use internally for diarrhea, clinical studies are lacking. This treatment is not recommended until safety and efficacy data are available.

References
Boulton, D.W., et al. "Extensive Binding of the Bioflavonoid Quercetin to Human Plasma Proteins," *J Pharm Pharmacol* 50:243-49, 1998.

Conquer, J.A., et al. "Supplementation With Quercetin Markedly Increases Plasma Quercetin Concentration Without Effect on Selected Risk Factors for Heart Disease in Healthy Subjects," *J Nutr* 128:593-97, 1998.

Dobelis, I.N., ed. *Magic and Medicine of Plants.* Pleasantville, N.Y.: Reader's Digest Association Inc., 1986.

Murakami, S., et al. "Inhibitory Effect of Tannic Acid on Gastric H+, K+, -ATPase," *J Natl Prod* 55:513-16, 1992.

OATS

GROATS, HAVER, HAVER-CORN, HAWS, OATMEAL

Taxonomic class
Poaceae

Common trade names
Aveeno Cleansing Bar, Aveeno Colloidal, Aveeno Dry, Aveeno Lotion, Aveeno Oilated Bath, Aveeno Regular Bath, Oats and Honey, Oat Bran, Oat Straw Tea, Quaker Oat Bran

Common forms
Tablets: 850 mg, 1,000 mg
Whole grains, cereals, wafers: 750 mg
   Also available as bath preparations, gels, lotions, powders, soaps, and teas.

Source
Oat extracts are derived from the grains of *Avena sativa*. Oats are culti-vated mainly in the United States, Russia, Canada, and Germany.

Chemical components
Oats contain saponins, carotenoids, gluten, polyphenols, monosaccha-rides, oligosaccharides, various minerals (such as iron, manganese, and zinc), fiber, and cellulose.

Actions
Oat products have emollient properties when applied topically to dry and pruritic skin. Oat bran cereals and oatmeal contain significant quantities of soluble and insoluble fiber. Dietary fiber is believed to lower cholesterol levels by binding bile acids and cholesterol in the in-testines, thus preventing their absorption. Although insoluble fiber is less effective, both forms of dietary fiber appear to reduce serum cho-lesterol levels.

Reported uses
Oat extracts have long been used as topical treatments for minor skin irritations and pruritus associated with common skin disorders. Oat-herb teas are claimed to be valuable as antigout agents and sedatives.
   Several trials suggest that regular intake of dietary fiber from oats can lower serum cholesterol levels in patients with elevated or normal serum cholesterol levels. When combined with other fiber-rich foods, these reductions are further increased (Van Horn et al., 1986). Four tri-als (Gerhardt and Gallo, 1998; Romero et al., 1998; Onning et al., 1998; Onning et al., 1999) have provided additional clinical support for the value of oats or oat-derived products in treating hyperlipidemia. A ran-domized, controlled, 6-week comparison of rice bran and oat bran demonstrated statistically significant reductions in cholesterol and LDL levels of about 13% and 17%, respectively (Gerhardt and Gallo, 1998).

Bold italic type indicates that reaction may be life-threatening.

No beneficial effects were noted for triglyceride or HDL levels. Rice bran performed in a manner similar to that of oat bran but to a lesser degree. In a trial of both normal and hypercholesterolemic Mexican men (Romero et al., 1998), an 8-week regimen of oat bran cookies produced a significant reduction in LDL levels of about 26%, as compared with that of a psyllium group (23%) and a control group (8%). Both active treatments were found to lower cholesterol levels in normal and hypercholesterolemic subjects. No effects were noted for HDL levels, but surprisingly, triglyceride levels were reduced about 28% by the oat bran cookies. Trials conducted by Onning and coworkers (1998 and 1999) demonstrate cholesterol-reducing properties of a novel formulation of oat milk. It has been suggested that the beta-glucans present in oat milk are responsible for the beneficial effects on the lipid profile (Onning et al., 1998). These trials also failed to document a significant effect of oat products on serum triglyceride or HDL levels.

Epidemiologic evidence supports a relation between oat bran intake and CV risk as measured by body mass index, blood pressure, and HDL levels (He et al., 1995). Oat extracts and oat bran bread products also appear to lower blood glucose and insulin levels as well as cholesterol levels (Pick, 1996; Hallfrisch et al., 1995), but the effects on glucose metabolism have not been consistently demonstrated.

Oat derivatives, such as green oat decoction (tea), may be useful in treating chemical addictions (Anand, 1971a), and the extract is being evaluated in smoking cessation programs (Anand, 1971b; Bye et al., 1974).

Dosages
For lowering cholesterol, studies used 50 to 100 g of dietary fiber from oat bran P.O. daily.
For topical use, apply once or twice daily.

Interactions
None reported.

Adverse reactions
GI: bloating, increased urgency of defecation (colonic bacteria and lipids contribute to increase in stool weight; Chen, 1998), flatulence, fullness, perianal irritation.
Skin: contact dermatitis (oat flour).

Contraindications and precautions
Oats have been considered to be contraindicated in patients with celiac disease, as are wheat, rye, and barley. Some information suggests that this may not necessarily be the case (Hallert et al., 1999). Certain oat products may be contaminated with wheat and, therefore, would remain contraindicated for patients with this disorder. Use cautiously in patients with bowel obstruction or other bowel dysmotility syndromes or constipation.

Special considerations
• Advise the patient taking oat bran to regulate bowel habits and drink plenty of fluids.
• Advise the patient using colloidal oat products for baths to avoid contact with the eyes and acutely inflamed areas. The products should be washed off with water.
• Inform the patient that increased bowel movements and flatulence can occur with ingestion of oat products.

Points of interest
• As with other grains, sometimes oats have been contaminated with aflatoxin, a fungal toxin linked with some cancers.

Commentary
Oats provide an important source of soluble dietary fiber and should be consumed (as with other grains and fibers) regularly as part of a healthy diet. Evidence supports the use of oat extracts and oat products as dietary supplement adjuncts to reduce CV risk factors, but long-term studies examining outcomes are needed. Beneficial effects on total cholesterol and LDL levels are small to moderate, and data on positive effects on HDL levels are lacking. Effects on glucose metabolism are inconsistent. Oatmeal baths may be useful for minor skin irritations, but clinical data supporting this therapeutic application are sparse.

References
Anand, C.L. "Treatment of Opium Addiction," *Brit Med J* 3:640, 1971a.

Anand, C.L. "Effect of *Avena sativa* on Cigarette Smoking," *Nature* 233:496, 1971b.

Bye, C., et al. "Lack of Effect of *Avena sativa* on Cigarette Smoking," *Nature* 252:580, 1974.

Chen, H.L. "Mechanisms by Which Wheat Bran and Oat Bran Increase Stool Weight in Humans," *Am J Clin Nutr* 68(3):711-19, 1998.

Gerhardt, A.L., and Gallo, N.B. "Full-fat Rice Bran and Oat Bran Similarly Reduce Hypercholesterolemia in Humans," *J Nutr* 128(5):865-69, 1998.

Hallert, C., et al. "Oats Can Be Included in Gluten-free Diet," *Lakartidningen* 96(30-31):3339-40, 1999.

Hallfrisch, J., et al. "Diets Containing Soluble Oat Extracts Improve Glucose and Insulin Responses of Moderately Hypercholesterolemic Men and Women," *Am J Clin Nutr* 61:379-84, 1995.

He, J., et al. "Oats and Buckwheat Intakes and Cardiovascular Disease Risk Factors in an Ethnic Minority of China," *Am J Clin Nutr* 61:366-72, 1995.

Onning, G., et al. "Effects of Consumption of Oat Milk, Soya Milk, or Cow's Milk on Plasma Lipids and Antioxidative Capacity in Healthy Subjects," *Ann Nutr Metab* 42(4):211-20, 1998.

Onning, G., et al. "Consumption of Oat Milk for 5 Weeks Lowers Serum Cholesterol and LDL Cholesterol in Free Living Men with Moderate Hypercholesterolemia," *Ann Nutr Metab* 43(5):301-9, 1999.

Pick, M.E. "Oat Bran Concentrate Bread Products Improve Long-term Control of Diabetes: A Pilot Study," *J Am Diet Assoc* 96:1254-61, 1996.

Romero, A.L., et al. "Cookies Enriched with Psyllium or Oat Bran Lower Plasma LDL Cholesterol in Normal and Hypercholesterolemic Men from Northern Mexico," *J Am Coll Nutr* 17(6):601-8, 1998.

Van Horn, L.V., et al. "Serum Lipid Response to Oat Product Intake with a Fat-modified Diet," *J Am Diet Assoc* 86:759-64, 1986.

OCTACOSANOL

ISOPOLICOSANOL, 1-OCTACOSANOL, 14C-OCTACOSANOL, N-OCTACOSANOL, OCTACOSYL ALCOHOL, OCTOCOSONOL, POLICOSANOL

Common trade names
Octacosanol Concentrate, Super Octacosanol, Wheat Germ Oil

Common forms
Capsules: 3,000 mcg, 8,000 mcg
Capsules (softgel): 3,000 mcg
Tablets: 1,000 mcg, 6,000 mcg

Source
Policosanol, and subsequently octacosanol, can be isolated from sugar cane wax, other vegetable waxes, and wheat germ oil. Octacosanol has also been isolated from *Eupolyphaga sinensis*, some *Euphorbia* species, *Acacia modesta*, *Serenoa repens*, and other plants.

Chemical components
Octacosanol is primarily a 28-carbon long-chain alcohol. The term has also been used to describe other long-chain 8- to 36-polycarbon alcohols. Octacosanol is the chief component of policosanol.

Actions
Octacosanol is taken up by muscle tissue, the liver, and the digestive tract. One study suggested that octacosanol increased muscle endurance in exercising rats because of higher stores of the agent in exercised rather than resting muscle. These researchers also suggested enhanced lipolysis in muscle and suppressed lipid accumulation in adipose tissue by octacosanol (Kabir and Kimura, 1995). In another study, some lipoprotein lipase activity was enhanced in rats fed octacosanol and a high-fat diet (Kato et al., 1995). Significant lipid-lowering effects, mostly of LDL levels, were found in rabbits fed policosanol (Arruzazabala et al., 1994). Earlier studies in animals suggest that the agent has androgenic effects and improves exercise tolerance.

There may also be a role for octacosanol in CV disorders. Varying doses of policosanol inhibited some mechanisms of platelet activation and aggregation in rats (Arruzazabala et al., 1993). In a drug-induced model of a myocardial infarction, pretreatment with policosanol promoted significant reductions in infarct size and decreased the number of polymorphonuclear cells and mast cells compared with control rats.

Evidence from one animal study suggests a role in cerebrovascular disorders (Molina et al., 1999). Policosanol, at a dose of 200 mg/kg, appeared to reduce mortality, cerebral edema, swelling, and necrosis of the

RESEARCH FINDINGS

Octacosanol in Parkinson's disease

Octacosanol was evaluated in patients with mild to moderate idiopathic parkinsonism because of its apparent ability to improve muscle endurance. Ten patients received 5 mg of octacosanol in a wheat germ oil base P.O. three times a day or placebo for 6 weeks. The patients rated themselves weekly on activities of daily living (ADLs), mood, physical endurance, and parkinsonian symptoms.

Only three patients improved significantly by the study's end. Some responded slightly or didn't have disease progression during treatment. Although ADLs and mood improved significantly, changes in other measurements were not significant. One patient experienced mild positional nonrotational dizziness, and two others experienced exacerbation of dyskinesias. The investigators believed that the octacosanol dosage might have been excessive for these patients. They concluded that octacosanol may be beneficial for patients with mild Parkinson's disease, but the benefit is likely to be small and less than that exerted by existing antiparkinsonian drugs (Snider, 1984).

brain in gerbils after artificial induction of cerebral ischemia by way of carotid ligation as compared with control animals.

One trial in healthy sedentary human subjects suggests that both isopolicosanol and octacosanol exert favorable effects on reaction time (after prompted by specific stimuli) as compared with placebo (Fontani et al., 2000).

Reported uses

Although regular use of octacosanal is claimed to enhance athletic performance, there are no supporting data. In fact, in one study, investigators were unable to document an ergogenic effect for policosanol (Stusser et al., 1998).

Anecdotal reports of success in treating amyotrophic lateral sclerosis with octacosanol have not been achieved in research studies.

Octacosanol has also been evaluated in the treatment of Parkinson's disease. (See *Octacosanol in Parkinson's disease.*)

Forty-five patients with coronary disease underwent treadmill exercise ECG testing to examine the effects of policosanol supplementation on angina and cardiac ischemia (Stusser et al., 1998). Subjects were randomized into one of three treatment groups—policosanol 5 mg P.O. twice daily, policosanol 5 mg P.O. twice daily plus aspirin 125 mg P.O. once daily, or placebo plus aspirin 125 mg P.O. once daily—and followed for 20 months. Subject demographics were similar at baseline. Both investigators and subjects were blinded to treatment identity. At trial conclusion, beneficial effects were seen in terms of policosanol's influence on cardiac functional capacity, resting angina, exertional angina, and cardiac ischemia (as measured by ST changes). The investigators concluded that policosanol-treated patients experienced benefit, documented by ECG changes as a result of the amelioration of myocardial ischemia seen with or without the addition of aspirin to the treatment group.

Dosage
Some sources suggest 40 to 80 mg P.O. daily of octacosanol. Doses vary considerably. Policosanol has been dosed at 5 mg P.O. b.i.d.

Adverse reactions
CNS: exacerbation of dyskinetic movements, nervousness.
CV: orthostatic hypotension.

Interactions
Carbidopa-levodopa: May worsen dyskinesias. Avoid administration with octacosanol.

Contraindications and precautions
Avoid using octacosanol in pregnant or breast-feeding patients; effects are unknown.

Special considerations
• Monitor the severity and frequency of dyskinetic events in patients taking both octacosanol and carbidopa-levodopa.
• Inform the patient that no long-term clinical data for octacosanol use exist.
• Inform the patient that existing clinical data do not support a role for octacosanol as an ergogenic aid for athletes.
• Advise women to avoid using octacosanol during pregnancy or when breast-feeding.

Commentary
Although interesting, data examining octacosanol do not definitively support its use for any condition. It may be useful in CV disease or Parkinson's disease, but more research is needed. Long-term risks have not been adequately assessed.

References
Arruzazabala, M.L., et al. "Cholesterol-lowering Effects of Policosanol in Rabbits," *Biol Res* 27:205-8, 1994.
Arruzazabala, M.L., et al. "Effects of Policosanol on Platelet Aggregation in Rats," *Thromb Res* 69:321-27, 1993.
Fontani, G., et al. "Policosanol, Reaction Time and Event-related Potentials," *Neuropsychobiology* 41(3):158-65, 2000.
Kabir, Y., and Kimura, S. "Tissue Distribution of 8-14C-Octacosanol in Liver and Muscle of Rats After Serial Administration," *Ann Nutr Metab* 39:279-84, 1995.
Kato, S., et al. "Octacosanol Affects Lipid Metabolism in Rats Fed on a High-fat Diet," *Br J Nutr* 73:433-41, 1995.

Molina, V., et al. "Effect of Policosanol on Cerebral Ischemia in Mongolian Gerbils," *Braz J Med Biol Res* 32(10):1269-76, 1999.

Snider, S. "Octacosanol in Parkinsonism," *Ann Neurol* 16:723, 1984. Letter.

Stusser, R., et al. "Long-term Therapy with Policosanol Improves Treadmill Exercise-ECG Testing Performance of Coronary Heart Disease Patients," *Int J Clin Pharmacol Ther* 36(9):469-73, 1998.

OLEANDER

ADELFA, LAURIER ROSE, ROSA FRANCESA, ROSA LAUREL, ROSE BAY

Taxonomic class
Apocynaceae

Common trade names
Anvirzel (hot water extract)

Common forms
Available as leaf extract and tincture.

Source
Although active components are found in all parts of Nerium oleander, they are extracted primarily from the leaves. Oleander is cultivated mainly as an ornamental shrub. It is native to the Mediterranean and widely grown in the southern United States and California. The bush grows about 20' high; has long, narrow, pointed leaves; and produces small clusters of red, pink, or white blossoms.

Chemical components
Oleander contains several cardiac glycosides, including oleandrin, neriin, oleandroside, nerioside, neridiginoside, nerizoside, neritaloside, odoroside-H, neridienone, proceragenin, digitoxigenin, beta-anhydroepidigitoxigenin, neriumogenin-*A*-3beta-D-digitaloside, gentiobiosyloleandrin, and odoroside A. Other pharmacologically active compounds include folinerin, rutin, rosagenin, cornerine, and oleandomycin. The plant also contains hydrocyanic and ursolic acids and traces of vitamins A, K, and C.

Actions
The cardioactive glycosides in oleander act similarly to the cardiac glycosides used in treating heart failure. Their pharmacologic similarities suggest that these compounds enhance the force and velocity of myocardial contractions through inhibition of the sodium-potassium-adenosine triphosphate pump in the sarcolemmal membrane (Clark et al., 1991). The flavonal glycosides influence vascular permeability and have diuretic actions. Cornerine improved myocardial function in clinical trials and is effective in cardiac conditions.

Oleandrin, the principal cardiac glycoside, acts as a diuretic and stimulates the heart. In vivo analysis suggests that it lacks anticancer activity but retains weak macrophage-mediated cell toxicity and weak mi-

---

togenic activity. An in vitro study determined that oleandrin inhibits activation of nuclear transcription factor-kappaB and activator protein-1 and their associated kinases, suggesting the potential of oleandrin to act as an antitumorigenic agent (Manna et al., 2000).

Reported uses
Despite oleander's well-recognized toxicity, claims of its use center around asthma, cancer, cardiac illnesses, corns, dysmenorrhea, epilepsy, and rashes. Folk remedies claim actions as an abortifacient, a cardiotonic, a cathartic, a diuretic, an emetic, an insecticide, a menstrual stimulant, and a parasiticide. In Curaçao, the sap is applied to warts, added to beverages, and used as an anthelmintic. In Venezuela, the leaves are boiled and the steam inhaled to alleviate sinus problems. The leaves are also used as poultices for skin diseases and to kill skin parasites and maggots in wounds.

Dosage
No consensus exists. The ingestion of oleander is not recommended. A single ingested leaf may produce fatal poisoning in an adult (Howard and DeWolf, 1974).

Adverse reactions
CNS: depression, vertigo.
EENT: severe nasopharyngeal irritation.
GI: abdominal cramps and pain, anorexia, nausea, vomiting.
Metabolic: hyperkalemia.
Respiratory: severe irritation (smoke inhalation), tachypnea.
Skin: contact dermatitis.
Other: *death.*

Interactions
Digoxin, digitoxin: Increased risk of toxicity and fatal outcomes. Avoid administration with oleander.

Contraindications and precautions
Because of its extreme toxicity, warn patients to avoid using any form of oleander.

Special considerations
🞂 **ALERT** All parts of the oleander plant are toxic. Death has occurred in adults and children after ingestion of the flowers, leaves, and nectar and from using oleander twigs as skewers to roast foods. Fatalities have also occurred after oral and rectal administration of the extract (Clark et al., 1991). Smoke from the burning wood and the water in which the plant has been immersed can also be toxic.
● The cross-reactivity between digoxin and oleander glycosides enables radioimmunoassays to measure serum digoxin levels in oleander poisoning. Assays for serum digoxin levels may not reflect the severity of the toxicity.

❦ ALERT Symptoms of oleander toxicity may mimic those of digitalis toxicity and include anorexia, colic, bloody diarrhea, dizziness, drowsiness, heart block, hyperkalemia, mydriasis, nausea, slow and irregular pulse rate, seizures, syncope, ventricular tachycardia or fibrillation, and vomiting. Death usually results from heart failure or respiratory paralysis (Tracqui et al., 1998). A canine model suggests that digoxin antibody fragments (such as Digibind) may be valuable in treating oleander toxicity (Clark et al., 1991). Additional studies in dogs also suggest a role for fructose-1,6-diphosphate in treating oleander toxicity (Markov et al., 1999).

❦ ALERT Manage oleander toxicity aggressively and treat as for digitalis toxicity. Treatment includes gastric lavage and administration of activated charcoal and emetics. Monitor serum potassium levels and ECG tracings. Systemic hyperkalemia induced by the plant can worsen cardiac function and can be treated with potassium exchange resins. Treat conduction deficits with antiarrhythmics, atropine, pacemakers, or phenytoin. Do not use digitalis preparations for oleander poisoning (Clark et al., 1991).

• Monitor heart rate and rhythm.
• Monitor serum potassium levels.
• Caution the patient to keep the plant and its products out of the reach of children and pets.
• Advise the patient to take precautions to prevent accidental ingestion.
• Advise the patient to avoid burning oleander branches or other plant parts in poorly ventilated areas to avoid toxic smoke.

Points of interest
• Birds may die from consuming less than 1 g of the plant. A fatal dose in a large animal such as a cow or horse may be 10 to 20 g.
• High-pressure liquid chromatography–mass spectrophotometry appears to be the method of choice to detect toxic levels of oleandrin (Tracqui et al., 1998).

Commentary
Oleander's extreme toxicity precludes any therapeutic use. Although it has been used in traditional medicine, no clinical trials support the efficacy and safety of this herb.

References
Clark, R.F., et al. "Digoxin-specific Fab Fragments in the Treatment of Oleander Toxicity in a Canine Model," *Ann Emerg Med* 20:1073-77, 1991.

Howard, R.A., and DeWolf, G. P., Jr. *Poisonous Plants Arnoldia* 34:73, 1974. Reprint.

Manna, S.K., et al. "Oleandrin Suppresses Activation of Nuclear Transcription Factor-kappaB, Activator Protein-1 and c-Jun NH2-Terminal Kinase," *Cancer Res* 60(14):3838-47, 2000.

Markov, A.K., et al. "Fructose-1,6-diphosphate in the Treatment of Oleander Toxicity in Dogs," *Vet Hum Toxicol* 41(1):9-15, 1999.

Tracqui, A., et al. "Confirmation of Oleander Poisoning by HPLC/MS," *Int J Legal Med* 111(1):32-34,1998.

OLIVE LEAF
LUCCA, OLEAE FOLIUM, OLEA EUROPA, OLIVIER

Taxonomic class
Oleaceae

Common trade names
None known.

Common forms
Available as fluidextracts, tincture, and teas.

Source
Most of the products consist of fresh or dried leaves of *Olea europaea*.

Chemical components
The olive leaf contains iridoide monoterpenes, triterpenes, flavanoids, and chalcones.

Actions
The touted mechanisms of actions of olive leaf are antihypertensive and hypoglycemic. Vasodilatory effects of olive leaf were thought to be derived from a substance called oleuropeoside. A study in male Wistar rats confirmed that lyophilized olive leaf decoction (2.5 mg/kg) administered I.V. showed hypotensive effects at doses of 25 to 50 mg/kg (Zarzuelo et al., 1991). The trial also found that oleuropeoside is not the sole antihypertensive component of olive leaf because the relaxant activity of the decoction was independent of the vascular epithelium's integrity.

Hypoglycemic activity was assessed in both normoglycemic and diabetic female Wistar rats (Gonzalez et al., 1991). The maximum hypoglycemic activity in normoglycemic rats was seen at doses of 0.5 mg/kg administered in February. The highest percentage yield of oleuropeoside occurred in the winter months, which suggests that it is responsible for the hypoglycemic activity. Significant hypoglycemia was seen at doses of 16 and 32 mg/kg at both 90 minutes and 150 minutes. Oleuropeoside also increased peripheral glucose uptake and potentiated the glucose-induced insulin resistance. However, in a 12-week study of male Swiss albino rats with and without streptomycin-induced diabetes, olive leaf showed no hypoglycemic effects in any rat group (Onderoglu et al., 1999).

Reported uses
Olive leaf has been used most commonly as an antidiabetic, an antihypertensive, and a diuretic. No clinical trials conducted in humans were found in the medical literature.

Dosage
Dosage has not been established.

Adverse reactions
CV: hypotension.
GI: irritation of stomach lining.
Metabolic: hypoglycemia.

Interactions
Antidiabetic drugs: May cause additive hypoglycemic effects. Monitor the patient closely.
Antihypertensives: May cause additive hypotensive effects. Use together cautiously.
Drugs used in hypotension or shock: May counteract hypertensive effects of these drugs. Avoid administration with olive leaf.

Contraindications and precautions
Olive leaf is contraindicated in patients with gallstones because olive leaf may cause colic. Also avoid its use in pregnant or breast-feeding patients because its safety has not been established. Use cautiously in hypertensive or diabetic patients because olive leaf could cause hypotension or hypoglycemia.

Special considerations
• Advise the patient to consult a health care provider before using herbal preparations because a treatment that has been clinically researched and proved effective may be available.
• Advise the patient to take olive leaf with a meal or snack to avoid GI irritation.
• Monitor for hypoglycemia.
• Monitor the patient's blood pressure.

Points of interest
• The German E Commission, which oversees drug use in Germany, considers olive leaf an unapproved product.
• Do not confuse olive leaf with olive oil.

Commentary
Olive leaf has been used for several years for its hypotensive and hypoglycemic properties. Conflicting reports of these effects have been noted in animals. The safety and efficacy of olive leaf in humans need further investigation before recommendations regarding its use can be made.

References
Gonzalez, M., et al. "Hypoglycemic Activity of Olive Leaf," *Planta Med* 58:513-15, 1991.
Onderoglu, S., et al. "The Evaluation of Long-term Effects of Cinnamon Bark and Olive Leaf on Toxicity Induced by Streptozocin Administration to Rats," *Pharm Pharmacol* 51:1305-12, 1999.
Zarzuelo, A., et al. "Vasodilator Effect of Olive Leaf," *Planta Med* 57:417-19, 1991.

OREGANO

MOUNTAIN MINT, ORIGANUM, WILD MARJORAM

Taxonomic class
Lamiaceae

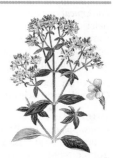

Common trade names
Multi-ingredient preparations: Oil of Oregano,
Oregamax, Oregano

Common forms
Capsules: 450 mg
Oil: 0.45 fl oz
   Also available as a spice.

Source
Oregano is derived from dried aboveground parts of *Origanum vulgare*,
a member of the mint family. It should not be confused with its close
relative, marjoram (*O. majorana*).

Chemical components
The plant contains hydrolyzable tannins, including gallic acid, an iron-
binding phenolic substance, and tocopherols.

Actions
Oregano may have significant antioxidant properties that may be attributed to the high levels of tocopherol. An oregano extract showed
antimutagenic activity against a dietary carcinogen (Kanazawa et al.,
1995). Gamma-tocopherol also occurs in high concentrations. This
tocopherol homologue is reported to be most active next to alpha-
tocopherol regarding antioxidant activity (Lagouri and Boskou, 1996).
   Phenolic compounds (such as gallic acid in oregano) may bind with
iron and decrease oregano's absorption in the gut (Brune et al., 1989).
Oregano inhibited mycelial growth of *Aspergillus parasiticus*, a common
food mold (Tantaoui-Elaraki and Beraoud, 1994).
   Oregano oil at concentrations of 2% or less inhibited many common
pathogenic gram-negative (bacilli) and gram-positive (cocci) organisms
(Hammer et al., 1999).

Reported uses
Herbalists have used oregano as a diaphoretic, a menstrual stimulant,
and a mild tonic. It is also used as a flavoring agent and preservative.
The antibacterial and antioxidant properties of oregano have led modern herbalists to recommend its use for superficial and systemic infections.
   In a small, uncontrolled study of 14 patients (Force et al., 2000),
600 mg of emulsified oregano oil administered daily for 6 weeks was associated with a clearing of intestinal parasites in more than one-half of
the 14 patients. Concerns exist with respect to the study design of this
clinical trial.

Dosage

As a dietary supplement, 2 capsules P.O. once or twice daily, preferably with meals, or a few drops of oil of oregano added to milk or juice.
For topical use, apply oil of oregano directly to affected region once or twice daily. As a shampoo, add a small amount of oil of oregano to commercial shampoo. After shampooing, allow the mixture to remain on the hair for a few minutes and then rinse. Add to pump soaps and use during showering and hand washing as an antiseptic cleanser.

Adverse reactions

Other: *hypersensitivity reaction.*

Interactions

Iron supplements: May reduce iron absorption. Separate administration of oregano by at least 2 hours when taken with iron supplements or iron-containing foods.

Contraindications and precautions

Oregano is contraindicated in patients who are hypersensitive to oregano or other herbs of the Lamiaceae family. Use cautiously in patients with anemia secondary to iron deficiency.

Special considerations

◆ ALERT Hypersensitivity reaction manifested by dysphagia, dysphonia, facial edema, pruritus, and upper respiratory tract distress has been described. Cross-sensitivity to plants in the Lamiaceae family (thyme, hyssop, basil, marjoram, mint, or sage) can occur (Benito et al., 1996).
• Instruct the patient to discontinue use of oil of oregano if a rash or irritation occurs.
• Instruct the patient to avoid taking oregano within 2 hours of iron-containing foods or supplements.

Points of interest

• Oregano is a wild, coarse plant with sprawling stems, pink or white flowers, and a balsamic aroma.
• The Greeks crowned newlyweds with the herb and planted it on graves. In ancient times, the herb was used as a remedy for narcotic poisonings and seizures.
• Samples of oregano from Mexico have been shown to harbor significant colonies of enterotoxigenic *Clostridium perfringens* (Rodriguez-Romo et al., 1998).

Commentary

Oregano shows some promise as an antifungal, an antioxidant, an antiseptic, and, perhaps, an anthelmintic. Because clinical human data are lacking, its use for these indications is not recommended.

References

Benito, M., et al. "Labiatae Allergy: Systemic Reactions Due to Ingestion of Oregano and Thyme," *Ann Allergy Asthma Immunol* 76:416-18, 1996.

Bold italic type indicates that reaction may be life-threatening.

Brune, M., et al. "Iron Absorption and Phenolic Compounds: Importance of Different Phenolic Structures," *Eur J Clin Nutr* 43:547-58, 1989.

Force, M., et al. "Inhibition of Enteric Parasites by Emulsified Oil of Oregano In Vivo," *Phytother Res* 14(3):213-14, 2000.

Hammer, K.A., et al. "Antimicrobial Activity of Essential Oils and Other Plant Extracts," *J Appl Microbiol* 86(6):985-90,1999.

Kanazawa, K., et al. "Specific Desmutagens in Oregano Against a Dietary Carcinogen, Trp-P-2, Are Galengin and Quercetin," *J Agric Food Chem* 43:404-9, 1995.

Lagouri, V., and Boskou, D., "Nutrient Antioxidants in Oregano," *Int J Food Sci Nutr* 47:493-97, 1996.

Rodriguez-Romo, L.A., et al. "Detection of Entertoxigenic *Clostridium perfringens* in Spices Used in Mexico by Dot Blotting Using a DNA Probe," *J Food Prot* 61(2):201-4, 1998.

Tantaoui-Elaraki, A., and Beraoud, L. "Inhibition of Growth and Aflatoxin Production in *Aspergillus parasiticus* by Essential Oils of Selected Plant Materials," *J Environ Pathol Toxicol Oncol* 13:67-72, 1994.

OREGON GRAPE

HOLLY-LEAVED BARBERRY, MOUNTAIN GRAPE

Taxonomic class
Berberidaceae

Common trade names
Barberry, Blue Barberry, Creeping Barberry, Holly Barberry, Holly-Leaved Berberis, Holly Mahonia, Mountain Grape, Oregon Barbery, Oregon Grape Holly, Oregon Grape-Holly, Oregon Grape Root, Trailing Mahonia, Water Holly

Common forms
Capsules: 400 mg
Fluidextract (tincture): 1 oz, 2 oz
   Also available as an ointment, powder, chopped root, and tincture.

Source
Active components are obtained from the bark of the roots and stems of *Mahonia aquifolium,* a bushy shrub that is native to the western United States. *M. aquifolium* was also known as *Berberis aquifolium* and should not be confused with the common barberry, *B. vulgaris.*

Chemical components
Oregon grape contains several alkaloids. The major alkaloids that contribute to the herb's pharmacologic activity are berberine, berbamine, and oxyacanthine. The plant also contains other alkaloids (canadine, corypalmine, hydrastine, isocorydine, oxyberberine, corytuberine, columbamine, and mahonine), resin, and tannin.

Actions
Although most *Mahonia* alkaloids have antibacterial properties, berbine also possesses amebicidal and trypanocidal properties. This alkaloid has

anticonvulsant and uteronic actions and has shown hypotensive and sedative effects in animals. Alkaloids isolated from *M. aquifolium* have demonstrated strong lipoxygenase-inhibitory and antioxidant properties (Bezakova et al., 1996; Misik et al., 1995).

These compounds also exert antiproliferative properties, suggesting a possible therapeutic role in treating such diseases as psoriasis in which lipoxygenase is involved (Müller et al., 1995). Root extracts have exhibited antifungal properties (McCutcheon et al., 1994).

Reported uses

Oregon grapes are edible, dark purple berries that have been used in wines and brandies. Oregon grape is claimed to have antiseptic, aphrodisiac, astringent, bile-stimulating, cathartic, cleansing, diuretic, expectorant, fever-reducing, and tonic properties. The root has been used for diarrhea, dyspepsia, dysuria, fever, gallbladder diseases, leukorrhea, and renal calculi. The tincture has been claimed to be useful in treating acne, arthritis, bronchitis, congestion, eczema, hepatitis, herpes, psoriasis, rheumatism, syphilis, and vaginitis.

Dosage

Traditional uses suggest the following dosages:
Powder: 0.5 to 1 g P.O. t.i.d.
Tincture: 2 to 4 ml P.O. t.i.d.

Adverse reactions

Skin: burning, itching, skin irritation (topical application).
Other: allergic reaction (topical application).

Interactions

None reported.

Contraindications and precautions

Avoid using Oregon grape in pregnant or breast-feeding patients; effects are unknown. It is also contraindicated in patients who are hypersensitive to Oregon grape or related plant species.

Special considerations

• Inform the patient that clinical evidence for therapeutic claims is lacking.
• Urge the patient to avoid getting the preparation in the eyes. Instruct him to flush the eyes well with water If contact occurs.
• Caution the patient that intense pain can occur with skin contact.
🌢 **ALERT** Ingestion of greater than 500 mg of berberine has resulted in reports of cardiac damage, diarrhea, dyspnea, hemorrhagic nephritis, hypotension, kidney irritation, lethargy, nausea, nosebleed, respiratory spasm and arrest, skin and eye irritation, vomiting, and death.

Bold italic type indicates that reaction may be life-threatening.

Points of interest

● Oregon grape is similar to but should not be confused with the common barberry *(B. vulgaris)*. Several components found in Oregon grape also occur in goldenseal *(Hydrastis canadensis)*.

Commentary

Although some studies suggest that the active components of Oregon grape or *M. aquifolia* may be useful for psoriasis or other diseases that involve the products of lipoxygenase metabolism (antioxidation), human studies are needed. There is limited information regarding the safety and efficacy of this herb.

References

Bezakova, L., et al. "Lipoxygenase Inhibition and Antioxidant Properties of Bis-benzylisoquinoline Alkaloids Isolated from *Mahonia aquifolium," Pharmazie* 51:758-61, 1996.

Jellin, J.M., et al. *Natural Medicines Comprehensive Database.* Stockton, Calif.: Therapeutic Research Faculty, 1999.

McCutcheon, A.R., et al. "Antifungal Screening of Medicinal Plants of British Columbian Native Peoples," *J Ethnopharmacol* 44:157-69, 1994.

Misik, V., et al. "Lipoxygenase Inhibition and Antioxidant Properties of Proto-berberine and Aporphine Alkaloids Isolated from *Mahonia aquifolium," Planta Med* 61:372-73, 1995.

Müller, K., et al. "The Antipsoriatic *Mahonia aquifolium* and Its Active Constituents. Part I. Pro- and Antioxidant Properties and Inhibition of 5-Lipoxygenase," *Planta Med* 60:421-24, 1995.

Müller, K., et al. "The Antipsoriatic *Mahonia aquifolium* and Its Active Components. Part II. Antiproliferative Activity Against Cell Growth of Human Keratinocytes," *Planta Med* 61:74-75, 1995.

PANSY

<small>FIELD PANSY, HEARTSEASE, JOHNNY-JUMP-UP, JUPITER
FLOWER, LADIES'-DELIGHT, WILD PANSY</small>

Taxonomic class
Violaceae

Common trade names
None known.

Common forms
Available as an extract.

Source
Active components are obtained from the flowers of *Viola tricolor.*

Chemical components
The stems and leaves contain flavonoids, salicylate derivatives, terpenes and triterpenes, carbohydrate derivatives, sterines, a polysaccharide, and magnesium tartrate. Vitamin F and other fatty acids have also been detected (Pápay et al., 1987). Other compounds include violanthin, rutin, violaquercitrin, resin, saponin, gums, and mucilage.

Actions
Physiologic mechanisms of action are poorly described. Salicylates may be responsible for anti-inflammatory properties because of prostaglandin inhibition. Although not a major component of pansy, rutin has been shown to exert many pharmacologic effects, the most well known of which is its ability to affect capillary permeability. Herbs with high levels of rutin were thought to be useful for bleeding events. Other effects of rutin include inhibition of angiotensin II and prostaglandin E_2.

Reported uses
This agent is claimed to be useful in treating bronchitis, rheumatism, skin cancer, and whooping cough. One Hungarian study indicates its possible use in preventing heart spasms and as an anti-inflammatory (Pápay et al., 1987).

Dosage
Dosage is 2 to 4 ml of tincture or tea P.O. t.i.d.

Adverse reactions
GI: cathartic effects (seeds), diarrhea.

Interactions
Salicylates: Effects may be additive. Use cautiously.

Contraindications and precautions
Avoid using pansy in pregnant or breast-feeding patients; effects are unknown.

Special considerations
• Monitor the patient for diarrhea.
• Advise women to avoid using pansy during pregnancy or when breast-feeding.
• Inform the patient that no clinical data support the use of this herb for any medical condition.

Commentary
Without clinical data supporting the use of pansy for medical purposes, it cannot be recommended.

References
Pápay, V., et al. "Study of Chemical Substances of *Viola tricolor* L.," *Acta Pharm Hung* 157:153-58, 1987.

PAPAYA

MELON TREE, PAPAIN, PAWPAW

Taxonomic class
Caricaceae

Common trade names
Papaya Enzyme, Papaya Enzyme with Chlorophyll, Papaya Leaf

Common forms
Tablets: 5 mg
Tablets (chewable): 25 mg
　Also available as a tea.

Source
Components are usually extracted from the leaves, seeds, pulp, and latex of *Carica papaya,* which is native to Mexico and Central America but also grows in other tropical areas.

Chemical components
Papaya is composed primarily of proteolytic enzymes, including papain and chymopapain. Papain (also know as vegetable pepsin) occurs in the leaves and fruit latex. The alkaloid carpaine has also been isolated from the leaves. The seeds contain the glycosides caricin and myrosin.

Actions
Meat, seeds, and plant pulp of unripe papaya have demonstrated antioxidant properties and exerted weak bacteriostatic activity in vitro.

Latex from papaya sap has inhibited the growth of *Candida albicans* in culture (Giordani et al., 1996).

Reported uses

Papain is classified as a debriding agent for necrotic tissue. Chymopapain is approved for intradiskal injection in patients with herniated lumbar intervertebral disks who do not respond to conventional therapy.

Papaya was used for athletic injuries and showed improved anti-inflammatory response and speedy recovery (Holt, 1969). It was also helpful in reducing postoperative edema and ecchymosis after nasal plastic surgery (Vallis and Lund, 1969). In patients who had undergone head and neck surgery, papaya reduced postoperative edema slightly (Lund and Royer, 1969).

Papain is claimed to be useful as an anthelmintic and in treating digestive disorders. The latex has been effective against intestinal nematodes in mice.

Dosage

For inflammation, clinical trials suggest 10 mg P.O. q.i.d. for 7 days.

Adverse reactions

CNS: decreased CNS activity (carpaine), paralysis.
CV: decreased heart rate.
GI: perforation of the esophagus and severe gastritis (with ingestion of excessive papaya or papain).
Skin: carotenemia, dermatitis.
Other: *anaphylactic shock* (reported after injection of chymopapain), *hypersensitivity reactions* (plant parts, extracts).

Interactions

None reported.

Contraindications and precautions

Avoid using papaya in pregnant or breast-feeding patients; effects are unknown. Use cautiously in patients with a history of atopy or in those who are prone to contact dermatitis reactions from the herb.

Special considerations

• Monitor the patient with hypersensitivity for reactions to papaya.
• Caution the patient against prolonged use because of the risk of severe gastritis and hypersensitivity reactions. Explain that the latex in the plant may induce dermatitis.
• Advise women to avoid using papaya during pregnancy or when breast-feeding.

Points of interest

• Papaya is a source of flavoring used in candies and ice cream.
• Papain is used in some facial creams to soften skin and as a meat tenderizer.

Bold italic type indicates that reaction may be life-threatening.

Commentary

Human clinical trials suggest that papaya may be useful in treating inflammation caused by trauma or surgical procedures. In vitro studies have documented bacteriostatic effects against enteropathogens, but human clinical trials need to be conducted to verify these claims. Because allergic reactions have been caused by plant parts and extracts, papaya should be used cautiously in patients with a history of hypersensitivity reactions.

References

Giordani, R., et al. "Fungicidal Activity of Latex Sap from *Carica papaya* and Antifungal Effect of D(+)-Glucosamine on *Candida Albicans* Growth," *Mycoses* 39:103-10, 1996.

Holt, H. "*Carica papaya* as Ancillary Therapy for Athletic Injuries," *Curr Ther Res Clin Exper* 11:621-24, 1969.

Lund, M., and Royer, R. "*Carica papaya* in Head and Neck Surgery," *Arch Surg* 98:180-82, 1969.

Vallis, C., and Lund, M. "Effect of Treatment with *Carica papaya* on Resolution of Edema and Ecchymosis Following Rhinoplasty," *Curr Ther Res Clin Exper* 11:356-59, 1969.

PAREIRA

ICE VINE, PARIERA RADIX, PERIERA BRAVA, VELVET LEAF

Taxonomic class

Menispermaceae

Common trade names

Multi-ingredient preparations: Pareira Complex

Common forms

Available as dried roots and stems, granules, and powders. Pareira is commonly combined with other plant species in homeopathic preparations (such as Pareira Complex).

Tubocurarine chloride, an alkaloid present in pareira, is available as a prescription injectable in the United States and contains 3 mg/ml of active drug. Each 3 mg is equivalent to about 20 units of crude curare extract. This injectable drug should not be confused with dietary supplements that contain pareira.

Source

Pareira is obtained from the roots and stems of *Chondrodendron tomentosum*, a tropical, woody vine that is native to the rain forests of the upper Amazon, Ecuador, and Panama. Root and stem sections are cleaned, cut into transverse segments, and dried. Commercial supplies of pareira come mainly from Rio de Janeiro and Bahia, Brazil.

Chemical components

Pareira contains various alkaloids, including delta-tubocurarine (also referred to as *d*-tubocurine), *d*-chondrocurine, *d*-isochondrodendrine, *d*-isochondrodendrine dimethyl ether, *l*-curarine (also referred to as *l*-curine or *l*-bebeerine), chondrofoline, and cycleanine. Only tubocurarine has the physiologic activity characteristic of curare, a potent muscle relaxant.

Actions

Several actions have been reported for pareira, including analgesic, antarthritic, antiaggregant, anticonvulsant, anti-inflammatory, antimalarial, antipyretic, antitumorigenic, cytotoxic, dopamine-receptor inhibitor, ganglionic blocker, hepatoprotective, histaminic, hypotensive, and vagolytic. None of these actions is supported by clinical data regarding oral administration of pareira.

Reported uses

Traditional use of pareira by oral and topical routes appears less hazardous as long as it is not introduced into the bloodstream. The herb is bitter and slightly sweet. It is claimed to be an antiseptic, a diuretic, a mild laxative, and a tonic and reportedly acts to induce menstruation. It has also been used to relieve chronic inflammation of the urinary tubules and has been recommended for calculi, generalized edema, gonorrhea, jaundice, leukorrhea, and rheumatism. It is used in Brazil for snakebites.

Pareira extracts have long been used as arrow poisons. Tubocurarine's ability to cause muscle paralysis has been extensively researched, and this agent is now commonly used in Western medicine. Tubocurarine chloride is used mainly to produce skeletal muscle relaxation during surgery, after induction of general anesthesia. It may also be used to facilitate endotracheal intubation and increase pulmonary compliance during assisted or controlled respiration and as an adjunct during pharmacologically or electrically induced convulsive therapy (Osol and Farrar, 1955).

Dosage

For snakebites, infusion (tea) of the root taken P.O.; bruised leaves applied externally.
For other disorders, 2 to 4 ml of fluidextract P.O.; 10 to 20 grains of solid extract P.O.; or 1 to 4 fl oz of infusion P.O.

Adverse reactions

None reported for oral preparation. The following reactions may occur with tubocurarine injection:
CV: hypotension.
GI: decreased GI motility and tone (caused by ganglionic blockade).
Musculoskeletal: residual muscle weakness.
Respiratory: *apnea (prolonged)*, pulmonary effects (**bronchospasm,** wheezing).

Bold italic type indicates that reaction may be life-threatening.

Skin: cutaneous effects (erythema, flushing, pruritus, urticaria, wheal formation; associated with histamine release).
Other: *malignant hyperthermia* (with parenteral administration of tubocurarine chloride; rare).

Interactions
None reported for oral preparation. The following reactions may occur with tubocurarine injection:
Drugs known to cause or increase neuromuscular blockade (aminoglycosides, lidocaine, neuromuscular blockers, polymyxin antibiotics): Increased risk of paralysis. Avoid administration with pareira.

Contraindications and precautions
Tubocurarine is contraindicated in patients for whom histamine release may be hazardous, in those who are hypersensitive to the drug, and in those with oral, gastric, and duodenal ulcers. This herb is also contraindicated in pregnancy because it may induce menstruation. The same cautions and precautions should be taken with oral administration of pareira. Use cautiously in patients with respiratory depression and in those with hepatic, renal, endocrine, CV, or pulmonary dysfunction.

Special considerations
● **ALERT** Examine mucous membranes to ensure that they are intact before the patient takes pareira. If there are cuts or sores in the mouth, the potential exists for the tubocurarine components of the plant to enter the bloodstream, resulting in the physiologic activity characteristic of curare.
● **ALERT** Caution the patient about the symptoms of curare exposure, and advise him to seek emergency medical help immediately if needed. The first symptoms of muscle relaxation after parenteral administration of tubocurarine typically include blurred vision, bilateral drooping of the lids, heaviness of the face, and relaxation of the jaws; next, generalized weakness and heaviness of the neck muscles, inability to raise the head, and weakness or complete paresis of the spinal muscles, legs, and arms; and finally, shallow respiration.
● Urge the patient to use pareira only under supervision of a health care provider.
● Advise the patient to keep pareira away from injured skin or mucous membranes.
● Do not confuse this product with abuta (false pareira, pareira, *Cissampelos pareira*). Although commonly referred to as pareira or false pareira, this woody climbing vine belongs to the genus *Cissampelos* and is unrelated to true pareira. Abuta is commonly referred to as the "midwives' herb" because of its analgesic properties and its traditional use for various women's ailments.

Points of interest
● Pareira is famous for being the source of the arrow poison curare. The term "curare" comes from an Amazon Indian word for poison. Ama-

zonian and other South American Indians tipped a dart or spear with curare to paralyze game animals.

Commentary

As a prescription drug, tubocurarine has a definite role as a nondepolarizing neuromuscular blocker. Pareira lacks clinical data to substantiate its claims for topical and oral use or of its safety and efficacy. The potential risks associated with oral ingestion of the plant parts outweigh any potential and as yet unproven therapeutic benefits.

References

Osol, A., and Farrar, G.E. *Dispensatory of the United States of America,* 25th ed. Philadelphia: Lippincott-Raven Pubs., 1955.

PARSLEY

COMMON PARSLEY, GARDEN PARSLEY

Taxonomic class
Apiaceae

Common trade names
Multi-ingredient preparations: Insure Herbal, Parsley Herb, Parsley Leaves

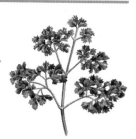

Common forms
Capsules: 430 mg, 450 mg, 455 mg
Liquid: 1 oz
　　Also available as teas.

Source

Leaves from *Petroselinum crispum* are most commonly used for parsley, but the roots, seeds, and oil are also used. The plant grows wild in parts of the Mediterranean but is cultivated in herb gardens worldwide. Germany, France, Belgium, Hungary, and California are the largest producers of parsley oils. Sometimes the plant is labeled as *Apium petroselinum, Carum petroselinum,* or *P. sativum.*

Chemical components

Parsley contains several vitamins and minerals, such as calcium, iron, vitamin A, a significant amount of B vitamins, and vitamin C. It also contains glycosides (apigenin and luteolin), furanocoumarins (bergapten, methoxypsoralen, psoralen, oxypeucedanin), proteins, carbohydrates, and an oleoresin. The volatile oil contains apiol, myristicin, tetramethoxyallylbenzene, terpene aldehydes, ketones, and alcohols.

Actions

In animals, parsley has demonstrated a significant hypotensive effect (Petkov, 1979; Opdyke, 1975); an increase in smooth-muscle tone in the bladder, uterus, and intestines (Opdyke, 1975); and stimulation of hepatic regeneration (Gershbein, 1977). Myristicin, a component of the

---

chemical that shares structural similarity with sympathetic amines, is thought to exhibit MAO inhibitor-like properties. When given to pregnant women, parsley oil has been reported to increase the levels of circulating plasma proteins and serum calcium and to increase diuresis (Buchanan, 1978). Aprolol and myristicin are uterine stimulants.

Reported uses
During the Middle Ages, parsley was claimed to be useful in treating asthma, edematous conditions, GI complaints, hepatic and renal dysfunctions, and the plague. In folk medicine, it has been used as an antiflatulent, an antimicrobial, an antirheumatic, an antispasmodic, a digestive aid, a diuretic, an expectorant, and a menstrual stimulant.

Parsley is a popular phytotherapy agent for hypertension in regions of Morocco (Ziyyat et al., 1997). It is also reportedly been prescribed for women with bladder problems.

Dosage
Traditional uses suggest the following dosages:
Liquid extract (1:1 in 25% alcohol): 2 to 4 ml P.O. t.i.d.
Tea: 2 to 6 g P.O. of the leaf or root.

Adverse reactions
CV: arrhythmias, hypotension.
Skin: contact dermatitis and photosensitivity (psoralen components).
With parsley seed oil:
GI: fatty liver, GI bleeding, ***hepatotoxicity*** (apiole and myristicin components).
GU: renal epithelial cell damage (apiole component), smooth-muscle contraction (bladder, uterus, intestine).
Respiratory: pulmonary vascular congestion.

Interactions
Antihypertensives: May increase hypotensive effects of these drugs. Monitor the patient.
MAO inhibitors in combination with certain antidepressants (selective serotonin reuptake inhibitors, some tricyclics), dextromethorphan, lithium, narcotic analgesics (meperidine): May promote or produce serotonin syndrome. Avoid administration with parsley.

Contraindications and precautions
Avoid using parsley in pregnant or breast-feeding patients; effects are unknown. Use parsley oil with extreme caution, if at all, in pregnant patients because of the risk of increased uterine contractions. Use cautiously in patients who are prone to arrhythmias, coronary insufficiency, heart failure, hepatic disease, hypotension, peptic ulcer disease, or renal failure. Also use cautiously in patients receiving other agents known to precipitate serotonin syndrome.

Special considerations
• Inform the patient with multiple health problems to avoid using parsley.
• Counsel the patient receiving drugs that may interact with parsley to avoid using this herb.
• Inform the patient that there is little clinical evidence to support any medicinal use of parsley.
• Advise women to avoid using parsley during pregnancy or when breast-feeding.

Points of interest
• Parsley is well known as a garnish for various culinary dishes. Parsley and parsley oils are used in small quantities in various baked goods, sauces, stews, packaged meats, soups, and other processed foods. The highest quantity (1.5%) is found in processed vegetables.
• In ancient Greece, parsley was commonly used at funerals. Wreaths for graves were made from parsley, and it is said that before the advent of embalming, the corpses were sprinkled with parsley to mask the smell.

Commentary
Although parsley has shown some useful actions in animals, until human clinical trials are available to support these claims, consumption of parsley beyond that normally found in food is not recommended.

References
Buchanan, R.L. "Toxicity of Spices Containing Methylenedioxybenzene Derivatives: A Review," *J Food Safety* 1:275-93, 1978.
Gershbein, L.L. "Regeneration of Rat Liver in the Presence of Essential Oils and Their Components," *Food Cosmet Toxicol* 15:171-81, 1977.
Opdyke, D.L.J. "Parsley Seed Oil," *Food Cosmet Toxicol* 13(Suppl):897-98, 1975.
Petkov, V. "Plants with Hypotensive, Antiatheromatous and Coronarodilating Action," *Am J Chin Med* 7:197-236, 1979.
Ziyyat, A., et al. "Phytotherapy of Hypertension and Diabetes in Oriental Morocco," *J Ethnopharmacol* 58:45-54, 1997.

PARSLEY PIERT

FIELD LADY'S MANTLE, PARSLEY BREAKSTONE, PARSLEY PIERCESTONE

Taxonomic class
Rosaceae

Common trade names
Multi-ingredient preparations: Parsley Piert

Common forms
Liquid extract: 1:1 in 25% alcohol
Tincture: 1:5 in 45% alcohol
    Also available as dried herb.

Source
Aphanes arvensis (also known as *Alchemilla arvensis* and *Alchemilla microcarpa)*, a low-growing, hairy annual growing to 4" (10 cm), is native to Europe, North Africa, and North America. The aerial parts of the herb are harvested when the flower is in bloom in the summer and are used either fresh or dried.

Chemical components
A related species, *Alchemilla vulgaris* (lady's mantle), is reported to contain 6% to 8% tannins. Although the exact composition is unknown, it is claimed to contain an astringent compound (Newall et al., 1996).

Actions
Parsley piert is claimed to have diuretic and astringent properties. Tannins are highly astringent compounds that act locally by precipitating proteins. Tannic acid coagulates protein and exerts an astringent action on the mucous membranes of the GI tract.

Reported uses
The herb has been used to treat kidney and bladder disorders, especially calculi, dysuria, and edema of renal and hepatic origin. It is also claimed to be a useful remedy for cystitis and recurrent urinary tract infections. No clinical studies with parsley piert have been reported.

Dosage
Dried herb: 2 to 4 g P.O. or by infusion P.O. t.i.d.
Liquid extract: 2 to 4 ml P.O. t.i.d.
Tea: A handful of the herb is mixed in 1 pt of boiling water; 3 or 4 cups are taken daily.
Tincture: 2 to 10 ml P.O. t.i.d.

Adverse reactions
None reported.

Interactions
None reported.

Contraindications and precautions
No known contraindications. Avoid using parsley piert in pregnant or breast-feeding patients; effects are unknown.

Special considerations
• Inform the patient that no clinical data support the use of parsley piert for any medical condition.
• Advise women to avoid using parsley piert during pregnancy or when breast-feeding.
• Do not confuse parsley piert with parsley (*Petroselinum crispum*) or fool's parsley (*Aethusa cynapium*).

Commentary
There is little, if any, chemical or clinical information on parsley piert. The herb cannot be recommended for use until safety and efficacy data are available.

References
Newall, C.A., et al. *Herbal Medicines: A Guide for Healthcare Professionals.* London: Pharmaceutical Press, 1996.

PASSION FLOWER

APRICOT VINE, CORONA DE CRISTO, FLEISCHFARBIGE, FLEISCHFARBIGE PASSIONBLUME, FLEUR DE LA PASSION, FLOR DE PASSION, GRANADILLA, GRANDILLA INCARNATA MEDIC, GRENADILLE, JAMAICAN HONEYSUCKLE, MADRE SELVA, MAYPOP, PASIONARI, PASSIFLORA, PASSIFLORAE HERBA, PASSIFLORE, PASSIFLORINA, PASSIONARIA, PASSIONBLUME, PASSIONBLUMENKRAUT, PASSION FRUIT, PASSION VINE, PURPLE PASSION FLOWER, WATER LEMON, WILD PASSION FLOWER

Taxonomic class
Passifloraceae

Common trade names
Multi-ingredient preparations: Actisane Nervosite, AM Plus (Brain 111 Formula), Ana-Sed, Anevrase, Anevrasi, Anti-Depression Support, Anti-Stress Support, Anxiety Control, Anxoral, Aranidorm-S, A.S.A.P., Astressane, Atri-Nerv, Atri-PMS, Aureal, Avedorm, B12 Nervinfant, Becalm, Belladonna Valobonin, Better Body Energy for Life, Bio Notte Baby, Bio Strath, Bio Strath #8, Biocarde, Biosedon S, Biral, Blandonal, BLF #30 Head-X, BLF #35 Sleep Like A Baby, BLF #48 Anti-Stress, Brevilon, Bunetten, Calmactiv, Calm Aid Formula, Calman, Calmo, Cardaminol, Chill Out, Chondroitin Plus, Cold Care P.M., Coreplex, Dicalm, Diet Pep, Dipect, Dormeasan, Dormo-Sern, Dormoverlan, Dream Sleep, Easy Now, Epanal, Epizon, Esten, Euphorbia Complex, Euphytose, Eupronerv, Euvegal N, Executive B, Female Advantage, Fiorlin, GABA-Val, Gabisedil, Gerard 99, Goodnight Formula, Good-Nite, Happy Camper, Herbal Anxiety Formula, Herbal-F, Herbal Fem, Herbal Gold Cigarettes, Herbal Insomnia Tablets, Herbal Nightcap, Herbal Pain Relief, Herbal Sleep Well, Infant Calm, Kalm-Assure, Kava 30%, Kavatrol Capsule, LaxActin, Lifesystem Herbal Plus Formula 2 Valerian, Liga-Pane, Liquid Kalm with Kava Kava Rot Extract, Magic Cigarettes, Melatonin PM Complex, Melissa Tonic, Melval, Men's PM Multi, Menopause, Modrenal GF, Mood Enhancer, Moradorm, Motherwort Compound, Musclease, Nardyl, Natisedine, Natracalm, Natudor, Natural Quiet, Naturest, Nervinfant, Neuropax, NightTime Complex with Melatonin, Nighty Night, NutraSleep, Nutrilite Passionflower with Chamomile, Nyton Herbal, Pain Less, Passiflora

---

Bold italic type indicates that reaction may be life-threatening.

Complex, Passiflorine, Passional, Passionflower Plus, Phytocalm, Plantival, PMT Formula, PoweRelief, Pronervon, Purple Blast, Quiet Life, Quiet Night, Quiet Nite, Quite Tyme, Quietan, Relax & Ease Tension ProHerbs, Relaxaplex, Relax & Sleep Formula 2, Relaxir, Relax B, Relax-O-Comp, Relax-U, Relax Now, Reliv RibRestore, Restful, SAF for Kids, Salusan Herbal Rest, Sedantol, Sedaselect, Sedatol, Sedinal, Sedinfant, Sediomed, Sedonerva, Serenity, Shi-Assure, Sleep-Assure, Slumber, SlumberActin, Snooze, Sominex, Soporin, Spasmocarbine, St. John's Complex, Stress-End, Stress Away, Stress Essentials, Super Mega B+C, T-EC, T-ER, T-SS, Trimax, Ultimate Sleep System, Ultra Diet Pep, Valerian Compound, Valerian Plus, Valerian-Primrose Virtue, Val-Plus, Vitaglow Herbal Stress, Wild Rose Nerve Formula, Women's Guardian, Women's PM Multi, #75 N3 Anti-Tensive

Common forms

Liquid extract: 1:1 in 25% alcohol
Tincture: 1:8 in 45% alcohol or containing 0.7% flavonoids

Also available as chewing gum, crude extract, dried herb, and in several homeopathic remedies. It is commonly used in combination with other sedative herbs.

Source

Active components are extracted from dried flowering and fruiting tops of *Passiflora incarnata,* a perennial climbing vine found in tropical and subtropical areas of the Americas. This plant should not be confused with its close relative, the cultivated blue passion flower (*P. caerulea*), which does not contain cyanogenic glycosides (Hegnauer, 1993).

Chemical components

Passion flower contains 2% to 3.9% flavonoids, including lucenin, orientin, isoorientin, passiflorine, saponarin, schaftoside, isoscoparin, swertisin, vitexin, isovitexin, and vicenin. It also includes harman (harmala) alkaloids, such as harman, harmaline, harmine, and harmalol. A pyrone derivative, maltol, has also been found in the plant. Small amounts of gynocardin, a cyanogenic glycoside, have been found in the leaf, although the evidence is conflicting. The coumarins umbelliferone and scopoletin have been detected in the root. Fatty acids and steroids have also been found in the plant.

Actions

The agent exerts both stimulatory and depressant CNS effects. The harman alkaloids are known to stimulate CNS activity through MAO inhibition. The sedative effects of maltol can mask the stimulatory effects of the alkaloids. A depressant effect and other sedative actions were seen when injected in mice, possibly because of constituents binding to central benzodiazepine receptors (Aoyagi et al., 1974). For maltol and its derivatives, anticonvulsant effects and reductions in spontaneous motor activity have been documented in mice (Aoyagi et al., 1974; Kimura et al., 1980).

Reported uses

Passion flower is claimed to be effective as an anxiolytic and a sedative and is approved in Germany to treat nervousness. It is also used to treat nervous GI complaints, pediatric excitability, and sleep disorders. Passion flower has been part of an inpatient detoxification protocol for benzodiazepine withdrawal, possibly because of its anxiolytic and sedative properties and certain constituents that act as ligands at the benzodiazepine–gamma-aminobutyric acid receptor complex (Rasmussen, 1997). A combination product containing passion flower signficantly improved anxiety as compared with placebo in 182 outpatients (Bourin et al., 1997).

Passion flower has also been used for asthma, climacteric symptoms, colic, diarrhea, dysentery, dysmenorrhea, epilepsy, hemorrhoids, herpes zoster, hypertension, hysteria, morphinism, neuralgia, neuralgia neurosis, ophthalmia, pain, palpitations and other cardiac rhythm abnormalities, Parkinson's disease, pediatric attention deficit disorders, postherpetic neuralgia, rashes, generalized seizures, spasms, and nervous tachycardia.

Passion flower is used topically for burns, hemorrhoids, inflammation, and bath preparations. Its extract is used as a flavoring in foods and beverages. (See *History of passion flower.*)

Dosage

Traditional uses suggest the following dosages:
For Parkinson's disease, 10 to 30 gtt P.O. (0.7% flavonoids) t.i.d.
Dried herb: 0.25 to 2 g P.O. t.i.d. The German Commission E monographs lists 4 to 8 g of dried above-the-ground parts or equivalent *Passiflora* preparations daily.
Liquid extract: 0.5 to 1 ml P.O. t.i.d
Tea: 4 to 8 g (3 to 6 tsp) P.O. daily in divided doses.
Tincture: 0.5 to 4 ml P.O. t.i.d. or q.i.d.
Pediatric: 1 tbsp of dried herb infused in 1 cup of boiling water for 5 minutes; 1 to 3 cups P.O. daily for excitability, depending on child's age.
Topical for hemorrhoids: Simmer 20 g of dried herb in 20 ml of water, strain, and cool; apply topically as needed.

Adverse reactions

CNS: CNS depression (with large doses), altered consciousness.
CV: hypersensitivity vasculitis.
Respiratory: *occupational asthma* and rhinitis (in workers preparing herbal formulations that contain passion flower; Giavina-Bianchi et al., 1997).

Interactions

Anticoagulants, antiplatelet drugs: May potentiate effects. Monitor the patient.
MAO inhibitors: May potentiate action. Monitor the patient.
Other CNS depressants: Effects may be additive. Use cautiously.

Bold italic type indicates that reaction may be life-threatening.

FOLKLORE
History of passion flower

The name *Passiflora* was adapted from the Italian *fior della passione*, a name applied to the flower and indicating its supposed resemblance to the elements surrounding the crucifixion of Christ. The corona found in the center of the blossom is said to represent the crown of thorns, the 3 styles are said to resemble the 3 nails, the ovary is the hammer, the 5 stamens represent the wounds of Christ, the 10 petals and sepals represent the 10 *true* apostles (excluding Peter and Judas), and the white and bluish purple colors represent purity and heaven. The fruit of the plant is the size of a hen's egg and is sweet and aromatic. The juice of the leaves was traditionally used by the Brazilians for fever.

Contraindications and precautions
Passion flower is contraindicated in pregnant or breast-feeding patients; harman (harmala) alkaloids and cyanogenic glycosides have shown uterine stimulant activity in animal models. It is also contraindicated in patients who are hypersensitive to passion flower.

Special considerations
• Monitor for adverse CNS effects.
• Urge women to report planned or suspected pregnancy.
• Advise women to avoid using passion flower during pregnancy or when breast-feeding.
• Caution the patient to avoid hazardous activities until the herb's CNS effects are known.
• Nausea, vomiting, drowsiness, prolonged QT interval, and episodes of nonsustained ventricular tachycardia have been reported in a 34-year-old woman (Fisher et al., 2000).
• Intraperitoneal administration to mice resulted in decreased spontaneous activity and respiratory and heart rate, tremorlike symptoms, and death (Aoyagi et al., 1974).

Points of interest
• In the United States, passion flower is collected almost entirely for export (Ramstad, 1959).
• The herb was patented in chewing gum form in Romania in 1978.
• Passion flower is found in sedative-hypnotic drug mixtures in Europe.
• The herb is listed by the Council of Europe as a natural food flavoring.

Commentary
Passion flower appears to exert mild sedative effects. Animal data support the use of passion flower as a sedative, but clinical data in humans are limited. Additional trials are needed to establish safety and efficacy.

Insufficient reliable information is available to support the use of passion flower for other claims.

References

Aoyagi, N., et al. "Studies on *Passiflora incarnata* Dry Extract. Part I. Isolation of Maltol and Pharmacological Action of Maltol and Ethylmaltol," *Chem Pharm Bull* 22:1008-13, 1974.

Bourin, M., et al. "A Combination of Plant Extracts in the Treatment of Outpatients with Adjustment Disorder with Anxious Mood: Controlled Study Versus Placebo," *Fundam Clin Pharmcol* 11(2):127-32, 1997.

Fisher, A., et al. "Toxicity of *Passiflora incarnata* L." *Clin Toxicol* 38(1):63-66, 2000.

Giavina-Bianchi, P., et al. "Occupational Respiratory Allergic Disease Induced by *Passiflora alata* and *Rhamnus purshiana*," *Ann Allergy Asthma Immunol* 79:449-54, 1997.

Hegnauer, R. *Chemotaxonomie der Planzen*, Vol 5: 295. Cited in Tyler, V., *The Honest Herbal*, 3d ed. Binghamton, N.Y.: Pharmaceutical Products Press, 1993, p. 238.

Kimura, R., et al. "Central Depressant Effects of Maltol Analogs in Mice," *Chem Pharm Bull* 28:2570-79, 1980.

Ramstad, E. *Modern Pharmacognosy.* London: McGraw-Hill, 1959.

Rasmussen, P. "A Role for Phytotherapy in the Treatment of Benzodiazepine and Opiate Drug Withdrawal," *Eur J Herbal Med* 3(1):11-21, 1997.

PAU D'ARCO

IPE, IPE ROXO, IPES, LA PACHO, LAPACHO, LAPACHO COLORADO, LAPACHOL, LAPACHO MORADO, PURPLE LAPACHO, RED LAPACHO, ROXO, TAHEEBO, TAJIBO, TRUMPET BUSH, TRUMPET TREE

Taxonomic class
Bignoniaceae

Common trade names
Multi-ingredient preparations: Advance Defense System Tablets, Brazilian Herbal Tea, Candistroy, Cat's Claw Defense Complex, Cellguard Coq 10 Nac, Healthgard with Echinacea, Immuno-Nourish, Pau D'arco, Pau D'arco Inner Bark, Ultra Multiple Vitamin, Wellness Formula Vitamin, Wellness Multiple Max Daily, Women's Ut Formula

Common forms
Available as capsules (460 mg), extracts, salve, tablets, and teas.

Source
Pau d'arco products are made from the bark of *Tabebuia impetiginosa* (also known as *Tabebula avellanedae* or *Tecoma curialis*). These evergreen flowering trees belong to the bignonia family and are native to Florida, the West Indies, Mexico, and Central and South America.

Chemical components
About 15 quinone compounds have been found in the heartwood of *T. impetiginosa*, including lapachol, B-lapachone (both naphthoquinones),

and tabebuin (an anthroquinone). *Tabebuia* naphthoquinones are extracted from plant material with organic solvents. Lapachol or xyloidone (dehydro-B-lapachone) wasn't found in the bark of *T. impetiginosa*, the part of the tree usually sold as pau d'arco, but both were present in the heartwood of related species. An analysis of 12 taheebo products available in Canada revealed that only one contained lapachol (Awang, 1988).

Actions

Lapachol and xyloidone have been extensively investigated for antimicrobial activity. Xyloidone was found to be active against only *Brucella* and *Candida* (Awang, 1988). Gram-positive bacteria were sensitive to lapachol and its isomer lapachone, but only *Pseudomonas aeruginosa* and *Brucella melitensis* were sensitive among the gram-negative organisms (Guiraud et al., 1994).

Although lapachol and B-lapachone are both fungistatic, the presumed mechanisms of action suggest that these compounds may be too toxic for medical use (Guiraud et al., 1994). Aqueous pau d'arco extracts have shown no activity against *Candida* cultures. Lapachol also has some effect as an antimalarial (Awang, 1988) and antischistosomal agent.

Human clinical trials have been inconclusive regarding the use of lapachol as an anticancer agent (Block et al., 1974; Awang, 1988). In vitro studies showed antineoplastic activity, but this action was inhibited by vitamin K_1 (Dinnen and Ebisuzaki, 1997). The anti-inflammatory properties have also been demonstrated for a rat paw edema model. Several lapacho compounds, particularly naphtho[2,3-b]furan-4.9-diones, demonstrated in vitro activity as antiproliferative agents in human keratinocytes and may provide the basis for developing new agents to treat psoriasis (Muller et al., 1999).

Reported uses

Tabebuia species have been used in Latin American and Caribbean folk medicine as aphrodisiacs and for treating anemia, backache, bedwetting, boils, colds, dysentery, dysuria, fever, gonorrhea, headache, incontinence, snakebite, sore throat, syphilis, toothache, and external wounds. The tea or topical extracts are claimed to be useful for *Candida albicans* infections, despite evidence that they are ineffective (Awang, 1988).

Other therapeutic claims include treatment of AIDS, allergies, cancer, diabetes, hepatic disease, hernia, infection, inflammation, lupus, rheumatism, smoker's cough, ulcers, and warts. The agent has also been touted as a blood purifier, with the ability to cleanse the blood of pathogens and chemical contaminants; clinical evidence in support of these claims is lacking.

Dosage

The quantity of pau d'arco contained in the product is not listed on the packaging for some preparations. Traditional uses suggest the following dosages:

Capsules: 1 or 2 capsules P.O. b.i.d. (with water or as a tea) at meals, or 3 or 4 capsules t.i.d. for no longer than 7 days.

Lapachol (unspecified product): 1 to 2 g/day P.O.
Lapachol tea: 15 to 20 g of bark steeped in 16 oz of boiling water for 10 minutes to make a tea with a lapachol content of about 3%.

Adverse reactions
GI: nausea, vomiting.
GU: pink urine.
Hematologic: reversible anticoagulant effects.

Interactions
Anticoagulants: May potentiate effects. Avoid administration with pau d'arco.

Contraindications and precautions
Pau d'arco is contraindicated in patients who are receiving drugs that interfere with blood clotting and in those with coagulation disorders (such as hemophilia, severe hepatic disease) or other hemorrhagic diseases (such as von Willebrand's disease and thrombocytopenia). It is also contraindicated in pregnant or breast-feeding patients and in children under age 18; effects are unknown.

Special considerations
• Caution the patient against using pau d'arco instead of conventional medical treatment.
• Monitor the patient for increased bleeding and bruising.
• Advise women to avoid using pau d'arco during pregnancy or when breast-feeding.

Points of interest
• *Taheebo* is a South American Indian word for the hard, durable wood of these trees from which the Indians made bows for hunting. The Portuguese, who first colonized Brazil, named the tree pau d'arco, meaning bow stick. The Spanish name for these trees is *lapacho* (Awang, 1988).

Commentary
There are no clinical data to support the use of pau d'arco for any medical condition. Besides lapachol and xyloidone, other chemical components of pau d'arco have not been studied. Because hydroquinone compounds are known to possess toxic effects, this herb should be considered potentially toxic. Therefore, its use cannot be recommended.

References
Awang, D.V.C. "Commercial Taheebo Lacks Active Ingredient," *Can Pharm J* 5:323-26, 1988.
Block, J.B., et al. "Early Clinical Studies with Lapachol (NSC-11905) Part 2," *Cancer Chemother Rep* 4:27-28, 1974.
Dinnen, R.D., and Ebisuzaki, K. "Search for Novel Anticancer Agents: A Differentiation-based Assay and Analysis of a Folklore Product," *Anticancer Res* 17:1027-34, 1997.
Guiraud, P., et al. "Comparison of Antibacterial and Antifungal Activities of Lapachol and B-Lapachone," *Planta Med* 60:373-74, 1994.

Bold italic type indicates that reaction may be life-threatening.

Muller, K., et al. "Potential Antipsoriatic Agents: Lapacho Compounds as Potent Inhibitors of HaCaT Cell Growth," *J Nat Prod* 62:1134-36, 1999.

PEACH

AMYGDALIN, *AMYGDALIS PERSICA*, LAETRILE, OLEUM PERSICORUM, PEACH OIL, *PERSICA VULGARIS*, PERSIC OIL, VITAMIN B_{17}

Taxonomic class
Rosaceae

Common trade names
Laetrile, Vitamin B-17

Common forms
Available as persic oil, peach kernel oil, peach bark, leaves, and seeds. Crushed seeds are marketed as cancer remedies, health foods, and vitamin supplements. None of these preparations is standardized as to the amount of active ingredient.

Source
Active components are obtained from the leaves, bark, and seeds or kernels of the fruit of *Prunus persica,* a fruit tree belonging to the rose family. The fruit (peach) is fleshy and succulent and surrounds a hard, deeply pitted stone or pit, which in turn envelops a seed or kernel. The leaves are typically gathered in the summer and dried. The bark is harvested from young trees in the spring and dried. Peach kernel oil is expressed from the kernels or seeds of the pit. The oil is also referred to as persic oil; persic oil may be obtained from either the peach kernel or the apricot kernel (*P. armeniaca*).

Chemical components
The leaves, seeds, flowers, and bark contain amygdalin, which on hydrolysis yields hydrocyanic acid. Phloretin is found in the bark and leaves. Numerous other minerals and compounds have been isolated from the bark, flower, fruit, leaf, seed, and root.

Actions
Peach kernel oil is used as a pharmaceutical oil; it has also demonstrated in vitro fungicidal properties (Mishra and Dubey, 1990). Various parts of the peach tree are claimed to irritate and stimulate the GI tract. Phloretin from the bark and leaves is an antibiotic that is effective against gram-positive and gram-negative bacteria. Leaves and bark also have diuretic, expectorant, laxative, sedative, and soothing actions. Amygdalin is known to be a highly toxic cyanogenic glycoside.

Reported uses
Traditionally, peach leaves and bark have been used as an analgesic, an anthelmintic, an antitussive, an astringent, a cathartic, a demulcent, a diuretic, an expectorant, and a sedative. They have been used topically

for blisters, boils, bruises, burns, eczema, warts, and minor wounds. They have also been used to treat bronchitis, constipation, dysentery, dysmenorrhea, dyspepsia, earache, generalized edema, halitosis, headache, hemorrhage, herpes zoster, hypertension, pneumonia, scurvy, sore throat, and tetanus.

Laetrile, also called amygdalin or vitamin B_{17}, has commonly been promoted as a cancer preventive and cure. It is obtained from the kernels of apricots, peaches, plums, cherries, nectarines, apples, and almonds. Extensive testing by the National Cancer Institute has failed to confirm the drug's anticancer effect (Moertel et al., 1982). Moreover, laetrile has been banned by the FDA because of the risk of poisoning from its cyanide content.

Dosage
Tea: ½ oz of dried bark or 1 oz of dried leaves steeped in 1 pt of boiling water for 15 minutes; take P.O. t.i.d.

Adverse reactions
Skin: allergic reaction (to outer skin of the fruit).

Interactions
None reported.

Contraindications and precautions
Peach is contraindicated in pregnant or breast-feeding patients because its risk profiles are still uncertain.

Special considerations
• Advise the patient to wear gloves if he is hypersensitive to the fruit and handling is necessary.
• There is one report of diarrhea, progressive proximal muscle weakness, and nephrotic syndrome after ingestion of a combination product containing peach pit.
◗ **ALERT** Caution the patient to avoid consuming pits or kernels because of the risk of cyanide poisoning. Cyanogenic glycosides are poisonous and are found in the seeds, leaves, flowers, and bark of the peach tree. The peach pit contains about 2.6 mg of hydrocyanic acid per gram of seed. A lethal dose of hydrocyanic acid is 50 to 60 mg in adults (equivalent to about 20 g of peach seeds; Holzbecher et al., 1984). Several fatalities have been reported from peach pit consumption. Symptoms of cyanide poisoning include sudden, severe vomiting and epigastric pain followed by coma, lethargy, seizures, and syncope. Chronic consumption of plants high in cyanogenic glycosides has resulted in ataxia, clonus, nerve deafness, peripheral neuropathy optic atrophy, and spastic paraparesis.
• Caution the patient to keep the dangerous parts of the peach (pits, kernels) away from children and pets.

Commentary

Although there are several anecdotal reports of the use of peach leaves or bark tea, clinical safety and efficacy data are lacking. Therefore, this treatment cannot be recommended. Consumption of peach kernels is potentially fatal, and there are no valid clinical studies documenting the effectiveness of hydrocyanic acid in the prevention or treatment of cancer. The potential risks associated with the consumption of peach kernels outweigh any potential benefits, and their use should be discouraged.

References

Holzbecher, M.D., et al. "The Cyanide Content of Laetrile Preparations, Apricot, Peach, and Apple Seeds," *Clin Toxicol* 22:341-47, 1984.

Mishra, A.K., and Dubey, N.K., "Fungitoxic Properties of *Prunus persica* Oil," *Hindustan Antibiot Bull* 32:91-93, 1990. Abstract.

Moertel, C.G., et al. "A Clinical Trial of Amygdalin (Laetrile) in the Treatment of Human Cancer," *N Engl J Med* 306:201-6, 1982.

PENNYROYAL

AMERICAN PENNYROYAL, EUROPEAN PENNYROYAL, MOSQUITO PLANT, SQUAWMINT

Taxonomic class
Lamiaceae

Common trade names
Multi-ingredient preparations: Aloe Herbal Horse Spray, Miracle Coat Spray-On Dog Shampoo, Pennyroyal, Pennyroyal Essential Oil

Common forms
Available as dried leaves, flowers, and oil.

Source
Active components are obtained from the dried leaves and flowering tops of American pennyroyal (*Hedeoma pulegioides*) and European pennyroyal (*Mentha pulegium*). Both belong to the mint family.

Chemical components
The leaves and flowering tops of *H. pulegioides* are the main source of pennyroyal oil. The oil consists chiefly of a monoterpene (pulegone), which ranges from 9% in Brazilian varieties to 16% to 30% in American varieties and 80% to 94% in European varieties. Other components of pennyroyal oil are hedeomal, tannins, alpha-pinene, beta-pinene, limonene, 3-octanone, *p*-cymene, 3-octylacetate, 3-octanol, 1-octen-3-ol, 3-methylcyclohexanone, menthone, piperitenone, and paraffins. Dried seeds of *H. pulegioides* contain protein, fat, ash, and small amounts of calcium, sodium, and potassium.

Actions
Pulegone is thought to be responsible for the toxic organ effects of pennyroyal oil in animals and humans. It is metabolized by the cytochrome P-450 enzyme system to form a toxic metabolite, methofuran. The monoterpene is also oxidized to several other metabolites that may be involved in toxicity. Once formed, methofuran, other pulegone metabolites, and unchanged pulegone can deplete hepatic glutathione, leading to hepatic failure. Pulegone is a potent liver toxin. It also acts as an insect repellent.

Pennyroyal oil is most commonly known for its abortifacient properties. It is believed that the oil causes irritation of the uterus with resultant uterine contractions (Sullivan et al., 1979). These effects are not consistent, and sometimes the use of pennyroyal oil as an abortifacient has resulted in hemorrhaging and even death.

Reported uses
Pennyroyal has been used for several ailments, most notably as an abortifacient. The whole plant was once used for fibroids and indurations of the uterus. The root, ground with vinegar, has also been used to treat tumors.

The plant has a strong, pungent odor similar to that of spearmint. The oil has a scent of citronella and has been used for scenting soaps and detergents and as an insect repellent. Some herbalists use pennyroyal oil to induce menstruation and to treat symptoms of premenstrual syndrome. As a hot infusion (tea), this herb has also been used to treat colds, fevers, and the flu because it promotes sweating. Other uses of pennyroyal include management of chest congestion, colic, and toothache.

Dosage
Oil: 1 to 8 gtt (for topical use only, as an insect repellent or in aromatherapy).
Tea: 1 or 2 tsp of dried pennyroyal leaves steeped in 1 cup of boiling water for 10 to 15 minutes, or mix 1 tbsp of dried herb with 1 cup of warm water. Drink up to 2 cups daily.

Adverse reactions
CNS: *coma,* confusion, dizziness, hallucinations, lethargy, malaise, rigors, *seizures.*
GI: abdominal cramps, hematemesis, nausea, vomiting.
GU: *renal failure.*
Hepatic: *hepatic failure.*
Respiratory: *respiratory depression.*
Other: *death.*

Bold italic type indicates that reaction may be life-threatening.

RESEARCH FINDINGS
Pennyroyal poisoning

Pennyroyal poisoning continues to occur regularly and with relatively small doses; as little as 1 tbsp of the oil has been reported to cause death. Other toxic effects, including seizures, have been reported after ingestion of less than 1 tsp of the oil. Because 50 to 100 g of leaves are needed to produce 1 ml of oil, 1 tsp may be equivalent to 0.5 kg of leaves (Mack, 1997).

One case report described a 24-year-old woman who repeatedly ingested extracts of pennyroyal and black cohosh root for 2 weeks to induce abortion. The patient experienced abdominal cramps, chills, vomiting, syncope, rigors, and difficulty walking. About 7.5 hours after ingestion, the patient was in cardiopulmonary arrest. On arrival in the emergency department, physical examination revealed coma and a rigid abdomen. A computed tomographic scan of the abdomen suggested a ruptured ectopic pregnancy. Throughout the initial 12 hours of hospitalization, the patient's course was marked by hemodynamic shock, decreased hematocrit, hepatic failure, and a clinical picture consistent with disseminated intravascular coagulation. The patient died 46 hours after her last pennyroyal ingestion (Anderson et al., 1996).

In another case, a 12-week-old infant died after being given acetaminophen, a brompheniramine-phenylpropanolamine cold remedy, and 4 oz of pennyroyal tea. In some of the other toxicity cases reported, individuals did not exceed the "recommended" doses.

Interactions
Inhibitors of the cytochrome P-450 system (amiodarone, azole antifungals, cimetidine, macrolide antibiotics, omeprazole): May alter rate of formation of toxic metabolites of pennyroyal. Monitor the patient.

Contraindications and precautions
Pennyroyal is contraindicated in pregnant or breast-feeding patients; abortive effects have been documented. It is also contraindicated in children, in patients with seizure disorders, and in those with renal or hepatic insufficiency. Use with extreme caution because of the lack of data and the risk of toxicity.

Special considerations
◤ ALERT Pennyroyal oils and teas continue to be promoted for several ailments. These products are potentially toxic and should not be ingested except under medical supervision of a health care provider. (See *Pennyroyal poisoning.*)

• Hepatotoxicity may be prevented by early administration of acetylcysteine (Anderson et al., 1996).

• Pennyroyal induces abortion in lethal or near-fatal doses. Therefore, it should never be used as an abortifacient.

• Caution the patient not to take the oil internally.

• Inform the patient who wants to take pennyroyal not to exceed recommended doses and to avoid taking it for longer than 1 week.

• Caution the patient to stop using the herb if unusual symptoms occur.

• Advise women to avoid using pennyroyal during pregnancy or when breast-feeding.

• Advise the patient to keep pennyroyal preparations out of the reach of children and pets.

Points of interest

• In ancient times, pennyroyal was hung in the rooms of convalescents and was believed to hasten recovery. Worn around the head, garlands of pennyroyal were also claimed to alleviate dizziness and headache. Use of pennyroyal as an abortifacient dates back to ancient Rome, at the time of Pliny the Elder (A.D. 23-79).

• Pennyroyal's scientific name stems from the Latin term for flea, *pulex*, which refers to the plant's use as an insect repellent. People have reportedly rubbed the leaves on their clothes or skin for this effect.

Commentary

Although pennyroyal has many therapeutic claims, there are no clinical data to support the use of this herb. Together with the herb's toxicity, the medicinal use of pennyroyal cannot be recommended.

References

Anderson, I.B., et al. "Pennyroyal Toxicity: Measurement of Toxic Metabolite Levels in Two Cases and Review of the Literature," *Ann Intern Med* 124:726-34, 1996.

Mack, R.B. "'Boldly They Rode...Into the Mouth of Hell': Pennyroyal Oil Toxicity," *NC Med J* 58:456-57, 1997.

Sullivan, J.B., et al. "Pennyroyal Oil Poisoning and Hepatotoxicity," *JAMA* 242:2873-74, 1979.

PEPPER, BLACK

BIBER, FILFIL, HU-CHIAO, KPSHO, KRISHNADI, LADA, PEPE, PEPER, PFEFFER, PHI NOI, PIMENATA, PJERETS, POIVRE, THE MASTER SPICE, THE KING OF SPICES

Taxonomic class

Piperaceae

Common trade names

Multi-ingredient preparations: Curry powder, Galat daga, Garam masala, Lowrey, McCormick, Panch phoron, Quatre epices, Ras El hanout, Sambaar podi, Trikatu

---

Bold italic type indicates that reaction may be life-threatening.

Common forms

Available as powder (ground into different grades of coarseness).

Sources

Piper nigrum, the pepper plant, is a woody vine that grows up to 20' tall and is indigenous to Southeast Asia. First cultivated by Indian colonists in Indonesia, it has been transplanted to many equatorial climates, notably Brazil, Malaysia, Sumatra, and China.

Slow drying of the unripe fruit creates black pepper, whereas quick drying creates green pepper. White pepper is obtained by washing the ripe fruit down to the seed core and then drying.

Chemical components

The main active ingredients in pepper are the alkaloids, particularly piperine. Other alkaloids include piperlongumine, piperyline, piperanine, piperidine, and piperettine. These alkaloids, along with chavicin, give pepper its pungent qualities.

Essential oils give pepper its aromatic qualities. Most of these oils consist of monoteroenes, terpenes (sabien, carvone, alpha and beta pinene, myrcene, limonene, borneol, carvacrol, and linalool), and sesquiterens (beta-caryophyllene, humelene, and beta-biasbolone). Other substances include safrol, myristicine, eugenol, beta-sitosterol, and five phenolic amides.

Actions

Pepper increases gastric secretions and bile flow and stimulates diuresis. Five phenolic amides have been identified, and all have greater antioxidant activity than alpha-tocopherol in vitro.

Minor anti-infective activity has been shown against several infectious agents by *Piper* species.

Black pepper's carcinogenic properties have also been studied. Safrol and tannic acids, both found in black pepper, cause tumors in several organs when given to mice. When another component of black pepper was added, the carcinogenicity of the other two substances was reduced. Therefore, it appears that black pepper might have its own built-in protectant. Black pepper may also have a protectant effect in the colon. Black pepper reduces the activity of *B*-glucoronidase and mucinase (Nalini et al., 1998), which may reduce the number of toxins reaching the mucosa of the colon. Mucinase inhibition reduces the loss of protectant mucins, and inhibition of *B*-glucoronidase stops the release of toxins that have been processed by the liver for excretion.

Black pepper extracts have been shown to stimulate melanocyte growth and differentiation in culture medium. This appears to have been achieved by stimulating protein kinase C (Lin et al., 1999). It will be important to see if this stimulation takes place in hair root sheath melanocytes because most other agents used to help depigmentation use ultraviolet light, which has a potential cancer risk.

The anti-inflammatory activity of piperine has been shown, although the mechanism wasn't clear (Mujumdar et al., 1990). Black pepper might have the ability to block pain impulses and cause pain relief.

Abortive and antifertility qualities were also shown in pregnant mice given piperine. It inhibited and delayed labor, exhibited abortive action (depending on the period of gestation), reduced uterine contractions, and caused bloody discharge. Fetal mortality was significantly increased.

Pipeline's ability to affect hepatic enzyme systems and increase drug bioavailability has been reported (Bano et al., 1991). Other studies have confirmed it to be a noncompetitive inhibitor of cytochrome P-450 mixed oxidase systems.

Reported uses
Claims include use as an antiflatulent and a digestive aid and to increase gastric juices, stimulate appetite and diuresis, and treat abdominal pain, colic, constipation, diarrhea, dysentery, heartburn, indigestion, and ulcers. A product called Trikatu, which contains black pepper, is popular in India for treating digestive ailments and for cold and flu symptoms, congestion, diabetes, obesity, rhinorrhea, and tumor control.

The oil vapors have helped to stop the craving for cigarettes in heavy smokers compared with placebo or a menthol-dispensing product. Somatic symptoms of anxiety have also been significantly reduced (Rose and Behm, 1994). Black pepper is thought to clear phlegm and mucous in respiratory conditions, but no studies are available to support these claims.

The herb is used also in muscular conditions and for arthritis, pain, rheumatism, sprains, and stiffness. Pain relief with black pepper is being studied in animals and humans.

Black pepper is used as an aromatic stimulant in weakness caused by cholera, coma, or vertigo and to clear the mind, improve memory, alleviate mental exhaustion, and lift the spirits. No studies were found analyzing the aromatic oil's effect on mental status.

Dosage
No consensus exists.

Adverse reactions
Respiratory: *fatal apnea* (in children when a handful of pepper was ingested).
Other: carcinogenic activity (safrol and tannins are known carcinogens). More information is needed because of conflicting studies and the possibility that protectant components may negate the carcinogenic potential.

Interactions
Drugs metabolized by the cytochrome P-450 system: Piperine is a nonspecific inhibitor of the cytochrome P-450 system and been proved to affect the metabolism of a few drugs. Use caution regarding the amount

---

Bold italic type indicates that reaction may be life-threatening.

ingested in patients taking drugs that have a narrow therapeutic index (such as theophylline and warfarin).

Smoking cessation aids: Additive effects. Monitor patient response.

Contraindications and precautions

Use black pepper cautiously in pregnant or breast-feeding patients; effects are unknown.

Special considerations

• Monitor the patient for changes in effects of drugs he may be taking that are metabolized by the P-450 system.

• Moderate doses generally do not produce many adverse reactions. The FDA has given this herb generally recognized as safe status.

• Inform the patient that the evidence for smoking cessation is inadequate to support therapeutic application in this regard. Refer him to an appropriate smoking cessation program.

Points of interest

• The common form of black pepper is a result of drying the unripe fruit (berries) slowly and grinding into different grades of coarseness. Also used are the essential oils, ground root, and ethanol extracts, which are then ground into a powder and mixed with other types of pepper.

• Peppers used to be named according to the port from which they were shipped, giving some hint as to the quality and potency of the product. Malabar used to indicate the best peppercorns in India. Also, Tellicherry was a particularly bold version of Malabar pepper. All Indian pepper is now called Malabar.

• Black pepper has been used for medicinal purposes worldwide since the time of Hippocrates, but nowhere is it used more medicinally than in India, where it occurs in almost every preparation.

• Black pepper is used as an insecticide, as a flavoring in brandy, and in perfumes and has a tremendous value as a spice in food, drinks, and desserts.

Commentary

Black pepper is the most widely used spice in the world and does have some pharmacologic properties. Although most claimed uses lack supporting evidence, studies in animals may indicate validity to some of these claims. It may hold promise as an aid for smoking cessation or as a vehicle for enhancing drug bioavailability. Studies in humans are needed before any anecdotal claim can be seriously considered.

References

Bano, G. et al. "Effect of Piperine on Bioavailability and Pharmacokinetics of Propranolol and Theophylline in Healthy Volunteers," *Eur J Clin Pharmacol* 41:615-17, 1991.

Lin, Z., et al. "Stimulation of Mouse Melanocyte Proliferation by *Piper nigrum* Fruit Extract and Its Main Alkaloid, Piperine," *Planta Med* 65: 600-603, 1999.

Mujumdar, A.M., et al. "Anti-inflammatory Activity of Piperine," *Jpn J Med Sci Biol* 43:95-100, 1990.

Nalini, N., et al. "Influence of Spices on the Bacterial (Enzyme) Activity in Experimental Colon Cancer," *J Ethnopharm* 62:15-24, 1998.

Rose, J.E., and Behm, F.M. "Inhalation of Vapor from Black Pepper Extract Reduces Smoking Withdrawal Symptoms," *Drug Alcohol Depend* 34:225-92, 1994.

PERIWINKLE

Taxonomic class
Apocynaceae

Common trade names
Blue Buttons, Cezayirmeneksesi, Common Periwinkle, Cut Finger, Flower of Immortality, Greater Periwinkle, Ground Ivy, Hundred Eyes, Joy-of-the-Ground, Pennywinkle, Pucellage, Sorcerer's Violet, True Periwinkle, Vencapervinc, Virgin Flower

Common forms
Available as dried herb for tea or infusion, fluidextract, and tincture.

Source
Periwinkle is derived from the dried aerial portions of the perennial plant *Vinca major*. The plant is native to southern Europe.

Chemical components
Various constituents have been reported to be isolated from the *V. major* plant, including terpenes and indole alkaloids (Chatterjee et al., 1975). Among the various alkaloids, vincamine has been reported to have some medicinal effects.

Actions
Periwinkle has been reported to have many effects—mainly antihemorrhagic and astringent properties—but the exact mechanism of action has not been clearly defined. It has also been claimed to have analgesic, antidiabetic, antimicrobial, anti-inflammatory, cardiotonic, diuretic, hypotensive, sedative, and spasmolytic properties. Specifically, vincamine is said to improve blood flow. Its antidiarrheal properties result from a reduction in fluid or blood loss combined with the toning of the membranes.

Reported uses
Periwinkle has been used internally and externally as an astringent in treating hemorrhage and excessive menorrhagia. Antihemorrhagic usage includes the treatment of hematuria, hemorrhoids, and uterine bleeding. Historically, the leaves of the periwinkle plant have been applied locally in the nostrils to decrease nosebleeds, to the gums to decrease bleeding, and topically to the extremities to relieve cramping. As an infusion, it has been reported to be useful as a decongestant and has been used as a gargle to reduce inflammation and pain in pharyngitis.

Periwinkle is reported to be used by herbalists as a substitute for insulin in treating diabetes, a controversial claim that has not been shown

---

Bold italic type indicates that reaction may be life-threatening.

to be valid in other periwinkle plants, particularly Madagascar periwinkle (Swanston-Flatt et al., 1989). Periwinkle has been claimed to be useful in improving blood flow in cerebral arteriosclerosis after a stroke. Early animal studies have been conducted in the use of periwinkle for treating atherosclerosis, hypertension, and ischemic heart disease (Petkov, 1979).

Dosage
Traditional uses suggest the following dosages:
Dried herb: 2 to 4 g or by infusion P.O. t.i.d.
Infusion: 1 tsp of dried herb combined with 1 cup of boiling water. Infuse for 10 to 15 minutes and then ingest as a tea t.i.d.
Liquid extract (1:1 in 25% alcohol): 2 to 4 ml t.i.d.
Tincture: 1 to 2 ml P.O. t.i.d.

Adverse reactions
GI: constipation.

Interactions
None reported.

Contraindications and precautions
Periwinkle should be avoided in patients with constipation.

Special considerations
• Periwinkle should be used only as a treatment for acute, short-term need; it may be dangerous if used regularly, with some resources claiming its limited availability because of its unspecified toxicity profile.
• Advise the patient to consult a health care provider before using herbal preparations because a treatment that has been clinically researched and proved effective may be available.
• This herb is reported to have an intensely bitter taste.
• Although no known chemical interactions have been reported in clinical studies, consideration must be given to the pharmacologic properties of the herbal product and the potential for exacerbation of the intended therapeutic effect of conventional drugs.

Points of interest
• Other plants commonly known as periwinkle include lesser periwinkle (*Vinca minor*), which has some reported use in treating dementia and tinnitus, and Madagascar periwinkle (*Catharanthus roseus*), which is extensively known as the source for the cytotoxic drugs vinblastine and vincristine.

Commentary
Although periwinkle (*V. major*) has many therapeutic claims, none has been verified using randomized, controlled trials. Until more research is conducted to better understand the activity of periwinkle and identify active components, if any, the use of periwinkle for any indication can't be recommended.

References

Chatterjee, A., et al. "Monoterpenoid Alkaloid from *Vinca major,*" *Planta Med* 28(2):109-11, 1975.

Duke, J.A. *The Green Pharmacy.* Emmaus, Pa.: Rodale Press, 1997.

Greive, M., and Leyel, C.F. *A Modern Herbal.* New York: Barnes & Noble Books, 1996.

Ody, P. *The Complete Medicinal Herbal.* New York: Dorling Kindersley, 1993.

Petkov, V. "Plants and Hypotensive, Antiatheromatous and Coronarodilatating Action," *Am J Chin Med* 7(3):197-236, 1979.

Swanston-Flatt, S.K., et al. "Glycaemic Effects of Traditional European Plant Treatments for Diabetes. Studies in Normal and Streptozotocin Diabetic Mice," *Diabetes Res* 10(2):69-73, 1989.

PEYOTE

ANHALONIUM, BIG CHIEF, BUTTONS, CACTUS, MESC, MESCAL, MESCAL BUTTONS, MESCALINE, MEXC, MOON, PAN PEYOTE, PEYOTE BUTTONS

Taxonomic class
Cactaceae

Common trade names
None known.

Common forms
Basic pan peyote: chloroform extract of ground peyote
Button: 45 mg of mescaline
Mescaline hydrochloride or sulfate: 375 mg of hydrochloride salt equals 500 mg of the sulfate salt
Soluble peyote: hydrochloride extract of basic pan peyote used for injection
Tincture: 70% alcohol extract of peyote

Source
The crude drug is obtained from the dried tops or whole plants of *Lophophora williamsii,* a small cactus that is native to Mexico and south Texas. Mescaline, the chief active ingredient, has been synthesized.

Chemical components
Several chemical compounds have been isolated and may play a role in the hallucinogenic actions of this plant. The main active constituent is the alkaloid mescaline, or 3,4,5-trimethoxyphenylethylamine. Other components include *N*-methylmescaline, *N*-formylmescaline, *N*-acetylmescaline, 3-demethylmescaline, *N*-formyl-3-demethylmescaline, *N*-acetyl-3-formylmescaline, *N*-acetylanhalamine, anhaladine, and anhalanine.

Actions
Mescaline achieves its affect by stimulating adenylate cyclase activity at central dopaminergic receptors in the anterior limbic structures. It

---

specifically acts on the pons and pontine raphe nuclei, decreasing neuronal firing and serotonin turnover. It also acts on the catecholamine and indolamine systems. It has been suggested that it may inhibit cholinergic neuromuscular transmission by blocking release of acetylcholine and affecting potassium conductance. Mescaline is also thought to have an affinity for 5-HT1A, 5-HT2A, and 5-ht2C receptors (Ghansah et al., 1993: Monte et al., 1997).

Reported uses
Peyote has long been used in Native American religious ceremonies. It has also reportedly been used as an antibiotic, a cardiotonic, a hallucinogenic, an intoxicant, a narcotic, a poison, a psychedelic, a sedative, and a tonic. Folk remedies involve the use of the herb for alcoholism, angina, fever, headache, heatstroke, paralysis, rheumatism, snakebite, and throat irritation and as a pain-killer for arthritis, backache, burns, and corns.

Until the 1960s, mescaline was used to induce a model of psychosis for researchers. The psychiatric community is pushing to reintroduce the use of hallucinogenics as a model for acute psychosis. Also, there have been three anecdotal reports of hallucinogenic drugs helping to alleviate the symptoms of obsessive-compulsive disorder (OCD). It is thought that these drugs, which are serotonin agonists, cause a downregulation of the serotonin receptors, causing a stabler situation for the OCD patient. Tolerance to the psychedelic aspects developed quickly in these patients while their symptoms continued to be relieved. Several patients had complete remission of symptoms that continued for some time even after discontinuation of the hallucinogenic.

Mescaline and lysergic acid diethylamide (LSD) were used years ago in many studies to attempt to treat alcoholism. The studies were not well controlled and had a wide range of methodologies and no consistent criteria for success. No inferences can be drawn from the results of these studies, but they may be pertinent in shaping the direction future research takes if these agents reappear.

Dosage
Use is not recommended. Mescaline doses of 5 mg/kg P.O. produce physical effects and hallucinations.

Adverse reactions
CNS: anxiety, ataxia, emotional liability, paranoia, tremor.
CV: hypertension, mild tachycardia.
EENT: mydriasis, nystagmus, photophobia.
GI: nausea, vomiting (within 30 to 60 minutes after ingestion).
Musculoskeletal: hyperreflexia, muscle fasciculations.
Other: diaphoresis; auditory hallucinations, visual hallucinations, and intensified color and texture perception (peaking at about 4 to 6 hours and lasting up to 14 hours). Visual hallucinations usually include complex geometric patterns that seem to follow the user (Giannini et al., 1986).

Interactions

Other drugs that act on the CNS (alcohol, marijuana, narcotic analgesics, psychedelics): May potentiate or aggravate effects. Avoid concomitant use.

Contraindications and precautions

Avoid using peyote in pregnant or breast-feeding patients; effects are unknown. Use cautiously in patients with CNS disorders. Peyote may be mixed with phencyclidine (PCP or angel dust) or other illicit drugs that may worsen the patient's condition.

Special considerations

• Mescaline and peyote are considered Schedule I controlled substances. Because of this designation, peyote is considered to have no accepted medical use and a high abuse potential. Native Americans use peyote in sacramental rites and are, therefore, exempt from prosecution under the Controlled Substance Act.

• Peyote is not thought to cause physical dependence, and it is not known if it can cause psychological dependence. Tolerance does occur and can cross over to effect LSD and DMT (dimethyltryptamine).

• Bradycardia, hypotension, respiratory depression, and vasodilation have occurred with mescaline doses over 20 mg/kg.

• Death from high doses is less common than traumatic fatalities resulting from altered perception.

• Treatment is supportive until the effects have worn off. Place the patient in a semidarkened room and "talk him down," if necessary. Diphenhydramine or a mild tranquilizer, such as diazepam, can be given if needed. Avoid using antipsychotics because psychosis resolves spontaneously.

Commentary

Besides the fact that peyote is illegal, it has no established medicinal use but is likely to reappear in future clinical psychiatric research literature.

References

Ghansah, E., et al. "Effects of Mescaline and Some of Its Analogs on Cholinergic Neuromuscular Transmission," *Neuropharmacology* 32:169-74, 1993.

Giannini, A.J., et al. "Contemporary Drugs of Abuse," *Am Fam Phys* 33:207-16, 1986.

Monte, A.P., et al. "Dihydrobenzofuran Analogues of Hallucinogens. Part 4. Mescaline Derivatives," *J Med Chem* 40:2997-3008, 1997.

Pedro, L. et al., "Hallucinogens, Serotonin and Obsessive-Compulsive Disorder," *J Psych Drugs* 30:359-65, 1998.

PHYLLANTHUS

PHYLLANTHUS AMARUS (SHO-SAIKO-TO, TJ-9, XINO-CHAI-HU-TANG), *PHYLLANTHUS NIRURI* (BUDHATRI, CHANCA PIEDRA, DERRIERE DOS, DES DOS, DUKONG ANAK, MEMENIRAN, MENIRAN, NIRURI, PITRISHI, SACHA OR SASHA FOSTER, SHATTER STONE, STONEBREAKER, TAMALAKA, TURI HUTAN)

Taxonomic class
Euphorbiaceae

Common trade names
None known.

Common forms
Capsules: 200 mg, 250 mg, 300 mg (dried powder)

Source
The entire plant of several species of *Phyllanthus*, excluding the roots, has been dried and blended into powder form.

Chemical components
Chanca piedra (*Phyllanthus niruri*) contains many phytochemicals, including 3,5,7-trihydroxyflavonal-4'-*o*-alpha-l-(-)-rhamnopyranoside, 4-methoxy-norsecurinine, 4-methoxy-securinine, 5,3',4'-trihydroxyfla-vonone-7-*o*- alpha-l- (-)-rhamnopyranoside, astragalin, brevifolin-carboxylic-acid, cymene, hypophyllanthin, limonene, lintetralin, lupa-20 (29)-ene-3-beta-ol, lupa-20(29)-ene-3-beta-ol-acetate, lupeol, methyl-salicylate, niranthin, nirtetralin, niruretin, nirurin, niruriside, phyllan-thin, phyllochrysine, phyltetralin, quercetin, quercetin-heteroside, quercetol, quercitrin, rutin, saponins, triacontanal, and tricontanol.

Actions
Phyllanthus species have shown antihepatotoxic activity in rats (Prakash et al., 1995), inhibition of endogenous DNA polymerase of hepatitis B virus (HBV) in animals and humans (Thyagarajan et al., 1988), and de-creased virion production along with down-regulation of hepatitis B surface antigen mRNA transcription in vitro (Ott et al., 1997).

Reported uses
Phyllanthus is used in many areas of the world, including South America and India, as an antibacterial, an antihepatotoxic, an anti-inflammatory, an antispasmodic, an antiviral, a choleretic, a digestive aid, a diuretic, an emmenagogue, a febrifuge, a hepatotonic, a hypoglycemic, a hypotensive, an immunostimulant, and a laxative.

Dosage
Dosage in studies ranged from 200 to 900 mg P.O. t.i.d. The traditional remedy consists of 1 to 3 ml of a 4:1 tincture or 1,000 to 2,000 mg P.O. b.i.d.

Adverse reactions
None reported.

Interactions
None reported.

Contraindications and precautions
Unknown.

Special considerations
• Because of claims of hypoglycemic activity, chanca piedra should be avoided or blood glucose levels monitored closely in diabetic patients.
• Advise the patient to consult a health care provider before using herbal preparations because a treatment that has been clinically researched and proved effective may be available.
• Although no known chemical interactions have been reported in clinical studies, consideration must be given to the pharmacologic properties of the herbal product and the potential for exacerbation of the intended therapeutic effect of conventional drugs.

Commentary
Although some clinical studies supported the use of *Phyllanthus* for HBV carriers, subsequent studies have not reproduced the same clinical findings (Leelarasamee et al., 1990). Much controversy exists on the use of *Phyllanthus* for this indication (Brook, 1988; Thyagarajan et al., 1990). Evidence to support other claims is lacking. More research is needed before definitive recommendations can be put forward.

References
Brook, M.G. "Effect of *Phyllanthus amarus* on Chronic Carriers of Hepatitis B Virus," *Lancet* 2(8618):1017-18, 1988. Letter.

Leelarasamee, A., et al. "Failure of *Phyllanthus amarus* to Eradicate Hepatitis B Surface Antigen from Symptomless Carriers," *Lancet* 13(336:8720):949-50, 1990. Letter.

Ott, M., et al. "*Phyllanthus amarus* Suppresses Hepatitis B Virus by Interrupting Interactions Between HBV Enhancer I and Cellular Transcription Factors," *Eur J Clin Invest* 27:11:908-15, 1997.

Prakash, A., et al. "Comparative Hepatoprotective Activity of Three Species, *P. urinaria, P. niruri, P. simplex,* on Carbon Tetrachloride Induced Liver Injury in the Rat," *Phytother Res* 9(8):594-96, 1995.

Thyagarajan, S.P., et al. "Effect of *Phyllanthus amarus* on Chronic Carriers of Hepatitis B Virus," *Lancet* 2(8614):764-66, 1988.

Thyagarajan, S.P., et al. "*Phyllanthus amarus* and Hepatitis B," *Lancet* 336(8720):949-50, 1990. Letter.

PILL-BEARING SPURGE

ASTHMA WEED, CATSHAIR, EUPHORBIA, GARDEN SPURGE,
MILKWEED, QUEENSLAND ASTHMAWEED, SNAKE WEED

Taxonomic class
Euphorbiaceae

Common trade names
Multi-ingredient preparations: As-Comp, Ephedra Plus, Euphorbia,
Sinus and Catarrh Complex

Common forms
Available as capsules, dried plant (powder), liquid extract, tablets, and
tincture.

Source
The crude drug is obtained from the dried plant of *Euphorbia pilulifera*
(also called *E. hirta* or *E. capitata*). It is an annual herb that is native to
India and Australia. In the United States, it occurs from Texas to Arizona.

Chemical components
The plant contains choline, shikimic acid, flavonoids (quercitrin, quercetin, leuococyanidin), triterpenes (taraxerol, taraxerone esters, alpha-
and beta-amyrin), sterols (campesterol, euphosterol, sitosterol), alkanes
(hentriacontane), phenolic acids, *l*-inositol, sugars, and resins. Tannins
have also been reported.

Actions
Rodents given an extract of *E. hirta* intraperitoneally exhibit dose-
dependent analgesic, anti-inflammatory, and antipyretic effects. Higher
doses produce sedative effects, whereas lower doses exert anxiolytic effects (Lanhers et al., 1991). These plant extracts may have antibacterial
activity, and in vitro amebicidal activity against *Entamoeba histolytica*
has also been reported. Shikimic acid has shown mutagenic activity in
mice.

Choline is a cholinergic agonist similar to acetylcholine but with less
activity. Shikimic acid is the precursor of phenylalanine, tyrosine, tryptophan, and several plant alkaloids. In guinea pigs, choline administration results in contraction of the ileum, whereas shikimic acid relaxes
the ileum. Quercetin, the aglycone of quercitrin, showed antidiarrheal
properties in mice (Galvez et al., 1993). Quercetin also decreases
platelet aggregation in humans.

Reported uses
Therapeutic claims for pill-bearing spurge include treatment of asthma,
bronchitis, coughs, diarrhea, dysentery, gonorrhea, hay fever, intestinal
amebiasis, ophthalmic disorders, snakebites, and thrush (Watt and
Breyer-Brandwijk, 1962).

Dosage
Traditional uses suggest the following dosages:
Dried plant: 120 to 300 mg P.O. or by infusion P.O. t.i.d.
Liquid extract (1:1 in 45% alcohol): 0.12 to 0.3 ml P.O. t.i.d.
Tincture (1:5 in 60% alcohol): 0.6 to 2 ml P.O t.i.d.

Adverse reactions
GI: emesis, gastric irritation.
Skin: contact dermatitis.
Other: cholinergic symptoms (with overdose).

Interactions
ACE inhibitors: May potentiate antihypertensive effects. Use together cautiously.
Anticholinergics (atropine, ipratropium, scopolamine, other belladonna-type alkaloids): Choline may decrease effects of these drugs. Use together cautiously.
Anticoagulants: May potentiate effects. Use together cautiously.
Barbiturates: May potentiate central hypnotic effects. Use together cautiously.
Disulfiram: Disulfiram reaction can occur if herbal form contains alcohol. Avoid administration with pill-bearing spurge.
Muscarinic agonists (arecoline, methacholine, muscarine), cholinesterase inhibitors (donepezil, edrophonium, physostigmine): Additive effect when combined and increased risk of toxicity. Use together cautiously.
Other drugs metabolized by CYP3A enzymes (cyclosporine, erythromycin): May inhibit cytochrome P-450-3A enzymes. Use together cautiously.

Contraindications and precautions
Pill-bearing spurge is contraindicated in pregnant or breast-feeding patients because it causes both contraction and relaxation of smooth muscle. Use cautiously with patients receiving anticoagulants and in those with bleeding disorders because platelet aggregation may be reduced.

Special considerations
• Toxic symptoms associated with excessive cholinergic stimulation include bradycardia, hypotension, lacrimation, salivation, sweating, and vomiting. Instruct the patient to stop using pill-bearing spurge if they occur.
• Advise the patient with allergies that dermatologic reactions can result from handling products that contain *E. hirta*.
• Caution the patient taking disulfiram not to take a form of the herb that contains alcohol.

Points of interest
• Pill-bearing spurge is not recognized by the FDA as being safe and effective for certain OTC use, such as asthma.

Bold italic type indicates that reaction may be life-threatening.

Commentary

Although this herb has shown possible analgesic, anti-inflammatory, antipyretic, anxiolytic, and sedative activity in animals and antibacterial action against certain strains of *Shigella* species, human clinical data are lacking. The FDA has ruled that products that contain *E. hirta* are neither safe nor effective for treating asthma; therefore, the herb should not be used to treat respiratory conditions. Because of the risk of drug interactions, use cautiously if taking concurrently with prescription drugs.

References

Galvez, J., et al. "Antidiarrheic Activity of *Euphorbia hirta* Extract and Isolation of an Active Flavonoid Constituent," *Planta Med* 59:333-36, 1993.

Lanhers, M.C., et al. "Analgesic, Antipyretic, and Anti-inflammatory Properties of *Euphorbia hirta*," *Planta Med* 57:225-31, 1991.

Watt, J.M., and Breyer-Brandwijk, M.G. *The Medicinal and Poisonous Plants of Southern and Eastern Africa*, 2nd ed. Edinburgh and London: E and S Livingston Ltd., 1962.

PINEAPPLE

ANANAS, GOLDEN ROCKET, SMOOTH CAYENNE PINEAPPLE

Taxonomic class
Bromeliaceae

Common trade names
Ananase

Common forms
Available as candy, extracts, juices, syrups, and whole fruit.

Source
Active components are derived from the juice and fruiting portion of *Ananas comosus*, a member of the bromeliad family that is native to South America. Pineapple is widely cultivated in tropical regions, especially Hawaii and Thailand.

Chemical components
The fruit contains citric acid, malic acid, vitamin A, and ascorbic acid. The leaves contain a steroidal compound, and a volatile oil contains aromatic compounds. All plant parts contain bromelain and several other proteolytic enzymes.

Actions
Juice from unripe pineapples reportedly produces violent cathartic action. The root and ripe fruit are claimed to have diuretic activity. Bromelain is moderately well absorbed from the intestine after oral administration. Bromelain's actions are reported to enhance serum fibrinolytic activity, inhibit fibrinogen synthesis, degrade fibrin and fibrinogen, and influence prostaglandin synthesis. It is also reported to lower serum tissue levels of kininogen and bradykinin (Lotz-Winter, 1990)

and functions as a novel inhibitor of T-cell signal transduction (Mynott et al., 1999). Consumption of pineapple juice reduces endogenous production of nitrogenous compounds in humans, implying a reduction in the risk of cancer (Helser et al., 1992).

Reported uses

Claims for pineapple include treatment of constipation, jaundice, and obesity and prevention of ulcers. Bromelain has been claimed to be useful in reducing local inflammation and edema after topical application. It may also hasten wound healing (Rowan et al., 1990).

Dosage

No consensus exists.

Adverse reactions

With excessive amounts of juice
EENT: angular stomatitis.
GI: diarrhea, nausea, vomiting.
GU: uterine contractions.
Skin: rash (dermal sensitization).

Interactions

ACE inhibitors: May antagonize effects on bradykinin. Do not administer with pineapple.
Anticoagulants: May prolong bleeding time. Avoid administration with pineapple.

Contraindications and precautions

The consumption of pineapple juice in large quantities is contraindicated in pregnant or breast-feeding patients.

Special considerations

• Advise the patient to consult a health care provider before using herbal preparations because a treatment that has been clinically researched and proved effective may be available.
• Advise the patient to avoid consuming excessive amounts of juice because significant GI distress can occur.
• Advise the pregnant patient to avoid consuming large quantities of juice (sometimes used in fad diets) because it may promote uterine contractions.

Points of interest

• Bromelain is used as a meat tenderizer in the food industry.
• The use of bromelain for treating burns and stings has declined because of the lack of documented support for this use.

Commentary

Pineapple is a reasonable source for obtaining bromelain, a useful proteolytic enzyme, but there are insufficient data to support therapeutic uses for the plant. Ingestion of quantities above that normally obtained in foods is not recommended.

Bold italic type indicates that reaction may be life-threatening.

References

Helser, M.A., et al. "Influence of Fruit and Vegetable Juices on the Endogenous Formation of *N*-Nitrosoproline and *N*-Nitrosthiozolidine-4-Carboxylic Acid in Humans on Controlled Diets," *Carcinogenesis* 13:2277, 1992.

Lotz-Winter, H. "On the Pharmacology of Bromelain: An Update with Special Regard to Animal Studies on Dose-dependent Effects," *Planta Med* 56:249, 1990.

Mynott, T.L., et al. "Bromelain, from Pineapple Stems, Proteolytically Blocks Activation of Extracellular Regulated Kinase-2 in T Cells," *J Immunol* 163(5):2568-75, 1999.

Rowan, A.D., et al. "Debridement of Experimental Full-thickness Skin Burns of Rats with Enzyme Fractions Derived from Pineapple Stem," *Burns* 16:243, 1990.

PINE BARK

Taxonomic class
Pinaceae

Common trade names
Oligomeric proanthocyanidins (OPCs), procyanidolic oligomers (PCOs), Pycnogenol

Common forms
Available in 50-mg and 100-mg tablets.

Source
Pycnogenol is a mixture of flavonoid compounds extracted from the bark of pine trees, most commonly the French maritime pine (*Pinus maritima*).

Chemical components
Active constituents of pycnogenol are mainly the flavonoids procyandins and phenolic acids. Interestingly, pycnogenol displays greater biological effect as a mixture than its purified components do individually, indicating that the components interact synergistically.

Actions
Pycnogenol and the proanthocanidins are primarily antioxidants (Packer et al., 1999). Pycnogenol has also been shown to possess anti-inflammatory, antimutagenic, and antitumorigenic effects by modulating cellular responses to oxidative challenges (Nardini et al., 2000) and to protect neuronal cells in vitro from glutamate-induced cytotoxicity (Kobayashi et al., 2000) and selectively induced cell death in human mammary cancer cells (Huynh et al., 2000).

Reported uses
The popularity of pycnogenol has only begun, with most of the interest focusing on its antioxidant properties. Most of the studies have been animal and in vitro, with few, if any, controlled human clinical trials. The most common indication for pycnogenol use is chronic venous insufficiency. It has also been advocated as a neuroprotectant in cases of dementia, especially if caused by cerebral ischemia. Promising in vitro

studies in the treatment of breast cancer have not been reported in humans, but it is a potential indication. Pycnogenol has also been reported to have CV benefits, such as vasorelaxant activity and ACE-inhibiting properties (Packer et al., 1999).

Dosage
There are no standard guidelines, but 50 to 100 mg/day P.O. is considered a reasonable supplemental level.

Adverse reactions
None reported.

Interactions
None reported.

Contraindications and precautions
Avoid using pine bark during pregnancy; effects are not known.

Special considerations
• Because pycnogenol is a water-soluble nutrient, excess intake is excreted in the urine.
• Caution the patient not to self-treat symptoms of venous insufficiency or dementia before seeking appropriate medical evaluation because this may delay diagnosis of a serious medical condition.
• Advise the patient to consult a health care provider before using herbal preparations because a treatment that has been clinically researched and proved effective may be available.

Commentary
The effects and benefits of antioxidants are just beginning to be understood, so the optimal levels are still unknown. Pycnogenol appears to be safe and a good source of antioxidant activity, but further human trials are needed to define its therapeutic role. The potential for use of pycnogenol in breast cancer is also exciting, but once again, controlled clinical trials are needed before its role can be defined.

References
Huynh, H.T., et al. "Selective Apoptosis in Human Mammary Cancer Cells (MCF-7) by Pycnogenol," *Anticancer Res* 20(4): 2417-20, 2000.

Kobayashi, M.S., et al. "Antioxidants and Herbal Extracts Protect HT-4 Neuronal Cells Against Glutamine-induced Cytotoxicity," *Free Radic Res* 32(2):115-24, 2000.

Nardini, M., et al. "In Vitro Inhibition of the Activity of Phosphorylase Kinase, Protein Kinase C, and Protein Kinase A by Caffeic Acid and a Procyandin-rich Pine-bark (*Pinus marittima*) Extract," *Biochim Biophys Acta* 1474(2):219-25, 2000.

Packer, L., et al. "Antioxidant Activity and Biologic Properties of a Procyandin-rich Extract from Pine (*Pinus maritima*) Bark, Pycnogenol," *Free Radic Biol Med* 27(5-6):704-24, 1999.

PIPSISSEWA
GROUND HOLLY, PRINCE'S PINE, SPOTTED WINTERGREEN,
WINTERGREEN

Taxonomic class
Ericaceae

Common trade names
Pipsissewa Fresh Upper Leaves

Common forms
Available as crude extracts and dried herb and in homeopathic preparations.

Source
Active components are obtained from the dried leaves of *Chimaphila umbellata*, a creeping perennial herb belonging to the heath family that is native to Eurasia and northern North America.

Chemical composition
Pipsissewa contains arbutin, chimaphilin, chlorophyll, ericolin, minerals, pectic acid, tannins, and urson. Isohomarbutin, reinfolin, homogentisic acid, toluquinol, avicularin, hyperoside, kaempferol, beta-stiosterol, taraxasterol, nonacosane, methyl salicylate, resins, gums, starches, and sugars have also been identified.

Actions
Pipsissewa is reported to have hypoglycemic action in animals (Segelman and Farnsworth, 1969). Arbutin and chimaphilin reportedly act as urinary antiseptics. Pipsissewa reportedly increases renal circulation and stimulates renal tubular function.

Reported uses
Therapeutic claims for pipsissewa include its use as an anticonvulsant, an antispasmodic, an astringent, a diaphoretic, and a diuretic; for nervous disorders; and, externally, for sores and ulcers. Tea made from pipsissewa has also shown antidiuretic properties. Pipsissewa, alone or in combination with other herbs, is used in homeopathic remedies for treating benign prostatic hyperplasia and urinary tract infections. Tannins make the herb potentially useful for treating diarrhea.

Dosage
No consensus exists.

Adverse reactions
GI: diarrhea, GI irritation, nausea, vomiting.
Skin: rash.

Interactions

Minerals, including iron-rich foods and supplements: Reduced mineral absorption. Pipsissewa should be taken 2 hours before or after meals or mineral supplements because tannins may form complexes with these agents.

Contraindications and precautions

Avoid using pipsissewa in breast-feeding patients; effects are unknown. Use cautiously or avoid use in patients with GI disorders (gastroesophageal reflux disease, gastric or duodenal ulcers, ulcerative colitis), iron deficiency, and malabsorptive disorders.

Special considerations

• Inform the patient that there is insufficient evidence to recommend use of pipsissewa.
• Advise the patient to consult a health care provider before using herbal preparations because a treatment that has been clinically researched and proved effective may be available.
• Caution the patient taking pipsissewa to immediately report unusual signs and symptoms and to stop using the herb.

Commentary

Because this herb lacks clinical evidence on safe doses and therapeutic claims, it should not be consumed.

References

Segelman, A.B., and Farnsworth, N.R. "Biological and Phytochemical Evaluation of Plants. Part IV. A New Rapid Procedure for the Simultaneous Determinatin of Saponins and Tannins," *Lloydia* 32:5695, 1969.

PLANTAIN

BLOND PLANTAGO, BROADLEAF PLANTAIN, BUCKHORN, CART TRACT PLANT, COMMON PLANTAIN, ENGLISH PLANTAIN, FLEA SEED, FRENCH PSYLLIUM, GREATER PLANTAIN, INDIAN PLANTAGO, LANTEN, NARROWLEAF PLANTAGO SEED, PLANTAIN SEED, PSYLLIUM, RIBWORT, RIPPLEGRASS, SNAKEWEED, SPANISH PSYLLIUM, TRACT PLANT, WAY-BREAD, WHITE MAN'S FOOT, WILD PLANTAIN, WILD SASO

Taxonomic class

Polygonaceae

Common trade names

Cenat (Spain), Effer-Syllium, Hydrocil, Konsyl, Metamucil, Perdeim

Common forms

Available as psyllium supplied as seeds or as powder or tablets. Also available as liquid extracts (1:1 in 25% alcohol) and tincture (1:5 in 45% alcohol) of the leaves of other plantain species.

Source

Active components are derived from leaves of *Plantago lanceolata* and *P. major* and from seeds and husks of *P. psyllium* and *P. ovata*. These plants are members of the buckwheat family and distributed world-wide.

Chemical components

Various plantain species contain plant acids, alkaloids, amino acids, and flavonoids. Sugars and polysaccharides have been found in the mucilaginous layer of the seed coat, including galactose, glucose, xylose, arabinose, and rhamnose. Protein, fiber, oil (oleic, linoleic, and linolenic acids), tannins, and iridoids can be found in the seeds. Polysaccharides have been found in leaf mucilage. Psyllium, commonly used as a bulk laxative, is produced from the outer coat or husk of the plantain seed. This outer coat contains 10% to 30% of mucilage or hydrocolloid.

Actions

The pharmacologic effects of many plantain extracts have been studied. Topical application of two phenylethanoids from *P. lanceolata* (acteoside and plantamajoside) has been found to have significant anti-inflammatory activity on mouse ear edema (Murai et al., 1995). Ursolic acid, a chemical isolated from a hexane extract of *P. major*, was found to have significant inhibitory effects on cyclooxygenase-2, although somewhat greater inhibition by the compound was reported for cyclooxygenase-1 (Ringbom et al., 1998). Antinephritic and immunosuppressive effects have also been reported with acteoside.

Diuretic effects of several Vietnamese herbal remedies, including *P. major,* given alone and in combination, were found not to have significant activity (Du Dat et al., 1992).

Clinical trials have shown psyllium to have a modest effect on lowering total cholesterol and LDL levels (Chan and Schroeder, 1995).

At least 16 antigens have been found in *P. lanceolata,* 6 of which are potentially allergenic (Baldo et al., 1982).

Minor antibacterial activity in vitro and weak bronchodilatory effects in animals have been documented. Hypotensive activity has been shown in dogs. Other preliminary data discuss spasmolytic and immunostimulant effects (Wegener and Kraft, 1999).

Reported uses

Leaf extracts of *P. major* and *P. lanceolata* have been used topically as an astringent for burns and wounds, for treatment of poison ivy, and for inflammation of mucous membranes and skin. Decoctions of the leaves and seeds have been used orally to treat chronic diarrhea and dysentery, for cough, as a gargle for throat irritation, as a diuretic, for upper respiratory tract infections (Germany), and for urinary tract disorders. Also, there have been some reports of extracts of *P. major* and *P. lanceolata* having anticancer or immunotropic activity.

Psyllium, derived from the seeds of *P. psyllium* and *P. ovata,* is used primarily as a bulk laxative and to lower serum cholesterol levels. One preliminary foreign trial lends support to the application of plantago for chronic bronchitis (Koichev, 1983).

Five grams of *P. psyllium* orally three times daily was shown to yield significantly beneficial effects ($P \leq .05$ for all) for both lipid (LDL, total cholesterol, triglycerides, and HDL) and glucose homeostasis (fasting plasma glucose) over that of placebo in a randomized, controlled, 6-week trial of 125 patients with type 2 diabetes (Roderiguez-Moran et al., 1998). In a smaller, related study, *P. psyllium* was shown to reduce the glycemic index of bread in type 2 diabetics (Frati Munari et al., 1998). This effect was demonstrated to be greater with *P. psyllium* than with either of the other treatments, acarbose or placebo.

One variety of plantain has been studied with favorable results in inflammatory bowel disease. (See *Plantain seeds in ulcerative colitis.*)

Dosage
Leaf extracts or decoctions have been used orally and topically. Traditional uses suggest the following dosage:
As a laxative, 7.5 g plantain seeds P.O. with large amounts of water.

Adverse reactions
CV: hypotension.
GI: abdominal distention, diarrhea, flatulence, GI obstruction.
Skin: dermatitis.
Other: *anaphylaxis, hypersensitivity reactions.*

Interactions
Carbamazepine, lithium: Psyllium seed has been reported to inhibit GI absorption of these drugs. Avoid administration with plantain.
Cardioactive drugs (beta blockers, calcium channel blockers, digitalis): Risk of increased digitalis effects. Avoid administration with plantain.

Contraindications and precautions
Plantain is contraindicated in pregnant or breast-feeding patients because of reported urotonic activity in vitro. It is also contraindicated in patients with a history of intestinal obstruction. Use plantain-derived products cautiously in patients with a history of allergy to other weed pollens or a history of occupational exposure to plantain.

Special considerations
• Studies have shown that many patients with a positive skin prick test reaction to weed pollens also react positively to plantain pollen extracts.
◗ **ALERT** Anaphylaxis to psyllium seed has been reported in people who had no previous allergy and in those with a history of occupational exposure to plantain (Lantner et al., 1990; Ford et al., 1992).
• Monitor the patient for signs of allergic reactions (dermatitis, rash).
• A patient with anorexia or bulimia may abuse laxatives, including this agent.
• Advise the patient to separate consumption of this herb from other drugs to avoid changes in absorption.

Bold italic type indicates that reaction may be life-threatening.

RESEARCH FINDINGS
Plantain seeds in ulcerative colitis

Preliminary evidence suggests that either relative deficiencies or impaired use of short-chain fatty acids (acetate, butyrate, and propionate) may play a role in the pathogenesis and development of ulcerative colitis. In vitro data suggest that these fatty acids, particularly butyrate, may function as anti-inflammatory agents for the bowel. Because fermentation of *Plantago ovata* seeds (dietary fiber) in the colon yields butyrate, an open-label, randomized, controlled multicenter clinical trial was pursued to determine if supplementation of the diet with *P. ovata* seeds might be beneficial in ulcerative colitis (Fernandez-Banares et al., 1999). Investigators from the Spanish Group for the Study of Crohn's Disease and Ulcerative Colitis identified 105 patients who were in remission from ulcerative colitis before enrollment. Subjects were randomly assigned to one of three treatment groups: (1) 10 g twice daily orally of *P. ovata* seeds, (2) 500 mg three times daily orally of mesalamine, or (3) both (at same doses). They were then followed for 12 months. Compliance with the study drug was monitored and ensured. The diagnosis of a relapse of ulcerative colitis was made by standard criteria, including information collected from all clinical, endoscopic, histologic, and radiologic tests. Exclusion criteria included no consent, uncooperative patient, significant renal or hepatic disease, allergy to salicylates or mesalamine, chronic intake of NSAIDs, and pregnancy.

Study Results
At trial conclusion, 102 patients were available for study. Treatment groups were not statistically different, except that more left-sided colitis patients were enrolled into the *P. ovata* seeds (only) group. Most notably, there was no difference in the probability of maintained remission over 1 year among the three treatment groups (Mantel-Cox test, $P=.67$; Breslow test, $P=.58$). Mean times to treatment failure were also statistically similar. GI adverse effects were the most common complaints recorded in the treatment groups using *P. ovata* seeds. Because this trial failed to identify a significant difference between the treatment groups, the investigators concluded that *P. ovata* seeds might be as effective as mesalamine in maintaining remission of ulcerative colitis, but a true test of treatment equivalence would have included treatment groups with at least 217 patients in each arm.

• Urge the patient to use more standard forms of bulk laxatives than plantain.
• Inform the patient with heart disease that some plantain dietary supplements contain cardiac glycosides that may interact with other drugs that he is taking.

Points of interest
• The FDA has reported that some dietary supplements that contain plantain are contaminated with cardiac glycosides (*Digitalis lanata;* Slifman et al., 1998).

Commentary
Plantain species have been claimed to be useful for many disorders, including inflammation of the skin and mucous membranes and as therapies for GI and urinary tract disorders. Psyllium mucilage has long been accepted for use as a gentle bulk laxative and may well achieve modest reductions in serum cholesterol and blood glucose levels with frequent oral administration. Additional clinical data are needed to identify its place in therapy in these areas. Interestingly, *P. ovata* seeds may be an effective alternative for patients who cannot tolerate the traditional salicylate-based anti-inflammatory agents used in ulcerative colitis. The data are preliminary, and confirmation from larger clinical trials is needed. Notably, plantain and any derived products should be used cautiously in patients with a history of allergy to plants or, especially, other weed pollens.

References
Baldo, B.A., et al. "Allergens from Plantain (*Plantago lanceolata*)," *Int Arch Allergy Appl Immunol* 68:295-304, 1982.

Chan, E.K., and Schroeder, D.J. "*Psyllium* in Hypercholesterolemia," *Ann Pharmacother* 29:625-27, 1995.

Du Dat, D., et al. "Studies on the Individual and Combined Diuretic Effects of Four Vietnamese Traditional Herbal Remedies (*Zea mays, Imperata cylindrica, Plantago major,* and *Orthosiphon stamineus*)," *J Ethnopharmacol* 36:225-31, 1992.

Fernandez-Banares, F., et al. "Randomized Clinical Trial of *Plantago ovata* Seeds (Dietary Fiber) as Compared with Mesalamine in Maintaining Remission in Ulcerative Colitis," *Am J Gastroenterol* 94(2):427-33, 1999.

Ford, M.A., et al. "Delayed Psyllium Allergy in Three Nurses," *Hosp Pharm* 27:1061-62, 1992.

Frati Munari, A.C., et al. "Lowering Glycemic Index of Food by Acarbose and *Plantago psyllium* Mucilage," *Arch Med Res* 29(2):137-41, 1998.

Koichev, A. "Complex Evaluation of the Therapeutic Effect of a Preparation from *Plantago major* in Chronic Bronchitis," *Probl Vatr Med* 11:61-69, 1983.

Lantner, R.R., et al. "Anaphylaxis Following Ingestion of a Psyllium-Containing Cereal," *JAMA* 264:2534-36, 1990.

Murai, M., et al. "Phenylethanoids in the Herb of *Plantago lanceolata* and Inhibitory Effect on Arachidonic Acid-induced Mouse Ear Edema," *Planta Med* 61:479-80, 1995.

Roderiguez-Moran, M., et al. "Lipid- and Glucose-lowering Efficacy of *Plantago psyllium* in Type II Diabetes," *J Diabetes Complications*12(5):273-78, 1998.

Ringbom, T., et al. "Ursolic Acid from *Plantago major*, a Selective Inhibitor of Cyclooxygenase-2 Catalyzed Prostaglandin Biosynthesis," *J Nat Prod* 61(10):1212-15, 1998.

Slifman, N.R., et al. "Contamination of Botanical Dietary Supplements by *Digitalis lanata*," *N Engl J Med* 17;339(12):806-11, 1998.

Wegener, T., and Kraft, K. "Plantain (*Plantago lanceolata*): Anti-inflammatory Action in Upper Respiratory Tract Infections," *Wien Med Wochenschr* 149(8-10):211-16, 1999.

POKEWEED

CANCER JALAP, CANCER-ROOT, CHANGRAS, COAKUM, CROWBERRY, GARGET, PIGEON BERRY, POCAN, POKE BERRY, POKE SALAD, POKEWEED ROOT, RED-INK PLANT, REDWOOD, SCOKE, TXIU KUB NYUG, VIRGINIAN POKE

Taxonomic class
Phytolaccaceae

Common trade names
None known.

Common forms
Available as an extract (1:1 in 45% alcohol) and tincture.

Source
The active components occur in the roots, stems, leaves, and berries of *Phytolacca americana*. This weedy perennial shrub grows throughout eastern North America.

Chemical components
The toxic agents of pokeweed are glycoside saponins (such as phytolaccigenin), a glycoprotein mitogen consisting of five glycoproteins, phytolaccatoxin, triterpenes, asparagine, and oxalic acid. The root contains three mitogenic lectins. A tannin and a resin are found in the plant. Pokeweed shoots contain protein, fat, carbohydrate, ascorbic acid, niacin, beta-carotene equivalent, calcium, phosphorus, and iron.

Actions
In humans, pokeweed appears to induce central and peripheral cholinergic stimulation. Other pharmacologic actions reported include abortifacient, anti-inflammatory, antineoplastic, cardioinductive, and diuretic. The PL-B lectin has the highest amount of mitogenic and hemagluttinating activity, whereas the PL-C lectin has the least hemagluttinating activity. Phytolaccigenin, one of the primary saponins, acts as a powerful parasiticide.

An interesting study was conducted by Uckun and colleagues (1999). These investigators examined the effect of an antiviral protein known as TXU (anti-CD7)-pokeweed in chimpanzees infected with the HIV-1 virus. After 2 months of TXU-pokeweed infusions, the HIV-1 burden was reduced to below detectable levels in three of four chimps. Effective inhibition of HIV-1 did appear to correlate with attainment of certain concentrations of the TXU-pokeweed immunoconjugate. Adverse effects noted in this trial included transient elevations in ALT levels and decreased serum albumin levels.

Reported uses

Pokeweed is said to possess emetic and laxative effects and to be useful for itching and rheumatism (Roberge et al., 1986). Other therapeutic claims include its use for cough, laryngitis, mammary abscesses, mastitis, mumps, swollen glands, and tonsillitis and as a lymphatic system cleanser. The mitogens and a protein (pokeweed antiviral protein) are being studied as antineoplastic agents against certain leukemias and osteosarcomas (Jansen et al., 1992; Anderson et al., 1995; Myers et al., 1997).

Pokeweed has long been known and used as an edible green vegetable, but only the young shoots are safe to eat and only after boiling (Fernald and Kinsey, 1958).

An uncontrolled pilot study suggested the potential efficacy of a three-herb homeopathic combination (including pokeweed) for treating the signs and symptoms of acute tonsillitis (Wiesenauer, 1998).

Dosage

No consensus exists. Traditional uses suggest the following dosages:
Dried root: 60 to 300 mg P.O. as an emetic.
Extract: 0.1 to 0.5 ml P.O., as needed.

Adverse reactions

CNS: *coma,* confusion, dizziness, headache, *seizures*, syncope, tremor, weakness.
CV: *heart block* (Roberge et al., 1986; Hamilton and Shih, 1995), hypotension, tachycardia.
EENT: blurred vision, eye irritation, excessive salivation, sore throat, sneezing.
GI: diarrhea, elevated liver function test results (animal data; Uckun et al., 1999), nausea, vomiting.
GU: urinary incontinence.
Hematologic: B- and T-cell disruption, eosinophilia.
Metabolic: hypoalbuminemia (animal data; Uckun et al., 1999).
Respiratory: *respiratory depression.*
Skin: contact dermatitis.
Other: *death in children* (Roberge et al., 1986; Hamilton and Shih, 1995), sweating.

Interactions

CNS depressants: Additive effects. Avoid administration with pokeweed.
Disulfiram: Disulfiram reaction if patient takes herbal form that contains alcohol. Avoid administration with pokeweed.
Fertility drugs, oral contraceptives: May lead to menstrual cycle abnormalities and uterine stimulation. Avoid administration with pokeweed.

Contraindications and precautions

Pokeweed is contraindicated in pregnant or breast-feeding women because of possible teratogenicity. Use cautiously in patients with a history of atopy and in those who are prone to contact dermatitis.

Bold italic type indicates that reaction may be life-threatening.

Special considerations
• Caution the patient about the potential toxicity of this herb.
• Instruct the patient to wear gloves if the plant is to be handled because of its potential for systemic toxicity if it contacts abraded skin.
• Advise the patient to keep pokeweed and its preparations out of the reach of children and pets.
• Caution the patient taking disulfiram not to take an herbal form that contains alcohol.
• Caution the patient to avoid hazardous activities until the CNS effects of pokeweed are known.
• Instruct women to report planned or suspected pregnancy.
• Advise women to avoid using pokeweed during pregnancy or when breast-feeding.
• Inform the patient that there are no clinical data to support the use of pokeweed.

Points of interest
• The FDA has classified pokeweed as an herb of undefined safety because of its narcotic-like effects.

Commentary
Almost all parts of pokeweed appear to be toxic. The plant shows some promise as an anticancer agent and looks intriguing for potential application in HIV, but clinical data to support its use for any condition are insufficient.

References
Anderson, P.M., et al. "In Vitro and In Vivo Cytotoxicity of an Anti-osteosarcoma Immunotoxin Containing Pokeweed Antiviral Protein," *Cancer Res* 55:1321-27, 1995.

Fernald, M.L., and Kinsey, A.C., *Edible Wild Plants of Eastern North America.* New York: Harper & Row, 1958.

Hamilton, R.J., and Shih, R.D. "Mobitz Type I Heart Block After Pokeweed Ingestion," *Vet Human Toxicol* 37: 66-67, 1995.

Jansen, B., et al. "Establishment of a Human T(4;11) Leukemia in Severe Combined Immunodeficient Mice and Successful Treatment Using Anti-CD19 (B43)-Pokeweed Antiviral Protein Immunotoxin," *Cancer Res* 52:406-12, 1992.

Myers, D.E., et al. "Large Scale Manufacturing of TXU (Anti-CD7)-Pokeweed Antiviral Protein (PAP) Immunoconjugate for Clinical Trials," *Leuk Lymphoma* 27:275-302, 1997.

Roberge, R., et al. "The Root of Evil: Pokeweed Intoxication," *Ann Emerg Med* 15:470-73, 1986.

Uckun, F.M., et al. "Toxicity, Biological Activity, and Pharmacokinetics of TXU (anti-CD7)-Pokeweed Antiviral Protein in Chimpanzees and Adult Patients Infected with the Human Immunodeficiency Virus," *J Pharmacol Exp Ther* 291(3):1301-7, 1999.

Wiesenauer, M. "Comparison of Solid and Liquid Forms of Homeopathic Remedies for Tonsillitis," *Adv Ther* 15(6):362-71, 1998.

POMEGRANATE

GRANATUM

Taxonomic class
Punicaceae

Common trade names
None known.

Common forms
Available as the crude herb or extract.

Source
Active components are derived from the bark, root, stem, peel, and fruit of *Punica granatum,* a shrub that is native to northwestern India and cultivated in many tropical areas.

Chemical components
The plant contains alkaloids (pelletierine, methylpelletierine, pseudo-pelletierine, and isopelletierine), mannite, various phenols, ellagic acid, and gallic acid. The bark and rinds contain about 20% tannins, including punicalin, punicalagin, granatins A and B, gallagyldilactone, casuarinin, pedunculagin, tellimagrandin I, and corilagin.

Actions
In vitro studies have shown *P. granatum* to have notable antimicrobial activity against *Staphylococcus aureus, Pseudomonas aeruginosa,* and *Candida albicans* (Navarro et al., 1996). Other studies have shown similar activity against various GI pathogens, supporting the folkloric use of pomegranate to treat diarrhea. Also, studies in rats showed that a methanol extract of *P. granatum* seed inhibited experimentally induced diarrhea and slowed GI motility (Das et al., 1999).

Tannins from pomegranate have shown antiviral activity against the herpes simplex 2 virus. Pomegranate components also showed anthelmintic activity against *Entamoeba* species (Segura et al., 1990), and a uterine stimulant effect has been observed in animals (Farnsworth et al., 1975).

Additional preliminary work in animals revolves around the application of pomegranate parts to lower blood glucose levels (Jafri et al., 2000), minimize ethanol-induced gastritis (Khennouf et al., 1999), and inhibit atherogenesis and platelet aggregation (Aviram et al., 2000).

Reported uses
Pomegranate is claimed to be useful as an anthelmintic, and it is used as an antidiarrheal in Asia and South America. In vitro studies appear to support these uses, but human clinical trials are lacking.

Dosage
No consensus exists. Infusions (tea) or extracts of plant parts are often the source of pomegranate studied during in vitro evaluations.

Bold italic type indicates that reaction may be life-threatening.

Adverse reactions
GI: nausea, vomiting.
Hepatic: *hepatotoxicity* (related to high tannin component).
Other: *carcinogenicity, hypersensitivity reactions* (Gaig et al., 1999).

Interactions
None reported.

Contraindications and precautions
Pomegranate is contraindicated in pregnant or breast-feeding patients and in those with asthma or atopy. Use cautiously, if at all, in patients with hepatic disease.

Special considerations
• Monitor liver function test results in patients taking pomegranate.
• Caution the patient that continued use of pomegranate may increase the risk of certain cancers. Women in northern Iran have the highest rate of esophageal cancer, attributed to a local food called majum, or majoweh, used during pregnancy. Majum is a crushed mixture of sour pomegranate seeds, black pepper, dried raisins, and, sometimes, garlic. This mix of harsh ingredients appears to cause esophageal trauma. Other local practices, such as consuming foods at higher than usual temperatures and preserving food by sun-drying, as well as the relative lack of fruits and vegetables in the diet may also be factors (Ghadirian, 1987). Dried pomegranate peel has been shown to contain excessive amounts of aflatoxin B-1, a compound known to increase the risk of certain cancers (Selim et al., 1996).
• Advise women to avoid using pomegranate during pregnancy or when breast-feeding.
• Caution the patient with a history of atopy (allergic reactions) or asthma not to use pomegranate preparations.

Commentary
Information supporting the use of pomegranate as an antidiarrheal is increasing, but trials consist only of animal or in vitro evidence. Clinical application in humans is lacking. Other preliminary evidence suggests activity against fungi, viruses, and helminths. Again, little human clinical data exist. Because of a possible link with some cancers, pomegranate cannot be recommended for internal use until more data become available.

References
Aviram, M., et al. "Pomegranate Juice Consumption Reduces Oxidative Stress, Atherogenic Modifications to LDL, and Platelet Aggregation: Studies in Humans and in Atherosclerotic Apolipoprotein E-deficient Mice," *Am J Clin Nutr* 71(5):1062-76, 2000.

Das, A., et al. "Studies on Antidiarrheal Activity of *Punica granatum* Seed Extract in Rats," *J Ethnopharmacol* 68(1-3):205-8, 1999.

Farnsworth, N.R., et al. "Potential Value of Plants as Sources of New Antifertility Agents, Part I," *J Pharm Sci* 64:535-98, 1975.

Gaig, P., et al. "Allergy to Pomegranate," *Allergy* 54(3):287-88, 1999.

Ghadirian, P. "Food Habits of the People of the Caspian Littoral of Iran in Relation to Esophageal Cancer," *Nutr Cancer* 9:147-57, 1987.

Jafri, M.A., et al. "Effect of *Punica granatum* Linn. (Flowers) on Blood Glucose Level in Normal and Alloxan-induced Diabetic Rats," *J Ethnopharmacol* 70(3):309-14, 2000.

Khennouf, S., et al. "Effects of *Quercus ilex* L. and *Punica granatum* L. Polyphenols Against Ethanol-induced Gastric Damage in Rats," *Pharmazie* 54(1):75-76, 1999.

Navarro, V., et al. "Antimicrobial Evaluation of Some Plants Used in Mexican Traditional Medicine for the Treatment of Infectious Diseases," *J Ethnopharmacol* 53:143-47, 1996.

Segura, J.J., et al. "Growth Inhibition of *Entamoeba histolytica* and *E. invadens* Produced by Pomegranate Root," *Arch Invest Med* 21:235-39, 1990.

Selim, M.I., et al. "Aflatoxin B-1 in Common Egyptian Foods," *J AOAC Int* 79:1124-29, 1996.

POPLAR

AMERICAN ASPEN, BLACK POPLAR, QUAKING ASPEN, WHITE POPLAR

Taxonomic class
Salicaceae

Common trade names
None known.

Common forms
Available as dried powdered bark or liquid extract.

Source
Active components are obtained from the bark of white poplar *(Populus alba)*, quaking aspen *(Populus tremuloides)*, and black poplar *(Populus nigra)*. Exudates from poplar leaf buds have also been evaluated.

Chemical components
The phenolic glycosides salicin and the salicin benzoate salts (populin, tremuloidin, and tremulacin) are isolated from poplar species. Other components include tannins, triterpenes including fats, waxes, alpha- and beta-amyrin, glucose, fructose, and various trisaccharides. *P. nigra* also contains the lignan (+)-isolariciresinol mono-beta-D-glucopyranoside, and 3-methyl-but-2-enyl caffeate. *P. tremuloides* also contains flavonoids and ubiquiteric phenolic carboxylic acids, including *p*-coumaric acid.

Actions
Because salicin is a salicylate precursor, its actions are likely to be similar to those of other salicylates. These effects may be clinically relevant.

A compound found in exudates of poplar leaf buds is thought to have antiviral properties (Amoros et al., 1994).

Reported uses
Traditionally, poplar has been used as an anti-inflammatory and an antirheumatic. The herb is also claimed to be useful for treating the common cold, cystitis, diarrhea, and GI and hepatic disorders.

Dosage
Liquid extract (1:1 in 25% alcohol): 1 to 5 ml P.O. t.i.d.
Powdered bark: 1 to 5 g P.O. or by decoction t.i.d.

Adverse reactions
EENT: tinnitus.
GI: GI bleeding, GI irritation (similar to that with salicylates).
GU: renal dysfunction.
Hepatic: *hepatotoxicity* (related to tannin).
Respiratory: asthma.
Skin: contact dermatitis (propolis product), pruritus.

Interactions
Anticoagulants, other antiplatelet drugs: Increased risk of bleeding. Avoid administration with poplar.
Salicylates: May cause adverse GI reactions. Avoid administration with poplar.

Contraindications and precautions
Avoid using poplar in pregnant or breast-feeding patients; effects are unknown. Use cautiously in patients who have a history of bronchial asthma, GI bleeding, nasal polyps, peptic ulcer disease, plant allergies, renal disease, or salicylate hypersensitivity.

Special considerations
• Inform the patient that consumption of poplar may increase the risk of bleeding in peptic ulcer disease or if he is taking an anticoagulant or antiplatelet drug.
• Advise the patient not to use poplar for a viral illness because of the risk of developing Reye's syndrome.
• Instruct the patient not to use OTC preparations that contain aspirin while taking poplar.
• Advise the patient who is taking a prescription drug that contains aspirin to avoid using poplar.
• Advise women to avoid using poplar during pregnancy or when breast-feeding.

Points of interest
• Propolis, a resinous plant product collected by honeybees, is largely composed of 3-methyl-but-2-enyl caffeate. Bees collect this material from the bud exudates of various trees, especially the poplar species. It has been well established that topically applied propolis and poplar bud exudate can cause severe contact dermatitis (Hausen et al., 1987a, 1987b).

Commentary
Because of the lack of animal and human clinical data, medicinal use of poplar cannot be recommended.

References
Amoros, M., et al. "Comparison of the Anti-Herpes Simplex Virus Activities of Propolis and 3-methyl-but-2-enyl Caffeate," *J Natl Prod* 57:644-47, 1994.

Hausen, B.M., et al. "Propolis Allergy. Part 1. Origin, Properties, Usage, and Literature Review," *Contact Dermatitis* 17:163-70, 1987a.

Hausen, B.M., et al. "Propolis Allergy. Part 2. The Sensitizing Properties of 1,1,-dimethylallyl Caffeic Acid Ester," *Contact Dermatitis* 17:171-77, 1987b.

PRICKLY ASH

ANGELICA TREE, HERCULES' CLUB, NORTHERN PRICKLY ASH, SOUTHERN PRICKLY ASH, SUTERBERRY, TOOTHACHE TREE

Taxonomic class
Rutaceae

Common trade names
Multi-ingredient preparations: Prickly Ash Bark, Prickly Ash Herb, Propolis Herb Liquid

Common forms
Available as powdered bark (10 g), berry liquid extract (1:1 in 25% alcohol, 1 oz, 2 oz), and tincture (1:5 in 45% alcohol, 1 oz, 2 oz).

Sources
Active components are obtained from the bark of the northern prickly ash (*Zanthoxylum americanum*) and the southern prickly ash (*Zanthoxylum clava-herculis*). Both trees belong to the rue (citrus) family and are native to the United States.

Chemical components
Coumarin derivatives (xanthyletin, xanthoxyletin, allo-xanthoxyletin) have been isolated from the bark of *Z. americanum* but have not been found in *Z. clava-herculis*. Other components found in the bark include tannins, resins, an acrid volatile oil, and the alkaloids nitidine and laurifoline.

Actions
The pharmacologic activity of prickly ash is relatively unknown. Natural coumarins possess anticoagulant, diuretic, hepatotoxic, and vasodilatory properties.

Neuromuscular blocking effects have been observed in animals, caused by toxins isolated from *Z. clava-herculis*. Laurifoline has been reported to lower blood pressure, and magnoflorine has been associated with neuromuscular blocking activity (Newall et al., 1996).

Bold italic type indicates that reaction may be life-threatening.

Reported uses

Prickly ash has been used as an antiflatulent, an antipyretic, a circulatory stimulant, and a diaphoretic. The bark of prickly ash has been used in the past as a commercial product for treating rheumatism and as a GI stimulant.

Dosage

Decoction: 15 g of bark in 600 ml of water.
Tincture: up to 5 ml P.O. t.i.d.

Adverse reactions

Hematologic: risk of increased bleeding (coumarins).
Skin: photosensitivity.
Other: *toxicity* (in sheep and cattle).

Interactions

Anticoagulants: May potentiate effects. Avoid administration with prickly ash.
Aspirin, NSAIDs: Increased anticoagulant effect. Avoid administration with prickly ash.
Disulfiram: Disulfiram reaction if herbal form contains alcohol. Avoid administration with prickly ash.

Contraindications and precautions

Prickly ash is contraindicated in patients with allergies to this herb or related plant species. Also avoid its use in pregnant or breast-feeding patients; effects are unknown.

Special considerations

• Caution the patient taking disulfiram not to take an herbal form that contains alcohol.
• Urge the patient to watch for signs of unusual bruising or bleeding.
• Instruct the patient to discontinue using prickly ash and to notify a primary health care provider if unusual symptoms occur.
• Inform the patient that few safety and efficacy data exist on this herb.
• Advise women to report planned or suspected pregnancy.
• Advise women to avoid using prickly ash during pregnancy or when breast-feeding.

Points of interest

• Prickly ash is called the toothache tree in folk medicine because the bark is chewed to relieve toothache.
• Ingestion of parts of the northern prickly ash tree has been suspected of causing death in sheep and cattle in Indiana. Ingestion of the bark of the southern prickly ash tree has also caused death and symptoms of toxicosis (blindness, dysphagia, high-stepping gait, inability to drink water) in beef cattle in Georgia.

Commentary

Despite its many uses in folklore medicine, there is little clinical information to support the use of prickly ash in humans. Therefore, its use cannot be recommended for any condition.

References

Newall, C.A., et al., eds. *Herbal Medicines. A Guide for Health Care Professionals.* London: Pharmaceutical Press, 1996.

PRIMROSE, EVENING

Taxonomic class
Onagraceae

Common trade names
Multi-ingredient preparations: Efamol, Epogram, Evening Primrose Oil, Mega Primrose Oil, My Favorite Evening Primrose Oil, Primrose Power, Super Primrose Oil

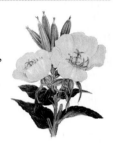

Common forms
Capsules: 50 mg, 500 mg, 1,300 mg
Gelcaps: 500 mg, 1,300 mg

Source
The oil is extracted from the seeds of *Oenothera biennis,* a biennial herb that is cultivated or grows wild in parts of North America and Europe.

Chemical components
Evening primrose oil is composed primarily of essential fatty acids, including linoleic acid, gamma linolenic acid, oleic acid, palmitic acid, and stearic acid.

Actions
The therapeutic action of evening primrose oil stems from essential fatty acids that are important as cellular structural elements and as precursors of prostaglandin synthesis. Linoleic acid cannot be manufactured by the body and, therefore, must be provided through dietary intake. The body relies on the metabolic conversion of linoleic acid (LA) to gamma linoleic acid (GLA). Deficient conversion, which has been observed in such disorders as cancer, CV disease, diabetes, hypercholesterolemia, skin conditions, and viral infections, affects prostaglandin E_1 and E_2 synthesis. It is claimed that LA and GLA supplementation from dietary sources maintains a balance between the inflammatory and noninflammatory prostaglandins that may, in turn, be useful in treating these disorders.

Reported uses

Evening primrose oil has been used as a vegetable with a peppery flavor. An infusion using the whole plant is reported to have astringent and sedative properties. Traditionally, it has been used for asthma, breast pain, asthmatic cough, diabetic neuropathy, eczema, GI disorders, hypercholesterolemia, multiple sclerosis, premenstrual syndrome (PMS), psoriasis, Raynaud's disease, rheumatoid arthritis, Sjögren's syndrome, and whooping cough and as an analgesic and a sedative (Barber, 1988; Briggs, 1986). Poultices made with evening primrose oil have been used to speed wound healing.

Patients with atopic dermatitis and eczema have an enzymatic defect for the conversion of LA to GLA. A meta-analysis of nine clinical trials showed an improvement in pruritic symptoms with GLA administration. Two large clinical trials have shown no evidence of benefit (Kleijnen, 1994).

Placebo-controlled studies have suggested that GLA is superior in treating breast pain and tenderness associated with PMS and benign breast disease (Briggs, 1986). Animal studies have shown that diabetic neuropathy can be prevented or reversed through GLA supplementation with evening primrose oil.

Evening primrose oil has been studied alone and with fish oils versus placebo in rheumatoid arthritis. These trials showed an improvement in the patient's symptoms, based on the reduced need for pain medication. There was no evidence, however, of evening primrose oil's having a disease-modifying action (Briggs, 1986).

Although LA can lower serum cholesterol levels, GLA's cholesterol-lowering activity is about 100 times that of LA. GLA has been reported to reduce hypertension and decrease platelet aggregation in both animals and humans.

Four clinical trials using evening primrose oil for treating schizophrenia have demonstrated promising results. Although the total number of participants is small (n=204), a moderately positive effect was noted by the researchers with few adverse reactions (Joy et al., 2000).

Hyperactive children are thought to have abnormal levels of essential fatty acids. Supplementation of evening primrose oil has produced controversial results. One trial saw no improvement in the behavioral patterns of children and serum fatty acid levels, but another study showed a calming effect in two-thirds of the children treated with evening primrose oil (Briggs, 1986).

Animal studies have indicated that evening primrose oil produced significant reductions in mammary tumors from baseline size. In vitro experiments found a dose-related inhibition of the growth rate in malignant tumors. High levels of essential fatty acids are toxic to several cancers but not lethal to normal cells. Human studies are under way to assess the effect of supplementation of essential fatty acids on cancer cell growth.

Dosage
The following dosages are based on a standardized GLA content of 8%:
For eczema, 320 mg to 8 g/day P.O. in adults. In children aged 1 to 12, 160 mg to 4 g/day P.O.; continue for 3 months.
For mastalgia, 3 to 4 g/day P.O.
   No consensus exists for other disorders.

Adverse reactions
CNS: headache, ***temporal lobe epilepsy*** (especially in schizophrenic patients or those taking epileptogenic drugs such as phenothiazines).
GI: nausea.
Skin: rash.

Interactions
Phenothiazines: Increased risk of seizures. Avoid administration with evening primrose.

Contraindications and precautions
Avoid using evening primrose in pregnant patients; effects are unknown. Also use cautiously, if at all, in schizophrenic patients and in those taking epileptogenic drugs.

Special considerations
• Urge the patient with a seizure disorder to reconsider use of evening primrose.
• Caution parents to use this herb for a hyperactive child only under supervision of a primary health care provider.
• Immunosuppression, inflammation, and thrombosis can occur because of slow accumulation of tissue arachidonate after use of GLA for longer than 1 year (Kleijnen, 1994).

Commentary
Evening primrose oil is not approved for treating any specific condition. Although the underlying mechanisms of essential fatty acid metabolism in health and disease may justify its alleged therapeutic uses, more clinical studies are needed to confirm the value of this oil for treating these conditions.

References
Barber, H.J. "Evening Primrose Oil: A Panacea?" *Pharm J* 240:723-25, 1988.

Briggs, C.J. "Evening Primrose, La Belle de Nuit, The King's Cure-all," *Can Pharm J* 3:249-54, 1986.

Kleijnen, J. "Evening Primrose Oil," *Br Med J* 309:824-25, 1994.

Joy, C.B., et al. "Polyunsaturated Fatty Acid (Fish or Evening Primrose Oil) for Schizophrenia," *Cochrane Database Sys Rev* 2:CD001257, 2000.

Bold italic type indicates that reaction may be life-threatening.

PROPOLIS

BEE GLUE, BEE PROPOLIS, BEE WAX, PROPOLIO

Common trade names
Bee Propolis, BeeRich Propolis, Propolis Plus

Common forms
Capsules: 200 mg, 500 mg, 600 mg
Cream: In combination with aloe and other common skin cream ingredients
Extract: Propolis content not given
Tablets: 600 mg
    Also available in dental gum, lozenges, and propolis jelly (used to treat oily scalp).

Source
Propolis is a resin collected by *Apis mellifera* bees from plant and trees buds. In the hive, the resin is modified by the addition of saliva and wax to a gluelike substance used to give support to the hive structure and entomb invaders.

Chemical components
More than 160 constituents have been identified to date, more than 50% (by weight) of which include phenolic compounds and flavonoids, such as pinocembrin, galangin, pinobanksin, and pinobanksin-3-acetate. The latter group is thought to be responsible for the antibacterial, antifungal, and antiviral action of propolis. Other constituents include beeswax, resins, vitamins, and amino acids.

Actions
The mechanism of antimicrobial activity of propolis is not completely understood, but it is thought to be caused by a synergistic effect between the flavonoids and other phenolics. Much of the study of this activity has focused on bacteria involved in dental caries. Activity has been shown against *Actinomyces* spp., *Porphyroomonas gingivalis, Staphylococcus aureus, Candida albicans, Enterococcus faecalis,* and *Bacillus cereus.*
    Additional mechanisms may include activation of immune system components, including macrophages and complement.

Reported uses
As with most natural medicines, propolis has been claimed to be useful in a wide range of ailments. The tablets and capsules are reported beneficial for cystitis, digestive tract disorders, eczema, infections, and premenstrual stress. Topical products are used to prevent infections associated with abscesses, burns, cuts, and scrapes. The gum, liquid extract, and lozenges are used to treat gum disorders, mouth ulcers, sore throats, and toothaches.

Dosage
Capsules or tablets: 400 to 600 mg/day P.O. for maintenance. Some manufacturers recommend increasing the dose threefold when symptomatology is indicative of an infection.
Extract: 15 to 30 gtt mixed into warm water and taken P.O. 1 to 3 times per day.

Adverse reactions
Skin: mild rash (found in people who are allergic to tree resin).

Interactions
None reported.

Contraindications and precautions
Because of propolis's suspected stimulatory effect on the immune system, use in children under age 1 year is not recommended. Propolis is contraindicated in patients with asthma or a history of anaphylaxis because of the possibility of allergic reactions to tree resin.

Special considerations
• Inform the patient that few data exist to support therapeutic use of propolis.
• Advise the patient to consult a health care provider before using herbal preparations because a treatment that has been clinically researched and proved effective may be available.
• Caution the patient with a history of atopy about using propolis because of its allergic potential.
• Although no known chemical interactions have been reported in clinical studies, consideration must be given to the pharmacologic properties of the herbal product and the potential for exacerbation of the intended therapeutic effect of conventional drugs.

Commentary
As with a number of natural products, many clinical studies that have examined the use of propolis have been conducted in foreign countries, not been reported in peer-reviewed journals, and lack proper design. Although in vitro studies appear promising, many of the claims made by proponents of propolis remain unsupported by scientific evidence. When warranted, conventional antimicrobial therapy should be used.

References
Amoros, M., et al. "Comparison of the Anti-Herpes Simplex Virus Activities of Propolis and and 3-methyl-but-2-enyl caffeate," *J Nat Prod* 57:644-47, 1994.

Ivanovska, N., et al. "Immunomodulatory Action of Propolis. Part VI. Influence of a Water Soluble Derivative on Complement Activity In Vivo." *J Ethnopharmacol* 47:145-47, 1995.

Koo, H., et al. "In Vitro Antimicrobial Activity of Propolis and *Arnica montana* Against Oral Pathogens," *Arch Oral Bio* 45:141-48, 2000.

PULSATILLA

ANEMONE PULSATILLA, CROWFOOT, EASTER FLOWER, KUBJELLE, MEADOW ANEMONE, PASQUE FLOWER, PRAIRIE ANEMONE, PULSATILLA AMOENA, PULSATILLAE HERBA, PULSATILLA VULGARA, *PULSATILLA VULGARIS*, SMELL FOX, STOR, WINDFLOWER

Taxonomic class
Ranunculaceae

Common trade names
Multi-ingredient preparations: Ana-Sed, Biocarde, Calmo, Cicaderma, Cirflo, DermaSlim TD, Eviprostat, Eviprostat N, Female Remedy, Hemoluol, Histo-Fluine P, Lifesystem Herbal Formula 4 Women's Formula, Mensuosedyl, Motion Sickness Remedy, Nytol Herbal, Premantaid, Proflo, Pulsatilla Med Complex, Pulsatilla 6X, Pulsatilla 30C, Pulsatilla Vitex Compound, Viburnum Complex, Women's Formula Herbal Formula 3, Yeast-X, #483 Oxox Cell Activator

Common forms
Available as a dried herb, liquid extract, and tincture and in homeopathic remedies.

Source
Active components are derived from the dried leaves, stems, and flowers of *Anemone pulsatilla* (also known as *Pulsatilla vulgaris*), a perennial plant that is native to southern Europe.

Chemical components
Ranunculin is a lactonic glucoside present in the undamaged, fresh plants. When the plants are crushed, the aglycone protoanemonin is enzymatically liberated. Protoanemonin dimerizes to form anemonin, anemoninic acid, and anemonic acid. Anemonin is highly volatile, and much of it is lost during drying. Other plant components include saponins, tannins, volatile oil, chelidonic and succinic acids (as calcium salts), flavonoids, and glucose. Delphinidin and pelargonidin glycosides occur in the flowers.

Actions
Protoanemonin causes stimulation followed by paralysis of the CNS in animals. In the fresh plant, it has antibacterial and local irritant properties; the dimer anemonin lacks these actions. Pulsatilla can be a powerful CNS and cardiac depressant. Protoanemonin-containing plants have caused abortions and teratogenic effects in grazing animals.

Reported uses
Pulsatilla has traditionally been claimed as useful for circulatory, gynecologic, and nervous disorders; earaches; spasmodic disorders of the genitourinary tract; and as an analgesic, a diuretic, an expectorant, a

menstrual stimulant, and a sedative. It has also been used internally to treat inner eye conditions such as cataract, glaucoma, iritis, retinal disorders, and scleritis. Its use in homeopathic medicine ranges from coughs and colds to digestive and gynecologic disorders.

Although pulsatilla and other homeopathic remedies have been claimed as superior to conventional treatments for otitis media in children (Friese et al., 1997), several design flaws make the data suspect.

In France, pulsatilla is used in the symptomatic treatment of nervous disorders, especially minor sleep disorders, and coughs. The German Commission E monographs list the potential uses of pulsatilla as disorders of genital organs, the GI tract, and the urinary tract; inflammatory and infectious diseases of the skin and mucosa; migraine headache; neuralgia; and general restlessness.

Dosage
Traditional uses suggest the following dosages:
Dried herb: 0.1 to 0.3 g in infusion P.O. t.i.d. Alternatively, ½ tsp of dried herb added to 1 cup of boiling water, steeped for 10 to 15 minutes, and taken P.O. t.i.d.
Liquid extract (1:1 in 25% ethanol): 0.1 to 0.3 ml P.O. t.i.d.
Tincture (1:10 in 25% ethanol): 0.5 to 3 ml P.O. t.i.d.

Adverse reactions
EENT: burning of the throat and tongue (if chewed).
GI: gastroenteritis, vomiting (large doses).
GU: albuminuria and hematuria (from kidney irritation), urinary tract irritation.
Skin: severe irritation (caused by direct contact of the fresh plant parts with the skin or mucous membranes).

Interactions
None reported.

Contraindications and precautions
Pulsatilla is contraindicated in pregnant or breast-feeding patients because of abortive and teratogenic effects in animals.

Special considerations
• Caution the patient not to use or handle fresh plant parts.
• Advise the patient to immediately report unusual symptoms, such as painful urination and blood in the urine.
◆ **ALERT** Pulsatilla is a potential poison. Symptoms in animals include abdominal pain, blisters, diarrhea, dizziness, hyperpigmentation, mouth and throat ulcers, nose and throat irritation, paralysis, polyuria, renal damage, excessive salivation, seizures, sneezing, painful urination, vision changes, vision loss, and vomiting.
• Advise women to avoid using pulsatilla during pregnancy or when breast-feeding.

Bold italic type indicates that reaction may be life-threatening.

FOLKLORE
History of *Anemone pulsatilla*

The scientific name for *Pulsatilla* comes from Greek legends. Windflower, the English term for anemone, refers to the flowers of the plant that appear to be blown open by the wind. Greek legends held that Anemos, god of winds, sent anemones to herald his coming in early spring. The name pasque flower, a synonym of pulsatilla, is derived from the Old French pasque, or Easter, and refers to various floral emblems of Easter as *Anemone patens*, *A. pratensis*, and *A. pulsatilla*.

The anemone was once regarded by various cultures as an ill omen; the Chinese called it the "Flower of Death." Other cultures regarded it as a charm against disease (Dobelis, 1986).

Pulsatilla has been used for centuries in traditional medicine. Dioscorides (A.D. 40 to 90), a well-known Roman physician, used pasque flower to treat ocular conditions. Native Americans have used pulsatilla for several conditions: they prepared a poultice of crushed, fresh leaves for rheumatism and neuralgia; inhaled the dried, pulverized leaves for headaches; and took a decoction of the root for pulmonary problems.

The sepals of the flower open wide in sunshine but close and fold over the stamens when evening approaches or rain threatens. This folding of the sepals has been likened to a tent; various legends have held that fairies used these "tents" for shelter from the elements.

Points of interest
• Pulsatilla has a long history of use in many cultures. (See *History of* Anemone pulsatilla.)

Commentary
Until clinical studies are performed documenting the safety and efficacy of pulsatilla in humans, this plant cannot be recommended for use. The potential for adverse effects outweighs any therapeutic benefit.

References
Dobelis, I.N., ed. *Magic and Medicine of Plants.* Pleasantville, N.Y.: Reader's Digest Association, Inc., 1986.

Friese K.H., et al. "The Homoeopathic Treatment of Otitis Media in Children— Comparisons with Conventional Therapy," *Int J Clin Pharmacol Ther* 35:296-301, 1997.

PUMPKIN

CUCURBITA, PEPONEN, PUMPKINSEED OIL, VEGETABLE MARROW

Taxonomic class
Cucurbitaceae

Common trade names
Multi-ingredient preparations: Action Super Saw Palmetto Plus, Hain Pumpkin Seed Oil Caps, Max Nutrition System, Mega Men Men's Vitapak, Men's Multiple Formula, Proleve 40, Prost-Answer Alcohol-Free, Pumpkin Seed Shield, Saw Palmetto Formula, Saw Palmetto Pygeum Plus, Ultimate Oil

Common forms
Available as seeds (whole or crushed), seed extract or oil, tablets, and tea.

Source
The seeds of various species of the *Cucurbita* genus, commonly known as pumpkin, squash, or gourd, are used. *C. pepo* (pumpkin, pepo, or vegetable marrow), *C. maxima* (autumn squash or red gourd), and *C. moschata* (crookneck squash, Canadian pumpkin, or Indian gourd) have been cultivated not only for medicinal use but also for nutritional and other practical uses. *C. pepo*, the pumpkin, seems to be used most often to prepare medicinal products that are available in the United States.

Chemical components
Cucurbitin, or (-) 3-amino-3-carboxypyrrolidine, a water-soluble amino acid, has been isolated as the pharmacologically active component of pumpkin seeds (Mihranian and Abou-Chaar, 1968). *Cucurbita* seed oil has been found to contain unsaturated fatty acids, including about 25% oleic acid and 55% linoleic acid. The presence of these fatty acids and phytosterols may account for effects on prostatic hypertrophy, but scientific evidence is lacking. Pumpkin seed oil has also been found to contain beta-carotenes, lutein, gamma- and beta-tocopherols, and selenium. These unsaturated fatty acids and antioxidants may also have a beneficial effect on lowering serum cholesterol levels and blood pressure when used in combination with more conventional therapeutic agents (Al-Zuhair et al., 1997 and 2000).

Actions
Cucurbitin inhibits the growth of immature *Schistosoma japonicum* in vivo (Mihranian and Abou-Chaar, 1968). Extracts of seeds and fruit of several pumpkin relatives show anthelmintic activity against pinworms and tapeworms in mice (Elisha et al., 1987).

The beneficial effects of pumpkin seeds on the prostate gland are commonly attributed to the unsaturated fatty acid content, claimed to

---

Bold italic type indicates that reaction may be life-threatening.

have a diuretic effect that increases urine flow and lessens the appearance of urinary retention without reducing prostatic enlargement. Curbicin, a preparation of pumpkin seeds and dwarf palm plants, was evaluated in patients with symptoms of benign prostatic hyperplasia (BPH) and found to significantly improve urinary flow, micturition time and frequency, and residual urine compared with controls (Carbin et al., 1990). However, another study found no evidence of inhibitory effect on further prostate growth (Bracher, 1997).

One study (Al-Zuhair et al., 1997) showed a potential additive or synergistic effect of pumpkin seed oil in combination with simvastatin to reduce serum cholesterol levels, with a reduction in LDL and an increase in HDL levels in hypercholesterolemic rabbits. This combination also decreased the aortic contractile response to norepinephrine. Pumpkin seed oil was also shown to decrease reflex tachycardia when used in combination with felodipine and to potentiate the antihypertensive effects of felodipine or captopril in hypertensive rats (Al-Zuhair et al., 2000). These beneficial effects were attributed to the antioxidant effects of tocopherols and selenium, and the linoleic and linolenic fatty acids, as nitric oxide (endothelium-derived relaxing factor), have been shown to be inactivated by superoxide radical in vitro. These beneficial effects haven't been proved in human studies, but the addition of pumpkin seed oil or other antioxidant dietary supplements may help to prevent or reduce lipoprotein oxidation in hypercholesterolemia and free radical–mediated endothelial dysfunction in hypercholesterolemia and hypertension.

Reported uses
Pumpkin has been used in the symptomatic treatment of BPH. For centuries, the seeds have been used to expel tapeworms and other intestinal worms and parasites, but large doses are required for anthelmintic activity to occur. Because cucurbitin content varies among species and even within species, pumpkin seeds are ineffective for treating *Taenia* infections. The availability of more reliable and effective medical treatments has resulted in a decreased use of pumpkin for this purpose. Some epidemiological reports have suggested a decreased incidence of hypertension and atherosclerosis in populations in which the seed oil is regularly consumed.

Dosage
For anthelmintic activity, some sources report 60 to 500 g of pumpkin seed in three divided doses, as tea or emulsion of the crushed seeds, in powdered sugar and milk or water (Elisha et al., 1987). In many cultures, daily consumption of small amounts of seed is recommended to prevent worm infestations. In Bulgaria, Turkey, and Ukraine, the daily consumption of a handful of pumpkin seeds is popular for treating BPH.

Adverse reactions
Metabolic: potential electrolyte loss from diuretic effects.

Interactions
Diuretics: Increased effects. Use together cautiously.

Contraindications and precautions
Pumpkin is contraindicated in patients when the cause of BPH is unknown. It is also contraindicated in pregnant or breast-feeding patients; effects are unknown.

Special considerations
• Monitor the patient for adverse diuretic effects, such as electrolyte loss.
• Monitor response to pumpkin if it is used as an anthelmintic.
• Advise the patient to seek medical attention for proper diagnosis and treatment of BPH. Symptoms may herald more serious disease, including other GI disorders, infection with intestinal parasites, or prostate cancer. Urinary tract outflow obstruction may also result in serious complications, including acute renal failure.
• Advise the patient to seek medical attention for the proper diagnosis and treatment of hypertension or hypercholesterolemia. Published human studies showing benefit of pumpkin seed oil for treating these conditions are lacking, and serious complications, including myocardial infarction and stroke, may result from failure to adequately control blood pressure.

Points of interest
• *Cucurbita* seeds and the oils and extracts made from them are sold throughout the world for medicinal purposes; the roasted seeds are commonly sold as snacks.
• OTC drugs for treating prostate enlargement were banned by the FDA in 1990 because of the risk of serious adverse reactions and complications.

Commentary
Although several small studies indicate a potential benefit of pumpkin seeds, seed extracts, and oils, these products vary widely in their active ingredients. Treatment failure can occur because a large dose is needed for anthelmintic activity and even supplements contain only trace amounts of active component.

These agents have not been proved to have a significant effect on BPH. It is advisable to check the ingredients for other toxic compounds before use.

Dietary supplementation with pumpkin seed oil or other preparations containing antioxidants may be of some benefit when added to a conventional medical treatment regimen for the long-term control of elevated blood pressure and serum cholesterol levels.

References
Al-Zuhair H., et al. "Efficacy of Simvastatin and Pumpkin-seed Oil in the Management of Dietary-induced Hypercholesterolemia," *Pharmacol Res* 35:403-8, 1997.
Al-Zuhair H., et al. "Pumpkin-seed Oil Modulates the Effect of Felodipine and Captopril in Spontaneously Hypertensive Rats," *Pharmacol Res* 41:555-63, 2000.

Bold italic type indicates that reaction may be life-threatening.

Bracher, F. "Phytotherapy of Benign Prostatic Hyperplasia," *Urologe A* 36:10-17, 1997. In German; abstract used.

Carbin, B.E., et al. "Treatment of Benign Prostatic Hyperplasia with Phytosterols," *Br J Urol* 6:639-41, 1990.

Elisha, E.E., et al. "The Anthelmintic Activity of Some Iraqi Plants of the Cucurbitaceae," *J Crude Drug Res* 25:153-57, 1987.

Mihranian, V.H., and Abou-Chaar, C.I. "Extraction, Detection and Estimation of Cucurbitin in Cucurbita Seeds," *Lloydia* 31:23-29, 1968.

PYGEUM

AFRICAN PLUM, AFRICAN PRUNE

Taxonomic class
Rosaceae

Common trade names
Pronitol, Provol, Tadenan

Common forms
Standardized extracts are available in capsules, softgels, and tablets. Dried bark for preparation of infusions is occasionally available in the United States.

Source
The bark of the *Prunus africana* (previously known as *Pygeum africanum*) tree, an evergreen that is native to Africa.

Chemical components
The bark contains three phytosterols (beta-sitosterol, beta-sitosterone, and campesterol); ferulic acid esters such as *n*-docosanol and *n*-tetracosanol; and the triterpenes oleanolic, crataegolic, and ursolic acid.

Actions
Pygeum extract or individual components have been found to inhibit prostaglandin formation and fibroblast proliferation within the prostate, inhibit enzymes destructive to connective tissue, increase prostatic secretions, improve composition of seminal fluid, and normalize glandular epithelium. Initiation of hyperplasia may occur by means of antiestrogenic effects. Pygeum does not have anticholinergic effects (Andro and Riffaud, 1995; Breza et al., 1998; McCutcheon, 2000).

Animal studies have shown decreases in levels of prolactin, luteinizing hormone (LH), and testosterone, but in one human study using pygeum extract, levels of LH, follicle-stimulating hormone, estrogens, and testosterone weren't affected, but *n*-docosanol is known to reduce LH and testosterone levels. Animal studies have demonstrated reduced excitability of the detrusor muscle by way of a decrease in sensitivity to electrical and chemical stimulation (Andro and Riffaud, 1995). Return of contractile function is associated with a normalization of myosin isoforms within the muscle (Gomes et al., 2000).

RESEARCH FINDINGS
A sampling of pygeum trials

This table includes examples of some of the better pygeum trials. Comparisons among trials are difficult because of differences in design and outcome measures.

Trial	Number	Length (days)	Formulation and dose (mg/day)
Chatelain et al., 1999	235	60*	Tadenan, 100
Breza et al., 1998	85	60	Tadenan, 100
Barlet et al., 1990	263	60	Tadenan, 100
Bassi et al., 1987	40	60	Pigenil, 100
Blitz et al., 1985	57	42	Tadenan, 100
Rigatti et al., 1985	49	60	Tadenan, 100
Dufour et al., 1983	120	42	Tadenan, 100
Gagliardi et al., 1983	40	30	Tadenan, 100
Donkervoort et al., 1977	20	84	Tadenan, 100
Carretero Gonzalez et al., 1973	100	90	Pronitol, 100

Tadenan = standardized *P. africanum* extract (Inverni della Beffa, Italy).

Pigenil = standardized *P. africanum* extract (Laboratoires DEBAT, France).

Pronitol = standardized *P. africanum* extract (Inofarma, Spain).

Reported uses

Traditionally, pygeum has been used as an aphrodisiac and as a treatment for stomachaches, "madness," fever, and general urinary troubles (McCutcheon, 2000). Today, pygeum is used primarily to decrease symptoms of benign prostatic hyperplasia (BPH). Evidence to support this claim is promising but not yet definitive.

Twelve double-blinded, placebo-controlled trials of pygeum for symptoms of BPH have demonstrated benefit greater than placebo. Also, the majority of 34 open-label, uncontrolled trials demonstrated some reduction of symptoms. Five small trials of pygeum extract or isolated components of pygeum compared treatment with other botanical therapies, NSAIDs, or anti-infectives with equivalent or superior results. The total patient exposure of these trials is about 2,600 subjects. Several additional trials have examined individual constituents of pygeum, such as beta-sitosterol and *n*-docosanol (Andro and Riffaud, 1995).

Although most results are positive in favor of pygeum, these trials all have methodological limitations, indicating that the treatment needs further investigation.

Design	Control	Subjective results	Objective results
RCDB	q.d. vs b.i.d.	+	+
0	None	+	+
RCDB	Placebo	+	+
RCDB	Placebo	+	+
RCDB	Placebo	+	NA
RCDB	NSAID	NA	+
RCDB	Placebo	+	+
RCDB	Anti-infective	+	+
RCDB	Placebo	-	-
0	None	+	+

*With 10-month follow-up period on 100 mg/day.

R = randomized. C = controlled. DB = double-blind. O = open label.

"+" = result showed benefit greater than comparator. "-" = no difference between treatment and comparator. NA = not assessed.

The trials that did show benefit generally noted improvement of symptoms according to a rating system such as the International Prostate Symptom Score and objective measures of urinary flow rate, frequency, and volume. Prostate volume, when tested, was either not changed or minimally affected. The longest controlled trials to date are only 3 months, and one open-label trial monitored patients for 10 months (Chatelain et al., 1999). (See *A sampling of pygeum trials.*)

Dosage
Extract (standardized to 14% total sterols): 100 to 200 mg/day P.O. in divided doses b.i.d.
Dried bark: 5 to 20 g/day P.O. (This form has not been tested in any clinical trials and is not recommended; McCutcheon, 2000).

Adverse reactions
GI: mild diarrhea (reported in one study; Barlet et al., 1990), indigestion.

Interactions
None reported.

Contraindications and precautions
No contraindications are known (McCutcheon, 2000; DerMarderosion, 2000). Prudence would recommend not using pygeum in conjunction with other treatments for BPH until studies assessing the safety of concomitant therapy have been completed.

Special considerations
• Urge the patient to seek medical attention for proper diagnosis to rule out prostate cancer before treating prostate symptoms.
• Advise the patient that pygeum may decrease urinary symptoms but will not shrink the enlarged prostate gland.
• Inform the patient that 6 to 8 weeks of therapy may be needed before benefits are observed.
• The products that have been most highly researched are generally not available in the United States except from some internet sources. Consumers should be careful to purchase standardized products that are as similar as possible to those used in trials.
• Short-term animal toxicity studies have examined doses up to 6 g/kg/day, and long-term studies have examined doses of 600 mg/kg/day for 11 months with no adverse effects (DerMarderosian, 2000).

Points of interest
• Pygeum has a high hydrocyanic acid component that imparts the taste of almonds. Milk-based infusions of pygeum have been used as substitutes for almond milk.
• Pygeum is the most common treatment for BPH symptoms in France and is widely used in Italy.
• Increased demand for pygeum has led to overharvesting. The tree is now threatened and international trade is being monitored.

Commentary
Despite positive results in most trials, the question of efficacy has not been definitively answered because of methodological limitations that weaken their usefulness in an evidence-based decision-making process. The placebo effect seen in most of these trials is large, and many studies do not use standard outcome measures. Definitive studies comparing pygeum extract with standard BPH therapy, such as alpha blockers (Flomax, Hytrin, Cardura) and 5-alpha-reductase inhibitors (Proscar), are needed before pygeum can be recommended. Pygeum's effects on endocrine activity need to be more stringently characterized as well.

Many patients with mild or even moderate symptoms of BPH choose watchful waiting over surgery or prescription drug treatment. In these patients, considering the known safety and toxicity data, a trial of pygeum extract is a reasonable option.

Bold italic type indicates that reaction may be life-threatening.

References

Andro, M-C., and Riffaud, J-P. "*Pygeum africanum* Extract for the Treatment of Patients with Benign Prostatic Hyperplasia: A Review of 25 Years of Published Experience," *Curr Ther Res* 56:796-816, 1995.

Barlet, A., et al. "Efficacy of *Pygeum africanum* Extract in the Treatment of Micturational Disorders Due to Benign Prostatic Hyperplasia. Evaluation of Objective and Subjective Parameters." *Wein Klin Wochenschr* 102:667-73, 1990. English translation obtained by University of Missouri-Kansas City Drug Information Center, 2000.

Bassi, P., et al. "Estratto Standardizzazto di *Pygeum africanum* nel Trattamento dell'ipertrofia Prostatica Benigna. Studio Clinico Controllato versus Placebo," *Minerva Urol Nefrol* 39:45-50, 1987.

Blitz, M., et al. "Etude Contrôlée de l'Efficacité d'un Traitement Médical sur des Sujets Consultant Pour la Première Fois Pour un Adénome de la Prostate," *Lyon Meditérr Méd* 21:11, 1985.

Breza, J., et al. "Efficacy and Acceptability of Tadenan (*Pygeum africanum* extract) in theTreatment of Benign Prostatic Hyperplasia (BPH): A Multicentre Trial in Central Europe," *Curr Med Res Op* 14:127-39, 1998.

Carretero Gonzalez, P., et al. "Experimentacion Clinica Con el Pronitol en al Adenoma Prostatico," *N Engl J Med* (Spanish ed.) 7:40-42, 1973.

Chatelain, C., et al. "Comparison of Once and Twice Daily Dosage Forms of *Pygeum africanum* Extract in Patients with Benign Prostatic Hyperplasia: A Randomized, Double-blind Study, with Long-term Open Label Extension," *Urology* 54:473-78, 1999.

DerMarderosion, A., ed. Pygeum monograph, 1998. Review of Natural Products. St. Louis: Facts and Comparisons, 2000.

Donkevoort, T., el al. "A Clinical and Urodynamic Study of Tadenan in the Treatment of Benign Prostatic Hypertrophy," *Eur Urol* 3:218-25, 1977.

Dufour, B., et al. "Traitement symptomatique de l'Adénome Prostatique. Etude Clinique Contrôlée des Effets de l'Extrait de *Pygeum africanum*," *Gaz Méd F* 90:2338-40, 1983.

Gagliardi, V., et al. "Terapia Medica Dell'ipertrofia Prostatica. Sperimentazione Clinica Controllata," *Arch Ital Urol Nefrol Andrologia* 55:51-69, 1983.

Gomes, C.M., et al. "Improved Contractility of Obstructed Bladders After Tadenan Treatment Is Associated with Reversal of Altered Myosin Isoform Expression," *J Urol* 163:2008-13, 2000.

McCutcheon, A.R. "Pygeum," in *Herbs: Everyday Reference for Health Professionals.* Edited by Chandler, F. Ottawa: Canadian Pharmacists Association, 2000.

Rigatti, P., et al. "Valutazione Clinica e Ecografica dell'efficacia Terapeutica del Tandenan nell'ipertrofia Prostatica," *Atti Accad Med Lomb* 40:1-6, 1985.

PYRUVATE

Common trade names

Pyruvate, Pyruvate Fuel

Multi-ingredient preparations: Prolab Creavate, PyruBalance, Pyruvate Accelerator, SportPharma Pyruvex

Common forms

Available in capsule form.

Source

Pyruvate is a 3-carbon byproduct of glucose metabolism in all animal and plant systems, including microorganisms. It is formed during digestive processes and throughout the body when glucose is broken down in the formation of adenosinetriphosphate (ATP). It also occurs naturally in fruits and vegetables, notably red apples, which may contain up to 400 mg of pyruvate per fruit.

Chemical components

Pyruvate is a single-agent chemical, 2-oxopropanoate, most often marketed as the calcium but also as the potassium, sodium, or magnesium salt.

Actions

Endogenous pyruvate is formed when glucose is metabolized to form ATP. Pyruvate is also formed in vivo from the 3-carbon amino acids (alanine, serine, cysteine) and threonine metabolism. Besides its formation during glycolysis, it is formed in an intermediate step in gluconeogenesis, specifically during the conversion of lactate to glucose. Pyruvate is the link between glycolysis and the citric acid or Krebs' cycle and may be broken down to form acetyl CoA, an important component of the Krebs' cycle. Microorganisms use pyruvate in the biosynthesis of ethanol and lactate, and plants use pyruvate to concentrate carbon dioxide, thus increasing photosynthesis of ATP (Stryer, 1981). Scientifically, pyruvate has demonstrated antioxidant activity in vitro, but this has not been demonstrated in vivo (Borle and Stanko, 1996; DeBoer et al., 1993). Pyruvate has also been shown to decrease ethanol-induced fatty liver (Rao et al., 1984) and acrylamide-induced neuropathy (Sabri et al., 1989) in rats. These effects are presumably caused by the antioxidant activity of pyruvate. Hemodynamically, pyruvate has been shown to induce vasodilation without affecting arterial tone or ventricular contractility (Romand et al., 1995). Numerous small, clinical trials have suggested that pyruvate may promote weight loss, increase lean muscle mass, and increase endurance during exercise. These studies used a limited patient population under strict controls that poorly correlate with most clinical situations. Study design and control have been questioned as well on many of these papers. Therefore, these data must be viewed objectively. Subsequent well-controlled studies have provided similar results in weight loss (about 2 to 4 lb lost; Kalman et al., 1999). Laboratory data have indicated that chronic oral pyruvate supplementation increases endurance in rats, possibly by sparing muscle glycogen (Ivy, 1998).

Reported uses

Based on the limited studies that have been performed, many manufacturers and lay consumers have promoted pyruvate as a supplement to reduce free radical formation and reduce the risk of cancer, heart disease, and numerous other disease states. The major reported uses for pyruvate include weight loss and maintenance of weight loss and as an ergogenic

---

Bold italic type indicates that reaction may be life-threatening.

aid to increase endurance. Studies based on the role that pyruvate plays in energy utilization and fatty acid oxidation suggest the use of dietary pyruvate supplementation as a component of nutritional therapy to decrease serum free fatty acid levels in type 2 diabetes (McCarty, 2000) and improve skeletal muscle health (Constantin-Teodosiu and Greenhaff, 1999). However, human clinical studies have demonstrated no effect on physical endurance or performance (Morrison et al., 2000; Stone et al., 1999).

Dosage
Most manufacturers recommend 2 to 5 g of pyruvate daily P.O. in divided doses with meals. Many of the clinical studies used doses ranging from 15 to 20 g/day.

Adverse reactions
GI: bloating, diarrhea, flatulence.
Other: *death*.

Interactions
None reported.

Contraindications and precautions
Do not use in patients with cardiomyopathy; one case report details the death of an infant with cardiomyopathy who was administered parenteral pyruvate (Matthys et al., 1991).

Special considerations
● Inform the patient that few data support ingestion of pyruvate; most claims are unsubstantiated.
● Advise the patient to consult a health care provider before using herbal preparations because a treatment that has been clinically researched and proved effective may be available.
● Although no known chemical interactions have been reported in clinical studies, consideration must be given to the pharmacologic properties of the herbal product and the potential for exacerbation of the intended therapeutic effect of conventional drugs.

Points of interest
● Dark beers and red wines contain significant amounts of pyruvate.
● Pyruvate is not an essential nutrient and, therefore, not associated with a deficiency syndrome.

Commentary
The scientific and clinical data concerning the effects of pyruvate are conflicting at best. Some evidence suggests that pyruvate may aid in weight loss, improve lipid profiles, and increase endurance; these changes are relatively small and perhaps not clinically relevant. Descriptions of adverse effect and toxicity profiles of sustained pyruvate intake are notably lacking. Given the problems seen from overenthusiastic ingestion of other ergogenic aids (ephedra, gamma-butyrolactone) by both amateur and pro-

fessional athletes, pyruvate supplementation should probably not be recommended until more extensive laboratory and clinical data have been generated and interpreted.

References

Borle, A., and Stanko, R.T. "Pyruvate Reduces Anoxic Injury and Free Radical Formation in Perfused Rat Hepatocytes," *J Appl Physiol* 270:G535-40, 1996.

Constantin-Teodosiu, D., and Greenhaff, D.L. "The Tricarboxylic Acid Cycle in Human Skeletal Muscle: Is There a Role for Nutritional Intervention," *Curr Opin Clin Nutr Metab Care* 2(6):527-31, 1999.

DeBoer, L.W.V., et al. "Pyruvate Enhances Recovery of Rat Hearts After Ischaemia and Reperfusion by Preventing Free Radical Generation," *J Appl Physiol* 265:H1571-76, 1993.

Ivy, J.L. "Effect of Pyruvate and Dihydroxyacetone on Metabolism and Aerobic Endurance Capacity," *Med Sci Sports Exerc* 30(6):837-43, 1998.

Jellin, J.M., et al. "Maidenhair Fern," in *Pharmacist's Letter/Prescriber's Letter Natural Medicines Comprehensive Database.* Stockton, Calif.: Therapeutic Research Faculty, 1999.

Kalman, D., et al. "The Effects of Pyruvate Supplementation on Body Composition in Overweight Individuals," *Nutrition* 15(5):337-40, 1999.

Matthys, D., et al. "Fatal Outcome of Pyruvate Loading Test in Child with Restrictive Cardiomyopathy," *Lancet* 338(8773):1020-21, 1991.

McCarty, M.F. "Toward a Wholly Nutritional Therapy for Type 2 Diabetes," *Med Hypotheses* 54(3):483-87, 2000.

Morrison, M.A., et al. "Pyruvate Ingestion for 7 Days Does Not Improve Aerobic Performance in Well-trained Individuals," *J Appl Physiol* 89(2):549-56, 2000.

Rao, G.A., et al. "Fatty Liver by Chronic Alcohol Ingestion Is Prevented by Dietary Supplementation with Pyruvate or Glycerol," *Lipids* 19(8):583-88, 1984.

Romand, J.A., et al. "Hemodynamic Effects of Pyruvate Infusion in Dogs," *J Crit Care* 10(4):165-73, 1995.

Sabri, M.I., et al. "Effect of Exogenous Pyruvate on Acrylamide Neuropathy in Rats," *Brain Res* 483(1):1-11, 1989.

Stone, M.H., et al. "Effects of In-season (5 Weeks) Creatine and Pyruvate Supplementation on Anaerobic Performance and Body Composition in American Football Players," *Int J Sport Nutr* 9(2):146-65, 1999.

Stryer, L. *Biochemistry.* New York: W.H. Freeman & Co., 1981, pp. 264, 268-69, 277, 283, 290-94, 349-50, 411, 416, 449, 545.

QUEEN ANNE'S LACE

BEE'S NEST, BIRD'S NEST, DEVIL'S PLAGUE, MOTHER'S DIE,
OIL OF CARROT, WILD CARROT, WILD CARROT SEED

Taxonomic class
Apiaceae

Common trade names
None known.

Common forms
Available as a crude extract and in teas.

Sources
The active ingredients are obtained from the leaves, roots, and seeds of
the *Daucus carota* subspecies *sativas,* which typically grows wild in various parts of North America.

Chemical components
The fruits and leaves of *D. carota* contain aglycones and glycosides,
which are flavonoids (apigenin, chrysin, luteolin) and porphyrins. Furanocoumarins (methoxypsoralens) are also found in the plant. The volatile oil contains many components (pinenes, geraniol, limonene, ter-
pinens, carophyllene, carotol, daucol, and asarone). *D. carota* seeds consist predominantly of unsaturated fatty acids (oleic acid, linolenic acid,
and palmitic acid) and myristicin. *D. carota* contains choline, ethanol,
xylitol, coumarin, formic acid, and oxalic acid.

Actions
The tertiary base of the seeds has papaverine-like, nonspecific, antispasmodic activity. Only about one-tenth the antispasmodic activity of papaverine was found in animals (Gambhir et al., 1979). In vitro, spasmodic
actions have been observed in both smooth muscle and skeletal muscle
and have been attributed to the choline component of Queen Anne's lace.

The petroleum ether extract and fatty acids of *D. carota* seeds were
found to halt the normal estrogen cycle and decrease ovary weight in
adult mice (Majumder et al., 1997). Seed extracts produced weak estrogenic activity and inhibited implantation of embryo (Prakash, 1984).

Pretreatment of *D. carota* extract on carbon tetrachloride–induced
acute hepatic damage in mice showed decreased serum enzyme levels
of glutamate oxaloacetate transaminase, glutamate pyruvate transaminase, glutamate dehydrogenase, lactate dehydrogenase, alkaline phosphatase, and sorbitol and reduced elevated serum bilirubin and urea
levels (Bishayee et al., 1995).

Minimal antifungal activity has also been suggested. Terpinen-4-ol is a documented component of other plants and known to produce diuresis by renal irritation. Various CV effects of wild carrot have been noted in animal models (Gilani et al., 1994); other studies in animals have reported hypotensive and cardiac depressant effects and CNS and respiratory depression at high doses.

Reported uses
D. carota is claimed to be useful as an aphrodisiac, an abortifacient, a diuretic, and a hypoglycemic agent. It has been reported anecdotally to treat cancer, cardiac and renal disease, dysentery, dyspepsia, gout, menstrual abnormalities, night blindness, ulcers, uterine pain, and worms. No controlled clinical trials support these claims.

Dosage
No consensus exists.

Adverse reactions
CNS: CNS depression.
CV: cardiac depression, hypotension.
GU: diuresis, renal irritation (excessive doses).
Skin: contact dermatitis, photosensitization (especially with wet leaves because of methoxypsoralen content).

Interactions
Analgesics, anxiolytics, sedative-hypnotic drugs: Risk of increased CNS depression. Monitor the patient.
Anticoagulants, antiplatelets: Theoretical increased risk of bleeding. Monitor PT and INR.
Antihypertensives: Risk of increased hypotensive effect. Use cautiously.
Digoxin, other rate-controlling drugs: Risk of increased depressant effects on myocardium. Monitor vital signs.
Hormones: Excessive use can interfere with hormonal therapy. Monitor the patient for clinical response.
Muscle relaxants, other drugs that affect muscle function: Risk of altered musculoskeletal contraction. Monitor the patient.

Contraindications and precautions
Avoid using Queen Anne's lace in pregnant or breast-feeding patients; effects are unknown. The seeds may have abortifacient action (Farnsworth et al., 1975).

Special considerations
• Inform the patient that data supporting the use of Queen Anne's lace are insufficient.
⚫ ALERT Inform the patient that some poisonous plants appear similar to and may be confused with *D. carota,* including water hemlock (*Cicuta maculata*), poison hemlock (*Conium maculatum*), and fool's parsley (*Aethusa cynapium*).
• Advise women to report any planned or suspected pregnancy.

Bold italic type indicates that reaction may be life-threatening.

• Advise the patient to avoid hazardous activities until CNS effects are known.
• Encourage the photosensitive patient to avoid exposure to sunlight by wearing sunblock, a hat, sunglasses, and appropriate clothing.

Points of interest
• *D. carota* is known as Queen Anne's lace because of its intricately patterned, flat flower cluster.
• The herb is also known as mother's die because of the superstition, "If you bring it into your home, your mother will die."
• The orange root of *D. carota* subspecies *carota* (the cultivated carrot) is consumed either cooked or raw and is different from *D. carota* subspecies *sativas*.
• *D. carota* is used as a dye, fragrance, and flavoring agent.

Commentary
Data from studies in animals suggest that *D. carota* has antifungal, antispasmodic, antisteroidogenic, and hepatoprotective properties. No data support the therapeutic use of *D. carota* for these claims. Contact with the leaves has been associated with dermatitis, and neurologic effects occur when the seeds are taken in high doses. Additional data are needed to determine the therapeutic potential for components of *D. carota*.

References
Bishayee, A., et al. "Hepatoprotective Activity of Carrot (*Daucus carota* L.) Against Carbon Tetrachloride Intoxication in Mouse Liver," *J Ethnopharmacol* 47:69-74, 1995.

Farnsworth, N.R., et al. "Potential Value of Plants as Sources of New Antifertility Agents I," *J Pharm Sci* 64:535-98, 1975.

Gambhir, S.S., et al. "Antispasmodic Activity of the Tertiary Base of *Daucus carota*, Linn. Seeds," *Indian J Physiol Pharmacol* 23:225-28, 1979.

Gilani, A.H., et al. "Cardiovascular Actions of *Daucus carota*," *Arch Pharmacol Res* 17:150-53, 1994.

Majumder, P.K., et al. "Anti-steroidogenic Activity of the Petroleum Ether Extract and Fraction 5 (Fatty Acids) of Carrot (*Daucus carota* L.) Seeds in Mouse Ovary," *J Ethnopharmacol* 57:209-12, 1997.

Prakash, A.O. "Biological Evaluation of Some Medicinal Plant Extracts for Contraceptive Efficacy," *Contracept Deliv Syst* 5:9, 1984.

QUINCE

COMMON QUINCE, *CYDONIA VULGARIS*, GOLDEN APPLE, *PYRUS CYDONIA*

Taxonomic class
Rosaceae

Common trade names
None known.

Common forms
Available as decoctum cydoniae, B.P. (decoction from seeds), fruit syrup, and mucilage of quince seeds.

Source
The fruit and seeds of *Cydonia oblonga* are used in preparing the medicinal products of quince.

Chemical components
The seeds contain fixed oil, protein, and a small amount of amygdalin, and its coat contains mucilage. The fruit pulp contains malic acid. Beta-D-glucopyranosyl-(1,6)-beta-D-glucopyranoside of 3-hydroxy-beta-ionol has also been isolated in the fruit.

Actions
Tertiary literature suggests astringent, cardiac, demulcent, diuretic, emollient, and restorative effects. A decoction of *C. oblonga* has been shown in vitro to have a bactericidal effect against *Vibrio cholerae* (Guevara et al., 1994).

A German abstract describes a three-way crossover study examining varying strengths of a mixture of extracts from both *Citrus limon* and *C. oblonga* and their effects on nasal mucociliary clearance (Degen et al., 2000). The investigators failed to detect a change in nasal mucociliary clearance.

Reported uses
Traditionally, quince fruit syrup has been commonly added to beverages to treat diarrhea, dysentery, and sore throat. The decoction from the seeds is taken internally in the treatment of dysentery, gonorrhea, and thrush; it is also used as an adjunct in boric acid eye lotions and in skin lotions and creams. Anecdotal data exist for these uses; no clinical human data are available. The mucilage of quince seeds has been used as a suspending agent in such pharmaceutical and toilet preparations as mouthwashes for canker sores, gum problems, and sore throats. Although the quince seeds are thought to be useful in treating cancer (Moertel et al., 1982)—probably because of amygdalin's cyanogenetic action—no studies have confirmed this effect.

Dosage
For diarrhea, dysentery, gonorrhea, and thrush, large quantities of decoctum cydoniae (2 drams of quince seed boiled in 1 pt of water for 10 minutes) P.O.

No dosages have been reported for the external use of mucilage preparations.

Adverse reactions
None reported.

Interactions
None reported.

Bold italic type indicates that reaction may be life-threatening.

Contraindications and precautions
Avoid using quince in pregnant or breast-feeding patients; effects are unknown.

Special considerations
● Advise the patient taking quince for GI symptoms that other agents with known safety and efficacy data are available.
● **ALERT** Quince seeds are potentially toxic because of their amygdalin (laetrile) content.
● Caution the patient to keep quince out of the reach of children and pets.

Points of interest
● Other varieties of quinces, especially the Japanese quince, *Cydonia japonica*, are not used medicinally.
● Japanese quince is a popular ornamental plant that is grown all over the world.

Commentary
Preparations made from the fruit or the mucilage derived from the seed coat may provide minor relief from diarrhea and sore throat because of their astringent and demulcent properties. Although a quince decoction has been shown to have an in vitro bactericidal effect against *V. cholerae*, there are no clinical reports suggesting its value in treating cholera. The amygdalin (laetrile) component of quince is toxic and ineffective as a cancer treatment and should not be consumed.

References
Degen, J., et al. "The Effect of a Nasal Spray Consisting of a Standardized Mixture of *Citrus limon* (succus) and an Aqueous Extract of *Cydonia oblonga* (fructus) on Nasal Mucociliary Clearance," *Arzneimittelforschung* 50(1):39-42, 2000.

Guevara, J.M., et al. "The *In Vitro* Action of Plants on *Vibrio cholerae*," *Rev Gastroenterol Peru* 14:27-31, 1994.

Moertel, C.G., et al. "A Clinical Trial of Amygdalin (Laetrile) in the Treatment of Human Cancer," *N Engl J Med* 306:201-6, 1982.

RAGWORT

CANKERWORT, COCASHWEED, COUGHWEED, DOG
STANDARD, FALSE VALERIAN, GOLDEN RAGWORT, GOLDEN
SENECIO, LIFEROOT, RAGWEED, St. James wort,
STAGGERWORT, STAMMERWORT, STINKING NANNY, SQUAW
WEED, SQUAWROOT

Taxonomic class
Asteraceae

Common trade names
Tansy Ragwort

Common forms
Available as fresh and dried herb.

Source
The leaves, seeds, and flowers of *Senecio jacobaea* are commonly used.
Ragwort is a member of the daisy family and native to North America.

Chemical components
Limited information exists on the chemical composition of *Senecio*
species. The volatile oil has been described for some species (Dooren et
al., 1981). Pyrrolizidine alkaloids (floridanine, florosenine, otosenine,
and senecionine) are the chief components isolated from the leaves,
seeds, and flowers.

Actions
Several texts report that ragwort has an astringent, cooling, analgesic effect when applied topically or gargled. It is also claimed to have diuretic, weak expectorant, and uterine stimulant properties.

Reported uses
Emollient poultices have been made from leaves. Plant "juice" has been
used as a wash for bee stings, burns, rheumatism, and cancerous ulcers
and as a gargle for ulcerations in the mouth and throat. Claims for use
of the plant have also been made for treating functional amenorrhea
and menopausal neurosis. These claims lack sufficient clinical trial data
to validate their application.

Dosage
Only external use of the herb is recommended. Poultices are made by
applying the bruised, fresh plant directly on the affected area. Dried
herb can be used by soaking it in warm water before applying. A gargle
is made by soaking the plant in warm water and then straining.

Adverse reactions
GI: *hepatotoxicity,* nausea, vomiting.
Respiratory: *pulmonary edema or effusion.*

Interactions
Hepatotoxins: Increased risk of hepatotoxicity. Avoid administration with ragwort.

Contraindications and precautions
Ragwort is contraindicated in patients who are susceptible to hepatic dysfunction. Avoid its use in pregnant or breast-feeding patients; effects are unknown.

Special considerations
● Pyrrolizidine alkaloids are metabolized to hepatotoxic pyrrolic compounds. Death resulting from hepatic failure has been reported in animals and humans.
● Monitor liver function test results.
● Advise the patient to report signs and symptoms of hepatic dysfunction (abdominal pain, fatigue, fever, jaundice).
● Advise women to avoid using ragwort during pregnancy or when breast-feeding.

Points of interest
● In South Africa, some *Senecio* species are used as food.

Commentary
Because there are well-documented cases of human and animal poisonings, ragwort presents an unacceptable risk and should not be used for any medicinal purpose.

References
Dooren, B., et al. "Composition of Essential Oils of Some *Senecio* Species," *Planta Med* 42:385-89, 1981.

RASPBERRY

BLACK RASPBERRY (*RUBUS OCCIDENTALIS*), BLACKBERRY (*RUBUS FRUTICOSUS, RUBUS FRONDOSUS, RUBUS HISPIDUS, RUBUS MACROPETALUS*), BRAMBLE, BRAMBLE OF MOUNT IDA, HINDBERRY, RASPBIS, RED RASPBERRY (*RUBUS IDAEUS*), *RUBUS*

Taxonomic class
Rosaceae

Common trade names
Red Raspberry Leaves

Common forms
Capsules: 384 mg, 400 mg
Liquid: 1 oz, 2 oz

Source
The red raspberry comes from the *Rubus idaeus* plant; other raspberry species exist and are referred to mostly as blackberries. The berries are commonly red, but they may also be yellow. The leaves, berries, and, sometimes, the root are used for medicinal purposes.

Chemical components
The *R. idaeus* leaves contain tannin, gallic and ellagic acids, flavonoids, fragarin, organic acids, and vitamin C. The fruit of the raspberry plant contains pectin, fructose, aromatic compounds, and vitamin C (less than that found in the leaves).

Actions
The tannins contained in the leaves of the raspberry plant have an astringent action, whereas the leaves have been used in teas to treat diarrhea and dysentery.

The most common medical claim of the raspberry is its use in pregnancy and childbirth. A tea prepared from the leaves has been used to prevent miscarriage, ameliorate morning sickness, aid in childbirth, and relieve menstrual cramps because it has a slight oxytocic property (reportedly from the fragarin component), which is said to both relax and stimulate the uterus. Some sources recommend that pregnant women in their last trimester partake of the fruit to "ease and speed" delivery.

Raspberry has lowered blood glucose levels in animals (Briggs and Briggs, 1997).

Red raspberry extract has shown significant antimicrobial activity toward *Staphylococcus aureus* (Rauha et al., 2000).

Reported uses
The leaves of the raspberry plant are reported to have anti-inflammatory, diuretic, and expectorant properties. A tea made from the leaves has been used as a mouthwash and to clean wounds. Because of the acidity of the juice, the fruits are considered useful for treating urinary conditions and breaking up and aiding the expulsion of kidney stones and gallstones. When mixed with sugar and boiled into a syrup, the juice has also been used as a gargle for inflamed tonsils.

Because of the presence of tannic and gallic acids, the roots are claimed to have antibiotic action. A tea prepared from the roots may be used for sore throats and cankers and in wound cleansing. All these claims are based on traditional or anecdotal data; human clinical trial data are lacking. The fruit is most commonly used for culinary purposes.

Dosage
Dried red raspberry leaf powder or tablets: 4 to 8 g P.O. t.i.d.
Liquid extract (1 g of leaf/ml of 25% ethanol): 4 to 8 ml P.O. t.i.d.

Adverse reactions
None reported.

Interactions
Antidiabetic drugs: Increased effectiveness of hypoglycemic action. Use cautiously.
Disulfiram: Disulfiram reaction can occur if the herbal product contains alcohol. Do not use together.

Contraindications and precautions
Use the raspberry leaf or preparations made from it with caution during pregnancy because they may initiate labor.

Special considerations
● Monitor the blood glucose level in a patient with diabetes.
● Caution the patient taking disulfiram not to take any preparation that contains alcohol.
● Urge women to report planned or suspected pregnancy. Advise the patient who wants to become pregnant not to exceed moderate consumption of the fruit.

Points of interest
● Raspberry syrup is commonly used to mask the taste of bitter-tasting drugs.

Commentary
Because the raspberry fruit is a common food item, it appears to be harmless when consumed in moderation. Plant extracts or products containing the leaves should be used with caution and under medical supervision in pregnant women because of their oxytocic effects. Despite its common use as a food, there is no acceptable medicinal use of raspberry.

References
Briggs, C.J., and Briggs, K. "Raspberry," *Can Pharmaceutical J* 130:41-43, 1997.
Rauha, J.P., et al. "Antimicrobial Effects of Finnish Plant Extracts Containing Flavonoids and Other Phenolic Compounds," *Int J Food Microbiol* 56(1):3-12, 2000.

RAUWOLFIA

INDIAN SNAKEROOT, *RAUWOLFIA*, SNAKEROOT

Taxonomic class
Apocynaceae

Common trade names
Harmonyl (deserpidine, U.K.), Raudixin, Rauwiloid (alseroxylon fraction), Serpasil (reserpine)

Common forms

Injection (reserpine): 250 mg/ml
Tablets: 50 mg (Raudixin)
    Also available as crude root, liquid and powdered extract, and tea.

Source

Of more than 100 species of rauwolfia growing in India, Thailand, South America, Asia, and Africa, the root of *Rauwolfia serpentina* is notable for its medicinal effects.

Chemical components

More than 50 alkaloids are found in *R. serpentina;* reserpine has been extensively studied in clinical evaluations. Other alkaloids include rescinnamine, deserpidine, syrosingopine, ajmaline (rauwolfine), ajmalinine, ajmalicine, isoajmaline, serpentine, rauwolfinine, and sarpagine.

Actions

Reserpine is known to have depressant, hypotensive, and sedative properties. It produces a catecholamine-depleting effect in the brain and peripheral sympathetic neurons.

Reported uses

Rauwolfia alkaloids have been used to lower fevers, calm noisy babies, cure diarrhea and dysentery, and treat some psychiatric illnesses.
    Much evidence exists that proves the rauwolfia alkaloids' success in the treatment of hypertension and psychiatric conditions. Although the use of rauwolfia alkaloids in hypertensive patients has decreased significantly in the United States because of the adverse effects of the drugs, reserpine is still used in countries such as Spain—usually with a thiazide diuretic (Capella et al., 1983).

Dosage

For hypertension, daily doses of Raudixin 200 mg, Rauwiloid 4 mg, or reserpine 0.25 mg P.O. (100 mg of crude root corresponds to 2 mg alseroxylon fraction, which corresponds to 0.1 mg of reserpine). Average daily dose is 600 mg, which corresponds to 6 mg of total alkaloids.

Adverse reactions

The following adverse reactions of reserpine can occur with higher doses of rauwolfia:
CNS: depression, hallucinations, nightmares, suicidal ideations, unsteadiness and parkinsonian syndrome (rare).
CV: *bradycardia*, hypotension (more common with parenteral than oral), premature ventricular beats.
EENT: nasal congestion.
Endocrine: *breast cancer* (controversial; O'Fallon et al., 1975; Armstrong et al., 1976; Schyve et al., 1978).
GI: diarrhea, GI complaints, peptic ulcer disease.

Bold italic type indicates that reaction may be life-threatening.

GU: decreased libido.
Metabolic: edema, increased appetite, weight gain.

Interactions
Antihypertensives, nitrates: Additive hypotensive effects. Use cautiously.
Barbiturates, CNS depressants: Pronounced CNS effects and toxicity when rauwolfia alkaloids are used with barbiturates (Pfeifer et al., 1976). Avoid administration with rauwolifia.
Cardiac glycosides: Lowered heart rate. Monitor the patient.
Levodopa: Reduced effectiveness of levodopa. Avoid administration with rauwolfia.
NSAIDs, tricyclic antidepressants: May reduce hypotensive effects of rauwolfia derivatives. Monitor the patient.
Sympathomimetics: Initial increase in blood pressure. Monitor the patient.

Contraindications and precautions
Rauwolfia is contraindicated in active peptic ulcer disease and ulcerative colitis because it increases gastric acid secretion. Use cautiously in patients with current diagnosis or past history of breast cancer and during pregnancy.

Special considerations
• The patient should discontinue rauwolfia ingestion at least 2 weeks before undergoing electroconvulsive therapy.
• Monitor blood pressure.
• Counsel the patient with a history of or at risk for depression to avoid using rauwolfia derivatives.
• Several reports have attempted to link the development of breast cancer with consumption of rauwolfia derivatives. Many reports have failed to verify this association, but the issue remains controversial.
• Advise the patient with a history of cancer (especially breast cancer) or peptic ulcer disease to avoid using rauwolfia derivatives.
• Caution the patient to avoid hazardous activities until CNS and hypotensive effects of rauwolfia derivatives are known.
• Inform the patient that the adverse effects of rauwolfia alkaloids limit their use. Other proven agents exist for treating hypertension and psychiatric illnesses.

Commentary
Rauwolfia alkaloids have proved to be valuable for treating hypertension and some psychoses; the most popular and most studied is reserpine. Extensive application of rauwolfia derivatives is limited by the adverse reactions of the drugs. Other safe and equally effective agents are available.

References
Armstrong, B., et al. "Rauwolfia Derivatives and Breast Cancer in Hypertensive Women," *Lancet* 2:8-12, 1976.

Capella, D., et al. "Utilization of Antihypertensive Drugs in Certain European Countries," *Eur J Clin Pharmacol* 25:431-35, 1983.

O'Fallon, W.M., et al. "Rauwolfia Derivatives and Breast Cancer. A Case/Control Study in Olmsted County, Minnesota," *Lancet* 2:292-96, 1975.

Pfeifer, H.J., et al. "Clinical Toxicity of Reserpine in Hospitalized Patients: A Report from the Boston Collaborative Drug Surveillance Program," *Am J Med* 271:269-76, 1976.

Schyve, P.M., et al. "Neuroleptic-induced Prolactin Level Elevation and Breast Cancer; An Emerging Clinical Issue," *Arch Gen Psychiatry* 35:1291-1301, 1978.

RED CLOVER

BEEBREAD, COW CLOVER, MEADOW CLOVER, MISSOURI MILK VETCH, PURPLE CLOVER, TREFOIL, WILD CLOVER

Taxonomic class
Fabaceae

Common trade names
Multi-ingredient preparations: Red Clover Blend, Red Clover Blossoms, Red Clover Cleanser, Red Clover Combo, Red Clover Plus, Red Clover Tops

Common forms
Capsules: 200 mg, 280 mg, 354 mg, 375 mg, 395 mg, 430 mg, 454 mg
Liquid: 1 oz, 2 oz
Tablets: 100 mg
   Also available as a tea and in raw sprouts.

Source
The aerial parts of the plant, specifically the rose-colored flower head, are used. *Trifolium pratense,* or red clover, was naturalized to the United States from its native Europe.

Chemical components
More than 125 chemicals have been identified in the red clover plant. The notable components include the elemental constituents (aluminum, calcium, copper, iron, magnesium, manganese, potassium), several carbohydrates (arabinose, glucose, xylose, rhamnose), two coumarins (coumarin, medicagol), various flavonoids and isoflavonoids, saponins, coumaric acid, salicylic acid, clovamide compounds, and fats.

Actions
In animals, isoflavonoid components are thought to be responsible for estrogen-like actions (Kelly et al., 1979). Components of red clover have altered vaginal cytology, increased follicle-stimulating hormone, and altered luteinizing hormone serum levels in animal models (Wilcox et al., 1990; Zava et al., 1998).
   Preliminary information reported that red clover possessed a carcinogen-protective effect in vitro (Cassady et al., 1988).

Bold italic type indicates that reaction may be life-threatening.

Reported uses
Red clover is used as an estrogen replacement for postmenopausal women, to treat chronic skin diseases, and to suppress whooping cough.

Dosage
Traditional uses suggest the following dosages:
For skin diseases, apply compress b.i.d.
Tincture: 2 to 6 ml P.O. t.i.d.
   Infusion made by pouring hot water over 1 to 3 tsp of dried herb. Let stand for 10 to 15 minutes, and take P.O. t.i.d.

Adverse reactions
GU: estrogen-like effects (breast tenderness and enlargement, change in menses, weight gain and redistribution).
Other: infertility and growth disorders (with large doses; reported in animals), potentiated growth of estrogen receptor–positive *neoplasia.*

Interactions
Anticoagulants (heparin, warfarin), antiplatelet drugss (aspirin, clopido-grel, ticlopidine): Increased risk of bleeding. Red clover contains some coumarin and coumarin-like compounds. Monitor the patient closely.
Oral contraceptives: Increased effects by increasing estrogen components. Use cautiously.

Contraindications and precautions
Avoid using red clover in pregnant or breast-feeding patients; effects are unknown. Also avoid its use in patients with estrogen receptor–positive neoplasia. Use cautiously in patients who are susceptible to bleeding problems or in those taking anticoagulants.

Special considerations
• Monitor the patient for signs and symptoms of bleeding.
• Alert the pathology laboratory reviewing the Papanicolaou smear that the patient is taking red clover.
• Inform the patient that few data exist about the use of red clover in humans. Other proven estrogen products exist and should be pursued first.
• Counsel women to avoid using red clover if pregnancy is desired.
• Advise the patient with a history of estrogen receptor–positive cancer to avoid use of red clover.

Points of interest
• Red clover has long been implicated as a cause of infertility in livestock (Hoffman et al., 1997).

Commentary
Although many uses for red clover have been reported, only animal and in vitro data exist. Because efficacy evidence in humans is lacking and the toxicity of the herb is essentially undescribed, consumption of red

clover cannot be recommended. Numerous estrogen products are available; the need for the herb's estrogen-like effects is questionable.

References
Cassady, J.M., et al. "Use of a Mammalian Cell Culture Benzo(a)pyrene Metabolism Assay for the Detection of Potential Anticarcinogens from Natural Products: Inhibition of Metabolism by Biochanin A, an Isoflavone from *Trifolium pratense* L," *Cancer Res* 48:6257-61, 1988.

Hoffman, P.C., et al. "Performance of Lactating Dairy Cows Fed Red Clover or Alfalfa Silage," *J Dairy Sci* 80:3308-15, 1997.

Kelly, R.W., et al. "Formononentin Content of Grasslands Pawera Red Clover and Its Estrogenic Activity in Sheep," *NZ J Exp Agricult* 7:131-34, 1979.

Wilcox, G., et al. "Estrogenic Effects of Plant Foods in Postmenopausal Women," *Brit Med J* 301:905-6, 1990.

Zava, D.T., et al. "Estrogen and Progestin Bioactivity of Foods, Herbs, and Spices," *Proc Soc Exper Biol Med* 217:369-78, 1998.

RED POPPY

CORN POPPY, CORN ROSE, FIELD POPPY, FLANDERS POPPY, *PAPAVER RHOEAS*

Taxonomic class
Papaveraceae

Common trade names
None known.

Common forms
Available as capsules.

Source
Red poppy, *Papaver rhoeas*, is an annual plant that is native to Europe, North Africa, and temperate areas of Asia and has been naturalized in North America and South America. The bright red flowers are used.

Chemical components
Red poppy contains many alkaloids, including papaverine, rhoeadine, and isorhoeadine. It has been reported that the alkaloid content is similar to that of the opium poppy, *Papaver somniferum,* which contains morphine, noscapine, and codeine. Controversy exists regarding the presence of significant pharmacologically active narcotic constituents. Other constituents of red poppy include meconic acid, mekocyanin, mucilage, and tannin.

Actions
The actions of the various components of red poppy have not been studied in animals or humans.

Reported uses
Similar to opium poppy, red poppy is claimed to be mildly analgesic and sedative. It has been primarily used as a cough suppressant and ex-

---

Bold italic type indicates that reaction may be life-threatening.

pectorant, but its effectiveness for any use has not been evaluated in controlled clinical human trials.

Dosage
No consensus exists.

Adverse reactions
CNS: potential CNS depressant effects.
Skin: allergic contact dermatitis (Gamboa et al., 1997).

Interactions
Analgesics, CNS depressants: Risk of additive effects of these drugs. Avoid administration with red poppy.

Contraindications and precautions
Avoid using red poppy in pregnant or breast-feeding patients; effects are unknown. Also, avoid its use in patients who are hypersensitive to morphine or codeine. Use cautiously in patients with a history of allergic contact dermatitis.

Special considerations
• Advise the patient to consult a health care provider before using herbal preparations because a treatment that has been clinically researched and proved effective may be available.
• Monitor CNS effects.
• Advise the patient that few data exist with regard to red poppy.

Points of interest
• Members of the Papaveraceae family may contain potentially toxic alkaloids, such as morphine, codeine, papaverine, noscapine, and thebaine. Because red poppy contains unknown quantities of these substances, toxic doses of red poppy cannot be estimated.

Commentary
Unlike opium poppy, little information is available about the red poppy. Its components are not well characterized, and the actual quantities contained are unknown. Red poppy has not been demonstrated to be therapeutically useful, and its toxic potential is unclear. Therefore, its use cannot be recommended.

References
Gamboa, P.M., et al. "Allergic Contact Urticaria from Poppy Flowers (*Papaver rhoeas*)," *Contact Dermatitis* 37:140-41, 1997.

RED YEAST RICE
HONG QU, *MONASCUS PURPUREUS*

Taxonomic class
Monascaceae

Common trade names
Cholestin

Common forms
Available as a 600-mg capsule in the United States. In China, dried red yeast rice is either powdered (ZhiTai) or extracted with alcohol (XueZhiKang).

Source
Red yeast rice is a traditional Chinese substance made by fermenting a particular strain of yeast, called *Monascus purpureus,* over rice. The red yeast rice is produced in China and imported by Pharmanex, Inc., for packaging into gelatin capsules in the United States.

Chemical components
Red yeast rice contains 0.4% naturally occurring HMG-CoA reductase inhibitors. The most abundant HMG-CoA reductase inhibitor is mevinolin, or lovastatin. It also contains unsaturated fatty acids, including monounsaturated fatty acids, diene-, triene-, tetraene-, and pentaene-fatty acids. Other components include amino acids, protein, saccharides, beta-sitosterol, campesterol, stignasterol, isoflavone, saponin, and other trace elements.

Actions
Red yeast rice has cholesterol-reducing properties. It contains lovastatin and related mevinic acid compounds that competitively inhibit 3-hydroxy-3-methyl-glutaryl-coenzyme A (HMG-CoA) reductase. This blocks the synthesis of cholesterol in the liver and results in decreased LDL, VLDL, and triglyceride levels. It also increases HDL levels.

Reported uses
Red yeast rice has been used to maintain desirable cholesterol levels in healthy people and to reduce cholesterol levels in people with hypercholesterolemia. Chinese medicine uses this product for diarrhea and indigestion, for improving blood circulation, and for spleen and stomach health.

Animal and human studies to evaluate the effectiveness of red yeast rice in hypercholesterolemia have been performed primarily in China. Studies in rabbits and quail have demonstrated cholesterol lowering and decreased lipid accumulation in the liver with XueZhiKang (Li et al., 1988). Clinical studies performed with several formulations of *M. purpureus* have also shown cholesterol-lowering effects. Studies conducted in the United States (Heber et al., 1999; Rippe et al., 1999) included appropriate diet instructions or surveys for the patients.

Dosage
Capsules: Two 600-mg capsules P.O. b.i.d.
Extract: 0.6 g P.O. b.i.d.

Each gram of Cholestin contains 4 mg of HMG-CoA reductase inhibitors: 2 mg as lovastatin, 1 mg as lovastatin acid, and 1 mg as a mixture of

---

seven other statins. Therefore, the recommended dose of 1,200 mg b.i.d. would provide 7.2 mg of lovastatin and 2.4 mg of other statins (O'Mathuna, 1999). The product is standardized to contain 0.4% (9.6 mg) HMG-CoA reductase inhibitors and greater than or equal to 150 mg of unsaturated fatty acids per daily dosage.

Adverse reactions
CNS: dizziness.
GI: bloating, flatulence, heartburn.
Other: *anaphylaxis* (Wiiger-Alberti et al., 1999).

Interactions
Cytochrome P-450 inhibiting drugs: Increased serum lovastatin level and risk of adverse effects. Avoid administration with red yeast rice.
Food: Increased bioavailability of lovastatin. Red yeast rice may be taken with food.
Grapefruit juice: 15-fold increase in serum lovastatin levels; increased risk of adverse effects. Do not administer red yeast rice with grapefruit juice.
Levothyroxine: Concomitant use with lovastatin can cause thyroid function abnormalities. Avoid using together.
Other cholesterol-lowering drugs: Increased risk of adverse effects and toxicity. Avoid administration with red yeast rice.

Contraindications and precautions
Red yeast rice should be avoided in patients who are at risk for or who have active hepatic disease and in those with a history of hepatic disease. It is also contraindicated in people who consume more than two alcoholic beverages daily; in patients with a serious infection, disease, or physical disorder or who have had an organ transplant; and in anyone younger than age 20. Avoid use in female patients who are breast-feeding, pregnant, or planning to become pregnant.

Special considerations
● Red yeast rice may be taken with food to minimize adverse GI effects.
🕮 **ALERT** Anaphylaxis to red yeast rice has been reported.
● Natural constituents in red yeast rice (HMG-CoA reductase inhibitors) in much higher doses have been associated with some rare but serious adverse effects, including hepatic and skeletal muscle disease.
● Elevated liver enzyme and creatine kinase levels can occur.

Points of interest
● Cholestin is considered a dietary supplement.
● Red yeast rice has been used in China since A.D. 800 to make red rice wine, to preserve and enhance food, and as a medicinal substance.
● Written records from the Ming dynasty (1368-1644) show that red yeast rice was believed to improve blood circulation and reduce clotting.

Commentary
Red yeast rice appears to be well tolerated and effective in lowering cholesterol levels. It is sold in the United States as a dietary supplement.

Until more clinical studies are performed, red yeast rice should be treated as an HMG-CoA reductase inhibitor. This includes potential adverse effects, drug interactions, and precautions associated with this drug class. Studies to evaluate the long-term safety and efficacy of this supplement in larger populations are needed.

References

Heber, D., et al. "Cholesterol-lowering Effects of a Proprietary Chinese Red-Yeast-Rice Dietary Supplement," *Am J Clin Nutr* 69:231-36, 1999.

Li, C., et al. "*Monascus purpureus*-fermented Rice (Red Yeast Rice): A Natural Food Product That Lowers Blood Cholesterol in Animal Models of Hypercholesterolemia," *Nutr Res* 18:71-81, 1988.

O'Mathuna, D. "Cholestin for the Treatment of Hypercholesterolemia," *Alternative Medicine Alert* 2(4):37-41, 1999.

Rippe, J., et al. "A Multi-center, Self-controlled Study of Cholestin in Subjects with Elevated Cholesterol," American Heart Association, 39th Annual Conference on Cardiovascular Disease Epidemiology and Prevention. March 24-27, 1999. Orlando, Fla.

Wang, J., et al. "Multicenter Trial of the Serum Lipid-lowering Effects of a *Monascus purpureus* (Red Yeast) Rice Preparation from Traditional Chinese Medicine," *Curr Ther Res* 58:964-78, 1997.

Wiiger-Alberti, W., et al. "Anaphylaxis Due to *Monascus purpureus*-fermented Rice (Red Yeast Rice)," *Allergy* 54:1330-31, 1999.

Zhiwei, S., et al. "A Prospective Trial of Extract of *Monascus purpureus* (Red Yeast) in the Treatment of Primary Hyperlipidemia," *Natl Med J China* 76:156-57, 1996.

RHATANY

KRAMERIA ROOT, MAPATO, PERUVIAN RHATANY, PUMACUCHU, RAIZ PARA LOS DIENTES, RATANHIAWURZEL, RED RHATANY, RHATANIA

Taxonomic class
Krameriaceae

Common trade names
Echtrosept-GT, Encialina, Gengivario, Parodontax, Repha-OS

Common forms
Available as a lozenge, mouthwash, powder, solution, syrup, and tincture.

Source
The active ingredients are extracted from the dried root of *Krameria triandra*, also known as pumacuchu or mapato.

Chemical components
The agent is composed primarily of 10% to 20% tannins. Rhataniatannic acid, also known as krameria tannic acid, is the principal tannin extracted from the plant.

Actions
Rhatany is a tannin-containing herb that functions as an astringent. The primary mechanism of action for astringents is the coagulation of surface proteins of cells (Swinyard and Pathak, 1985), which decreases cell permeability and reduces secretions of inflamed tissues. The coagulated surface proteins function as a protective barrier on skin surfaces and help to promote growth of new tissue underneath. In areas of inflammation, astringents cause vasoconstriction and reduce blood flow. Astringents cool and dry skin surfaces when applied as wet dressings; they also clean the skin of surface exudates and debris.

Reported uses
Therapeutic claims for rhatany are derived from the plant's astringent properties. They are claimed to be useful in treating conditions that involve irritations of the skin, mucous membranes, and gingiva. Both internal and external preparations of rhatany are thought to have medicinal uses. Specific applications have included treatment of bleeding gums, bowel and bladder bleeding, canker sores, diarrhea, dysentery, inflammatory disorders of the oropharynx, pyorrhea, and urinary incontinence. Clinical trials supporting the safety and efficacy of rhatany in treating these conditions are lacking.

Dosage
Numerous doses involving several forms have been prepared, but clinical trials establishing standard doses of rhatany are lacking. The German Commission E recommends the decoction to be taken P.O. (1 g in 1 cup of water) or 5 to 10 gtt of tincture in 1 glass of water.
For topical use, apply b.i.d. or t.i.d.

Adverse reactions
GI: *acute hepatotoxicity* (with tannic acid).
Skin: allergic contact dermatitis (Goday Bujan et al., 1998).

Interactions
Disulfiram: Disulfiram reaction if the tincture product contains alcohol. Avoid administration with rhatany.

Contraindications and precautions
Rhatany is contraindicated in patients who are hypersensitive to products that contain the plant or its components. Avoid use of rhatany-containing products that have high concentrations of tannins. Tannic acid–containing products are generally considered unsafe and ineffective, and frequent ingestion of such products could result in absorption of tannic acid from the GI tract, increasing the risk of hepatotoxicity. Also, chronic topical administration may sufficiently denude mucosal surfaces and mucous membranes to cause damage.

Special considerations
• Monitor liver function test results.
• Caution the patient taking disulfiram not to take the tincture form of rhatany.
• Advise the patient to report signs and symptoms of hepatic dysfunction (fatigue, fever, jaundice).

Points of interest
• Only two astringent solutions—aluminum acetate and witch hazel—are considered safe and effective by the FDA for treating minor skin irritations (West and Nowakowski, 1996). The FDA has ruled that no ingredient in rhatany is generally recognized as safe and effective for use as an OTC oral wound-healing agent (Flynn, 1996).

Commentary
Rhatany is a tannin-containing plant that is claimed to have several medicinal applications as an astringent. Well-controlled clinical trials supporting its safety and efficacy are lacking. Internal and external use of rhatany are probably best avoided until more information is available.

References
Flynn, A.A. "Oral Health Products," in *Handbook of Nonprescription Drugs*, 9th ed. Edited by Covington, T.R., et al. Washington, D.C.: United Book Press, Inc., 1996.

Goday Bujan, J.J., et al. "Allergic Contact Dermatitis from *Krameria triandra* Extract," *Contact Dermatitis* 38(2):120-21, 1998.

Swinyard, E.A., and Pathak, M.A. "Locally Acting Drugs," in *Goodman and Gilman's: The Pharmacological Basis of Therapeutics*, 7th ed. Edited by Goodman, L.S., et al. New York: Macmillan, 1985.

West, D.P., and Nowakowski, P.A. "Dermatitis," in *Handbook of Nonprescription Drugs*, 9th ed. Edited by Covington, T.R., et al. Washington, D.C.: United Book Press, Inc., 1996.

ROSE HIPS

DOG ROSE FRUIT, DOG BRIER FRUIT, HIPBERRIES, WILD BRIER BERRIES

Taxonomic class
Rosaceae

Common trade names
Multi-ingredient preparations: Rose Hips, Vitamin C with Rose Hips

Common forms
Available as capsules, cream, extracts, syrup, tablets, teas, and tincture in combination with vitamin preparations.

Source
The rose hip, or fruit of *Rosa canina,* is usually dried and processed before use. The plant grows widely in North America after having been

---

naturalized from Europe and Asia. *R. canina* is the major source of rose hips, but other Rosaceae plants have also been used.

Chemical components
Rose hips contain significant vitamin C, tannins, pectins, and carotene (carotenoids).

Actions
The *R. canina* flower petal extract containing anthocyans was shown to have a protective effect on radiation-induced cell damage in Chinese hamster cells (Akhmadieva et al., 1993). The roots of *R. canina* showed anti-inflammatory effects in vitro. This anti-inflammatory activity was also exhibited by several plant extracts used in Turkish traditional medicine when they exerted effects on either tumor necrosis factor or interleukin-1 (Yesilada et al., 1997).

Although rose hips is claimed to have a diuretic effect, this effect was not seen in rats (Grases et al., 1992). An infusion of *R. canina* may have some benefit on calcium oxalate urolithiasis.

Reported uses
A natural source of vitamin C (Brand et al., 1982), rose hips has been claimed to be useful as a laxative, capillary strengthener, and boost to the immune system to prevent illness. Although vitamin C has been studied for these effects, studies on rose hips are lacking. Some herbal references claim that the leaves have been used as a poultice to heal wounds.

Dosage
No consensus exists.

Adverse reactions
GI: diarrhea.
GU: renal dysfunction (poorly documented).
Skin: skin irritation (from topical applications).
Other: allergic reaction (Kwaselow et al., 1990).

Interactions
Estrogens and oral contraceptives: Increased serum levels of these drugs. Monitor for adverse effects.
Iron: May enhance absorption of oral iron products. Monitor patient.
Warfarin: May antagonize effects of warfarin. Monitor concurrent therapy.

Contraindications and precautions
Avoid using rose hips in pregnant or breast-feeding patients; effects are unknown. Use cautiously in patients with atopy or plant allergies. Vitamin C supplements typically should be avoided in people with a

history of kidney stones because high doses of vitamin C may lead to increased urinary oxalate production and an increased risk of stone formation.

Special considerations
• In diabetic patients, high doses of rose hips may cause false-negative urine glucose determinations (due to vitamin C content).
• Advise the patient to take sources of vitamin C from reliable manufacturers; rose hips (after processing) may represent only a minor and variable source of vitamin C.
• Advise the patient with plant allergies to pursue other sources of vitamin C.
• Large doses of rose hips may cause false-negative results on stool occult blood and urine glucose tests. Instruct the patient to discontinue ingestion of rose hips at least 48 hours before taking stool occult blood test.

Points of interest
• Rose hips contain more vitamin C per milligram than many citrus fruits and raw broccoli. However, much of the vitamin C contained in rose hips (more than 50%) may be destroyed during processing. More than 100 g of actual rose hips may be needed to obtain 1,200 mg of vitamin C. Thus, many products that contain rose hips are supplemented with synthetically prepared vitamin C.
• Although a German monograph supported the use of rose hips for preventing colds and flu, the data seem questionable.

Commentary
Despite the herb's vitamin C content, large quantities of rose hips must be ingested to obtain commonly available amounts of vitamin C in tablet form.

References
Akhmadieva, A.Kh., et al. "The Protective Action of a Natural Preparation of Anthocyan (Pelargonidin-3,5-diglucoside)," *Radiobiologia* 33:433-35, 1993.

Brand, J.C., et al. "An Outstanding Food Source of Vitamin C," *Lancet* 16:873, 1982. Letter.

Grases, F., et al. "Effect of *Rosa canina* Infusion and Magnesium on the Urinary Risk Factors of Calcium Oxalate Urolithiasis," *Planta Med* 58:509-12, 1992.

Kwaselow, A., et al. "Rose Hips: A New Occupational Allergen," *J Allergy Clin Immunol* 85:704-8, 1990.

Yesilada, E., et al. "Inhibitory Effects of Turkish Folk Remedies on Inflammatory Cytokines: Interleukin-1alpha, Interleukin-1beta, and Tumor Necrosis Factor," *J Ethnopharmacol* 58:59-73, 1997.

ROSEMARY

COMPASS PLANT, INCENSOR, OLD MAN

Taxonomic class
Lamiaceae

Common trade names
Rosemary Oil

Common forms
Available as infusion, tea, or volatile oil and in bath
and toiletry products.

Source
The leaves, twigs, and flowering tops are typically
pursued for active medicinal components of
Rosmarinus officinalis. Rosemary is native to the
Mediterranean region but commonly cultivated indoors and
in mild climates of North America.

Chemical components
The leaves contain a volatile oil, from which several compounds have
been isolated (monoterpene hydrocarbons, camphor, borneol, and cineole). The leaves also contain the flavonoid pigments diosmin, diosmetin, and genkwanin. Numerous volatile and aromatic compounds
are also present.

Actions
Several pharmacologic effects have been described for rosemary or its
components. Antibacterial and antifungal properties have been demonstrated for the volatile oil. Various gram-positive and gram-negative organisms commonly responsible for food spoilage are inhibited by the
presence of rosemary oil. The antioxidant properties are attributed to
carnosol and ursol components of rosemary oil or rosmarinic acid and
caffeic acid.

Several sources report that diosmin reduces capillary permeability
and fragility, whereas a derivative of rosemaricine is capable of inducing
smooth-muscle relaxant and analgesic effects in vitro (al-Sereiti et al.,
1999). I.V. administration of rosemary oil has demonstrated spasmolytic action on the Oddi muscle sphincter of guinea pigs. Rabbit models of
septic shock have shown that I.V. rosmarinic acid suppresses endotox-
in-mediated activation of the sequence of steps leading to septic shock.
It also suppresses release of thromboxane A_2, formation of prostacyclin,
thrombocytopenia, and hypotension (Bult et al., 1985). Although these
effects are believed to be the result of the inhibitory effect of rosmarinic
acid on complement (a component of blood), other studies have suggested other mechanisms of anti-inflammatory activity (Parnham and
Kesselring, 1985).

Rosmarinic acid has also been touted as the component responsible for successful prevention of adult respiratory distress syndrome in rabbit models (Parnham and Kesselring, 1985). Additional rodent studies of rosemary oil and rosmarinic acid have demonstrated increased locomotor effects and antigonadotropic effects, respectively.

Rosmarinic acid has demonstrated inhibitory activity against HIV integrase (Kim et al., 1999).

A number of studies have been published that suggest potential anticancer properties of the plant. These preliminary studies suggest that rosemary components have the potential to decrease activation and increase detoxification of important human carcinogens. Rosemary components might have potential as chemoprotectants, but studies in humans are needed (Huang et al., 1994; Oxford et al., 1997, al-Sereiti et al., 1999).

Reported uses

The clinical effects of rosemary are not well known; few studies have been conducted in humans. Rosemary is widely used as a spice in cooking. It has been claimed to be of use in traditional medicine for its antiflatulent, antispasmodic, astringent, diaphoretic, and tonic properties.

Rosemary extract and the volatile oil have been used through the centuries to promote menstrual flow and as an abortifacient. Rosemary oil has been used topically and taken internally to improve chronic circulatory weakness and hypotension, although a few tertiary references warn against internal consumption of the undiluted volatile oil. Rosemary has also been used for indigestion and rheumatic disorders; efficacy is yet to be demonstrated.

A lotion consisting of rosemary has been suggested to stimulate hair growth and prevent baldness, although this has not been proved.

Dosage

Therapeutic doses of rosemary have not been defined, but the following have been promoted:

Liquid extract (1:1 in 45% alcohol): 1 to 4 ml P.O. t.i.d.

Tea: 1 to 4 g of the leaf as a tea P.O. t.i.d.

Essential oil in an ointment preparation may also be used externally.

Adverse reactions

GI: GI irritation (with large quantities of volatile oil).

GU: antifertility effects (rosemary oil may prevent implantation but does not appear to interfere with the normal development of the fertilized ova after implantation [Lemonica et al., 1996]), renal damage (with large quantities of volatile oil).

Skin: dermatitis and photosensitivity in hypersensitive people, erythema (possible with preparations meant for bathing).

Interactions

Disulfiram: Disulfiram reaction if herbal product contains alcohol. Do not use together.

Bold italic type indicates that reaction may be life-threatening.

Contraindications and precautions

Avoid using rosemary in pregnant or breast-feeding patients; effects are unknown. Use cautiously in patients who have experienced a plant sensitivity reaction.

Special considerations

• Inform the patient that therapeutic efficacy has not been demonstrated for rosemary or its components for any disease.
• Caution the patient that the undiluted oil should not be taken internally until its safety can be established.
• Caution women who wants to become pregnant to avoid consumption of this herb.
• Advise the patient taking disulfiram not to take a form of this herb that contains alcohol.

Points of interest

• German health authorities have approved rosemary for internal use for indigestion and as a supportive treatment for rheumatic disorders. It is also approved for external use for circulatory disorders.
• A review on the therapeutic potential of the pharmacologic constituents of *R. officinalis* has been published (al-Sereiti et al., 1999).
• Rosemary extract may function as an effective food preservative for meat products (Karpinska et al., 2000).

Commentary

Rosemary is widely used in both cooking and cosmetics. Several components of rosemary oil have been shown to possess pharmacologic activity. Enthusiasm for some interesting pharmacologic effects seen in animals must be interpreted in light of the fact that studies in humans are unavailable. Until studies are conducted in humans, this herb cannot be recommended for any therapeutic application. Future areas of research will probably focus on the potential of rosemary in treating acute inflammatory conditions, such as adult respiratory distress syndrome and septic shock, or as a chemotherapeutic agent.

References

Bult, H., et al. "Modification of Endotoxin-induced Hemodynamic and Hematologic Changes in the Rabbit by Methylprednisolone, F(ab')2 Fragments and Rosmarinic Acid," *Biochem Pharmacol* 35:1397-1400, 1985.

Huang, M.T., et al. "Inhibition of Skin Tumorigenesis by Rosemary and Its Constituents Carnosol and Ursolic Acid," *Cancer Res* 54:701-8, 1994.

Karpinska, M. et al. "Antioxidative Activity of Rosemary Extract in Lipid Fraction of Minced Meat Balls During Storage in a Freezer," *Nahrung* 44(1):38-41, 2000.

Kim, H.K., et al. "HIV Integrase Activity of *Agastache rugosa*," *Arch Pharm Res* 22(5):520-23, 1999.

Lemonica, I.P., et al. "Study of the Embryotoxic Effects of an Extract of Rosemary (*Rosmarinus officinalis* L.)," *Brit J Med Biol Res* 29:223-27, 1996. Abstract.

Oxford, E.A., et al. "Mechanisms Involved in the Chemoprotective Effects of Rosemary Extract Studied in Human Liver and Bronchial Cells," *Cancer Lett* 114:275-81, 1997.

Parnham, M.J., and Kesselring, K. "Rosmarinic Acid," *Drugs Future* 10:756-57, 1985.

al-Sereiti, M.R., et al. "Pharmacology of Rosemary (*Rosmarinus officinalis* L.) and Its Therapeutic Potentials," *Indian J Exp Biol* 37(2):124-30, 1999.

ROYAL JELLY

QUEEN BEE JELLY

Common trade names
Royal Jelly

Common forms
Available in ampules (100 mg), capsules (100 mg, 300 mg, 500 mg, 1,000 mg), topical cream, lotion, ointment, and soap.

Source
Royal jelly is a milky white secretion formulated by worker bees of *Apis melliferis* and fed to the queen bee to induce her growth and development.

Chemical components
Royal jelly consists of a mixture of complex proteins, sugars, fats, water, fatty acids, carbohydrates, and variable amounts of vitamins (A, B, C, and E) and minerals (potassium, calcium, zinc, iron, manganese, and acetylcholine). The B vitamins are especially prominent, with pantothenic acid expression predominating (Vittek, 1995). Royal jelly also provides about 20 amino acids and contains gamma globulin. A substance known as 10-hydroxy-trans-(2)-decanoic acid (HDA) has been identified and is thought to play an important role in bee growth and regulation.

Actions
Clinical trials have noted some antimicrobial activity in royal jelly, attributed to HDA and gamma globulin. The activity is found to be 25% less effective than penicillin and 20% less active than chlortetracycline.

Preliminary studies found antitumorigenic activity in experimental mouse leukemias using royal jelly. Published reports suggest that royal jelly may be effective in preventing atherosclerosis. It significantly influences lipid metabolism in rats and prevents atherosclerosis in rabbits fed cholesterol-rich diets.

Serum cholesterol levels were reduced up to 25% in humans. Because of an abundance of phytosterols (mainly beta-sitosterol), royal jelly is thought to decrease the resorption of cholesterol in the GI tract. (Both beta-sitosterol and cholesterol compete for binding sites.) Researchers have reported a significant reduction in serum total lipid and cholesterol levels and normalization of HDL and LDL levels (Vittek, 1995).

Reported uses
Queen bees are twice the size of worker bees, are fertile (worker bees are sterile), and live 5 to 8 years longer than worker bees, all of which may

---

Bold italic type indicates that reaction may be life-threatening.

contribute to the purported claims of royal jelly. Royal jelly does not provide any estrogenic effects that promote fertility, growth, or longevity. The agent's effectiveness in rejuvenating the skin and slowing the aging process (erasing wrinkles and facial blemishes) has not been substantiated.

Although there is no evidence for it, royal jelly has also been claimed to be useful for treating male-pattern baldness and menopause and for improving sexual performance. A cholesterol-lowering action has been reported in humans. Although royal jelly has demonstrated in vitro antimicrobial activity, no clinical trials have been reported for this indication.

Dosage
For cosmetic use, apply royal jelly topically b.i.d. or t.i.d.
For lowering cholesterol levels, 50 to 100 mg P.O. daily.

Adverse reactions
Metabolic: hyperglycemia.
Respiratory: *exacerbation of asthma; bronchospasm* in asthmatic patients.
Other: *allergic reaction.*

Interactions
Antidiabetics: May lead to loss of glycemic control in diabetic patients. Avoid administration with royal jelly.

Contraindications and precautions
Avoid use of royal jelly in pregnant or breast-feeding patients; effects are unknown. Use cautiously in patients who are susceptible to allergic reactions or asthma and in those taking antidiabetic drugs.

Special considerations
• Monitor blood glucose levels closely because royal jelly may contribute to loss of glycemic control in diabetic patients.
• Counsel the patient with atopy against using this agent. Royal jelly has been responsible for IgE-mediated anaphylaxis, leading to death in at least one person (Bullock et al., 1994; Harwood et al., 1996).
• Inform the asthmatic patient that life-threatening bronchospasm has occurred after ingestion of this agent.
• Advise women to report planned or suspected pregnancy.

Commentary
Death has occurred by bronchospasm with the use of royal jelly in asthmatic patients. The agent may reduce cholesterol levels in humans, but long-term evidence is lacking and the availability of clinically proven agents limits royal jelly's usefulness for this condition. Insufficient data and poorly documented risk profiles for royal jelly make it unsuitable for use.

References

Bullock, R.J., et al. "Fatal Royal Jelly Induced Asthma," *Med J Aust* 160:44, 1994.

Harwood, M., et al. "Asthma Following Royal Jelly," *N Z Med J* 23:325, 1996.

Vittek, J. "Effect of Royal Jelly on Serum Lipids in Experimental Animals and Humans with Atherosclerosis," *Experientia* 51:927-35, 1995.

RUE

HERB-OF-GRACE, HERBYGRASS, RUTA, RUTAE HERBA, VINRUTA

Taxonomic class
Rutaceae

Common trade names
Multi-ingredient preparations: Joint and Muscle Relief Cream, Rue-Fennel Compound, Rue Herb Liquid

Common forms
Available as astringent, capsules, creams, crude herb, and extracts.

Source
Rue, or *Ruta graveolens,* although cultivated in Europe, America, Asia, and Africa, is native to the Mediterranean region. This small evergreen shrub with blue-green foliage and small yellow conical flowers is generally considered to have a disagreeable odor. Both the leaves and the root have been used.

Chemical components
Numerous specific chemical entities have been isolated from *R. graveolens,* including 2-nonanone, 2-undecanone, chalepensin, quinoline alkaloids (arborinine, ribalinidin), furocoumarins (bergapten, xanthoxanthin, daphnoretin, rutamarin), gamma-eagarine, lignanes, (helioxanthine) volatile oils (geijerene), and psoralens.

Actions
Rue extracts have been shown to possess antimicrobial effects. On a cellular level, rue has demonstrated both mutagenic and cytotoxic actions in numerous models. Studies in mammals have demonstrated an antifertility action, mediated by decreased implantation in rodents (Ghandi et al., 1991). An abortifacient action has also been noted. Components of rue nonselectively block potassium and sodium channels in myelinated nerves (Bethge et al., 1991).

Rue has also demonstrated CV effects in rats. It exhibits positive chronotropic and inotropic effects in isolated rat atria (Chui and Fung, 1997). It acts as a hypotensive agent in normotensive animals, presumably through a direct vasodilatory mechanism. The alkaloids present in rue have demonstrated antispasmodic effects. Rue also exhibits analgesic properties in mice proved by the acetic acid and hot plate para-

---

digms (Atta and Alkofahi, 1998). Methanolic extracts of rue have been shown to increase nerve growth factor activity as well (Li et al., 1999).

Reported uses

Rue has traditionally been promoted as an abortifacient and a spasmolytic. It has also been used for its sedative effects and to promote lactation. Based on anecdotal data and studies in animals, the herb is being promoted for treating arthritis, bruising, sports injuries, sprains and strains, and other joint and muscle disorders. No human clinical trial data are available for these uses.

Many herbal preparation manufacturers also promote rue for use in amenorrhea, digestive disorders, dysmenorrhea, earache, edema, eye strain, and neuralgia and as an anthelmintic. Rue has also been used by Chinese herbalists for snake and insect bites. These claims also lack supporting data.

Dosage

No clinical studies establish a safe dose for rue. Some references recommend the following:

For earache, a few drops of infused oil on a cotton plug placed over the ear.

Capsule: 1 capsule P.O. t.i.d. with water and food.

Cream: applied as needed.

Extract: ¼ to 1 tsp P.O. t.i.d. with water and food.

Adverse reactions

CV: hypotension.

Skin: allergic skin reactions (erythema, hyperpigmentation, and severe blistering) with topical use, photosensitivity.

Other: increased risk of spontaneous abortion.

Interactions

Antihypertensives: May increase vasodilatory effects. Use with caution.

Digoxin, dobutamine: Increased inotropic effects and negative chronotropic effects. Use with caution.

Fertility drugs: May counteract therapy. Avoid administration with rue.

Warfarin: May potentiate effects of warfarin and other anticoagulants. Monitor coagulation parameters more intensively (Heck et al., 2000).

Contraindications and precautions

Avoid using rue in pregnant patients because of the risk of abortion. Use cautiously in patients with a history of heart failure or arrhythmias and in those receiving antihypertensives.

Special considerations and precautions

- Monitor for cumulative effects in patients taking antihypertensives.
- Rue is thought to be a powerful antidote at low doses; larger doses are toxic.
- Inform the patient that there is insufficient information regarding the effects of rue in humans. The risks of use outweigh the benefits.

• Advise women to report planned or suspected pregnancy.
• Instruct the patient to discontinue use of the herb and to notify the health care provider of allergic skin reactions.

Commentary

Preliminary studies in animals show that rue has many interesting pharmacologic effects. Insufficient testing in humans makes any therapeutic application premature. The strong potential for contact dermatitis severely restricts topical use of this agent. In Germany, rue is considered ineffective and unsafe. Rue cannot be recommended for any use.

References

Atta, A.H., and Alkofahi, A. "Anti-nociceptive and Anti-inflammatory Effects of Some Jordanian Medicinal Plant Extracts," *J Ethnopharmacol* 60:117-24, 1998.

Bethge, E.W., et al. "Effects of Some Potassium Channel Blockers on the Ionic Currents in Myelinated Nerve," *Gen Physiol Biophys* 10:225-44, 1991.

Chui, K.W., and Fung, A.Y. "The Cardiovascular Effects of Green Beans (*Phaseolus aureus*), Common Rue (*Ruta graveolens*), and Kelp (*Laminaria japonica*) in Rats," *Gen Pharmacol* 29:859-62, 1997.

Ghandi, M., et al. "Post-coital Antifertility Action of *Ruta graveolens* in Female Rats and Hamsters," *J Ethnopharmacol* 34:49-59, 1991.

Heck, A.M., et al. "Potential Interactions Between Alternative Therapies and Warfarin," *Am J Health Systems Pharm* 57(13):1221-27, 2000.

Heskel, N.S., et al. "Phytophotodermatitis Due to *Ruta graveolens*," *Contact Dermatitis* 9(4):278-80, 1983.

Li, P., et al. "Enhancement of the Nerve Growth Factor-meditaed Neurite Outgrowth from PC12D Cells by Chinese and Paraguayan Medicinal Plants," *Biol Pharm Bull* 22(7):752-55, 1999.

Paulini, H., et al. "Mutagenic Compounds in an Extract from *Rutae herba* (*Ruta graveolens* L.)," *Mutagenesis* 2(4):271-73, 1987.

Schempp, C.M., et al. "Bullous Photoxic Contact Dermatitis Caused by *Ruta graveolens* L. (garden rue), *Rutaceae*. Case Report and Review of Literature," *Hautarzt* 50(6):432-34, 1999.

Stashenko, E.E., et al. "High Resolution Gas-Chromatographic Analysis of the Secondary Metabolites Obtained by Subcritical-Fluid Extraction from Colombian Rue," *J Biochem Biophys Methods* 43(1-3):379-90, 2000.

Trovato, A., et al. "In Vitro Cytotoxic Effect of Some Medicinal Plants Containing Flavonoids," *Boll Chim Farm* 135(4):263-66, 1996.

Tyler, V.E. "Rue," in *The Honest Herbal*, 3rd ed. New York: Pharmaceutical Products Press, 1993.

Wessner, D., et al. "Phytophotodermatitis Due to *Ruta graveolens* Applied as Protection Against Evil Spells," *Contact Dermatitis* 41(4):232, 1999.

Wolters, B., and Eilert, U. "Antimicrobial Substances in Callus Cultures of *Ruta graveolens*," *Planta Med* 43(2):166-74, 1981.

Bold italic type indicates that reaction may be life-threatening.

SAFFLOWER

AMERICAN SAFFRON, AZAFRAN, BASTARD SAFFRON,
BENIBANA, DYER'S SAFFRON, FAKE SAFFRON

Taxonomic class
Asteraceae

Common trade names
Multi-ingredient preparations: Safflower Oil, Saffron

Common forms
Available as capsules (390 mg), extracts, liquid (8.5 oz), oil (12 oz,
16 oz), and tea.

Source
Carthamus tinctorius is indigenous to the Middle East but cultivated
throughout Europe and the United States for its edible oil, which is obtained from the seeds.

Chemical components
The oil consists of unsaturated fatty acids, including linoleic acid
(75%), oleic acid (13%), palmitic acid (6%), stearic acid (3%), and a
mixture of saturated fatty acids. The flowers of the plant contain a dye,
carthamin. Seven antioxidant compounds have been isolated from *C.
tinctorius.*

Actions
Safflower oil, considered a long-chain triglyceride, may exert an effect
on the reticuloendothelial system. The linoleic acid portions of the oil
(polyunsaturated fatty acids) are converted into immunosuppressants,
prostaglandin E_2, and prostaglandin I_2 within the prostaglandin pathway (Sax, 1990).

Rats that were fed a diet high in safflower oil appeared to become in-
sulin-resistant (Ellis et al., 2000).

Reported uses
Safflower is used to treat constipation and fever. The oil has been compounded with glycerin, rose oil, polysorbate 80, benzyl alcohol, and water to produce an external massage lotion. The topical administration of
safflower oil in patients with essential fatty acid deficiency failed to
show improvement in critically ill patients, but previous studies have
supported this use in stable outpatients and chronically ill patients
(Sacks et al., 1994).

A diet high in safflower oil has been shown to reduce total cholesterol and LDL levels in some cases (Wardlaw et al., 1991; Herbel et al., 1998).

In Chinese herbal medicine, safflower has been used to treat menstrual disorders.

A 6-month study designed to determine the clinical benefit, if any, of dietary intervention with omega-3 fatty acids (fish oil capsules + canola oil and margarine) or omega-6 fatty acids (safflower oil capsules + sunflower oil and margarine) on asthma severity in 39 children failed to identify a significant difference between the two types of dietary interventions. Notably, no placebo group was included in the study (Hodge et al., 1998).

Dosage
Dried flower: 2 to 3 g P.O. t.i.d.
Extract: 3 g of dried flower in 15 ml of alcohol and 15 ml of water P.O. t.i.d.
Fresh flower: 1 or 2 tbsp P.O. t.i.d.

Adverse reactions
None reported.

Interactions
Immunosuppressants (azathioprine, cyclosporine, tacrolimus): Safflower oil may enhance the immunosuppressive effects of these drugs. Monitor the patient closely if administered together.
Vaccines: May cause immunosuppressive effects. Avoid concurrent use.

Contraindications and precautions
Use safflower cautiously in immunosuppressed patients, especially burn or septic patients and transplant recipients. Avoid excessive consumption of safflower in pregnant or breast-feeding patients. Murine models have shown safflower to be a uterine stimulant (Shi et al., 1995). Dietary intake of fatty acids in the form of safflower oil has been shown to rapidly increase (within hours) fatty acid concentrations in human breast milk (Francois et al., 1998). The significance of this effect is unknown.

Special considerations
• Do not administer vaccines to patients who are using safflower because of its potential immunosuppressive effects.
• Inform the patient that with the exception of cholesterol reduction, most studies have failed to support therapeutic applications for safflower oil.
• Counsel the patient using safflower oil for its lipid-lowering effects to change to other, more effective and universally proven cholesterol-lowering therapies.

Points of interest
• Safflower oil or linoleic acid may be a component of commercially available lipid emulsions.

Bold italic type indicates that reaction may be life-threatening.

● Safflower (*C. tinctorius*) should not be confused with true saffron (*Crocus sativus*).

Commentary

Safflower is used primarily as a source of edible polyunsaturated oil. It has been used in teas to reduce fever by inducing sweating and as a laxative, but there is no supporting evidence for these uses. Although a diet rich in safflower oil has been shown to lower cholesterol levels, it has not been proven to reduce the incidence of CV mortality; therefore, safflower oil remains an adjunct to other, proven therapies.

References

Ellis, B.A., et al. "Long-chain Acyl-CoA-Esters as Indidators of Lipid Metabolism and Insulin Sensitivity in Rat and Human Muscle," *Am J Physiol Endocrinol Metab* 279(3):E554-60, 2000.

Francois, C.A., et al. "Acute Effects of Dietary Fatty Acids on the Fatty Acids of Human Milk," *Am J Clin Nutr* 67(2):301-8, 1998.

Herbel, B.K., et al. "Safflower Oil Consumption Does Not Increase Plasma Conjugated Linoleic Acid Concentrations in Humans," *Am J Clin Nutr* 67(2):332-37, 1998.

Hodge, L., et al. "Effect of Dietary Intake of Omega-3 and Omega-6 Fatty Acids on Severity of Asthma in Children," *Eur J Respir J* 11(2):361-65, 1998.

Sacks, G.S., et al. "Failure of Topical Vegetable Oils to Prevent Essential Fatty Acid Deficiency in a Critically Ill Patient Receiving Long-term Parenteral Nutrition," *JPEN* 18:274-77, 1994.

Sax, H.C. "Practicalities of Lipids: ICU Patient, Autoimmune Disease, and Vascular Disease," *JPEN* 14:223S-25S, 1990.

Shi, M., et al. "Stimulating Action of *Carthamus tinctorius* L., *Angelica sinensis*, (Oliv) Diels and *Leonurus sibiricus* L. on the Uterus," *Chung Kuo Chung Yao Tsa Chih* 20:173-75,192, 1995.

Wardlaw, G.M., et al. "Serum Lipid and Apolipoprotein Concentrations in Healthy Men on Diets Enriched in Either Canola Oil or Safflower Oil," *Am J Clin Nutr* 54:104, 1991.

SAFFRON

INDIAN SAFFRON, KESAR, KUM KUMA, TRUE SAFFRON, ZAFFRON

Taxonomic class

Iridaceae

Common trade names

None known.

Common forms

Available as crude powder.

Source

Saffron is derived from the dried stigmas and tops of styles of *Crocus sativus*, which is indigenous to southern Europe and Asia Minor.

Chemical components

Saffron contains several compounds, including carotenoids such as crocines, crocetins, picrocrocin, and dimethyl-crocetin. Hydrolysis of the agent results in the production of safranal and glucose. An essential oil may also be produced.

Actions

The components of saffron have been shown to be cytotoxic in vitro to human carcinoma, sarcoma, and leukemia cells (Escribano et al., 1996; Nair et al., 1995). This effect is believed to be dose-dependent and attributed to the carotenoid components, specifically dimethyl-crocetin. The crocetin component of saffron appears to increase the diffusion of oxygen in plasma, possibly by as much as 80% (Grisolia, 1974). This action may prevent atherosclerosis secondary to vascular wall hypoxia and a subsequent decrease in RBC diffusion of oxygen. Antioxidant properties were later described in humans in a study of 20 patients (Verma and Bordia, 1998). Fifty-milligram doses of saffron dissolved in milk and given twice daily significantly reduced mean lipoprotein oxidation susceptibility for 10 healthy patients and 10 patients with existing coronary disease as compared with their own baseline data. The ultimate clinical significance of this effect is unknown.

Saffron also is reported to have immunomodulating effects, but supporting data are lacking.

Reported uses

Saffron has been used as a diaphoretic, an expectorant, and a sedative. In some parts of Asia, it has been made into a paste and used to treat dry skin. It is also thought to have some aphrodisiac effects. Clinical trials supporting these claims do not exist. Its use is primarily as a coloring and flavoring agent.

Dosage

No consensus exists. Saffron may be ingested by mixing the powder with food or brewing it as a tea.

Adverse reactions

None reported with culinary doses (under 1.5 g). The following reactions have been documented with doses above 5 g:
CNS: vertigo.
CV: *bradycardia.*
EENT: epistaxis.
GI: vomiting.
GU: menorrhagia (less frequent).
Skin: facial flushing.
Other: spontaneous abortion (rare).

Interactions

None reported.

Bold italic type indicates that reaction may be life-threatening.

Contraindications and precautions
Saffron is contraindicated in pregnant women because of the risk of spontaneous abortion. Avoid using this compound in breast-feeding patients; effects are unknown.

Special considerations
• Recommend that the patient maintain doses of less than 5 g daily to minimize the risk of adverse reactions.
• Instruct the patient to immediately report unusual signs or symptoms to his primary health care provider.
• Inform the patient that evidence to support therapeutic applications for saffron is insufficient and that its risks are not well described.

Points of interest
• A combination of saffron with quinine and opium has received a patent in Germany for inhibiting premature ejaculation.

Commentary
Although saffron has been used safely as a food additive for many years, its use as a medicinal agent remains to be determined. Until adequate human trials can be conducted, the use of saffron to prevent or treat cancer or CV conditions cannot be recommended.

References
Escribano, J., et al. "Crocin, Safranal, and Picrocrocin from Saffron (*Crocus sativus* L.) Inhibit the Growth of Human Cancer Cells In Vitro," *Cancer Lett* 100:23-30, 1996.
Grisolia, S. "Hypoxia, Saffron and Cardiovascular Disease," *Lancet* 7871:41, 1974.
Nair, S.C., et al. "Saffron Chemoprevention in Biology and Medicine: A Review," *Cancer Biother* 10:257-64, 1995.
Verma, S.K., and Bordia, A. "Antioxidant Property of Saffron in Man," *Indian J Med Sci* 52(5):205-7, 1998.

SAGE

DALMATIAN, GARDEN SAGE, MEADOW SAGE, SCARLET SAGE, TREE SAGE

Taxonomic class
Lamiaceae

Common trade names
None known.

Source
Active components are extracted from the *Salvia officinalis* plant. A perennial plant with violet-blue flowers, it is native to southern Europe but now cultivated in North America.

Chemical components
Components include caffeic acid, carnosol, chlorogenic acid, ellagic, ferulic acid, rosemarinic, tannins, picrosalvin, and salvin. About 1% to

2.8% of the plant is composed of volatile oil, and 30% to 50% of that oil is either alpha- or beta-thujones.

Actions

Sage extract and oil have been shown to have antispasmodic activity in the guinea pig ileum, CNS depressant effects in mice, and hypotensive activity in cats (Todorov et al., 1984). The herb's antimicrobial activity in vitro is attributed to the alpha- and beta-thujone component. The antimicrobial action was evident for *Bacillus subtilis, Escherichia coli, Klebsiella ozanea, Salmonella* species, *Shigella sonnei,* and various fungi species (Meier et al., 1994).

One study conducted in rabbits showed a hypoglycemic effect from sage ingestion (Cabo et al., 1985).

Reported uses

Sage has been used as an antioxidant, an antispasmodic, and an astringent. It is also claimed to be therapeutic for diarrhea, dysmenorrhea, galactorrhea, gastritis, gingivitis, and sore throat. Clinical trial data are lacking to support these claims.

A preliminary study conducted in Italy lends some support to the notion that sage might be valuable as a therapy for postmenopausal women who suffer from estrogen deprivation. In 20 of 30 (67%) postmenopausal Italian women, such symptoms as dizziness, headache, hot flashes, insomnia, and palpitations resolved after daily therapy with a combination of sage and alfalfa extracts. The remaining 10 women demonstrated partial response to therapy. Prolactin levels were significantly elevated as well, suggesting a dopaminergic blocking–like effect. Definitive conclusions cannot be drawn because questions exist with respect to study design (De Leo et al., 1998).

Sage has been used for many years as a food flavoring and fragrance for soaps and perfumes.It is listed by the Council of Europe as a natural source of food flavoring.

Dosage

For menstrual disorders, 1 to 4 ml of leaf extract (1:1 in 45% alcohol) P.O. t.i.d.
For sore throat, 1 to 4 g of leaf as a gargle P.O. t.i.d.

Adverse reactions

CNS: *tonic-clonic seizures.*
EENT: cheilitis, stomatitis (with high doses or long-term use).
Other: local irritant.

Interactions

Anticonvulsants: Lowered seizure threshold. Avoid administration with sage.
Disulfiram: Disulfiram reaction if sage product contains alcohol. Do not use together.
Insulin, oral antidiabetic drugs: Antagonized glycemic control, necessitating dose adjustment. Monitor blood glucose levels closely.

Bold italic type indicates that reaction may be life-threatening.

Contraindications and precautions

Avoid using sage in pregnant patients because it may cause spontaneous abortion. Use cautiously in patients who are prone to hypoglycemia (such as diabetics) and in those who are receiving anticonvulsants because seizure control may be diminished.

Special considerations

• Caution the diabetic patient against using sage because it may worsen his condition and promote loss of glycemic control.

• Advise the epileptic patient to avoid using sage because it may worsen his condition and lower his seizure threshold.

• Caution the patient taking disulfiram not to take a sage product that contains alcohol.

Commentary

Little clinical information is available to recommend the medicinal use of sage. More evidence is needed in postmenopausal women. Animal data and toxicology information suggest that consumption of sage may reduce glycemic control in diabetic patients and lessen control of seizures in epileptic patients.

References

Cabo, J., et al. "Accion hipoglucemiante de prepardos fitoterapicos que contienen especies del genero salvia," *Ars Pharmaceutica* 26:239-49, 1985.

De Leo, V., et al. "Treatment of Neurovegetative Menopausal Symptoms with a Phytotherapeutic Agent" (Italian), *Minerva Ginecol* 50(5):207-11, 1998.

Meier, S., et al. "The Antimicrobial Activity of Essential Oils and Essential Components Towards Oral Bacteria," *Oral Microbiol Immunol* 9:202-8, 1994.

Todorov, S., et al. "Experimental Pharmacological Study of Three Species from Genus *Salvia*," *Acta Physiol Pharmacol Bulg* 10:13-20, 1984.

SAM-E

ADEMETIONINE, S-ADENOSYL-L-METHIONINE, S-ADENOSYLMETHIONINE, SAMe, SAMMY

Common trade names

AdoMet (Sweden), Nature Made

Common forms

Available as 200-mg tablets.

Source

SAM-e is synthesized in many mammalian cells, including the brain, but most of SAM-e's metabolic generation occurs in the liver, where it uses more than 70% of dietary methionine (Cantoni, 1953).

Chemical components

S-adenosyl-L-methionine is an unstable intermediate compound related to the amino acid methionine, produced during the conversion of methionine to cysteine. SAM-e functions as a methyl donor in the synthesis of taurine, glutathione, and other polyamine compounds (Cantoni, 1975). This biochemical conversion takes place in the presence of methionine-adenosyl-transferase and ATP.

Actions

SAM-e functions as a primary methyl group ($-CH_3$) donor for a broad range of compounds (catecholamines, neurotransmitters, proteins, membrane phospholipids, fatty acids, nucleic acids, porphyrins, choline, carnitine, and creatine). After liberation of its methyl group, SAM-e is converted to S-adenosylhomocysteine, a competitive inhibitor of SAM-e–mediated methylation reactions. SAM-e crosses the blood-brain barrier and has been shown to increase homovanillic acid and 5-hydroxyindolacetic acid levels (Bell et al., 1994). SAM-e lowers luteinizing hormone and prolactin levels (Fava et al., 1990). It displays a weak, inconsistent effect on MAO type B receptors as well (Bottiglieri et al., 1984). Rat data suggest that tissue levels of SAM-e decline sharply after birth and continue to diminish as the organism ages, despite the presence of an intact SAM-e enzyme synthesizing system (methionine-adenosyl-transferase; Eloranta, 1977).

One particular trial in rats that has received significant attention in the medical literature is the study conducted by Laudanno (1987). In this trial, 30 male Wistar rats were randomly allocated to treatment with SAM-e 100 mg/kg (0.2 ml/100 g of body weight) by gastric lavage, misoprostol 100 mcg/kg subcutaneously, or only the vehicles for both agents 30 minutes before exposure with absolute ethanol. Twenty minutes after exposure to ethanol, the rats were killed and their gastromucosal surfaces examined for damage and necrosis. The breadth and severity of GI injury were then assessed by blinded investigators. Similar study designs were enlisted with other rats for evaluating aspirin-induced damage and physical stress–induced (immobilization) gastromucosal injury. At trial conclusion, both SAM-e and misoprostol functioned similarly, appearing to protect rodent GI tissue significantly better than the vehicles used alone for all three types of gastromucosal injury ($P<.01$ for all comparisons). The investigators theorized that the gastroprotective effect of SAM-e was probably related to increased synthesis of nonprotein sulfhydryl compounds at the gastric level.

Animal studies have suggested a potential for hepatoprotection from various toxins, including acetaminophen, carbon tetrachloride, cyclosporin A, D-galactosamine, ethanol, and lead.

SAM-e is poorly absorbed and has poor bioavailability, supposedly related to a first-pass effect. Peak plasma levels are attained 3 to 6 hours after oral administration of 400 mg (Stramentinoli, 1987). The half-life of the injectable formulation is about 80 minutes. A study examining a 400-mg SAM-e single dose calculated a half-life of 1.7 ± 0.3 hours (Loehrer et al., 1997). The volume of distribution of SAM-e is reported to be 0.4 L/kg (Osman et al., 1993). Most of SAM-e is metabolized by the liver, with 24% of an administered dose excreted in feces and less than 20% excreted in urine.

Reported uses

Many potential therapeutic claims exist for SAM-e. The rationale for general therapeutic application of SAM-e stems from the philosophy that exogenous administration of SAM-e may restore "youthful" levels of this metabolite and thereby induce beneficial changes in the person whose problems are at least in part related to a relative deficiency of the compound.

Trials in patients with depression

The vast majority of clinical trial evidence surrounds the application of SAM-e for various depressive disorders.

Almost 40 clinical trials have pursued the use of SAM-e for therapeutic potential in some kind of depressive syndrome. Sample sizes of these trials vary considerably, ranging from 7 to 86 patients. The dose used has also varied considerably. Studies have used either parenteral (range 45 to 400 mg/day) or oral SAM-e (1,600 mg/day) and a combination of the two. Several reviews and at least two meta-analyses have examined the available evidence surrounding SAM-e in the therapy for depression for trials completed before 1994 (Andreoli, 1992; Bressa, 1994). The most recent meta-analysis (Bressa, 1994) concluded that SAM-e was superior to placebo in treating depressive disorders and about as effective as standard tricyclic antidepressants. Other recent studies appear to support the therapeutic application of SAM-e in depression but have some notable deficiencies in study design (Criconia et al., 1994; Agricola et al., 1994). SAM-e was also evaluated in depressed patients with Parkinson's disease (this trial was not included in the meta-analysis conducted by Bressa in 1994; Carrieri et al., 1990). This double-blind, randomized, placebo-controlled trial used a twice-daily dose of 200 mg I.M. and 400 mg P.O. in 21 patients. Assessment occurred at 2-week intervals. After 30 days, patients were washed out (2 weeks) and then crossed-over to the opposite course of therapy. At the close of the trial, averaged results of scoring for the Hamilton Rating Scale for Depression (HRSD) and Beck's Self-Depression Inventory (BSDI) favored SAM-e treatment over placebo ($P<.01$ for HRSD and $P<.05$ for BSDI). Parkinsonism symptoms were unchanged. Despite notable deficiencies in many early studies, taken altogether, there appears to be significant evidence to support the efficacy of SAM-e therapy in depression.

Trials in patients with depression from fibromyalgia

Fibromyalgia, a nonarticular rheumatoid disorder, is characterized by general and chronic pain in the skeletal muscle along with well-defined "tender points" and occurs in about 15% of the general population. Many patients with fibromyalgia experience depression associated with their disorder. At least seven trials have attempted to describe a role for SAM-e in fibromyalgia. In general, SAM-e did appear to reduce tender point pain in several studies (Grassetto and Varotto, 1994; Ianniello et al., 1994; DiBenedetto et al., 1993). Notably, some of these trials might be criticized for using subjective measurements and lacking placebo controls, but as might be suggested from clinical trials in depression, depressive symptoms associated with fibromyalgia appeared to respond well to therapy with SAM-e.

Trials in patients with various conditions
SAM-e has been evaluated substantially in patients with osteoarthritis. (See *SAM-e trials in patients with osteoarthritis.*)

SAM-e has been pursued and thought to be of some limited benefit in treating Alzheimer's disease, epilepsy, HIV-related neurologic complications, metabolic defects, migraine headaches, multiple sclerosis, Parkinson's disease, and spinal cord disease.

Mato and colleagues (1999) evaluated SAM-e supplementation (AdoMet, 1,200 mg/day P.O.) in 123 patients with alcoholic cirrhosis in a randomized, placebo-controlled, double-blind manner. Histologic confirmation of disease was available in more than 80% of patients enrolled in the trial. Patients were randomized to either SAM-e or placebo for 2 years. No significant differences in baseline demographics were seen between the two groups. At trial termination, when compared with the placebo group, treatment with SAM-e produced an almost 50% reduction in the combined outcome parameter of overall mortality and liver transplantation (30% versus 16%, *P*=NS), but this was not statistically significant. On further subgroup analysis (removal of Child class C patients), a statistically significant effect was seen favoring SAM-e over placebo in the same parameter (29% versus 12%, *P*=.025). The combined parameter of time to death or liver transplantation for this subgroup was also found to be statistically significant favoring SAM-e supplementation. The investigators concluded that long-term treatment with SAM-e may improve survival or delay liver transplantation for patients with less advanced hepatic disease.

SAM-e was studied in a small group of women (*N*=18) with respect to its ability to relieve intrahepatic cholestasis caused by pregnancy (Frezza et al., 1984). After 10 and 20 days of therapy, statistically significant declines in serum ALT, AST, conjugated bilirubin, and total bile acid levels were noted as compared with baseline data (*P*<.05 for all) for the 800-mg dose of SAM-e. The same parameters were found to be significantly different statistically in favor of the 800-mg SAM-e dose when compared with the saline-only infusion. This was not the case for the 200-mg SAM-e dose.

Adverse reactions
CNS: cognitive impairment, dizziness, headache, insomnia, psychoactivation to hypomania ("switch" phenomenon).
GI: diarrhea, heartburn, nausea, vomiting (these reactions are usually mild but some have been severe enough to warrant hospitalization).
Metabolic: elevated alkaline phosphatase levels.
Other: *anaphylaxis,* pain at injection site.

Interactions
Antidepressants, other mood-altering agents: Serotonin syndrome has been described in a patient taking I.M. S-adenosylmethionine and

---

Bold italic type indicates that reaction may be life-threatening.

RESEARCH FINDINGS

SAM-e trials in patients with osteoarthritis

Osteoarthritis (OA), a common affliction of elderly people, is characterized by a loss of cartilage in affected joints and hypertrophic changes in neighboring bone structures. This irregularity exists, at least in part, because of a malfunction in proteoglycan synthesis. In vitro studies of SAM-e suggest that it may favorably affect proteoglycan synthesis, thereby potentially restoring the imbalance that occurs in these patients (Harmand et al., 1987). The presence of SAM-e aided in the reversal of detrimental effects to fibronectin and proteoglycans induced by tumor necrosis factor-α (Barcelo et al., 1987; Gutierrez et al., 1997). Interestingly, in a study of the effects of SAM-e on depression, some of the subjects with OA noted marked improvement in their joint disease (Di Padova, 1987).

An extensive review of clinical trial data published between 1980 and 1987 includes information from 12 studies and more than 22,000 patients on the use of SAM-e in OA (Di Padova, 1987). In these trials, SAM-e doses ranged from 400 to 1,200 mg P.O. daily, with treatment courses from 3 weeks to 2 years. The author concluded that clinical trials thus far had shown that SAM-e improves symptoms of OA better than placebo but equivalent to nonsteroidal anti-inflammatory drugs (NSAIDs). In comparisons of SAM-e with various NSAIDs—ibuprofen (Capretto et al., 1985; Marcolongo et al., 1985), indomethacin (Vetter, 1987), naproxen (Domljan et al., 1989; Caruso and Pietrogrande, 1987), and piroxicam (Maccagno et al., 1987)—it appears that the beneficial therapeutic effect may lag behind that of the NSAIDs at 2 weeks but SAM-e achieves equal efficacy at 4 weeks and longer (Di Padova, 1987; Vetter, 1987; Domljan et al., 1989; Caruso and Pietrogrande, 1987; Maccagno et al., 1987).

Although this report summarizes an impressive array of clinical data from a large number of subjects, 95% of the study subject population information was gathered from open-label studies. The author of this review was a researcher affiliated with a manufacturer of SAM-e during the 1970s and 1980s.

More recently, Bradley and colleagues (1994) conducted a 28-day trial in 81 patients with OA. This study, one of the few conducted in the United States and carried out at two joint research centers, was a randomized, double-blind trial comparing SAM-e (400 mg I.V. every day for 5 days and then 200 mg P.O. three times a day for 23 days) with placebo in patients with OA of the knee. After randomization to treatment, patients were evaluated by way of the Stanford Health Assessment Questionnaire (disability and pain scales). They were also questioned in regard to the

SAM-e trials in patients with osteoarthritis
(continued)

duration of joint stiffness in the morning and overall activity of their arthritis. Patients were assessed for joint swelling and tenderness, and a goniometer was used to measure range of motion. Patients were appraised by how quickly they were able to walk 50 feet. Beck's Self-Depression Inventory (BSDI) and the Face Scale of Lorish and Maisiak were also administered. Throughout the study, acetaminophen use was allowed but monitored closely. Because randomization to both research centers yielded unevenly paired patient groups, the data were evaluated at each site, rather than as an aggregate.

At site A, the only parameter that resulted in a statistically significant difference between the two groups was rest pain. Interestingly, no significant differences were noted between SAM-e and placebo for the BSDI or the Face Scale, suggesting that any improvements in joint function were not related to mood alteration. At site B, only the patient's estimate of walking distance tolerance favored SAM-e over placebo (P=.05). Nonsignificant trends favoring SAM-e were explained by the investigators as possibly being attributed to increased acetaminophen usage in the SAM-e group.

The investigators suggested that further investigation with SAM-e was warranted because of benefits observed in this study and in other reports and because ideal pharmacotherapy for OA is lacking. In summary, it appears that earlier trial data (pre-1988) and laboratory work may have supported a role for SAM-e in OA, but more recent investigational evidence seems to place that suggestion in doubt.

clomipramine (Iruela et al., 1993). Avoid administration with SAM-e. *Glucocorticoids:* Rat studies show that SAM-e supplementation increases plasma corticotropin and glucocorticoid levels (Baldessarini, 1987; Chawla et al., 1990). May have implications for patients who are taking corticosteroids or increase the risk of adrenal crisis after the supplement is withdrawn in those taking it chronically. Avoid administration with SAM-e.

MAO inhibitors: Until the effect of SAM-e on MAO receptors is clarified, patients should avoid consuming foods that have a high tyramine content, such as aged foods, wines, and cheeses, and certain opioid derivatives, such as meperidine and dextromethorphan, because of the potential for a dangerous interaction. Avoid administration with SAM-e.

Bold italic type indicates that reaction may be life-threatening.

Contraindications and precautions

Information surrounding the use of SAM-e in patients who are pregnant or breast-feeding is severely limited. In a small trial by Frezza and colleagues (1984), no untoward effects, as defined by normal Apgar scores, were documented in the newborns of 12 women who received I.V. formulations of SAM-e during their pregnancies.

Hyperhomocysteinemia (elevated plasma homocysteine level) is a relatively rare disorder. It has been associated with a dramatically increased risk of thrombosis and premature CV disease (Alfthan et al., 1997). Because SAM-e participates in the transsulfuration pathway of methionine, there appears to be a theoretical but potentially dangerous risk with SAM-e supplementation in those individuals who are susceptible to elevated homocysteine levels (that is, patients with defective or absent cystathionine beta-synthase or patients with deficiencies or partial deficiencies of vitamin B_6 or B_{12}). Early data obtained from SAM-e trials led investigators to believe that SAM-e supplementation might be a protective factor against the development of coronary disease related to hyperhomocysteinemia. Some data, however, appear conflicting. Whether SAM-e supplementation might lead to elevated homocysteine levels, promoting an increased risk of coronary disease, peripheral arterial occlusive disease, cerebrovascular disease, or thrombosis, is yet to be resolved.

Special considerations

• Monitor the patient with a history of bipolar (manic) disorder because he may be at risk for a manic or hypomanic episode when instituting or continuing supplementation with SAM-e.
• Monitor serum alkaline phosphatase levels periodically.
• Inform the patient with hyperhomocysteinemia of the potential risks associated with using SAM-e.
• Review established, proven pharmacotherapeutic options with the patient who wants to begin therapy with SAM-e.
• Advise women to avoid using SAM-e during pregnancy or when breast-feeding until more is known.

Points of interest

• Some discussion places the overall incidence of adverse reactions at 20% (Friedel et al., 1989). Most reactions are associated with the GI tract.
• Some early data suggested a possible relation between SAM-e serum levels and success in treating depression. Despite the availability of a sensitive assay for SAM-e, no definitive therapeutic range for SAM-e serum levels has been documented.
• SAM-e (200-mg tablet) retails at about $20 for 20 tablets. The cost of a 30-day supply ($120 for 800 mg/day and $240 for 1,600 mg/day) may exceed that of traditional antidepressants by several dollars, depending on the drug selected.
• In the July 5, 1999, issue of *Newsweek,* it was suggested that SAM-e is one of the 25 most popular dietary supplements in the United States (Cowley and Underwood, 1999).

Commentary
Studies have evaluated SAM-e supplementation in depression of various origins (depression alone; depression associated with Parkinson's disease, fibromyalgia, alcoholism, and menopause). Notably, a few reasonably well-designed studies seem to support the effectiveness of SAM-e in depression. Larger-scale placebo-controlled trials and comparative trials comparing SAM-e with selective serotonin-reuptake inhibitors or other, newer-generation antidepressants are needed before definitive conclusions can be drawn regarding SAM-e's place in the pharmacotherapy for depression. Enthusiasm for its immediate therapeutic application in depression should be tempered with the fact that SAM-e's risk-benefit profile is not nearly as well described as those of contemporary antidepressants.

SAM-e therapy for fibromyalgia and perhaps osteoarthritis deserves further consideration and investigation because of some promising early clinical trial data, but no definitive recommendations regarding these potential applications can be made at this time. All other potential therapeutic applications are quite preliminary.

Although many studies have documented adverse events—some severe—related to SAM-e supplementation, further study, especially long-term evaluation, is needed in this area. Of concern is the theoretical risk of artificially elevating homocysteine levels in patients who are prone to hyperhomocysteinemia, a rare but established risk factor for coronary disease and thrombosis.

References
Agricola, R., et al. "S-Adeonsyl-L-Methionine in the Treatment of Major Depression Complicating Chronic Alcoholism," *Curr Ther Res* 55(1):83-91, 1994.

Alfthan, G., et al. "Plasma Homocysteine and Cardiovascular Disease Mortality," *Lancet* 349:397, 1997.

Andreoli ,V. "S-Adenosyl- Methionine (SAMe) as Antidepressant," *New Trends Clin Neuropharmacol* 6:11-18, 1992.

Baldessarini, R.J. "Neuropharmacology of S-Adenosyl-L-methionine," *Am J Med* 83:(S-5a):35-42, 1987.

Barcelo, V.A., et al. "Effect of S-Adenosylmethionine on Experimental Osteoarthritis in Rabbits," *Am J Med* 83(S-5A):55-59, 1987.

Bell, K.M., et al. "S-Adenosylmethionine Blood Levels in Major Depression: Changes with Drug Treatment," *Acta Neurol Scand* 154:15-18, 1994.

Bottiglieri, T., et al. "S-Adenosylmethionine Influences Monoamine Metabolism," *Lancet* 2:224, 1984. Letter.

Bradley, J.D., et al. "A Randomized, Double-blind, Placebo-controlled Trial of Intravenous Loading with S-Adenosylmethionine (SAM) Followed by Oral SAM Therapy in Patients with Knee Osteoarthritis," *J Rheumatol* 21(5):905-11, 1994.

Bressa, G.M. "S-Adenosyl-L-methionine (SAMe) as Antidepressant: Meta-analysis of Clinical Studies," *Acta Neurol Scand* (S-154):7-14, 1994.

Cantoni, G.L. "S-Adenosylmethionine: A New Intermediate Formed Enzymatically from L-Methionine and Adenosine-triphosphate," *J Biol Chem* 204:403-16, 1953.

Cantoni, G.L. "Biological Methylation: Selected Topics," *Ann Rev Biochem* 44:435-51, 1975.

Capretto, C., et al. "A Double-blind Controlled Study of S-Adenosyl-methionine (SAMe) vs Ibuprofen in Gonarthrosis, Coxarthrosis, and Spondylarthrosis," *Clin Trials J* 22:15-24, 1985.

Carrieri, P.B., et al. "S-Adenosylmethionine Treatment of Depression in Patients with Parkinson's Disease," *Curr Ther Res* 48(1):154-60, 1990.

Caruso, I., and Pietrogrande, V. "Italian Double-blind Multicenter Study Comparing S-Adenosylmethionine, Naproxen, and Placebo in the Treatment of Degenerative Joint Disease," *Am J Med* 83(S-5A):66-71, 1987.

Chawla, R.K., et al. "Biochemistry and Pharmacology of S-Adenosyl-L-methionine and Rationale for Its Use in Liver Disease," *Drugs* 40(3):98-110, 1990.

Cowley, G., and Underwood, A. "What Is SAMe?" *Newsweek,* July 5, 1999, 46-50.

Criconia, A.M., et al. "Results of Treatment with S-Adenosyl-L-Methionine in Patients with Major Depression and Internal Illnesses," *Curr Ther Res* 55(6):666-74, 1994.

DiBenedetto, P., et al. "Clinical Evaluation of S-adenosylmethionine Versus Transcutaneous Electrical Nerve Stimulation in Primary Fibromyalgia," *Curr Ther Res* 53(2):222-29, 1993.

Di Padova, C. "S-Adenosylmethionine in the Treatment of Osteoarthritis; Review of Clinical Studies," *Am J Med* 83:(S-5A):60-65, 1987.

Domljan, Z., et al. "A Double-blind Trial of Adenosylmethionine vs Naproxen in Activated Gonoarthrosis," *Int J Clin Pharmacol Ther Toxicol* 7:329-33, 1989.

Eloranta, T.O. "Tissue Distribution of S-Adenosylmethionine and S-Adenosylhomocysteine in the Rat," *Biochem J* 166:521-29, 1977.

Fava, M., et al. "Neuroendocrine Effects of S-Adenosyl-L-methionine, a Novel Putative Antidepressant," *J Psychiatric Res* 24:177-84, 1990.

Frezza, M., et al. "Reversal of Intrahepatic Cholestasis of Pregnancy in Women After High Dose S-Adenosyl-L-methionine Administration," *Hepatology* 4(2):274-78, 1984.

Friedel, H.A., et al. "S-Adenosyl-L-Methionine. A Review of Its Pharmacological Properties and Therapeutic Potential in Liver Dysfunction and Affective Disorders in Relation to Its Physiological Role in Cell Metabolism," *Drugs* 38:389-416, 1989.

Grassetto, M., and Varotto, A. "Primary Fibromyalgia Is Responsive to S-Adenosylmethionine," *Curr Ther Res* 55(7):797-806, 1994.

Gutierrez, S., et al. "SAMe Restores the Changes in the Proliferation and in the Synthesis of Fibronectin and Proteoglycans Induced by Tumor Necrosis Factor Alpha on Cultured Rabbit Synovial Cells," *Br J Rheum* 37:27-31, 1997.

Harmand, M.F., et al. "S-Adenosylmethionine on Human Articular Chondrocyte Differentiation: An In-Vitro Study," *Am J Med* 83(s-5a):48-54, 1987.

Ianniello, A., et al. "S-Adenosyl-L-methionine in Sjogren's Syndrome and Fibromyalgia," *Curr Ther Res* 55(6):699-706, 1994.

Iruela, L.M., et al. "Toxic Interaction of S-Adenosylmethionine and Clomipramine," *Am J Psychol* 150:522, 1993. Letter.

Laudanno, O.M. "Cytoprotective Effect of S-Adenosylmethionine Compared with That of Misoprostol Against Ethanol-, Aspirin- and Stress-induced Gastric Damage," *Am J Med* 83(S-5A):43-47, 1987.

Loehrer, F.M.T., et al. "Influence of Oral S-Adenosylmethionine on Plasma 5-Methyl-tetrahydrofolate, S-Adenosylhomocysteine, Homocysteine and Methionine in Healthy Humans," *J Pharmacol Exp Therap* 282(2):845-50, 1997.

Maccagno, A., et al. "Double-blind Controlled Clinical Trial of Oral S-Adenosylmethionine Versus Piroxicam in Knee Osteoarthritis," *Am J Med* (S-5A):83:72-77, 1987.

Marcolongo, N., et al. "Double-blind Multicenter Study of the Activity of S-Adenosylmethionine in Hip and Knee Osteoarthritis," *Curr Ther Res* 37:82-94, 1985.

Mato, J.M., et al. "S-Adenosylmethionine in Alcoholic Liver Cirrhosis: A Randomized, Placebo-controlled, Double-blind, Multi-center Clinical Trial," *J Hepatol* 30:1081-89, 1999.

Osman, E., et al. "S-Adenosyl-L-methionine: A New Therapeutic Agent in Liver Disease?" *Aliment Pharmacol Ther* 7:21-28, 1993. Review.

Stramentinoli, G. "Pharmacologic Aspects of S-Adenosylmethionine: Pharmacokinetics and Pharmacodynamics," *Am J Med* 83(s-5A):35-42, 1987.

Vetter, G. "Double-blind Comparative Clinical Trial with S-Adenosylmethionine and Indomethacin in the Treatment of Osteoarthritis," *Am J Med* 83(s-5a):78-80, 1987.

SANTONICA

LEVANT WORMSEED, SEA WORMWOOD, SEMEN CINAE, SEMEN SANCTUM, WORMSEED

Taxonomic class
Asteraceae

Common trade names
None known.

Common forms
Available as dried, powdered santonin and oral tablets.

Source
The flowers and seeds of *Artemisia cina* (a distinct variety of *Artemisia maritima)* are found in most parts of Asia.

Chemical components
Santonin, the active ingredient, is a lactone glycoside extracted from unopened flowers. It is bitter-tasting and odorless and occurs as a colorless to white crystalline powder. Other ingredients include artemisin and a volatile oil.

Actions
Some references claim that this herb has anthelmintic properties and is effective against roundworms and threadworms but not tapeworms.

Reported uses
Santonica has been used anecdotally throughout history as an anthelmintic for adults and, especially, children. Russia exported the crude powder to the United States during World War II, until the United States was able to produce a domestic supply itself (Pratt and Youngken, 1951). Santonica was used for pertussis in the 1700s (Hocking, 1997).

Dosage
Oral lozenges, powder, tablets: 2 to 5 grains P.O. in varying dosages.

Bold italic type indicates that reaction may be life-threatening.

Adverse reactions
CNS: *epileptiform seizures*, headache.
EENT: visual disturbances (including aberrations of color vision).
GI: nausea, vomiting.

Interactions
Anticonvulsants: May lower seizure threshold. Avoid administration with santonica.

Contraindications and precautions
Avoid using santonica in pregnant or breast-feeding patients; effects are unknown. Use cautiously in patients who are prone to seizures.

Special considerations
• Advise the patient not to take santonica without medical supervision.
• Caution the patient to avoid performing hazardous activities until CNS effects of santonica are known.
• Advise women to report planned or suspected pregnancy.
🕭 **ALERT** Deaths have resulted from poisonings.
• Caution the patient to keep santonica out of the reach of children and pets.

Commentary
Historically, santonica has been widely used as an anthelmintic. It was an official product in the National Formulary and British Pharmacopeia into the 1950s. Its value cannot be discounted, but more contemporary anthelmintics are probably less toxic and more effective against a wider range of worm infestations.

References
Hocking, G.M. *A Dictionary of Natural Products.* Medford, N.J.: Plexus Publishing, Inc., 1997.
Pratt, R., and Youngken, H.W. *Pharmacognosy: The Study of Natural Drug Substances and Certain Allied Products,* 3rd ed. Philadelphia: Lippincott-Raven Pub., 1951.

SARSAPARILLA

ECUADORIAN SARSAPARILLA, HONDURAN SARSAPARILLA, JAMAICAN SARSAPARILLA, MEXICAN SARSAPARILLA, RABBIT ROOT, SALSAPARILHA, SALSEPAREILLE, SARSA, SARSAPARILLA ROOT, SMILAX

Taxonomic class
Smilacaceae

Common trade names
Multi-ingredient preparations: Sarsaparilla, Sarsaparilla Root Extract

Common forms
Available as capsules (425 mg, 520 mg), dried root powder, liquid (30 ml), solid root extract, tablets, and teas.

Source

The dried roots and rhizomes of various *Smilax* species (*S. aristochiifolia, S. regelii, S. febrifuga, S. ornata*) are used in commercial products. *Smilax* species are cultivated in Mexico, Jamaica, and South America.

Chemical components

Saponins constitute 1% to 3% of the chemical components of sarsaparilla, with the three main saponins being sarsaponin (parillin), smilasaponin (smilacin), and sarsaparilloside. Other saponins include sarsapogenin (parigenin), smilagenin, diosgenin, tigogenin, aspergenin, and laxogenin. Phytosterols, such as beta-sitosterol, may contribute to an anti-inflammatory effect. Resins, starch, trace volatile oils, and cetyl alcohol constitute the remainder of the compound.

Actions

Sarsaparilla's pharmacologic effects have been attributed to the saponins, which are claimed to be blood purifiers or tonics that supposedly remove unwanted toxins from the body. This idea might have arisen from sarsaparilla's supposed diaphoretic and diuretic effects. Other purported effects of saponins include an ability to bind serum cholesterol in the GI tract and a hemolytic effect if administered I.V. These pharmacologic effects are not well documented.

Sarsaparilla has shown in vitro activity against common dermatophytes (*Epidermophyton floccosum, Trichophyton rubrum, Trichophyton mentagrophytes*; Caceres et al., 1991). Significant anti-inflammatory activity and prevention of chemically induced hepatocellular damage have been noted in rodents (after pretreatment with sarsaparilla; Ageel et al., 1989; Rafatullah et al., 1991). Sarsaparilla was found not to have any beneficial effects for improving the healing of bone fractures in rats.

Reported uses

Sarsaparilla root is claimed to be useful for treating renal disease, rheumatism, and skin diseases such as psoriasis and eczema. Older research attempts to substantiate sarsaparilla for use in psoriatic disease.

The most notable trial involved patients with psoriasis vulgaris who received sarsaponin (a major component of sarsaparilla) or placebo (Thermon, 1942). Although the study showed favorable results in terms of improved symptoms, duration of benefit, and reduced disease exacerbations, problems with study design led to questions regarding the final conclusions reached.

Because of its steroidal components, sarsaparilla has also been touted as an athletic performance–enhancing agent. These steroids have not been proven to be anabolic, and therefore, this claim remains unsubstantiated. Sarsaparilla has been promoted as an appetite and digestion aid and as a diuretic. Its extract has been evaluated as adjunctive therapy in leprosy (Rollier, 1959).

The 1992 German Commission E monograph advocates the use of sarsaparilla in treating psoriasis, renal disease, and rheumatic complaints and for diaphoresis and diuresis.

Sarsaparilla is accepted by the FDA as a flavoring agent.

Dosage
For psoriasis, 1 to 4 g of dried root, 8 to 30 ml of concentrated sarsaparilla compound decoction, or 8 to 15 ml of liquid extract P.O. t.i.d. has been suggested.

Adverse reactions
CV: hypotension.
GI: diarrhea, GI irritation.
GU: renal dysfunction.
Hematologic: hemolysis (I.V. use).
Metabolic: electrolyte imbalances.
Respiratory: *asthma* (inhalation of root dust).

Interactions
Bismuth: May increase absorption or elimination or both. Avoid administration with sarsaparilla.
Certain hypnotic drugs: Increased elimination. Monitor for lack of effectiveness.
Digitalis: Increased absorption. Do not use together.
Oral drugs: Saponins may affect absorption of other drugs. Other drugs should be taken 2 hours before or after taking sarsaparilla.

Contraindications and precautions
Avoid using sarsaparilla in pregnant or breast-feeding patients; effects are unknown.

Special considerations
• Inform the patient that therapeutic claims for sarsaparilla are weakly substantiated.
• Advise the patient with asthma to avoid inhaling sarsaparilla root dust or root particles.
• Caution the patient who is already taking a diuretic about excessive diuretic effects, fluid and electrolyte imbalances, and hypotension.

Points of interest
• Since the 16th century, sarsaparilla was thought to be an effective treatment for syphilis. It gained popularity in the Old West of the United States and was the drink of choice for cowboys. It was even listed for such uses in the USP from 1820 to 1910. Activity against syphilis has not been pharmacologically substantiated.

Commentary
The use of sarsaparilla for any condition needs further research. Mechanisms and properties are not clearly documented or adequately researched. The most notable clinical trial evaluated the herb's use in

psoriasis, but poor study design and the presence of confounding variables placed the conclusions in question.

References

Ageel, A..M., et al. "Experimental Studies on Antirheumatic Crude Drugs Used in Saudi Traditional Medicine," *Drugs Exp Clin Res* 15:369-72, 1989.

Caceres, A., et al. "Plants Used in Guatemala for the Treatment of Dermatophytic Infections," *J Ethnopharmacol* 31:263-76, 1991.

Rafatullah, S., et al. "Hepatoprotective and Safety Evaluation Studies on Sarsaparilla," *Int J Pharmacognosy* 29:296-301, 1991.

Rollier, R. "Treatment of Lepromatous Leprosy by a Combination of DDS and Sarsaparilla (*Smilax ornata*)," *Int J Leprosy* 27:328-40, 1959.

Thermon, F.M. "The Treatment of Psoriasis with a Sarsaparilla Compound," *N Engl J Med* 227:128-33, 1942.

SASSAFRAS

AGUE TREE, BOIS DE SASSAFRAS, CINNAMON WOOD, FENCHELHOLZ, LIGNUM FLORIDUM, LIGNUM SASSAFRAS, ROOT BARK, SALOOP, SASSAFRASHOLZ, SAXIFRAX

Taxonomic class
Lauraceae

Common trade names
None known.

Common forms
Available as crude bark, liquid extract, oil, powder, and tea.

Source
The sassafras tree, *Sassafras albidum,* is native to the eastern region of North America. The oil and teas are extracted from the roots and bark of the sassafras tree.

Chemical components
Sassafras alkaloids include isoquinoline-type 0.02%, aporphine, benzylsoquinoline derivatives, boldine, isoboldine, norboldine, cinnabolaurine, norcinnamolaurine, and reticuline. Other components include volatile oils, safrole (a highly aromatic oil), anethole, apiole, asarone, camphor, elemicin, eugenol, menthone, myrisicin, pinene apiole, thujone, magnolol, isomagnolol, tannins, resins, mucilage, and wax. The pleasant-tasting oil is a 2% portion of the roots and 6% to 9% component of the root bark.

Actions
Most studies have focused on the investigation of sassafras toxicity. Sassafras root bark is 5% to 9% safrole. Safrole has been demonstrated to be hepatocarcinogenic in rodents (Borchert et al., 1973). Sassafras has also been shown to induce hepatic enzymes P-450 and P-488. The

---

oil has been used to relieve flatulence and, topically, as an antiseptic and a pediculicide.

Reported uses

Sassafras has been used primarily as a tonic or performance-enhancing agent. Tea prepared from the bark has also been used as a diaphoretic and a diuretic to treat cachexia, dermatologic conditions, rheumatism, sexually transmitted diseases, and visceral obstruction. The herb was originally recommended as a cure for syphilis, but its effectiveness has never been demonstrated. Traditionally, sassafras has been favored as a remedy for cutaneous eruptions, gout, and rheumatic pain.

Dosage

For dermatologic conditions and sexually transmitted diseases, dosages vary with formulation.

Bark: 2 to 4 g P.O. by infusion t.i.d.

Extract (1:1 in 25% alcohol): 2 to 4 ml P.O. t.i.d.

Oil: apply topically.

Powder: tea is prepared by adding ½ tsp of powder to 1 cup (8 oz) of boiling water and infusing for 15 minutes.

Adverse reactions

CNS: ataxia, CNS depression, hallucinogenic effects, paralysis, stupor.

CV: *CV collapse,* hot flashes.

EENT: ptosis.

GI: increased risk of liver cancer, nausea, vomiting.

GU: spontaneous abortion.

Metabolic: hypothermia.

Musculoskeletal: muscle spasm.

Skin: dermatitis, diaphoresis, hypersensitivity to touch.

Interactions

Drugs metabolized by P-450 and P-488 enzyme systems (including some antidepressants, cardiac drugs, and immunosuppressants: May increase toxicity of these drugs. Sassafras is an inducer of hepatic microsomal enzymes, and its component safrole is a potent inhibitor of certain hepatic microsomal enzyme systems (Opdyke, 1974). Monitor patient closely if used together.

Contraindications and precautions

Avoid using sassafras in pregnant or breast-feeding patients; effects are unknown.

Special considerations

🍃 **ALERT** Death has resulted in adults who have ingested 1 tsp of sassafras oil and in children who have ingested a few drops of oil (Craig, 1953).

🍃 **ALERT** Caution the patient to avoid prolonged internal or external use (longer than 2 weeks) of sassafras. Safrole, the major constituent of

the oil of sassafras, is a hepatic carcinogen; even some safrole-free extracts have been reported to produce tumors in animal models.
• Monitor for hepatic dysfunction in patients using sassafras.
• Caution the patient regarding known adverse reactions, particularly CNS effects when performing activities that require alertness.
• Inform the patient about sassafras's carcinogenic effects.
• Advise patients, especially pregnant or breast-feeding women, to avoid internal and external use of sassafras.
• Inform the patient that consumption of sassafras may interfere with the elimination of other drugs being taken.

Points of interest
• The volatile oil and safrole were banned by the FDA for use as food additives or flavor-enhancing agents. A safrole-free sassafras extract is approved for food use in the United States.
• Many adverse reactions are attributed to the safrole component.

Commentary
Sassafras has traditionally been used for several conditions, including dermatologic and rheumatic illnesses, and as a flavoring agent in select beverages. Despite extensive evidence of toxicity and carcinogenesis as well as legal restrictions, sassafras continues to be readily available in natural product stores and other facilities in the United States. The herb may influence the metabolism of many prescription drugs. Therefore, the use of sassafras or its components cannot be recommended.

References
Borchert, P., et al. "The Metabolism of the Naturally Occurring Hepatocarcinogen Safrole to 1'-Hydroxysafrole and the Electrophilic Reactivity of 1'-Acetoxysafrole," *Cancer Res* 33:575-89, 1973.

Craig, J.O. "Poisoning by the Volatile Oils in Childhood," *Arch Dis Child* 28:475-83, 1953.

Opdyke, D.L.J. "Safrole," *Food Cosmet Toxicol* 12:983-86, 1974.

SAVORY

BEAN HERB, WHITE THYME

Taxonomic class
Labiatae

Common trade names
None known.

Common forms
Available as fresh and dried leaves for teas and tonics and as infusion, oil, and tincture.

Source
Medicinal formulations are extracted from the fresh leaves and dried leaves and stems of *Satureja hortensis* L. An oil is made through steam

---

distillation of the entire dried herb. Savory is native to Europe but also grown in North America.

Chemical components
The medicinal components of savory are thought to be the volatile oil and the astringent tannin.

Actions
Dried savory contains a volatile oil that features mild antibacterial and antifungal properties in vitro. Savory also contains an astringent tannin and an expectorant called cineole.

Reported uses
Savory is primarily used to improve digestion and treat diarrhea, but claims have also been made about its use as treatment for GI discomforts, such as abdominal cramps, flatulence, and indigestion. It has also been recommended for treating chest congestion, cough, and sore throat.

In ancient Rome, savory was thought to increase sexual drive.

None of these effects have been demonstrated in controlled clinical trials and are based primarily on folklore and a few animal studies.

Dosage
No consensus exists.
Infusion: 4 tsp of herb per cup of water P.O. t.i.d. (1 to 2 tsp of herb per cup for children).
Tincture: 1 tsp P.O. t.i.d. (½ tsp for children).

Adverse reactions
None reported.

Interactions
None reported.

Contraindications and precautions
Avoid using savory in pregnant or breast-feeding patients; effects are unknown.

Special considerations
• Inform the patient that little information exists about savory.
• Monitor liver function test results periodically.
• Advise the patient who wants to take savory for its purported effects on the GI tract that there are alternative, established pharmacologic treatments.
• Undiluted oil applied to the backs of mice was fatal for 50% within 48 hours.

Points of interest
• The FDA places savory on the generally recognized as safe list.

Commentary

Savory has traditionally been used to treat symptoms associated with digestive disorders. Although no human clinical trials are available, savory appears to be safe at recommended doses. Because of the availability of more effective drugs, savory cannot be recommended for any indication.

References

Hajhashemi, V., et al. "Antispasmodic and Anti-diarrheal Effect of *Satureja hortensis* L. Essential Oil," *J Ethnopharmacol* 71(1-2):187-92, 2000.

SAW PALMETTO

AMERICAN DWARF PALM TREE, CABBAGE PALM, IDS 89, LSESSR, SABAL

Taxonomic class

Arecaceae

Common trade names

Permixon, Propalmex, Strogen

Common forms

Available as berries (fresh or dried), capsules (80 mg, 160 mg, 300 mg, 320 mg, 380 mg, 460 mg, 500 mg, 540 mg, 580 mg, 600 mg), liquid extract (4 oz), tablets, and teas.

Source

The brownish black berry of the American dwarf palm, also known as *Serenoa repens* or *Sabal serrulata*, is used to extract active compounds. The berries contain about 1.5% of an oil. Until a fat-soluble purified extract was produced, it was believed that the plant extracts had little effect because they were poorly absorbed.

Chemical components

The active ingredient in commercial preparations is the *n*-hexane liposterolic extract of *S. repens* (LSESR). This extract contains a complex mixture of various compounds, including fatty acids (primarily lauric acid), phytosterols, and polysaccharides. Two biologically active monacylglycerides were also isolated.

Actions

The precise mechanism of action of saw palmetto is not defined. Most research involves animal and human models, using prostate tissue or cell lines. Several pharmacodynamic effects have been described in in vitro studies. LSESR has been shown to inhibit 5-alpha-reductase, the enzyme responsible for conversion of testosterone to dihydrotestosterone (DHT; Weisser et al., 1996).

Although controversial, LSESR is believed to have greater potency and to inhibit both subtypes of 5-alpha-reductase, whereas finasteride

---

Bold italic type indicates that reaction may be life-threatening.

selectively inhibits type 2 5-alpha-reductase. LSESR also appears to have an inhibitory effect on the binding of DHT to androgen receptors in the prostate. Other data suggest that LSESR also has an anti-inflammatory effect and inhibits prolactin and growth factor–induced prostatic cell proliferation (Paubert-Braquet et al., 1996, 1998). Other authors have theorized that saw palmetto might have spasmloytic properties (Gutierrez et al., 1996).

In one study, LSESR inhibited hormonally induced prostate enlargement in rats (Paubert-Braquet et al., 1996); this effect was greatest after 60 days of treatment. Decreased levels of DHT and antiestrogenic activity after 3 months of LSESR treatment occurred in men with benign prostatic hyperplasia (BPH; DiSilverio et al., 1992).

Reported uses
Saw palmetto tea is claimed to be effective in managing such genitourinary problems as BPH; in increasing sperm production, breast size, and sexual vigor; and in acting as a mild diuretic. (See *LSESR to treat benign prostatic hyperplasia*, page 698.)

Dosage
For BPH, clinical studies in humans have used 320 mg P.O. in divided doses b.i.d. Duration of treatment has usually been 3 months, but both shorter and longer trials (up to 6 months) have been conducted. Other recommendations include 1 to 2 g of fresh saw palmetto berries or 0.5 to 1 g of dried berry in decoction P.O. t.i.d.

Adverse reactions
CNS: headache.
CV: hypertension.
GI: abdominal pain, constipation, diarrhea, nausea.
GU: decreased libido, dysuria, impotence, urine retention.
Musculoskeletal: back pain.

Interactions
None reported.

Contraindications and precautions
Saw palmetto is contraindicated during pregnancy and in women of childbearing age because of its potential hormonal effects. Use cautiously in patients with conditions other than BPH because data regarding its effects are lacking.

Special considerations
• Saw palmetto apparently does not alter the size of the prostate. Initially, there was concern that the herb causes a false-negative prostate-specific antigen (PSA) result, but subsequent reports have demonstrated no effect on PSA. Baseline PSA may be suggested before starting treatment.
• Saw palmetto should be taken with food to minimize GI effects.

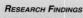

RESEARCH FINDINGS

LSESR to treat benign prostatic hyperplasia

The effectiveness of the lipidosterolic extract of *Serenoa repens* (LSESR) in the treatment of benign prostatic hyperplasia (BPH) has been studied in several human noncomparative, placebo-controlled trials as well as comparative trials with other drugs (Plosker and Brogden, 1996). Most trials involved men between ages 60 and 70 and used doses of 320 mg daily for 1 to 3 months. Of seven placebo-controlled clinical trials, four included at least 50 patients. Three of the larger trials showed that *S. repens* was superior to placebo in reducing nighttime and daytime urinary frequency and increasing peak flow rate. Significant symptomatic improvement compared with placebo was reported in one study (Champault et al., 1984).

In another, well-conducted, large, double-blind, randomized, comparative trial involving 1,098 men, *S. repens* and finasteride demonstrated similar efficacy (Carraro et al., 1996).

No significant difference was found in patient-reported quality of life or objective measures as defined by the International Prostate Symptom Score. *S. repens* had little or no effect on prostate size and prostate-specific antigen levels, suggesting a mechanism other than its proposed antiandrogenic effect. Patients receiving *S. repens* had significantly better sexual function scores compared with those receiving placebo.

A more recent small, randomized, placebo-controlled trial supported a slight advantage of saw palmetto over placebo, but the difference was not statistically significant (Marks et al., 2000).

S. repens has also been compared with alfuzosin and prazosin in two smaller, double-blind, randomized trials. Such objective results as urinary frequency, postvoid residuals, and mean urinary flow favored the alpha$_1$-receptor antagonist in both studies, but the results were not statistically significant.

Published reviews of this herb include those by Gerber (2000) and by McPartland and Pruitt (2000).

• Inform the patient who wants to use saw palmetto for BPH to do so only after a diagnosis has been made and only on the advice of his primary health care provider.
• Advise women to avoid using saw palmetto during pregnancy or when breast-feeding.

Points of interest

• Saw palmetto tea was included in the USP and National Formulary from 1906 to 1950 for urogenital ailments.

Bold italic type indicates that reaction may be life-threatening.

Commentary

Saw palmetto, specifically LSESR, appears to be well tolerated and has shown greater efficacy than placebo and equal efficacy to finasteride in improving subjective and objective symptoms of BPH. Its use is supported by many in vitro, in vivo, and clinical studies involving humans. Although LSESR appears to be a safe and effective alternative agent, more placebo-controlled comparative studies involving alpha$_1$-receptor antagonists are needed to further delineate the herb's role in managing BPH.

References

Carraro, J.C., et al. "Comparison of Phytotherapy (Permixon) with Finasteride in the Treatment of Benign Prostate Hyperplasia: A Randomized International Study of 1,098 Patients," *Prostate* 29:231-40, 1996.

Champault, G., et al. "A Double-blind Trial of an Extract of the Plant *Serenoa repens* in Benign Prostatic Hyperplasia," *Br J Clin Pharmacol* 18:461-62, 1984.

DiSilverio, F., et al. "Evidence that *Serenoa repens* Extract Displays an Antiestrogenic Activity in Prostatic Tissue of Benign Prostatic Hypertrophy Patients," *Eur Urol* 21:309-14, 1992.

Gerber, G.S. "Saw Palmetto for the Treatment of Men with Lower Urinary Tract Symptoms," *J Urol* 163(5):1408-12, 2000.

Gutierrez, M., et al. "Mechanisms Involved in the Spasmolytic Effect of Extracts from *Sabal serrulata* Fruit on Smooth Muscle," *Gen Pharmacol* 27(1):171-76, 1996.

Marks, L.S., et al. "Effects of a Saw Palmetto Herbal Blend in Men with Symptomatic Benign Prostatic Hyperplasia," *J Urol* 163(5):1451-56, 2000.

McPartland, J.M., and Pruitt, P.L. "Benign Prostatic Hyperplasia Treated with Saw Palmetto: A Literature Search and an Experimental Case Study," *J Am Osteopath Assoc* 100(2):89-96, 2000.

Paubert-Braquet, M., et al. "Effect of *Serenoa repens* Extract (Permixon) on Estradiol/Testosterone-induced Experimental Prostate Enlargement in the Rat," *Pharmacol Res* 34:171-79, 1996.

Paubert-Braquet, M., et al. "Effect of the Lipodosterolic Extract of *Sernoa repens* (Permixon) and Its Major Components on Basic Fibroblast Growth Factor-induced Proliferation of Cultures of Human Prostate Biopsies," *Eur Urol* 33:340-47, 1998.

Plosker, G.L., and Brogden, R.N. "*Serenoa repens* (Permixon). A Review of Its Pharmacology and Therapeutic Efficacy in Benign Prostatic Hyperplasia," *Drugs Aging* 9:379-95, 1996.

Weisser, H., et al. "Effects of the *Sabal serrulata* Extract IDS 89 and Its Subfractions on 5 Alpha-reductase Activity in Human Benign Prostatic Hyperplasia," *Prostate* 28:300-6, 1996.

SCENTED GERANIUM

Taxonomic class

Geraniaceae

Common trade names

None known.

Common forms
Available as essential oil, potpourri, and tea flavoring. Scented geranium is commonly used as a house plant.

Source
There are six genera in the Geraniaceae family: *Erodium, Geranium, Hypseocharis, Monsonia, Pelargonium,* and *Sarcocaulon.* The scented geraniums are derived from *Pelargonium,* the largest of the genera. True geranium are found on all continents, but the *Pelargonium* occur predominantly in South Africa.

Chemical components
Flavonoids and tannins (geraniin) are the active ingredients in many geranium species.

Actions
Although scented geranium has limited documented use in medical literature, several geranium species appear to have antibacterial, antifungal, antioxidative, antiviral, and pesticidal qualities.

Geranium viscossissimum var. *viscossissimum* has been found to release ellagic and gallic acids on hydrolysis; these acids exhibit significant growth-inhibiting activity against larvae of the polyphagous pest insect *Heliothis virescens* (Gegova et al., 1993). Geraniin (tannin from *Geranium thunbergii*) was found to be protective against oxidative damage in the mouse ocular lens. One study found that phagocytosis of yeast was induced by geraniin isolated from peritoneal macrophages with geraniin, isolated from *G. thunbergii* (Ivancheva et al., 1992).

The polyphenolic complex of *Geranium sanguineum* L. showed efficacy against herpes simplex, HIV-1, influenza, and vaccinia in in vitro cell cultures, with its anti-influenza effect being most pronounced (Serkedjieva, 1997).

Reported uses
Scented geranium is reportedly useful as a pesticide. It is also reported to be an antiviral, but no clinical data support this claim.

Dosage
No consensus exists. The leaves are commonly used in tea or potpourri preparations, and the essential oils may be used to make tablets and creams.

Adverse reactions
Skin: contact dermatitis.
Other: allergic reaction.

Interactions
None reported, but scented geranium may interact with flu vaccines. Avoid using together.

Bold italic type indicates that reaction may be life-threatening.

Contraindications and precautions
Avoid using scented geranium in pregnant or breast-feeding patients; effects are unknown. Use cautiously in atopic patients.

Special considerations
- Inform the patient that periodic testing of hepatic and renal function and hematologic profile may be required.
- Inform the patient who wants to use scented geranium for its antimicrobial effects that other antimicrobial drugs exist whose risk-benefit profiles are well described.
- Advise the atopic patient of the potential for adverse skin reactions.

Points of interest
- Scented geraniums are used as ornamental plants in the United States and as natural pesticides in gardens.
- Essential oils obtained from *Pelargonium* species have been identified for their potential to act as food preservatives.

Commentary
Most of the information available for the medicinal use of scented geranium comes from foreign language journals and is based on in vitro data and trials in animals. Insufficient data exist to support any therapeutic application of scented geranium in humans. More data are needed to determine the safety of this plant.

References
Gegova, G., et al. "Combined Effect of Selected Antiviral Substances of Natural and Synthetic Origin. Part 2. Anti-influenza Activity of a Combination of a Polyphenolic Complex Isolated from *Geranium sanguineum* L. and Rimantadine In Vivo," *Acta Microbiol Bulg* 30:37-40, 1993.

Ivancheva, S., et al. "Polyphenols from Bulgarian Medicinal Plants with Anti-infectious Activity," *Basic Life Sci* 59:717-28, 1992.

Serkedjieva, J. "Antiinfective Activity of a Plant Preparation from *Geranium sanguineum* L.," *Pharmazie* 52:799-802, 1997.

SCHISANDRA

GOMISHI, OMICHA, SCHIZANDRA, TJN-101, WU-WEI-ZU

Taxonomic class
Schisandraceae

Common trade names
Schisandra Extract, Sheng-mai-san

Common forms
Available as capsules (100 mg), dried fruit, and liquid.

Source
The active components of *Schisandra chinensis* may be extracted using ethanol. Active components are isolated through petroleum ether ex-

traction of the fruit, stems, or kernel. Schisandra is native to China, Russia, and Korea.

Chemical components
The extracts of seeds and fruit are composed of numerous lignans (schizandrins, schizandrols, and schisantherins); malic, tartaric, nigranoic, and citric acids; resins; pectin; vitamins A, C, and E; sterols; and tannins. The fruit contains a volatile oil.

Actions
Schisandra has exhibited antioxidant activity in animals. Studies on the myocardium of rats suggest some protective benefit against hypoxia and reperfusion injuries (Li et al., 1996). Schisandrin A (TJN-101) showed some inhibition of leukotrienes and decreased artificially induced hepatic damage in rats. Oral dosages of TJN-101 decreased hepatic injury and mortality in a dose-dependent manner. The proposed mechanism of benefit may result from nonspecific hepatoprotection rather than toxin inhibition. Specifically, schisandra may promote protective effects by stimulating hepatic metabolism and inhibiting leukotriene formation through augmentation of the hepatic glutathione antioxidant and detoxification system (Ko et al., 1995). Another study in mice demonstrated that schisandrin B had a hepatoprotective effect against carbon tetrachloride–induced toxicity (Ip et al., 2000).

A component of schisandra has been found to inhibit reverse transcriptase in vitro (Sun et al., 1996).

An in vitro study showed that a water extract of *S. chinensis* acted as a scavenger of the hydroxyl radical (Ohsugi et al., 1999).

Reported uses
Schisandra is claimed to be of benefit in preventing hepatic injury, although only studies in animals have been conducted. Antioxidant properties may contribute to this action.

This herb has long been used in Chinese medicine for treating hepatic, pulmonary, and renal disorders. It is also claimed to be useful for treating ocular disorders, but clinical trials are lacking. Advocacy literature suggests that schisandra has adaptogenic properties (helps the body deal with stress), but this also remains unproven.

Dosage
Dosage of 100 mg of extract P.O. b.i.d. has been suggested.

Adverse reactions
CNS: profound CNS depression (rare).

Interactions
Drugs predominantly eliminated by the liver: Schisandra extracts may enhance elimination of hepatically metabolized drugs. Monitor patient closely.

Bold italic type indicates that reaction may be life-threatening.

Contraindications and precautions
Avoid using schisandra in pregnant or breast-feeding patients; effects
are unknown. Use cautiously in patients taking drugs that are extensively metabolized by the liver.

Special considerations
• Inform the patient that little information exists regarding schisandra's
safety and efficacy.
• Advise women to avoid using schisandra during pregnancy or when
breast-feeding.
• Advise the patient that drugs eliminated through the liver may interact with schisandra. Urge him to inform his health care provider about
any drugs (prescription and OTC) that he is taking.

Points of interest
• The Chinese name *wu-wei-zu* means five-flavored herb (or seeds),
which refers to the sweet, sour, pungent, bitter, and salty taste of schisandra.

Commentary
Schisandra has shown a protective effect on the liver in some animals,
but human data regarding its safety and efficacy are lacking. Claims for
treating pulmonary and renal conditions have also not been adequately
proven. Little is known about the adverse effects and dosage range of
schisandra extracts; therefore, this herb cannot be recommended for
medicinal use.

References
Ip, S.P., et al. "Differential Effect of Schisandrin B and Dimethyl Diphenyl Bicarb-
    oxylate (DDB) on Hepatic Mitochondrial Glutathione Redox Status in Carbon
    Tetrachloride Intoxicated Mice," *Mol Cell Biochem* 205(1-2):111-14, 2000.
Ko, K.M., et al. "Effect of a Lignan-enriched Fructus Schisandrae Extract on Hepa-
    tic Glutathione Status in Rats: Protection Against Carbon Tetrachloride Toxic-
    ity," *Planta Med* 61:134-37, 1995.
Li, P.C., et al. "*Schisandra chinensis*-dependent Myocardial Protective Action of
    Sheng-Mai-San in Rats," *Am J Chin Med* 24:255-62, 1996.
Ohsugi, M., et al. "Active-oxygen Scavenging Activity of Traditional Nourishing-
    tonic Herbal Medicines and Active Constituents of *Rhodiola Sacra*," *J Ethno-
    pharmacol* 67(1):111-19, 1999.
Sun, H.D., et al. "Nigranoic Acid, a Triterpenoid from *Schisandra sphaerandra* That
    Inhibits HIV-1 Reverse Transcriptase," *J Nat Prod* 59:525-27, 1996.

SCULLCAP

HELMET FLOWER, HOODWORT, SKULLCAP

Taxonomic class
Lamiaceae

Common trade names
Scullcap Herb, Skullcap

Common forms

Capsules: 300 mg, 425 mg, 429 mg
Liquid extract: 1 oz, 2 oz
Powder: 10 oz

Source

The leaves and roots of the plants *Scutellaria laterifolia* and *Scutellaria baicalensis* are prepared as hot water or methanolic extracts. Scullcap is native to temperate regions of North America.

Chemical components

Scutellaria species contain flavonoids (apigenin, luteolin, hispidulin, scutellarein, scutellarin, baicalein, baicalin), an iridoid (catalpol), limonene, terpineol, carophyllene, cadinene, and other sesquiterpenes in the volatile oils. Wogonin, lignin, resin, and tannins are also present.

Actions

Scullcap is believed to have anticonvulsant and sedative actions. An aqueous extract was found to have mild anthelmintic properties in vitro. Other studies found bacteriostatic or bactericidal effects in vitro. One study showed that concomitant use of baicalin with several beta-lactam antibiotics lowered the minimum inhibitory concentrations when tested against MRSA (Liu et al., 2000).

A root extract of scullcap showed anti-inflammatory action by inhibiting interleukin-1 and inhibited the synthesis of prostaglandin E_2 and leukotriene B_4 (Chung et al., 1995). Another study noted the inhibitory effects of scullcap flavonoids on sialidase—an agent associated with certain cancers—in mice. Scullcap extracts decreased 5-fluorouracil and cyclophosphamide myelotoxicity as well as tumor cell viability in mice (Razina et al., 1987).

The extracts (flavonoids) of scullcap have demonstrated antiviral effects against the influenza virus and human T-cell leukemia virus type I. Investigators believe that the inhibitory effect of the extract is dose-dependent (Baylor et al., 1992). Another agent, baicalin, inhibited both HIV-1 infection and replication in human peripheral blood cells (Li et al., 1993). In vitro data suggest that scullcap may also inhibit Epstein-Barr virus early antigen activation.

Extracts from *S. baicalensis* decreased cardiomyocyte cell death after an ischemia-reperfusion experiment. The authors of the study suggested that baicalin's protective effect could be attributed to the flavonoid's ability to scavenge superoxide, hydrogen peroxide, and hydroxyl radicals (Shao et al., 1999).

Reported uses

Scullcap has been used traditionally as an anticonvulsant, an anti-inflammatory, a cholesterol-lowering agent, and an agent for movement disorders and spasticity. Little, if any, information exists to support the use of this herb in humans.

Bold italic type indicates that reaction may be life-threatening.

Scullcap has also been used as an antiviral and has demonstrated some efficacy in animal studies in vitro. One study found that the addition of scullcap to chemotherapy prompted an increase in serum immunoglobulin levels in patients with lung cancer who were theophylline-resistant (Smolianinov et al., 1997). In another study of patients receiving chemotherapy for lung cancer, the addition of a dry scullcap extract promoted hematopoiesis and an increase in the circulating precursors of erythroid and granulocyte colony-stimulating factors (Goldberg et al., 1997).

Other foreign reports in humans have suggested a role for scullcap in therapy of stroke and cerebral thromboembolism.

Dosage
Doses have been administered P.O., I.V., and I.M.
Dried herb: 1 to 2 g as a tea P.O. t.i.d.
Liquid extract (1:1 in 25% alcohol): 2 to 4 ml P.O. t.i.d.
Tincture (1:5 in 45% alcohol): 1 to 2 ml P.O. t.i.d.

Adverse reactions
GI: *hepatotoxicity.*

Excessive doses of tincture:
CNS: confusion, giddiness, *seizures*, stupor.
CV: *arrhythmias.*
Musculoskeletal: fasciculations.

Interactions
Disulfiram: Disulfiram reaction can occur if herbal form contains alcohol. Avoid concurrent use.
Immunosuppressants: May alter effect on serum immunoglobulin levels. Do not use with scullcap.

Contraindications and precautions
Avoid using scullcap in pregnant or breast-feeding patients; effects are unknown.

Special considerations
• Monitor liver function test results periodically.
• Advise the patient to avoid taking large doses of scullcap tincture because of possible toxicities.
• Inform the patient that commercial sources of scullcap have been found to be contaminated with other herbs.
• Inform the patient that insufficient evidence exists to recommend scullcap for any condition or disease.
• Advise women to avoid using scullcap during pregnancy or when breast-feeding.

Points of interest
• Scullcap has been demonstrated to be adulterated with *Teucrium* species. Some species of *Teucrium* (*T. chamaedrys*-Germander) have also been linked with hepatotoxicity.

Commentary

Although several animal and in vitro studies have demonstrated the inhibitory effects of scullcap on pathologic viruses, there is little, if any, clinical trial evidence to support this application in humans.

Furthermore, in vitro studies claiming antibiotic or cardioprotective properties have not been substantiated by human trials. Human studies have demonstrated some benefit of scullcap consumption in lung cancer, which points out the need for vigorous follow-up clinical investigation.

References

Baylor, N.W., et al. "Inhibition of Human T Cell Leukemia Virus by the Plant Flavonoid Baicalin (7-glucuronic acid, 5,6-dihydroxyflavone)," *J Infect Dis* 165:433-37, 1992.

Chung, C.P., et al. "Pharmacological Effects of Methanolic Extract from the Root of *Scutellaria baicalensis* and Its Flavonoids on Human Fibroblast," *Planta Med* 61:150-53, 1995.

Goldberg, V.E., et al. "Dry Extract of *Scutellaria baicalensis* as a Hemostimulant in Antineoplastic Chemotherapy in Patients with Lung Cancer," *Eksp Klin Farmakol* 60:28-30, 1997.

Li, B.Q., et al. "Inhibition of HIV Infection by Baicalin—A Flavonoid Compound Purified from Chinese Herbal Medicine," *Cell Mol Biol Res* 39:119-24, 1993.

Liu, I.X., et al. "Baicalin Synergy with Beta-lactam Antibiotics Against Methicillin-resistant *Staphylococcus aureus* and Other Beta-lactam-resistant Strains of *S. aureus*," *J Pharm Pharmacol* 52(3):361-66, 2000.

Razina, T.G., et al. "Enhancement of the Selectivity of the Action of the Cytostatics Cyclophosphane and 5-Fluorouracil by Using an Extract of the Baikal Skullcap in an Experiment," *Vopr Onkol* 33:80-84, 1987.

Shao, Z.H., et al. "Extract from *Scutellaria baicalensis* georgi Attenuates Oxidative Stress in Cardiomyocytes," *J Mol Cell Cardiol* 31(10):1885-95, 1999.

Smolianinov, D.A., et al. "Effect of *Scutellaria baicalensis* Extract on the Immunologic Status of Patients with Lung Cancer Receiving Antineoplastic Chemotherapy," *Eksp Klin Farmakol* 69:49-51, 1997.

SEA HOLLY

ERYNGO, SEA HOLME, SEA HULVER

Taxonomic class
Apiaceae

Common trade names
None known.

Common forms
Available as dried roots, extract, and tincture.

Source
The active components are derived from the dried roots of *Eryngium maritimum*. Sea holly is typically found along seashores in temperate regions.

Chemical components
Active components include saponins, coumarins, plant acids, and flavonoids.

Actions
Extracts of sea holly indicated possible anti-inflammatory action in rats, as demonstrated by decreased paw edema (Lisciani et al., 1984).

Reported uses
Sea holly is used primarily for urologic conditions; it is claimed to act as a diuretic when normal urine flow is inhibited by conditions that obstruct urinary flow, such as cystitis, kidney stones, enlarged or inflamed prostate, and urethritis. These reported uses are anecdotal and lack supporting evidence (Hiller et al., 1976).

Dosage
For diuretic action, sea holly may be taken as a decoction (tea) or tincture P.O. t.i.d.

Adverse reactions
None reported.

Interactions
Diuretics: May increase electrolyte loss. Monitor electrolyte levels closely.

Contraindications and precautions
Avoid using sea holly in pregnant or breast-feeding patients; effects are unknown.

Special considerations
• Inform the patient that little information exists regarding sea holly.
• Caution the patient receiving diuretics against using sea holly.
• Caution the patient that long-term use of sea holly may lead to electrolyte imbalance.
• Advise women to avoid using sea holly during pregnancy or when breast-feeding.

Commentary
Despite its longtime use as a urologic remedy, there is insufficient evidence to support the medicinal application of sea holly for any disease.

References
Hiller, K., et al. "Saponins of *Eryngium maritimum* L. 25. Contents of Various Saniculoideae," *Pharmazie* 31:53, 1976.
Lisciani, R., et al. "Anti-inflammatory Activity of *Eryngium maritimum* L. Rhizome Extracts in Intact Rats," *J Ethnopharmacol* 12:263-70, 1984.

SELF-HEAL

ALL HEAL, BRUNELLA, CONSUELDA MENOR, HSIA KU TS'AO, *PRUNELLA INCISA*, *PRUNELLA QUERETTE*, SICKLEWORT, XIA KU CAO

Taxonomic class
Lamiaceae

Common trade names
None known.

Common forms
Available as liquid and fresh plant.

Source
Prunella vulgaris is a perennial weed commonly found in fields, grassy areas, and woods of North America, Asia, and Europe. Various parts of the plant are used.

Chemical components
Components isolated from the whole herb include oleanolic acid, rutin, hyperoside, ursolic acid, caffeic acid, vitamins, tannins, carotenoids, essential oils, and alkaloids. The flowers contain the glycosides of delphinidin, cyanidin, *d*-camphor, *d*-fenchone, and ursolic acid. Prunellin, an aqueous extract of the herb, has been identified as an active antiviral compound.

Actions
Antiviral activity of prunellin against the HIV-1 virus has been shown in vitro. Prunellin was more effective than Retrovir (AZT) in inhibiting reverse transcriptase activity. Viral replication was abolished for up to 60 days after exposure in lymphoid and monocytoid cells. When the extract was added after viral adsorption, the aqueous extract achieved partial inhibition of HIV replication. Prunellin was also found to inhibit the binding of glycoprotein 120 to CD4 cells, which was concluded to be its primary mechanism for inhibiting HIV-1 infection (Yao et al., 1992).

Diluted and undiluted aqueous extracts of *P. vulgaris* provided complete coverage against HIV-induced cytotoxicity. Diluted *P. vulgaris* extract with zidovudine or didanosine provided protection of 69% to 74% compared with either agent alone (John et al., 1994). Additional data have documented similar effects; the components of *P. vulgaris* may possess a noncompetitive, HIV reverse transcriptase inhibitor that may be suitable for oral administration (Kageyama et al., 2000).

Patients with herpes simplex virus (HSV) type I keratitis were given an ophthalmic form of *P. vulgaris* extract and experienced clinical cure or improvement (Zheng, 1990). New evidence suggests that this anti-HSV activity is the effect of an anionic polysaccharide compound iso-

---

Bold italic type indicates that reaction may be life-threatening.

lated from *P. vulgaris*. The compound was not inhibitory toward cytomegalovirus, certain influenza strains, or poliovirus. In the concentration tested, it was found to be noncytotoxic to human cells and lacked any significant anticoagulant effect (Xu et al., 1999).

In vitro studies in human lung carcinoma and lymphocytic leukemia showed ursolic acid to have significant cytotoxic activity (Lee et al., 1988). Ursolic acid has shown marginal cytotoxic activity in human colon and mammary tumor cells.

Anti-inflammatory effects for some components of *P. vulgaris* have been documented (Ryu et al., 2000).

Reported uses
In Chinese folklore medicine, *P. vulgaris* is still used for such conditions as bacillary dysentery, cancer, infectious hepatitis, jaundice, pleuritis with effusion, and tuberculosis (Lee et al., 1988). Self-heal has been used for treating boils, colic, diarrhea, flatulence, hemorrhage, and sore throat. Its main use, as recommended by herbalists, is for GI upset and sore throat.

Dosage
Because most studies have been in vitro, standard doses are not known. The formulation of the herb appears to be an important aspect with regard to treatment. Aqueous extracts have the most antiviral activity (Yamasaki et al., 1996). An infusion of *P. vulgaris* has been used as a gargle and is prepared by mixing 1 g of the fresh plant in boiling water and then cooling.

Adverse reactions
None reported.

Interactions
None reported.

Contraindications and precautions
No known contraindications.

Special considerations
• Advise the patient that although *P. vulgaris* has been shown to be beneficial in suppression of HIV-1 retroviral activity, it should not be used as a substitute for conventional therapy.
• Caution the patient to use the herb cautiously because its effects on GI conditions and sore throat have not been evaluated.
• Although no known chemical interactions have been reported in clinical studies, consideration must be given to the pharmacologic properties of the herbal product and the potential for exacerbation of the intended therapeutic effect of conventional drugs.
• Advise the patient to notify the prescriber and pharmacist of any herbal or dietary supplement he is taking when filling a new prescription.

Points of interest

• *P. vulgaris* was originally called *Brunella vulgaris*, from the German word *bruen*, meaning quinsy. Quinsy is a disorder of the throat for which *Brunella* was considered a cure.

Commentary

P. vulgaris shows some benefit against HIV-1 retrovirus and certain cancers, but significant in vivo studies in animals or humans are lacking. Although *P. vulgaris* appears promising as a medicinal agent, more information is needed to determine its safety and efficacy in humans.

References

John, J.F., et al. "Synergistic Antiretroviral Activities of the Herb, *Prunella vulgaris*, with AZT, ddI and ddC," *Abstr Gen Meet Am Soc Microbiol* 94:481, 1994. Abstract S-27.

Kageyama, S., et al. "Extract of *Prunella vulgaris* Spikes Inhibits HIV Replication at Reverse Transcription In Vitro and Can Be Absorbed from Intestine In Vivo," *Antivir Chem Chemother* 11(2):157-64, 2000.

Lee, K.H., et al. "The Cytotoxic Principles of *Prunella vulgaris*, *Psychotrial serpens*, and *Hyptis capitata*: Ursolic Acid and Related Derivatives," *Planta Med* 54:308-11, 1988.

Ryu, S.Y., et al. "Anti-allergic and Anti-inflammatory Triterpenes from the Herb of *Prunella vulgaris*," *Planta Med* 66(4):358-60, 2000. Letter.

Xu, H.X., et al. "Isolation and Characterization of an Anti-HSV Polysaccharide from *Prunella vulgaris*," *Antiviral Res* 44(1):43-54, 1999.

Yamasaki, K., et al. "Anti-HIV-1 Activity of Labiatae Plants, Especially Aromatic Plants," *Int Conf AIDS* 11:65, 1996. Abstract Mo.A.1062.

Yao, X.J., et al. "Mechanism of Inhibition of HIV-1 Infection In Vitro by Purified Extract of *Prunella vulgaris*," *Virology* 187:56-62, 1992.

Zheng, M. "Experimental Study of 472 Herbs with Antiviral Action Against the Herpes Simplex Virus," *Chung His I Chieh Ho Tsa Chih* 10:39-41, 1990.

SENEGA

MILKWORT, MOUTAIN FLAX, NORTHERN SENEGA, *POLYGALA* ROOT, RATTLESNAKE ROOT, SENECA, SENECA ROOT, SENECA SNAKEROOT, SENEGA ROOT, SENEGA SNAKEROOT

Taxonomic class

Polygalaceae

Common trade names

Multi-ingredient preparations: Enhance, SN-X Vegitabs

Common forms

Available as dried powdered root, extract, lozenges, syrups (various concentrations), teas, and tinctures.

Source

The source of senega preparations is the dried root and rootstock of *Polygala senega,* a perennial herbaceous plant that is indigenous to

---

southern Canada and the United States. The plant is grown commercially in Canada and Japan.

Chemical components

The active ingredients in senega preparations are the root saponins. Senegin is a saponin that hydrolyzes to form the glycosides, presenegin, and then senegenin, a chlorine-containing triterpenoid. Other root saponins include various senegasaponins and polygalic acid, which may add to the irritant activity of senega. Other compounds include carbohydrates (arabinose, sucrose, and fructose among others), alphaspinasterol, polygalitol, resins, valeric acid ester, fatty acids, salicylic acid, and methyl salicylate.

Actions

Senega is claimed to have an expectorant effect through direct irritation of the upper respiratory tract mucosa. This causes secretion of fluid from mucosal cells within the bronchioles as a reflex response to the irritation. A few *Polygala* species have been shown to produce a sedative-like effect in rodents, probably attributed to the saponin components (Carretero et al., 1986). Pharmacokinetic studies in animals show poor oral absorption of senega saponins from the GI tract (Johnson et al., 1986). Senegin has shown an ability to decrease blood glucose levels by 250 to 300 mg/dl in both normal and diabetic mice (Kako et al., 1997) by a mechanism that may be insulin-dependent (Kako et al., 1996). Senegin has also demonstrated an ability to lower both triglyceride and cholesterol levels in normal and hyperlipidemic mice (Masuda et al., 1996). Senegasaponins have been shown to decrease the absorption of alcohol in rats (Yoshikawa et al., 1996, 1995). The saponins have also demonstrated an immunomodulatory action characterized by increases in immunoglobulin G, interleukin, and interferon gamma levels in both mice and hens exposed to antigens (Estrada et al., 2000).

Various saponins have apparently demonstrated an ability to regrow hair (Ishida et al., 1999).

Reported uses

Although Native Americans first used senega root for rattlesnake bites, evidence supporting this use is lacking. Despite laboratory evidence for antidiabetic, antihyperlipidemic, and other activities, the primary recommendations for senega continue to be respiratory in nature. Herbal practitioners recommend senega root as an expectorant for coughs and in asthma, chronic bronchitis, croup, pharyngitis, and pneumonia (Briggs, 1988). Other claims include its use as a diaphoretic, an emetic, and a sialogogue. Although senega was listed as an official drug in the National Formulary until 1960, no human clinical trials demonstrating its efficacy for these claimed uses are available. Patent documentation in France suggests that senega has activity toward the treatment of eczema, graft rejection, inflammation, multiple sclerosis, and psoriasis.

Dosage
For respiratory conditions, 2 tbsp of syrup P.O. every 4 hours as needed; 2.5 to 5 ml of tincture P.O.; 0.3 to 1 ml of extract P.O.; or 0.5 to 1 g of dried root P.O. t.i.d.

Adverse reactions
CNS: anxiety, mental dullness, vertigo.
EENT: mouth and throat pain, visual disturbances.
GI: abdominal pain, diarrhea, GI irritation, nausea, vomiting.
Hematologic: hemolysis (I.V. administration).

Interactions
Anticoagulants: May prolong bleeding time. Avoid administration with senega.
Antidiabetic drugs: Senega may counteract hypoglycemic therapy. Avoid administration with senega.
CNS depressants: May increase CNS effects. Avoid administration with senega.

Contraindications and precautions
Senega is contraindicated in patients with aspirin or salicylate hypersensitivity. Also avoid its use in pregnant or breast-feeding patients; effects are unknown.

Special considerations
• Inform the patient that inadequate data exist for any therapeutic use of senega.
• Instruct the diabetic patient to monitor for loss of glycemic control.
• Monitor the patient for increased bleeding.
• Advise women to avoid using senega during pregnancy or when breast-feeding.

Commentary
Senega root preparations have been used as expectorants for centuries. Although the herb's efficacy and safety have been widely reported in the lay press, controlled trials are lacking. Compared with other expectorant products, senega's significant adverse effects and unproven efficacy preclude it from being recommended for any therapeutic use. Laboratory data support further research into the components and actions of senega as an immunomodulator and for treating diabetes, hyperlipidemia, male-pattern baldness and, potentially, alcoholism. Ideally, it could prove to be a source of novel drugs for the treatment of these disease states, but the potential toxicity and adverse effect profile would not warrant the use of senega as a treatment option for those patients.

References
Briggs, C.J. "Senega Snakeroot —A Traditional Canadian Herbal Medicine," *Can Pharm J* 121:199-201, 1988.
Carretero, M.E., et al. "Etudes Pharmacodymiques Preliminaires de *Polygala micro-phylla* (L.), sur le Systeme Nerveux Central," *Planta Med Phytother* 20:148-54, 1986.

Bold italic type indicates that reaction may be life-threatening.

Estrada, A., et al. "Isolation and Evaluation of Immunological Adjuvant Activities of Saponins from *Polygala senega* L.," *Comp Immunol Microbiol Infect Dis* 23(1):27-43, 2000.

Ishida, H., et al. "Studies of the Active Substances in Herbs Used for Hair Treatment. Part III. Isolation of Hair-Regrowth Substances from *Polygala senega* var. *latifolia* TORR. et. GRAY," *Biol Pharm Bull* 22(11):1249-50, 1999.

Johnson, I.T., et al. "Influence of Saponins on Gut Permeability and Active Nutrient Transport *In Vitro*," *J Nutr* 116:2270-77, 1986.

Kako, M., et al. "Hypoglycemic Activity of Some Triterpinoid Glycosides," *J Natl Prod* 60(6):604-5, 1997.

Kako, M., et al. "Hypoglycemic Effect of the Rhizomes of *Polygala senega* in Normal and Diabetic Mice and Its Main Component, the Triterpinoid Glycoside Senegin-II," *Planta Med* 62(5):440-43, 1996.

Kako, M., et al. "Effect of Senegin-II on Blood Glucose in Normal and NIDDM Mice," *Biol Pharm Bull* 18(8):1159-61, 1995.

Masuda, H., et al. "Intraperitoneal Administration of Senega Radix Extract and Its Main Component, Senegin II, Affects Lipid Metabolism in Normal and Hyperlipidemic Mice," *Biol Pharm Bull* 19(2):315-17, 1996.

Yoshikawa, M., et al. "Bioactive Saponins and Glycosides. Part II. Senegae Radix. (2): Chemical Structures, Hypoglycemic Activity, and Ethanol Absorption-Inhibitory Effect of E-senegasaponin c, and Z-senegins II, III, and IV," *Chem Pharm Bull* 44(7):1305-13, 1996.

Yoshikawa, M., et al. "Bioactive Saponins and Glycosides. Part I. Senegae Radix. (1): E-senegasaponins a and b and Z-senegasaponins a and b, Their Inhibitory Effect on Alcohol Absorption and Hypoglycemic Activity," *Chem Pharm Bull* 43(12):2115-22, 1995.

Yoshikawa, M., et al. "E-senegasaponins A and B and Z-senegasaponins A and B, Z-senegins II and III, New Type Inhibitors of Ethanol Absorption in Rats from Senegae Radix, the Roots of *Polygala senega* L. var *latifolia* Torrey et Gray," *Chem Pharm Bull* 43(2):350-52, 1995.

SENNA

ADEN SENNA, CASSIA ACUTIFOLIA, CASSIA AUGUSTIFOLIA, CASSIA SENNA, MECCA SENNA, NUBIAN SENNA, TINNEVELLY SENNA

Taxonomic class
Fabaceae

Common trade names
Senekot, Senexon, Senna Leaves, Senokot-S, Senolax

Common forms
Capsules: 10 mg, 25 mg, 470 mg
Senna tea or infusion of senna: 100 g of senna leaves, 1,000 ml of distilled boiling water, and 5 g of sliced ginger or coriander
Syrup of senna: 218 minims of fluidextract of senna, 81 minims of coriander, and sufficient syrup (6.5 fluid drams)
Tablets: 187 mg
    Also available as fluidextract, granules, suppositories, syrup, and teas.

Source

Active compounds are derived from the leaves and pods (fruits) of many *Cassia* species *(C. acutifolia, C. augustifolia,* and *C. senna).* Other species used include *C. chamecrista, C. fistula, C. lanceolata, C. marilandica,* and *C. obovata.*

Chemical components

Many chemical components are isolated from senna. The leaves contain myricyl alcohol, a flavonol containing kaempferol and isormamnetin. Anthraquinone derivatives and their glycosides constitute 3% to 5% of senna.

Sennosides A and B are the major components characterized by a rhein-dianthrone aglycone. Sennosides C and D are characterized by rhein and aloe-emodin aglycone. The leaves also contain chrysophanol and free sugars (fructose, glucose, sucrose, and pinitol). The seeds do not contain anthraquinones. The plant also contains cathartic acid, cathartin, mucilage, phaeoretin, sennacrol, and sennapicrin.

C. augustifolia has a total anthracoid content of 2% to 3% compared with *C. senna,* which has 3.5% to 5%; thus, *C. augustifolia* must be used in higher doses to receive the same action (Dreessen and Lemli, 1982).

Actions

Senna is a prodrug that is cleaved into an active component by intestinal bacteria. *Bacteroides fragilis, Streptococcus faecalis,* and *S. faecium* have been found to hydrolyze and reduce the glycosides into their active laxative aglycone component (Dreessen and Lemli, 1982). Senna works primarily to increase peristaltic activity in the lower bowel. Its primary site of action is the intestinal wall. It also has antiabsorptive properties and stimulates secretions. Senna passes into the breast milk of breast-feeding women (Morton, 1977).

It is postulated that sennosides may exert part of their laxative action by stimulation of prostaglandin E_2, leading to stimulation of colonic fluid and electrolyte excretion (Beubler and Kollar, 1988).

Reported uses

Senna is valuable as a laxative. The herb is used to relieve constipation and cleanse the bowel before diagnostic procedures are performed. Both the leaves and the pods possess this activity.

A study comparing the efficacy of senna and lactulose in maintaining bowel regularity in a group of terminal cancer patients found the agents to be similar in efficacy. Senna was deemed to be favored only because of cost considerations (Agra et al., 1998).

Other uses are based on the *Cassia* species used. Claims include applying a paste of vinegar and powdered leaves *(C. alata)* for use in treating burns, psoriasis, and rashes (Morton, 1977). A combination of the leaves, flowers, and pods has been used to allay fever; the leaves have been mixed with rose petals as a purgative; the juice or the powdered leaves have been used for cancerous tumors; and the aloe-emodin and beta-sitosterol components are believed to be useful in various tumor types. Senna has also been used to help expel intestinal worms.

Dosage

For constipation, adult dose is 2 tablets (187 mg) P.O. at bedtime (maximum of 8 tablets/day); in children who weigh more than 60 lb (27 kg), 1 tablet at bedtime (maximum of 4 tablets/day).
Compound or aromatic syrup: 2 fluid drams P.O.
Concentrated solution: ½ to 1 dram P.O.
Fluidextract: ½ to 2 fluid drams P.O.
Powdered leaves: 1 dram P.O.

Adverse reactions

GI: abdominal cramps, cachexia, colic, pigmentation of the colon (with excessive use).
Skin: dermatitis (saponin).

Prolonged use:
GI: diarrhea, melanosis coli.
Metabolic: hypokalemia.
Musculoskeletal: tetany, clubbing of fingers.

Interactions

Calcium channel blockers, calmodulin antagonists, indomethacin: Blocked diarrheal effects. Avoid administration with senna.

Contraindications and precautions

Senna is contraindicated in patients with GI inflammatory conditions, hemorrhoids, and prolapses.

Long-term use of sennoside laxatives may cause pseudomelanosis coli. This phenomenon may be associated with an increased risk of colorectal cancer. Subsequently, senna ingestion has been associated with an increased risk of certain cancers. Although this is not definitively recognized, van Gorkom and colleagues (2000) and others (Joo et al., 1998) have found detrimental effects (acute massive cell loss) on the colons of patients who received single doses of the laxative. Also, an abstract from a German journal describes a retrospective study that identified a possible link between senna laxative use and urothelial cancers (Bronder et al., 1999).

Special considerations

• Inform the patient that senna may discolor urine.
• Instruct the patient to increase fluid intake and add bulk-containing foods to his diet (whole-grain breads, grains, fruits, vegetables) to assist in relieving constipation.
• Caution the patient not to use senna if intense abdominal pain or nausea occurs.
• Advise the patient not to take stimulant laxatives for longer than 1 week. When the condition resolves, senna should be discontinued.

• Inform the patient that there are differences in potency between herbal supplements that contain sennosides.

Points of interest
• Laxative abuse is a widespread problem for patients with eating disorders and for elderly patients who believe that they must have daily bowel movements. Adverse effects associated with excessive ingestion of senna include clubbing of the fingers, hypokalemia, and tetany (Prior and White, 1978).

Commentary
Senna is a widely used laxative that may be found in many OTC products. The leaves and pods have been used to relieve constipation; thus, herbal supplements that contain sennosides are believed to be safe and effective when used according to labeling. Many studies comparing senna products with other laxatives find it to be a useful agent for treating constipation. Because overuse of products that contain anthranoids has been shown to cause many adverse effects, besides possible links to certain cancers, these agents should be used only for temporary relief of constipation.

References
Agra, Y., et al. "Efficacy of Senna Versus Lactulose in Terminal Cancer Patients Treated with Opioids," *J Pain Symptom Manage* 15(1):1-7, 1998.

Beubler, E., and Kollar, G. "Prostaglandin-mediated Action of Sennosides," *Pharmacology* 36(Suppl.1):85-91, 1988.

Bronder, E., et al. "Analgetika und laxantien als risikofaktoren fur krebs der ableitenden Harnwege-Ergebnisse der Berliner Urothelkarzinom-Studie," *Soz Praventivmed* 44(3):117-25, 1999.

Dreessen, M., and Lemli, J. "Qualitative and Quantitative Interactions Between the Sennosides and Some Human Intestinal Bacteria," *Pharm Acta Helv* 57:350-52, 1982.

Joo, J.S., et al. "Alterations in Colonic Anatomy Induced by Chronic Stimulant Laxatives: The Cathartic Colon Revisited," *J Clin Gastroenterol* 26(4):283-86, 1998.

Morton, J.F. *Major Medicinal Plants—Botany, Culture and Uses.* Springfield, Ill.: Charles C. Thomas, Bannerstone House, 1977.

Prior, J., and White, I. "Tetany and Clubbing in Patients Who Ingested Large Quantities of Senna," *Lancet* 2:947, 1978.

Van Gorkom, B.A., et al. "Influence of a Highly Purified Senna Extract on Colonic Epithelium," *Digestion* 61(2):113-20, 2000.

SHARK CARTILAGE

Common trade names
Benefin Shark Cartilage, Carticin, Cartilade, GNC Liquid Shark Cartilage, Informed Nutrition Shark Cartilage, Natural Brand Shark Cartilage, Schiff Shark Cartilage

---

Bold italic type indicates that reaction may be life-threatening.

Common forms
Ampules: 10 ml (containing 80 mg/ml)
Capsules: 500 mg, 700 mg, 750 mg, 800 mg, 1,000 mg
Concentrate: 500 mg/15 ml
Powder: 8 oz
Tablets: 750 mg, 1,000 mg

Source
Cartilage is obtained from the spiny dogfish shark, *Squalus acanthias,* and the hammerhead shark, *Sphyrna lewini.*

Chemical components
Glycoproteins sphyrnastatin 1 and 2 are obtained from cartilage of the hammerhead shark.

Actions
Shark and other animal cartilage products have been used with success since the 1950s to promote wound healing and to treat chronic inflammatory and other nonneoplastic disorders (Prudden, 1965). It is known that certain isolates from shark cartilage possess antiangiogenic properties.

The growth and metastasis of malignant tumors are dependent on angiogenesis. Angiogenesis and antiangiogenesis are multifactorial and counteracting mechanisms that involve a number of stimulatory and inhibitory factors secreted by tumor cells.

Except for a few in vitro studies, little has been published in peer-reviewed scientific journals or presented at scientific meetings regarding the antitumorigenic activity of crude shark cartilage or shark cartilage isolates in animal xenograft models. No data are available on absorption, pharmacokinetics, bioavailability, stability, immunomodulation, dose escalation, synergy (or antagonism) with other anticancer agents, or toxicity in cancer patients treated with shark cartilage preparations because the nature of the antiangiogenic moiety in shark cartilage is unknown.

Cartilage composes 6% of the shark's total body weight, making it an abundant source of cartilage compared with mammalian sources (Hunt and Connelly, 1995).

Shark cartilage extract implanted into rabbit corneas that contained implanted tumors was found to significantly inhibit tumor neovascularization. The inhibitor did not appear to act directly on the tumor itself because the carcinomas continued to grow slowly (Hunt and Connelly, 1995).

Reported uses
A 16-week Cuban trial attempted to evaluate the efficacy of shark cartilage in 29 patients with cancer; 15 were deemed evaluable and 3 showed response to treatment. This trial had design flaws; the types of cancer, definition of response, and reasons for exclusion of some patients were not documented. The National Cancer Institute (NCI) Division of Cancer Treatment decided not to begin NCI-sponsored clinical trials

because of the incomplete and unimpressive data from this study (Hunt and Connelly, 1995).

In another study of cancer patients taking shark cartilage either rectally or orally, 10 of the 20 patients reported an improved quality of life—including decreased pain and increased appetite—after 8 weeks. Also, 4 of the 20 patients showed partial or complete response (50% to 100% reduction in tumor mass). Patient selection criteria, cartilage dose, concomitant antitumorigenic therapy, and the type of cancer studied were not presented (Mathews, 1993).

A 12-week trial on 60 patients with advanced cancer evaluated the safety and efficacy of shark cartilage. All patients were given 1 g/kg of powdered shark cartilage daily for 12 weeks. Of the 47 fully assessable patients, 5 were taken off study because of GI toxicity or intolerance to shark cartilage. Progressive disease occurred in 27 patients. Five patients died of progressive disease while undergoing shark cartilage therapy. No complete or partial responses were noted. Under the specific conditions of this study, shark cartilage as a single agent was inactive in patients with advanced-stage cancer and had no salutary effect on quality of life. Unanswered is whether shark cartilage in combination with conventional chemotherapy or as adjuvant therapy in early-stage disease is beneficial (Miller et al., 1998).

Dosage

For cancer treatment, typical doses of commercially available shark cartilage dietary supplements range from 500 to 4,500 mg/day P.O., depending on the type of preparation and the amount of "pure" shark cartilage contained. Many commercially available shark cartilage food supplements contain only binding agents or fillers. Without reliable dose-response data and bioavailability studies, it is difficult to determine if these products have true antiangiogenic activity.

The manufacturer of commercially available capsules and tablets recommends the dosing interval to be two to six times daily.
Ampules: 1 ampule P.O. daily.
Concentrates: 1 to 2 tbsp/day P.O.
Powder: 1 g in divided doses P.O. t.i.d.

Adverse reactions
Hepatic: *hepatitis.*

Interactions
None reported.

Contraindications and precautions
Use shark cartilage cautiously in patients with hepatic disease.

Special considerations
• Inform the patient that data supporting the use of shark cartilage for any cancer are inadequate.

Bold italic type indicates that reaction may be life-threatening.

RESEARCH FINDINGS
Shark cartilage–induced hepatitis

A case of shark cartilage–induced hepatitis was reported in a 57-year-old man with a 3-week history of anorexia, diarrhea, nausea, and vomiting. He took no prescription drugs but had begun taking shark cartilage dietary supplements 10 weeks before hospitalization. Because of a change in the odor of the supplements, he stopped taking them a few days before his symptoms began. He denied using alcohol or drugs and had no history of blood transfusions.

The patient's evaluation included ultrasonography of the right upper quadrant and computed tomographic scan of the abdomen, both of which yielded unremarkable results. Results of hepatitis serologic tests as well as tests for antinuclear antibody, ferritin, and acetaminophen levels were also unrevealing. The patient was discharged with a presumed diagnosis of drug-induced hepatitis. A follow-up examination performed 6 weeks after discharge showed normal liver function (Ashar and Vargo, 1996).

- Advise the patient to undergo periodic liver function testing if the use of shark cartilage is planned. (See *Shark cartilage–induced hepatitis*.)
- Inform the patient that commercially available forms of shark cartilage contain varying amounts of the active ingredient.

Points of interest
- After the publication of W. Lane's *Sharks Don't Get Cancer* in 1992, shark cartilage became the newest "cancer cure." Contributing to the media frenzy, a *60 Minutes* segment in February 1993 spotlighted shark cartilage as a promising treatment, and cancer information offices were swamped with calls about what some believed to be a new weapon against cancer.

Commentary
Because most macromolecules are usually not absorbed by the intestinal tract, it is questionable that oral administration of shark cartilage can release some compounds into the blood. No reliable dose-response data or bioavailability studies are available.

No well-controlled clinical studies have been published. The NCI began a trial of shark cartilage in 1994, but it was stopped because each batch of shark cartilage (provided by advocates) was contaminated. There is no evidence that shark cartilage offers any benefit to patients with cancer. The demonstration of efficacy requires randomized, controlled trials with shark cartilage versus the best supportive care or conventional salvage chemotherapy with or without shark cartilage. These issues may now be moot because of the identification of purified antiangiogenic factors (such as angiostatin and endostatin) and the anticipated or imminent initiation of phase I/II trials (Arnst, 1998).

References
Arnst, C. "Starving Tumors to Death," *Business Week*, 65-66, April 27,1998.

Ashar, B., and Vargo, E. "Shark Cartilage–induced Hepatitis," *Ann Intern Med* 125:780-81, 1996.

Hunt, T.J., and Connelly, J.F. "Shark Cartilage for Cancer Treatment," *Am J Health-Syst Pharm* 52:1756-60, 1995.

Mathews, J. "Media Feeds Frenzy Over Shark Cartilage as Cancer Treatment," *J Natl Cancer Inst* 85:1190-91, 1993.

Miller, D.R., et al. "Phase I/II Trial of the Safety and Efficacy of Shark Cartilage in the Treatment of Advanced Cancer," *J Clin Oncol* 16:3649-55, 1998.

Prudden, J. "The Clinical Acceleration of Wound Healing with Cartilage," *Surg Gynecol Obstet* 105:283-87, 1965.

SHEPHERD'S PURSE

CAPSELLA, CASE-WEED, MOTHER'S HEART, SHOVELWEED

Taxonomic class
Brassicaceae

Common trade names
None known.

Common forms
Available as dried herb and liquid extract (1 oz).

Source
The leaves and stems of *Capsella bursa-pastoris* are most commonly sought for their medicinal properties.

Chemical components
Shepherd's purse contains flavonoids (quercetin, diosmetin, luteolin, and hesperetin), their glycosides (rutin, diosmin, and hesperidin), various amines (acetylcholine, choline, histamine, and tyramine), volatile oils (predominantly camphor), carotenoids, fumaric acid, sinigrin (mustard oil glucoside), and vitamins C and K.

Actions
Shepherd's purse is claimed to have antihemorrhagic and urinary antiseptic properties. Some sources suggest that the seeds have skin-reddening properties. Ethanolic extracts of shepherd's purse have demonstrated anti-inflammatory and reduced vessel wall permeability effects. Also, intraperitoneal injection accelerated recovery of stress-induced gastric lesions in rats. Gastric acid secretion was unaffected (Kuroda and Takagi, 1969).

Hypotensive effects have been noted in several animal models. Negative inotropic and chronotropic effects have been seen, including effects causing coronary vasodilation (Jurisson, 1971).

Unidentified components have been shown to cause smooth-muscle contraction (intestine, uterine, tracheal) and sedative effects in animals (Jurisson, 1971). Weak and limited antibacterial and antineoplastic activities have also been demonstrated with some components of shepherd's purse (Kuroda, 1977; Moskalenko, 1986).

Reported uses
Shepherd's purse has been claimed to be popular therapy for diarrhea, hematemesis, hematuria, menorrhagia, and other bleeding disorders. Scientific evidence of these uses in humans is lacking.

Dosage
Dried plant: infusion of 1 oz of dried plant in 12 oz of boiling water; cool and take P.O. t.i.d.
Liquid extract: 1 tsp in 8 oz of water P.O. q.i.d.

Adverse reactions
CNS: ataxia, sedation.
CV: hypotension.
EENT: mydriasis.
Metabolic: hypothyroidism with thyroid enlargement (isothiocyanate component).
Respiratory: *respiratory paralysis* (in animals given toxic doses).

Interactions
Antihypertensives: May increase hypotensive effects. Do not use together.
Beta blockers, calcium channel blockers, digoxin: Added effects on myocardium. Avoid administration with shepherd's purse.
Hypnotic drugs, sedatives: Added CNS effects. Avoid administration with shepherd's purse.
Warfarin: Because the plant contains vitamin K, the potential to antagonize warfarin exists if ingested in sufficient quantity. Avoid administration with shepherd's purse.

Contraindications and precautions
Avoid using shepherd's purse in pregnant or breast-feeding patients; effects are unknown. Use cautiously in patients receiving heart rate–modifying drugs or CNS depressants and in those with heart or lung disease.

Special considerations
• Inform the patient that insufficient evidence exists to support a role for any therapeutic application of shepherd's purse.
• Suggest other, well-known and well-proven therapies to patients with significant heart or lung disease.

- Caution the patient not to self-treat symptoms of illness before seeking appropriate medical evaluation because this may delay diagnosis of a serious medical condition.
- Urge the patient to notify the prescriber and pharmacist of any herbal or dietary supplement he is taking when filling a new prescription.

Commentary
Most of the data regarding shepherd's purse come from in vitro models or animal studies. Few or no human clinical trial data exist to support a role for this herb in therapeutic applications. Shepherd's purse may be dangerous for patients with preexisting lung or heart disease.

Despite interesting pharmacologic effects in animals, human clinical data are needed before shepherd's purse can be recommended for use.

References
Jurisson, S. "Determination of Active Substances of *Capsella bursa-pastoris*," *Tartu Riiliku Ulikooli Toim* 270:71-79, 1971.

Kuroda, K. "Neoplasm Inhibitor from *Capsella bursa pastoris*," *Japan Kokai* 41:207, 1977.

Kuroda, K., and Takagi. K. "Studies on *Capsella bursa-pastoris.* Part II. Diuretic, Anti-inflammatory and Anti-ulcer Action of Ethanol Extracts of the Herb," *Arch Int Pharmacodyn Ther* 178:392-99, 1969.

Moskalenko, S.A. "Preliminary Screening of Far-Eastern Ethnomedicinal Plants for Antibacterial Activity," *J Ethnopharmacol* 15:231-59, 1986.

SKUNK CABBAGE

DRACONTIUM FOETIDUM, MEADOW CABBAGE, POLE-CAT CABBAGE, SKUNKWEED

Taxonomic class
Araceae

Common trade names
None known.

Common forms
Available as liquid extract, powdered root, and tincture.

Source
The rhizome and roots of the skunk cabbage plant (*Lysichitum americanum;* formerly *Symplocarpus foetidus)* are sought for their active ingredients in skunk cabbage.

Chemical components
Skunk cabbage consists of starches, gum-sugar, fixed and volatile oils, resin, tannin, an acrid principal, iron, large amounts of nonspecified alkaloids, phenolic compounds, and glycosides. There have been reports of high concentrations of oxalates or salts in the rhizome, consisting of calcium that forms insoluble calcium crystals. Some of these oxalates contain potassium, but these crystals are soluble (Konyukhov et al., 1970).

Actions
Little is known about the components of skunk cabbage and their pharmacologic activity. Few documented scientific studies about the pharmacologic and medicinal use of skunk cabbage in vitro or in animal or human models exist. One study suggests that some components may have antifungal properties (Hanawa et al., 2000).

Reported uses
Skunk cabbage has been used for chest tightness, irritable coughs, and other spasmodic respiratory tract disorders (asthma, bronchitis, and whooping cough).

It is also claimed to be useful in nervous disorders. Another claim as a diuretic is also unsubstantiated. The Micmac Indians crushed the leaves of skunk cabbage and inhaled the pungent oils to treat headaches.

Dosage
For coughs, 0.5 to 1 ml of extract (1:1 in 25% alcohol) P.O. t.i.d.; 2 to 4 ml of tincture (1:10 in 25% alcohol) P.O. t.i.d.; or 0.5 to 1 g of rhizome powder mixed with honey P.O. t.i.d.

Adverse reactions
CNS: dizziness, drowsiness, headache, vertigo.
EENT: burning of oral mucosa, stomatitis (when root is taken orally and calcium oxalate crystals may be embedded in mouth).
GI: nausea, vomiting (with overdose by inhalation).
GU: damaged renal tubules (where the crystals may lodge).
Skin: inflammation, pruritus, redness (contact with root).

Interactions
None reported.

Contraindications and precautions
Avoid using skunk cabbage in pregnant or breast-feeding patients; effects are unknown. Also avoid its use in patients who have a history of kidney stones because of its high oxalate concentration.

Special considerations
• Inform the patient that little information is available regarding skunk cabbage.
• Inform the patient about the available pharmaceutical therapies for treating asthma and bronchitis.
• Advise women to avoid using skunk cabbage during pregnancy or when breast-feeding.

Points of interest
• Skunk cabbage gets its name from the appearance of its leaf and from the distinctive, unpleasant odor it secretes when bruised.
• The root of skunk cabbage is bitter and acrid and has a disagreeable odor.

Commentary
Because of the lack of information regarding the components of skunk cabbage, its pharmacologic activities, and its safety and efficacy, its use as a medicinal therapeutic agent cannot be recommended.

References
Hanawa, F., et al. "Antifungal Nitro Compounds from Skunk Cabbage *(Lysichitum americanum)* Leaves Treated with Cupric Chloride," *Phytochemistry* 53(1):55-58, 2000.

Konyukhov, V.P., et al. "Dynamics of the Accumulation of Biologically Active Agents in *Lysichitum camtsochatcense* and *Symplocarpus foetidus*," *Uch Zap Khabarovsk Gos Pedagog Inst* 26:59-62, 1970.

SLIPPERY ELM

AMERICAN ELM, INDIAN ELM, MOOSE ELM, RED ELM, SWEET ELM

Taxonomic class
Ulmaceae

Common trade names
Slippery Elm Bark, Vegetarian Caps

Common forms
Available as powdered or shredded bark, capsules (375 mg, 400 mg), liquid extract (1:1 in 60% alcohol), and lozenges.

Source
The inner bark of *Ulmus rubra* Muhl. (*Ulmus fulva* Mich.) is used for medicinal purposes. Slippery elm can be found throughout North America. The pieces of bark are flat (2 to 4 mm thick) and oblong. The bark's outer surface is light yellow to reddish brown; the inner surface is much paler.

Chemical components
The major therapeutic component in slippery elm bark is a mucilaginous material that consists of hexoses, pentoses, methylpentoses, at least two polyuronides, glucose, galacturonic acid, *l*-rhamnose, *d*-galactose, and fructose (trace). Other components include tannins, phytosterols (phytositosterol, citrostadienol, dolichol), sesquiterpenes, calcium oxalate, and cholesterol.

Actions
Slippery elm has largely been used as a soothing agent. It has demulcent and emollient activity (Locock, 1997). The tannin components may impart some astringent activity.

Reported uses
Although this plant was once listed in the USP, no clinical study data are available to support its use. Its soothing effects have long been described

---

and been accepted by many herbalists. Slippery elm has, therefore, been used as an antitussive and a skin emollient and to soothe GI discomfort. Some pharmacognosy textbooks have added that a poultice of powdered slippery elm bark has been used for inflammation of the skin and GI tract.

Dosage

For GI discomfort, powdered bark as a 1:8 decoction of 4 to 16 ml P.O. t.i.d., or 4 g in 500 ml of boiling water P.O. t.i.d.; or 5 ml of liquid extract P.O. t.i.d.

For topical use as a skin emollient, poultice made of coarse powdered bark in boiling water.

Adverse reactions

GU: spontaneous abortion (with whole bark preparations).

Interactions

None reported.

Contraindications and precautions

Avoid using slippery elm in pregnant or breast-feeding patients and in those who are hypersensitive to slippery elm or its components.

Special considerations

● Inform the patient that insufficient data exist to describe the risks and benefits of slippery elm.

● Advise women to avoid using slippery elm during pregnancy or when breast-feeding.

● Caution the patient to avoid whole-bark preparations of slippery elm because little evidence exists to support the herb's use.

● Although no known chemical interactions have been reported in clinical studies, consideration must be given to the pharmacologic properties of the herbal product and the potential for exacerbation of the intended therapeutic effect of conventional drugs.

Points of interest

● Small quantities of powdered slippery elm bark have been included in the multiherbal decoction known as Essiac. Anecdotal reports supported the notion that this formulation had anticancer activity, but a clinical trial could not show any benefit.

Commentary

Insufficient published data are available to recommend internal use of this agent. Proven contemporary therapies should be used instead.

References

Locock, R.A. "Essiac," *Can Pharm J* 14:18-19, 1997.

SOAPWORT

BOUNCING BET, BRUISEWORT, CROW SOAP, FULLER'S HERB, LATHERWORT, SOAP ROOT, SWEET BETTY, WILD SWEET WILLIAM

Taxonomic class
Caryophyllaceae

Common trade names
None known.

Common forms
Available as a decoction, dried root and leaves, extract, fluidextract, inspissated juice, and root powder.

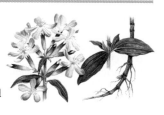

Source
Medicinal formulations are extracted from the root and leaves of *Saponaria officinalis,* which is indigenous to Asia and has become naturalized to eastern North America.

Chemical components
Chemical components of soapwort include saponin, sapotoxin, saponarin, several saporins (ribosome-inactivating proteins), resin, gum, woody fiber, and mucilage.

Actions
Soapwort is claimed to alter metabolism and have astringent, diaphoretic, and tonic effects. Saponins derived from *S. officinalis* have been shown to reduce the rate of bile salt absorption in vivo in rats. Dietary saponins may also be useful for controlling plasma cholesterol levels and nutrient absorption.

Saporins have been shown to be powerful cytotoxic agents in vitro, especially when conjugated to molecular targeting antibodies or protein ligands (Soria, 1989). Saporins, alone or with targeting molecules, have shown cytotoxic action in vitro to human breast cancer, leukemia, lymphoma, and melanoma cells (Gasperi-Campani et al., 1991; Siena et al., 1989; Tecce et al., 1991).

Reported uses
Soapwort has been used externally for its sudsing action as an ingredient in herbal shampoos. Historically, soapwort preparations were taken internally for itching associated with dandruff and dermatitis, gout, rheumatism, and cutaneous symptoms associated with syphilis. It has also been used for jaundice and intestinal problems. Human clinical trials are lacking for any medicinal uses.

Soapwort has been used as an expectorant and laxative in small doses and for such skin conditions as acne, boils, eczema, and psoriasis; human studies are lacking for these uses.

Bold italic type indicates that reaction may be life-threatening.

Dosage
Decoction: 2 to 4 fl oz P.O. t.i.d. or q.i.d.
Extract (or inspissated juice): 10 to 20 grains P.O. t.i.d. as needed.
Fluidextract: ¼ to 1 dram P.O. t.i.d. as needed.

Adverse reactions
CNS: *neurotoxicity* (Chan et al., 1995).
GI: GI ulceration, nausea, vomiting (oral administration); indigestion (severe).
GU: *nephrotoxicity.*
Hepatic: *hepatotoxicity* (Stripe et al., 1987).

Interactions
None reported.

Contraindications and precautions
Avoid using soapwort in pregnant or breast-feeding patients; effects are unknown. Because of the numerous toxicities associated with ingestion of soapwort, its use is contraindicated in many patients.

Special considerations
🕮 **ALERT** Some components of soapwort, notably saponin, sapotoxin, and the saporins, are potentially gastrotoxic; therefore, high doses of the herb for prolonged periods (longer than 2 weeks) should be avoided.
● Periodically monitor hepatic and renal function of patients who use soapwort.
● Advise the patient to avoid oral consumption of soapwort because of its strong cathartic effects.
● Although no known chemical interactions have been reported in clinical studies, consideration must be given to the pharmacologic properties of the herbal product and the potential for exacerbation of the intended therapeutic effect of conventional drugs.

Points of interest
● The Egyptian soapwort root, *Gypsophila struthium*, has seldom been used medicinally as a substitute for soapwort (*S. officinalis*). It contains saponin and some of the same components as *S. officinalis*.
● Saponins are known for their ability to produce foam or suds in solution. The term saponification refers to the process of making soap. The taste of plant products that contain high concentrations of saponin is said to be much like soap. Soapwort was once popular as a cleaning and sizing agent in the textile industry. This use, known as "fulling," is how soapwort came to be referred to as "fuller's herb."
● Soapwort is commonly included as an ingredient in herbal shampoos.

Commentary
Soapwort has traditionally been used to treat symptoms associated with syphilis and for treating jaundice and intestinal complaints. The presence of potentially toxic components makes this root and its preparations poor choices as a general tonic or for supportive therapy. Although

purified saponins have been shown to be cytotoxic to cancer cells in vitro, there is no clinical evidence for their use. Because of the availability of safer, more effective drugs, soapwort cannot be recommended for any indication.

References

Anger, R.T., et al. "Preferential Destruction of Cerebellar Purkinje Cells by OX7-Saporin," *Neurotoxicity* 21(3):395-403, 2000.

Barbieri, L., et al. "Polynucleotide Adenosine Glycosidase Activity of Saporin-L1 Effect on Forms of Mammalian DNA," *Biochem Biophys Acta* 1480(1-2):258-66, 2000.

Chan, T.Y., et al. "Neurotoxicity Following the Ingestion of a Chinese Medicinal Plant, *Alocasia macrorrhiza*," *Hum Exp Toxicol* 14:727-28, 1995.

Gasperi-Campani, A., et al. "Inhibition of Growth of Breast Cancer Cells In Vitro by the Ribosome-inactivating Protein Saporin 6," *Anticancer Res* 11:1007-11, 1991.

Siena, S., et al. "Activity of Monoclonal Antibody-Saporin-6 Conjugate Against B-Lymphoma Cells," *Cancer Res* 49:3328-32, 1989.

Soria, M. "Immunotoxins, Ligand-Toxin Conjugates and Molecular Targeting," *Pharmacol Res* 21(Suppl. 2):35-46, 1989.

Stripe, F., et al. "Hepatotoxicity of Immunotoxins Made with Saporin, a Ribosome-inactivating Protein from *Saponaria officinalis*," *Virchows Arch* 53: 259-71, 1987.

Tecce, R., et al. "Saporin 6 Conjugated to Monoclonal Antibody Selectivity Kills Human Melanoma Cells," *Melanoma Res* 1:115-23, 1991.

Ying, W., et al. "Anti-B16-f10 Melanoma Activity of a Basic Fibroblast Growth Factor—Saporin Mitotoxin," *Cancer* 74(3):848-53, 1994.

SORREL

BELGIAN-RED SORREL, CUCKOO'S MEATE, CUCKOO SORROW, DOCK, GARDEN SORREL, GREENSAUCE, GREEN SORREL, SHEEP SORREL, SOUR DOCK, SOURGRASS, SOUR SAUCE, SOURSUDS

Taxonomic class
Polygonaceae

Common trade names
Sheep Sorrel, Sheep Sorrel Burdock

Common forms
Available as dried plant liquid (1 oz), juice from fresh plants, liquid (1 oz), and teas.

Source
Garden sorrel is known as *Rumex acetosa;* the popular sorrel is the sheep sorrel (*R. acetosella*). All sorrel species are native to Europe and northern Asia and have been naturalized in North America. Several parts of the sorrel plant, such as the flowers, leaves, roots, and seeds, have been used for their medicinal value.

Chemical components

Oxalates, particularly potassium oxalate (a soluble oxalate salt), is a constituent of the sorrel plant. Although it occurs in the soluble oxalate form and especially in the leaves, the content of oxalates in the plant varies with geographic location and season. Other compounds include tartaric acid, anthracene, oxymethylanthraquinone, and tannins. Ascorbic acid has also been identified in high concentrations in the leaf and berry. The active chemical compounds have not been isolated.

Actions

Because of the poisonous nature of the soluble oxalates found in the plant, a wide range of toxicity in humans and animals has been described. Soluble oxalate salts are absorbed without irritating the mucosa. The onset of symptoms occurs from 2 to 48 hours after the ingestion of these salts (Sanz and Reig, 1992). Oxalates are excreted unchanged in the urine within 24 to 36 hours after ingestion.

Reported uses

Various claims for the therapeutic effect of sorrel have contributed to its medical use as an antiseptic and a diuretic and for treating scurvy. It has also been used in the treatment of diarrhea because of its astringent properties.

Dosage

No consensus exists. The flowers and leaves are made into a tea. Juice from the plant may be diluted with water and taken P.O.

Adverse reactions

CNS: brain damage (caused by soluble oxalate salts).
CV: myocardial damage (caused by soluble oxalate salts).
GI: gastroenteritis.
GU: renal damage.
Hepatic: hepatic dysfunction (caused by soluble oxalate salts).
Metabolic: hypocalcemia with resultant tetany.
Skin: dermatitis (with fresh herbal products).

Interactions

Diuretics: Additive effects. Avoid administration with sorrel.
Other renal or hepatotoxic drugs: Additive toxic effects. Avoid administration with sorrel.

Contraindications and precautions

Sorrel is contraindicated in children, in pregnant or breast-feeding patients, and in patients who are prone to developing or have a history of kidney stones.

Special considerations

• Urge the patient to change the water in which sorrel leaves are cooked at least once to decrease the herb's potency; otherwise, the herb is toxic.

🖤 **ALERT** After ingesting 500 g of garden sorrel in a soup, a patient experienced diarrhea, hypocalcemia, metabolic acidosis, and vomiting, leading to extensive liver necrosis and death (Farre et al., 1989).
• Advise the patient to use sorrel cautiously because the oxalates contained in the plant may be toxic.
• Instruct the patient to keep sorrel out of the reach of children and pets.

Points of interest
• The estimated fatal dose of oxalic acid is 15 to 30 g; as little as 5 g may cause death.
• The concentration of soluble oxalates in the leaves varies, depending on the season and geographic location of the sorrel plant.
• The herb was used in the 16th century for treating fevers. The medicinal value of sorrel was recognized through the 19th century, but concern over the plant's poisonous nature limited its use (Crellin and Philpott, 1990).

Commentary
Therapeutic claims for the use of sorrel to treat fevers and diarrhea and as a diuretic lack supporting evidence. There appear to be no data regarding efficacy in animals or humans. Toxicity and death in animals and humans have been documented in the literature.

References
Crellin, J.K., and Philpott, J. *A Reference Guide to Medicinal Plants: Herbal Medicine Past and Present.* Durham, N.C.: Duke University Press, 1990.
Farre, M., et al. "Fatal Oxalic Acid Poisoning from Sorrel Soup," *Lancet* 2:1524, 1989.
Sanz, P., and Reig, R. "Clinical and Pathological Findings in Plant Oxalosis: A Review," *Am J Forensic Med Pathol* 13:342-45, 1992.

SOUTHERNWOOD

APPLERINGIE, BOY'S LOVE, GOD'S TREE, LAD'S LOVE, MAIDEN'S RUIN, OLD MAN, *GARDE ROBE*

Taxonomic class
Asteraceae

Common trade names
None known.

Common forms
Available as extracts, oil, and teas.

Source
Artemisia abrotanum is a strongly aromatic, shrubby perennial that is native to southern Europe. The leaves, tops, shoots, and seeds are used.

Chemical components
The volatile oil of *A. abrotanum* is composed primarily of absinthol. Other components include abrotanin, adenosine, adenine, choline, caly-

---

canthosides, guanines, essential oils, malates, nitrates of potassium, isofraxidine, resin, scopolin, scopoletin, tannins, succinic acid, and umbelliferone.

Actions
The extraction process of *A. abrotanum* isolated four flavonols: three coumarins (umbelliferone, scopoletine, and isofraxidine) and one sesquiterpene (hydroxydavanone). These flavonols showed a dose-dependent relaxing effect on the carbacholine-induced contraction of guinea pig trachea. These components inhibit the cAMP phosphodiesterase and the spasmolytic flavone 7-*O*-methyleriodictyol. More studies and assays are needed to determine the extent of southernwood's spasmolytic effects. Human studies are needed to determine this herb's place in medicinal use (Bergendorff and Sterner, 1995).

One German abstract describes the choleretic effects of isofraxidine, scopoletine, and umbelliferone, with isofraxidine being the most potent (Nieschulz and Schmersahl, 1968).

Reported uses
Medicinal use of southernwood is limited and sparsely documented. Anecdotal claims include its use as an anthelmintic, a digestive aid, and a diuretic. Others include its use as an antiseptic detergent, a cure for fevers and wounds, and a uterine stimulant and to promote menstruation. The ash of southernwood mixed with an ointment is thought to promote hair regrowth in balding men. None of these claims is supported by published trials.

Dosage
Dried herb: 2 to 4 g added to hot water and taken P.O. t.i.d.
Extract (1:1 in 25% alcohol): 2 to 4 ml P.O. t.i.d.

Adverse reactions
None reported.

Interactions
None reported.

Contraindications and precautions
Pregnant or breast-feeding patients should not use this herb; effects are unknown.

Special considerations
• Inform the patient that little information exists regarding the benefits and dangers of southernwood.
• Advise the patient to consult his health care provider before using herbal preparations because a treatment that has been clinically researched and proved effective may be available.
• Although no known chemical interactions have been reported in clinical studies, consideration must be given to the pharmacologic proper-

ties of the herbal product and the potential for exacerbation of the intended therapeutic effect of conventional drugs.
• Advise women to avoid using southernwood during pregnancy or when breast-feeding.

Points of interest
• *Artemisia* is thought to come from Artemis, the Greek goddess of hunting and chastity. Artemis was identified with Diana, who is the goddess of nature, the forests, and the moon.
• There are more than 180 species of *Artemisia*, including *A. absinthium* (wormwood), *A. vulgaris* (mugwort), and *A. abrotanum* (southernwood).
• Southernwood's obnoxious odor fends off moths and insects, leading to the name *Garde Robe*. It has been placed in clothes and on the skin for this purpose. The branches and leaves produce a yellow dye used for coloring wool.

Commentary
There is little documentation in clinical trials supporting the use of southernwood for medicinal purposes. The emergence of other *Artemisia* species for use in herbal preparations has made southernwood a less favorable option. The most likely uses for this agent appear to be as a stimulant for menstruation and, possibly, a spasmolytic. The use of southernwood should be avoided until clinical studies support these therapeutic claims and the herb's safety and efficacy can be established.

References
Bergendorff, O., and Sterner, O. "Spasmolytic Flavonols from *Artemisia abrotanum*," *Planta Med* 61: 370-71, 1995.
Nieschulz, V.O., and Schmersahl, P. "Uber choleretische Wirkstoffe aus *Artemisia abrotanum* L.," *Arzneimittelforschung* 18:1330-36, 1968.

SOY

Common trade names
Multi-ingredient preparations: Estroven, Genisoy, Genistein, Isoflavone, Iso-Soy Protein, Maxilife, Novasoy, Soy Isoflavone, Ultrasoy

Common forms
Available in capsules (50 mg isoflavones), powder (to reconstitute into soy protein shakes), and tablets (various strengths, ranging from 20 to 50 mg isoflavones).

Source
Foods that contain soy include soy milk, roasted soybeans, textured vegetable protein, soyflour, tempeh, and tofu.

Chemical components
Soy contains isoflavones that are commonly referred to as phytoestrogens. The most noted isoflavones are daidzein, genistein, and equol.

Bold italic type indicates that reaction may be life-threatening.

Actions

Although isoflavones interact with estrogen receptors, they are not estrogens because they lack the steroidal nucleus; nor are they converted in the body to estrogens. Their ability to attach to estrogen receptors is thought to be due in part to the strategically placed hydoxyl groups in their structure. Isoflavone estrogenic effects of soy are weak and minimal in perimenopausal women because of the abundance of estrogen. When estrogen decreases at menopause, the isoflavones' effect is greater.

Reported uses

Soy products have been advocated for treating symptoms associated with menopause. With regular consumption, it is thought that the isoflavones (phytoestrogens) reduce hot flashes and vaginal dryness and have a positive effect on sleep difficulties and mood disorders (Scambia et al., 2000; Albertazzi et al., 1998). Epidemiologic evidence in Asian women, whose soy consumption is high, has shown that they experience fewer hot flashes than do European and Western women. Twenty-five percent of Japanese women complain of hot flashes compared with 85% of North American women and 80% of European women (*The Medical Letter*, 2000).

Other uses suggested for soy include the prevention of breast, colon, prostate, and uterine cancer and osteoporosis and the reduction of heart disease through lowering total cholesterol and LDL levels, blood pressure, and, possibly, the risk of atherosclerosis.

It is theorized that the isoflavones prevent cancer by inhibiting the growth of existing tumor cells. Although a definitive statement that soy reduces cancer risk cannot be made at this time, a review of in vitro and in vivo data at the National Cancer Institute provides evidence of a protective effect, which warrants continued investigation (Messina et al., 1991, 1994). Soy protein was evaluated for its cholesterol-lowering effects in 26 normocholesterolemic and hypercholesterolemic men. The results suggest that soy may enhance the hypocholesterolemic effects of a National Cholesterol Education Program Step 1 diet (Wong et al., 1998). Phytoestrogens may stabilize bone mineral density, thereby reducing osteoporosis and fractures (Cauley et al., 1995). Animal experiments in ovarian hormone–deficient rats demonstrated a reduction in bone loss with soy protein–based diets (Arjmandi et al., 1998). Preliminary results from human studies indicate that the benefit may not be as great in humans. The only positive effects of phytoestrogens on bone in postmenopausal women have been limited to the lumbar vertebrae (Anderson et al., 1998). One study did not support a preventive effect of low, unsupplemented dietary intake of phytoestrogen on postmenopausal cortical bone loss. No conclusion could be drawn about effects of higher doses of phytoestrogens (Kardinaal et al., 1998).

Dosage

Recommendations have been based on the daily average diet of Asian women, which contains 25 to 40 mg of isoflavones. Most commercial products provide this amount through measurement of the isoflavones genistein and daidzein.

Adverse reactions
GI: flatulence (minimized by slowly increasing ingested amount).
Other: intolerance to soy products and soybeans.

Interactions
None reported.

Contraindications and precautions
Soy is contraindicated in patients who are hypersensitive to soy products and in those with estrogen-dependent tumors (Hsieh et al., 1998).

Special considerations
• Inform the patient that soy contains some substances, besides the isoflavones, that may contribute to the proposed effects. Therefore, limiting intake to only isoflavones may not be beneficial.
• Inform the patient that isoflavones (phytoestrogens) are found in various food supplements, including wheat, barley, oats, sunflower seeds, peanuts, walnuts, almonds, cashews, apples, gooseberries, guava, yams, broccoli, cauliflower, green tea, black tea, wine, bourbon, and beer (Mazur, 1998).
• Advise the patient to consult a health care provider before using herbal preparations because a treatment that has been clinically researched and proved effective may be available.

Points of interest
• Various soy products are available commercially. Soy milk is an excellent alternative for patients with lactose intolerance or dairy allergies and those who require a gluten-free diet.

Commentary
Most of the evidence that soy products help to prevent cancer, heart disease, menopausal symptoms, and osteoporosis is in a preliminary stage. Rationale for the use of soy is based on epidemiologic evidence from Asian countries, suggesting that a diet high in isoflavones can reduce menopausal symptoms and cancer risks, prevent CV disease, and improve bone density. Women who are seeking alternatives to pharmaceutical hormone replacement therapy (HRT) because of a desire for more natural remedies, adverse reactions to HRT, or fear of breast or endometrial cancer often look to soy and the isoflavones as a substitute. There is some evidence implying soy's usefulness, but it is inadequate to recommend routine use or replacement of HRT regimens.

References
Albertazzi, P., et al. "The Effect of Dietary Soy Supplementation on Hot Flashes," *Obstet Gynecol* 91(1):6-11, 1998.
Anderson, J.J., et al. "Phytoestrogens and Bone," *Baillieres Clin Endocrinol Metab* 12(4):543-57, 1998.

Bold italic type indicates that reaction may be life-threatening.

Arjmandi, B.H., et al. "Bone-sparing Effect of Soy Protein in Ovarian Hormone-deficient Rats Is Related to Its Isoflavone Content," *Am J Clin Nutr* 68(6Suppl):1364S-68S, 1998.

Cauley, J.A., et al. "Estrogen Replacement Therapy and Fractures in Older Women. Study of Osteoporotic Fractures Research Group," *Ann Intern Med* 122(1):9-16, 1995.

Hsieh, C.Y., et al. "Estrogenic Effects of Genistein on the Growth of Estrogen Receptor-positive Human Breast Cancer (MCF-7) Cells In Vitro and In Vivo," *Cancer Res* 58(17):3833-38, 1998.

Kardinaal, A.F., et al. "Phyto-oestrogen Excretion and Rate of Bone Loss in Post-menopausal Women," *Eur J Clin Nutr* 52(11):850-55, 1998.

Mazur, W. "Phytoestrogen Content in Foods," *Bailliere's Clin Endocrinol Metab* 12(4):729-42, 1998.

Messina, M., et al. "The Role of Soy Products in Reducing Risk of Cancer," *J Natl Cancer Inst* 83:541-46, 1991.

Messina, M.J., et al. "Soy Intake and Cancer Risk: A Review of the In Vitro and In Vivo Data," *Nutr Cancer* 21(2):113-31, 1994.

Scambia, G., et al. "Clinical Effects of a Standardized Soy Extract in Postmeno-pausal Women: A Pilot Study," *J North Am Menopause Soc* 7(2):105-11, 2000.

The Medical Letter 42(1072):17-18, 2000.

Wong, W.W., et al. "Cholesterol-lowering Effect of Soy Protein in Normocholes-terolemic and Hypercholesterolemic Men," *Am J Clin Nutr* 686 (Suppl):1385S-89S, 1998.

SPIRULINA

BLUE-GREEN ALGAE, DIHE, TECUITLATL

Taxonomic class
Oscillatoriaceae

Common trade names
Spirulina

Common forms
Capsules: 420 mg, 500 mg, 750 mg
Powders: 20 mg
Supplemental fruit drinks: 20 mg
Tablets: 250 mg, 380 mg, 500 mg, 750 mg
   Also available as fresh plant for consumption as food.

Source
Spirulina belongs to the Oscillatoriaceae family of algae that occur in high-salt, alkaline waters in subtropical and tropical areas. There are about 35 *Spirulina* species. They appear blue-green because of the chlorophyll (green) and phycocyanin (blue) pigments in their cells and take the form of microscopic, corkscrew-shaped filaments.

Chemical components
Spirulina has a high nutritional content. Protein represents 60% to 70% of its sample, even in dry weight. The protein content includes 22 amino acids, 47% of which represent essential amino acids, such as phenylala-

nine. Although spirulina is one of the richest protein sources of plant origin, 15% of the crude protein is derived from nonprotein nitrogen. Spirulina also contains fats, carbohydrates, B complex vitamins (especially B_{12}), vitamins A and E, trace elements (manganese, selenium, and zinc), minerals (calcium, potassium, and magnesium), and iron. The bioavailability of the iron is 60% greater than in commercially available iron supplements. Spirulina also contains gamma-linolenic acid (GLA) and a sulfolipid fraction; GLA is a rich source of omega-6 essential fatty acid.

Actions

Because of its high nutritional content, spirulina has been used as a supplement for malnourished and starving adults and children. A study of malnourished children aged 5 to 12 months who were fed spirulina, milk, or soy milk found that despite a lower protein digestibility (spirulina 60% and soy 70%), nitrogen retention was higher with spirulina (40%) than with soy (30%; Dillon et al., 1995).

Because phenylalanine is thought to act on the brain's appetite center to alleviate hunger pangs, spirulina was used to promote weight loss. However, the FDA advisory committee on OTC drugs has ruled that phenylalanine lacks safety and efficacy data supporting its use in weight control (Popovich, 1982).

A sulfated polysaccharide called calcium spirulan has been formulated from the algae's lipid content, and it exhibits antiviral properties. The compound was found to have a high selectivity index for inhibiting the replication of all enveloped viruses, including human cytomegalovirus, herpes simplex virus, HIV-1, influenza A virus, measles virus, and mumps virus. Research is directed toward a detailed structure of the complex and the relation between molecular conformation and bioavailability (Hayashi et al., 1996).

Reported uses

Spirulina has been used in diet and weight-loss products for its high nutritional value and claimed action on appetite suppression. There are reports of its use instead of dietary supplements, but its cost does not justify its use in this manner. In developing countries, such as Peru, India, Vietnam, and Togo and other African countries, spirulina is used to help fight protein and vitamin A malnutrition. In industrialized countries, the GLA content is thought to contribute to the prevention of CV disease.

A double-blind, placebo-controlled, cross-over study was conducted to evaluate spirulina's effect on weight reduction (Becker et al., 1986). Sixteen patients already enrolled in an outpatient dietary self-help group took part in this 4-week trial. Patients were asked to ingest 14 spirulina tablets (Verum: spirulina 200 mg + synthetic vanilla) or placebo (spinach powder 200 mg + synthetic vanilla) immediately before each meal three times daily. Patients were evaluated for changes in body weight, biochemical variables, blood pressure, heart rate, and adverse effects of treatment (by questionnaire) at 2-week intervals. Each treatment phase lasted for 4 weeks with a 2-week washout between phases. At the end of the study, the spirulina group had dropped an average of

1.4 kg in weight, whereas the placebo group had dropped an average of 0.7 kg. The difference between the two groups was not statistically significant, but the investigators suggested that the results were sufficiently promising to warrant pursuit of a longer-term trial. Concerns exist with respect to the trial's study design (small sample size, unclear blinding and randomization techniques) and short duration.

Calcium spirulina (Ca-SP), a polysaccharide derived from spirulina, has demonstrated inhibition of replicating viral cells (similar to antiretroviral mechanistic activity) in vitro. An inhibition of heparin cofactor II–dependent antithrombin activities has been shown in vitro as well. Simultaneous treatment with Ca-SP and tissue plasminogen activator (tPA) results in a synergistic enhancement of tPA production (Hayakawa et al., 1997).

Other reported uses for spirulina include treatment of anemia, diabetes, glaucoma, hair loss, hepatic disease, peptic ulcers, pancreatitis, and stress. None of these uses has been supported through clinical trials.

Dosage
The usual dose is 3 to 5 g P.O. daily before meals. In malnourished infants, 3 to 15 g/day P.O. has resulted in rapid weight gain.

Adverse reactions
Hepatic: increased serum alkaline phosphatase level (Becker et al., 1986).
Metabolic: increased serum calcium level (Becker et al., 1986).

Interactions
Anticoagulants: Spirulina may interfere with these drugs. Monitor PT and INR.

Contraindications and precautions
Spirulina is contraindicated in patients in whom the risk of heavy metal poisoning is not outweighed by benefit of use. Use cautiously in pregnant or breast-feeding patients.

Special considerations
• Advise the patient that spirulina can contain significant amounts of mercury, depending on where it is grown. Daily consumption of 20 g of spirulina can produce a mercury concentration that is above the 180-mcg safety limit. Reported mean heavy metal levels include arsenic, cadmium, lead, and mercury.
• Inform the patient that spirulina may also contain minute amounts of radioactive divalent and trivalent metallic ions, depending on where the product was manufactured.
• Inform the patient that spirulina has a mild marine odor that is stronger than its taste.

Points of interest
• The GLA content in spirulina is 25% to 30% compared with 10% to 15% in other sources, such as evening primrose oil and black currant berry.

• Algae have long been regarded as promising sources of protein if food shortages occur in the future.

• In regions that are not familiar with its use, the algae's color may present a problem, especially when used in baby foods. Decolorizing the product can be accomplished conveniently.

Commentary

There is no question regarding the nutritional value of spirulina, but more economical means of providing protein and nutrients are available than through algae. Supplementation with commercially available vitamins does not exclude the risks of heavy metal poisoning and exposure to radioactive ions. Spirulina cannot be recommended for any medical use until clinical research details its benefits.

References

Becker, E.W., et al. "Clinical and Biochemical Evaluations of the Alga Spirulina with Regard to Its Application in the Treatment of Obesity. A Double-blind Cross-over Study," *Nutr Report Int* 33(4)565-73, 1986.

Dillon, J.C., et al. "Nutritional Value of the Alga Spirulina," *World Rev Nutr Diet* 77:32-46, 1995.

Hayakawa, Y., et al. "Calcium Spirulan as an Inducer of Tissue-type Plasminogen Activator in Human Fetal Lung Fibroblasts," *Biochem Biophys Acta* 1355(3):241-47, 1997.

Hayashi, T., et al. "Calcium Spirulan, an Inhibitor of Enveloped Virus Replication, from a Blue-Green Alga *Spirulina platensis*," *J Nat Prod* 59:83-87, 1996.

Popovich, N.G. "Spirulina," *Am Pharm* 22:8-10, 1982.

SQUAW VINE

CHECKERBERRY, DEERBERRY, MITCHELLA REPENS, MITCHELLA UNDULATA, ONE-BERRY, PARTRIDGE BERRY, RUNNING BOX, SQUAWBERRY, TWIN BERRY, TWO-EYED BERRY, TWO-EYED CHECKERBERRY, WINTER CLOVER

Taxonomic class

Rubiaceae

Common trade names

Mitchella repens, Partridge Berry, Squaw Vine

Common forms

Available as whole leaves, liquid extract (1 oz, 2 oz), dried plant (powder), and tincture.

Source

Squaw vine is the dried plant of *Mitchella repens* Linne, common to the woodlands of the central and eastern United States. The plant blooms in July and is usually harvested late in summer.

Chemical components
The leaves of the plant contain resin, wax, mucilage, dextrin, and tannin. The leaves are also thought to contain glycosides and saponins (Chevallier, 1996).

Actions
Tannic acid has local astringent properties that act on GI mucosa, which is thought to occur through binding and precipitation of proteins, and forms insoluble complexes with select heavy metal ions, alkaloids, and glycosides. It has also been shown to have antisecretory and antiulcerative effects within the GI tract because of an inhibitory action on the gastric enzyme system. Saponins are usually less toxic to humans after oral ingestion, but when administered I.V., they act as potent hemolytics (Budavari, 1996).

Reported uses
Squaw vine has been used as an astringent, a diuretic, and a tonic. Because its tonic properties are thought to work primarily on the uterus, squaw vine has been used extensively as an aid in labor and childbirth. Native Americans were the first to use the plant to make parturition safer and easier. It has also been used in cases of abdominal pain associated with menstruation, abnormal menstruation, and heavy bleeding (Chevallier, 1996). Other claims include its use as a remedy for amenorrhea, diarrhea, dysentery, dysuria, edema, gonorrhea, hysteria, kidney stones, polyuria, and vaginitis (Duke, 1985). Crushed squaw vine berries have been mixed with myrrh and used for sore nipples (Chevallier, 1996). The use of squaw vine is based on traditional and anecdotal reports, not on controlled human clinical trials.

Dosage
Liquid extract: ½ to 1 tsp P.O. t.i.d.
Squaw vine (dried): 30 to 60 grains (2 to 4 g) P.O.
Tincture: 1 to 2 ml P.O. t.i.d.

Adverse reactions
GI: heartburn, ***hepatotoxicity*** (rare).
Other: irritated mucous membranes.

Interactions
Alkaloid-related drugs (atropine, scopolamine), iron-containing products: Tannic acid may slow metabolic breakdown. Monitor the patient.
Cardiac glycosides: Risk of increased effect of these drugs. Use together cautiously.
Disulfiram: Disulfiram reaction can occur if herbal form contains alcohol. Do not use together.

Contraindications and precautions
Squaw vine is contraindicated during the first and second trimesters of pregnancy. Use cautiously in patients with preexisting hepatic disease or complications.

Special considerations
• Saponin glycosides have a bitter taste and are irritating to the mucous membranes.
• Monitor liver function test results. Advise the patient to immediately discontinue use of squaw vine if transaminase levels become elevated.
• Urge women to report planned or suspected pregnancy.
• Advise the patient to immediately report symptoms of hepatic dysfunction (fever, jaundice, right upper quadrant pain).
• Caution the patient taking disulfiram not to take an herbal form that contains alcohol.

Commentary
Although there appears to be widespread use of squaw vine as a medicinal herb, none of these claims has been studied or proved in animals or humans.

References
Budavari, S. *The Merck Index: An Encyclopedia of Chemicals, Drugs, and Biologicals,* 12th ed. Whitehouse Station, N.J.: Merck & Co., 1996.
Chevallier, A. *The Encyclopedia of Medicinal Plants.* New York: DK Publishing, Inc., 1996.
Duke, J.A. *CRC Handbook of Medicinal Herbs.* Boca Raton, Fla.: CRC Press, 1985.

SQUILL
EUROPEAN SQUILL, INDIAN SQUILL, MEDITERRANEAN SQUILL, RED SQUILL, SEA ONION, SEA SQUILL, WHITE SQUILL

Taxonomic class
Liliaceae

Common trade names
Not commercially available.

Common forms
Available as dried roots, extract, and tincture.

Source
The active components are derived from the bulbous portion of the base and the dried inner scales of the bulb of *Urginea maritima.*

Chemical components
The herb contains several steroidal cardioactive glycosides, including scillaren A and B, proscillaridin A, glucoscillaren, scillaridin A, and scilliroside as well as several flavonoids (von Wartburg et al., 1968).

Actions
Squill has shown peripheral vasodilatory and heart rate–lowering properties in rabbits. In humans, the herb exhibits inotropic and chronotropic effects on the heart that are similar to those of digitalis but less

---
Bold italic type indicates that reaction may be life-threatening.

potent (Stauch et al., 1977). In low doses, squill is a mucolytic (improves the flow of secretions), whereas at higher doses, it acts as an emetic by both centrally mediated and local gastric irritant mechanisms (Court, 1985).

Reported uses
The herb is well known for its cardiac effects, and before the discovery of the more effective cardiac glycosides, it was used to treat symptoms related to heart failure. It is also used for its diuretic and expectorant effects (Orita, 1996). Red squill rich in scilliroside is commercially known as a highly effective rat poison.

Dosage
Decoction: ½ to 1 tsp of dried root mixed with a pot of hot water and steeped for 10 to 15 minutes. Refrigerate and take 1 cup P.O. t.i.d.
Dried root: 0.06 to 0.25 g of P.O. t.i.d.
Tincture: ½ to 1 ml P.O. t.i.d.

Adverse reactions
CNS: CNS stimulation, *seizures* (if ingested in sufficient doses; Tuncok et al., 1995).
CV: *cardiotoxicity (heart block, arrhythmia, asystole)* if ingested in high doses (Tuncok et al., 1995).
GI: gastric irritation, vomiting.

Interactions
Antiarrhythmics, beta blockers, calcium channel blockers, digoxin: May increase cardiac effects and toxicity. Monitor the patient closely.
CNS stimulants: Risk of additive effects. Avoid administration with squill.
Disulfiram: Disulfiram reaction can occur if herbal product contains alcohol. Avoid use together.
Glucocorticoids, laxatives: May increase effects and adverse reactions. Avoid administration with squill.

Contraindications and precautions
Squill is contraindicated in pregnant or breast-feeding patients and in patients with potassium deficiency. Use cautiously in patients with cardiac disorders and in those receiving drugs that may interact with squill, such as antiarrhythmics, beta blockers, calcium channel blockers, and digoxin.

Special considerations
• Monitor the patient for adverse CNS reactions.
• Monitor vital signs, including heart rhythm, of patient who is also taking cardiac drugs.
ALERT One fatality has been reported in a patient who developed atrioventricular block, hyperkalemia, nausea, seizures, ventricular arrhythmias resembling those of digitalis toxicity, and vomiting after ingesting two bulbs from the *U. maritima* (squill) plant (Tuncok et al., 1995).

- Inform the patient that insufficient data exist to support the herb's use as a therapeutic agent.
- Caution the cardiac patient to avoid using squill because it may promote disease exacerbation or contribute to cardiotoxicity.
- Advise the patient to avoid hazardous activities until the herb's CNS effects are known.
- Caution the patient who is taking disulfiram against ingesting an herbal product that contains alcohol.
- Urge women to report planned or suspected pregnancy.
- Instruct the patient to keep squill out of the reach of children and pets.

Commentary

Squill extract is used primarily as an expectorant. Its use as a cardiac stimulant declined after the discovery of cardiac glycosides. Squill's use for cardiac effects cannot be recommended.

References

Court, W.E. "Squill—Anergetic Diuretic," *Pharm J* 235:194-97, 1985.

Orita, Y. "Diuretics," *Nippon Jinzo Gakkai Shi* 38:1-7, 1996.

Stauch, M., et al. "Effect of Proscillaridin-4í-methylether on Pressure Rise Velocity in the Left Ventricle of Patients with Coronary Heart Disease," *Klin Wochenschr* 55:705-6, 1977.

Tuncok, Y., et al. "*Urginea maritima* (Squill) Toxicity," *J Toxicol Clin Toxicol* 33(1):83-6, 1995.

Von Wartburg, A., et al. "Cardiac Glycosides from White Sea Onion or Squill. The Constitution of the Scilliphaeosides and Glucoscilliphaeosides," *Helv Chim Acta* 51:1317-28, 1968.

STEVIA

Azuca-caa, Caa-ehe, Ca-a-yupe, Honey Leaf, Kaa-he-e, sweet herb

Taxonomic class

Asteraceae

Common trade names

Clear Stevia Extract, Mr. Stevia, Stevia, Stevia—Alcohol Free, Stevia Power, Suncare (combination with other herbs), Symfre

Common forms

Available as capsules (57 mg), crude leaf, dried crude leaf extract, herbal powder (greenish), and liquid extract of Paraguayan leaves (4:1 in water) and in combination with other herbs. Some products may be standardized to a minimum of 90% steviosides.

Source

Originating in the highlands of Paraguay and Brazil, *Stevia rebaudiana* is only one of more than 300 *Stevia* species. Stevia is a small, shrubby perennial with small white flowers. Attempts have been made to establish the plant in other countries, but few have been successful. China remains one of the major producers of stevia. It is cultivated in lesser quantities in Israel, Thailand, and Central America.

Chemical components

Stevia is most known for its sweet diterpene glycoside components (stevioside, dulcoside, rebaudiosides A-E). The leaves can contain up to 10% stevioside, which accounts for the plant's sweetness. Stevioside is formed from three glucose molecules linked to steviol, a diterpenic carboxylic alcohol. Other constituents include jhanol, austroinulin, 6-*O*-acetylaustroinulin, 7-*O*-acetyl- austroinulin, triterpenes (amyrin acetate, lupeol), sterols (stigmasterol, beta-sitosterol), rutin, sterebins A-H, flavonoid glycosides (apigenin-4'-*O*-glucoside, luteolin-7-*O*-glucoside, kaempferol-3-*O*-rhamnoside, quercitrin, quercetin-3-*O*-glucoside, quercetin-3-*O*-arabinoside, and centaureidin), arabinose, and tannins. Major components of the essential oil are sesquiterpenes (carophyllene, carophyllene oxide, nerolidol, farnesene, humulene) and monoterpenes (linalool, terpinen-4-ol). Spathulenol and carophyllene oxide have been identified in stevia leaves.

Actions

Much work has centered around the use of stevia's glycosides as alternative sweetening agents. Stevioside appears to be 100 to 200 times sweeter than sucrose; rebaudioside A, 150 to 300 times sweeter; rebaudioside C, 50 times sweeter; and dulcoside A, 30 times sweeter (Phillips, 1989). The crude leaves and herbal powder are supposedly 10 to 15 times sweeter than table sugar. Bitter principles of the plant reportedly occur in the veins of the leaf. Oral stevioside is primarily excreted in the feces. The majority of stevioside is converted to steviolbioside, steviol, and glucose in the colon. Steviol is subsequently conjugated by the liver and then secreted back into the GI tract with bile.

A 5% solution of stevia acted as an antifertility agent in both male and female rats (Planas and Kuc, 1968). Attempts to duplicate this finding have failed. A study evaluating 2.5 mg/kg doses of stevioside from stevia leaves produced no abnormalities in either growth or reproduction in hamsters (Yodyingyuad and Bunyawong, 1991).

The mechanism for stevia's hypotensive effect is not agreed on. Some information suggests that it possesses diuretic-like effects, whereas other data suggest calcium channel blocking activity, producing a vasodilatory response.

Some data discuss a possible negative chronotropic effect of stevia.

Reported uses

Stevia has a substantial history of use as a natural sweetener in South America and Japan. Countries such as Taiwan, China, Malaysia, and South Korea use stevia in salty foods (pickled vegetables, dried seafood, soy sauce) to mask the pungency of table salt. Other claims involve stevia application as a contraceptive, a GI tonic, and a skin softener.

Some claims exist that tout stevia as a remedy for diabetes. Limited animal studies have not reliably proved a hypoglycemic effect for stevia

(White et al., 1994). Data in humans are limited. Anecdotal reports of hypoglycemia with the herb do exist. Early trials suffer from poor study design. The most often cited support for a hypoglycemic effect comes from a study that originated in Brazil (Curi et al., 1986). Sixteen normal volunteers were given a glucose tolerance test both before and after 20 g/day doses (5 g P.O. every 6 hours) of *S. rebaudiana*. A control group received a dose of 250 mg of arabinose on the same schedule as the stevia aqueous extract. Arabinose was chosen because of its predominance in the aqueous stevia extract. Blood glucose levels in the treatment group were statistically significantly lower than those in the control group at each time tested (including fasting glucose). The investigators postulated that an increase in the mitochondrial respiration rate or inhibition of gluconeogenesis was the most likely mechanism of stevia's hypoglycemic effect.

Stevioside was evaluated versus placebo in a multicenter, double-blind, randomized, placebo-controlled year-long trial of 106 Chinese patients with hypertension (Chan et al., 2000). Before enrollment, patients underwent a 30-day washout period. Both groups were similar in demographic, clinical, and biochemical characteristics. At study conclusion, stevioside had significantly lowered blood pressure as compared with placebo. Mean reductions in blood pressure were 12 mmHg for systolic and 8 mmHg for diastolic.

Dosage
No consensus exists. Stevia has commonly been used much like table sugar. The study in hypertension evaluated 250-mg capsules of stevioside given P.O. t.i.d. (Chan et al., 2000). Other manufacturers recommend dosing as often as 3 to 6 times daily.

Adverse reactions
CNS: asthenia, dizziness, headache.
GI: bloating (may be significant to cause discontinuation), nausea.
GU: *nephrotoxicity* (seen in hamsters; related to I.V. steviol administration; Toskulkao et al., 1997).
Musculoskeletal: myalgia.

Interactions
Antidiabetic drugs: May cause additive or exaggerated hypoglycemic effects. Monitor blood glucose levels closely, especially during initiation.
Antihypertensives (especially calcium channel blockers and diuretics): May increase hypotensive effects. Monitor blood pressure intensively.

Contraindications and precautions
Avoid using stevia in pregnant or breast-feeding patients until safety issues are resolved.

Special considerations
• Inform the patient that stevia's safety profile has not been routinely established.

Bold italic type indicates that reaction may be life-threatening.

• Advise the patient with labile blood pressure or who is prone to hypo-glycemia or nephrotoxicity to reconsider ingestion of stevia.
• Inform the patient about the many pharmacotherapeutic options available to control blood pressure or blood glucose levels. Emphasize that the risks and benefits for other allopathic agents are better docu-mented than those for stevia.

◖ ALERT Steviol, a potential metabolite of stevia glycosides, has been shown to be mutagenic (Pezzuto et al., 1985; Matsui et al., 1996), but the actual production of this activated metabolite in humans has not been confirmed. This issue remains controversial.

Points of interest
• Both stevia and rebaudioside A have been show to be stable to heat and changes in pH. Rebaudioside A is subject to degradation on long-term exposure to sunlight.
• Data have shown that stevioside and rebaudioside A, despite their sweetness, do not promote development of caries (Das et al., 1992).
• In 1987, the Japanese, considered the largest users of stevia, consumed more than 700 metric tons of stevia leaves. This figure is believed to have increased dramatically since that time. It has been used in Japanese versions of Wrigley's gums, yogurts, and diet Coke and in a host of con-fectioneries since 1975.
• The FDA (1995) considers stevia an unsafe food additive if used for technical effect (sweetener or flavorant). As a dietary supplement, it is not subject to any particular action under the provisions of the Food, Drug and Cosmetic Act, allowing consumption and marketing in the United States for this use.
• In Brazil, stevia tea and capsules are approved for sale for treating dia-betes.

Commentary
Despite some notable information documenting potential therapeutic application in hypertension or diabetes, the risk profile of stevia re-mains unclear. Because many pharmacotherapeutic options for these conditions exist, patients might be best served to remain with drugs whose safety and efficacy profiles are reasonably predictable and well documented. Large-scale studies in at-risk patient populations are needed before definitive recommendations (especially on dosing) re-garding the therapeutic application of stevia can be made.

References
Chan, P., et al. "A Double-blind, Placebo-controlled Study of the Effectiveness and Tolerability of Oral Stevioside in Human Hypertension," *Br J Clin Pharmacol* 50:215-20, 2000.

Curi, R., et al. "Effect of *Stevia rebaudiana* on Glucose Tolerance in Normal Adult Humans," *Brazilian J Med Biol Res* 19:771-74, 1986.

Das, S., et al. "Evaluation of the Carcinogenic Potential of the Intense Natural Sweeteners Stevioside and Rebaudioside A," *Caries Res* 26:363-66, 1992.

Matsui, M., et al. Evaluation of the Genotoxicity of Stevioside and Steviol Using Six In Vitro and One In Vivo Mutagenicity Assays," *Mutagenesis* 11:573-79, 1996.

Pezzuto, J.M., et al. "Metabolically Activated Steviol, the Aglycone of Stevioside, Is Mutagenic," *Proc Natl Acad Sci USA* 82:2478-82, 1985.

Phillips, K.C. *Stevia: Steps in Developing a New Sweetener. Developments in Sweeteners.* Edited by Grenby, T.H. London: Elsevier Applied Science, 1989, 1-443.

Planas, G.M., and Kuc, J. "Contraceptive Properties of *Stevia rebaudiana*," *Science* 162:1007, 1968.

Toskulkao, C., et al. "Acute Toxicity of Stevioside, a Natural Sweetener, and Its Metabolite, Steviol, in Several Animal Species," *Drug Chem Toxicol* 20:31-44, 1997.

White, J.R., et al. "Oral Use of a Topical Preparation Containing an Extract of *Stevia rebaudiana* and the Chrysanthemum Flower in the Management of Hyperglycemia," *Diab Care* 17(8):940, 1994.

Yodyingyuad, V., and Bunyawong, S. "Effect of Stevioside on Growth and Reproduction," *Hum Reprod* 6(1):158-65, 1991.

ST. JOHN'S WORT

AMBER, AMBER TOUCH-AND-HEAL, CHASSEDIABLE, DEVIL'S SCOURGE, GOATWEED, GOD'S WONDER PLANT, GRACE OF GOD, *HYPERICUM*, KLAMATH WEED, MELLEPERTUIS, ROSIN ROSE, SAINT JOHN'S WORT, WITCHES' HERB

Taxonomic class
Hypericaceae

Common trade names
Multi-ingredient preparations: Hypercalm, Hypericum, Kira, Mood Support, Nutri Zac, St. John's Wort, Tension Tamer

Common forms
Available as capsules, sublingual capsules, dried plant, oil (1 oz), tea, and liquid tinctures. Solid dosage forms are available as 250 mg (standardized to 0.14% hypericin) and 100 mg, 150 mg, 300 mg, 333 mg, 450 mg, and 500 mg (standardized to 0.3% hypericin).

Source
St. John's wort is obtained from the flowering tops of the perennial plant *Hypericum perforatum* L. The plant is endemic to Europe and Asia and was brought to the United States by European colonists.

Chemical components
The chemical composition of St. John's wort is related to the harvesting, drying process, and storage of plant material. The biological activity is probably attributable to several components rather than a single component. Active components include the naphthodianthrones (hypericin, pseudohypericin), flavonoids (hyperin, hyperoside, isoquercetrin, kaempferol, luteolin, quercetin, quercitrin, rutin), biflavonoids (amentoflavone, I3,II8-biapigenin), and phloroglucinols (adhyperforin, hyperforin). The above-ground plant parts contain tannin, which may account for wound-healing effects.

Actions

The exact mechanism of antidepressant effects has not been determined. Early in vitro studies demonstrated that hypericin inhibited type A and, to a lesser extent, type B MAO (Suzuki et al., 1984). A purer form of hypericin did not inhibit MAO (Cott, 1995). High concentration of St. John's wort affects serotonin reuptake in vitro (Perovic et al., 1995), but the level required was much higher than that achieved with usual therapeutic doses. Other studies have demonstrated that St. John's wort is a weak inhibitor of norepinephrine uptake and minimally inhibits catechol-O-methyltransferase. St. John's wort affects receptor affinity of adenosine, benzodiazepine, gamma-aminobutyric acid (GABA)-A, GABA-B, and inositol triphosphate in vitro (Chavez, 1997). One study found that hypericin has modest binding affinity for muscarinic cholinergic and nonselective sigma receptors (Raffs, 1998).

Other demonstrated biological activities include inhibition of stress-induced increased corticotropin-releasing hormone, corticotropin, and cortisol levels; increased nocturnal plasma melatonin levels; and modulation of cytosine expression, particularly interleukin-6. St. John's wort and hypericin also have antiviral activity, including action against retroviruses (Chavez, 1997).

Reported uses

St. John's wort has long been used to treat bronchial inflammation, burns, cancer, depression, enuresis, gastritis, hemorrhoids, hypothyroidism, insect bites and stings, insomnia, renal disorders, and scabies and has been used as a wound healing agent (Bombardelli et al., 1995; Chavez, 1997). Hypericin is being studied for treatment of HIV infection as well as topically for phototherapy of skin diseases, including Kaposi's sarcoma, cutaneous T-cell lymphoma, psoriasis, and warts (Chavez, 1997). St. John's wort is used to treat mild to moderate depression. (See *Studies of St. John's wort,* page 748.) St. John's wort has also been studied in obsessive-compulsive disorder (Taylor et al., 2000) and premenstrual syndrome (Stevinson et al., 2000).

Dosage

For burns and skin lesions, cream applied topically; strength is not standardized.

For depression, 300 mg of standardized extract preparations (standardized to 0.3% hypericin) P.O. t.i.d. for 4 to 6 weeks. Or, 2 to 4 g of tea that has been steeped in 1 to 2 cups of water for about 10 minutes and taken P.O. daily for 4 to 6 weeks.

Adverse reactions

CNS: dizziness, restlessness, sleep disturbances.
EENT: dry mouth.
GI: constipation, GI distress.
Skin: *phototoxicity.*
Other: allergic hypersensitivity.

RESEARCH FINDINGS
Studies of St. John's wort

A meta-analysis of 23 randomized clinical trials involving 1,757 outpatients with depressive disorders was published in the *British Medical Journal* (Linde et al., 1996). Sample size ranged from 30 to 162 patients, and the duration of treatment ranged from 4 to 12 weeks. Fifteen trials were placebo-controlled and eight trials compared St. John's wort with other drugs (amitriptyline, bromazepam, desipramine, diazepam, imipramine, and maprotiline). St. John's wort was found to be more effective than placebo and as effective as standard antidepressants. St. John's wort caused fewer adverse reactions than did standard antidepressants.

However, these trials had many flaws: inadequate diagnostic criteria, inclusion of patients with only mild to moderate depression, lack of information about the randomization process, lack of compliance control, variable dosage of St. John's wort, low dosage of antidepressants, short duration of treatment, lower placebo response rate than in other clinical trials, lack of statistical analysis information, and failure to perform an intent-to-treat analysis.

Another review evaluated 12 placebo-controlled trials, three of which compared St. John's wort with contemporary allopathic antidepressants for treating mild to moderate depression (Volz, 1997). Similar to the meta-analysis, most of the studies evaluated had methodologic flaws, and the author concluded that further studies are needed.

Interactions

Alcohol, MAO inhibitors, narcotics, OTC cold and flu medications, sympathomimetics, tyramine-containing foods: May increase MAO inhibition activity. Avoid administration with St. John's wort.

Cyclosporine: May decrease cyclosporine concentrations (Barone et al., 2000). Use cautiously together.

Digoxin: May decrease digoxin concentrations (Cheng, 2000). Monitor the patient and serum digoxin levels.

Drugs metabolized by the liver: St. John's wort may influence hepatic microsomal enzymes. Use with caution with these drugs.

Indinavir (HIV protease inhibitor): May decrease indinavir concentrations. Discourage concomitant use.

Paroxetine: May cause sedative-hypnotic intoxication with concurrent ingestion (Gordon, 1998). Avoid administration with St. John's wort.

Serotonergic drugs (amphetamines, serotonin reuptake inhibitors, trazodone, tricyclic antidepressants): Serotonin syndrome can occur when St. John's wort is used with these drugs. Use cautiously together.

Bold italic type indicates that reaction may be life-threatening.

Contraindications and precautions
St. John's wort is contraindicated in patients with a history of allergy to St. John's wort or its components. Avoid its use in children and in pregnant or breast-feeding patients; effects are unknown.

Special considerations
• The patient's depression should be evaluated by a health care provider. Conventional therapy may be prudent for a moderate to severe disorder.
• Instruct the patient to purchase herbs only from a reputable source because products and their contents vary among manufacturers.
• Caution the patient against using the herb with alcohol and OTC cold and flu medications.
🔺 **ALERT** Phototoxicity has occurred in grazing animals that consumed large amounts of St. John's wort. Until recently, phototoxicity had not been reported in humans. Systemic photosensitivity of recurring elevated erythematous lesions occurred in light-exposed areas in a woman who took an unknown dose of St. John's wort for 3 years (Golsch et al., 1997). Pure hypericin has resulted in phototoxicity when given I.V. and P.O. in clinical trials to patients with AIDS (Chavez, 1997) and depression (Schempp et al., 2000).
• Advise the patient to take precautions against sun exposure.

Points of interest
• In spring 1998, the National Institutes of Health began a 3-year, multicenter clinical study to investigate the efficacy of St. John's wort for treating major depressive disorders. The study included 336 patients and compared a standardized extract of St. John's wort with a selective serotonin reuptake inhibitor and placebo. After evaluating efficacy at 8 weeks, patients who responded were treated for an additional 18 weeks. The study included a 4-month follow-up period to assess long-term effects. Results of this study are not yet available.
• St. John's wort oil is prepared by extracting the flowers with olive oil.

Commentary
There are numerous case reports and clinical trials evaluating the safety and efficacy of St. John's wort. The herb is more effective than placebo for treating mild to moderate depression and as effective as standard antidepressants but causes fewer adverse effects. A study evaluated the efficacy of St. John's wort for severe depression and reported that St. John's wort is equally as effective as imipramine with significantly fewer adverse effects (Vorbach, 1997). Although most clinical trials contained design flaws, overall they indicate that St. John's wort may be valuable for treating depressive disorders. Additional, well-designed studies are needed. The USP expert advisory panel has determined that there is insufficient evidence in the scientific literature to support the use of St. John's wort for treating mild to moderate depression or any other medical condition.

References

Barone, G.W., et al. "Drug Interaction Between St. John's Wort and Cyclosporine," *Ann Pharmacother* 34(9):1013-16, 2000.

Bombardelli, E., et al. "*Hypericum perforatum,*" *Fitoterapia* 66:43-68, 1995.

Chavez, M.L. "Saint John's Wort," *Hosp Pharm* 32:1621-32, 1997.

Cheng, T.O. "St. Johns Wort Interaction with Digoxin," *Arch Intern Med* 160(16):2548, 2000. Letter.

Cott, J. "Medicinal Plants and Dietary Supplements: Sources for Innovative Treatments or Adjuncts?" *Psychopharmacol Bull* 31:131-37, 1995.

Golsch, S., et al. "Reversible Increase in Photosensitivity to UV-B Caused by St. John's Wort Extract," *Hautarzt* 48:249-52, 1997.

Gordon, J.B. "SSRIs and St. John's Wort: Possible Toxicity?" *Am Fam Physician* 57:950-53, 1998.

Linde, K., et al. "St. John's Wort for Depression: An Overview and Meta-analysis of Randomized Clinical Trials," *Br Med J* 313:253-58, 1996.

Perovic, S., et al. "Effect on Serotonin Uptake by Postsynaptic Receptors," *Arzneimittelforschung* 45:1145-48, 1995.

Raffs, R.B. "Screen of Receptor and Uptake-Site Activity of Hypericin Component of St. John's Wort Reveals Sigma Receptor Binding," *Life Sci* 62:265-70, 1998.

Schempp, C.M., et al. "Effect of Topical Application of *Hypericum perforatum* Extracts (St. John's Wort) on Skin Sensitivity to Solar Simulated Radiation," *Photodermatol Photoimmunol Photomed* 16(3):125-28, 2000.

Stevinson, C., et al. "A Pilot Study of *Hypericum perforatum* for the Treatment of Premenstrual Syndrome," *Br J Gynecol* 107(7): 870-76, 2000.

Suzuki, O., et al. "Inhibition of Monoamine Oxidase by Hypericin," *Planta Med* 50:272-74, 1984.

Taylor, L.H., et al. "An Open-label Trial of St. John's Wort *(Hypericum perforatum)* in Obsessive-compulsive Disorder," *J Clin Psychiatry* 61(8):575-78, 2000.

Volz, H.P. "Controlled Clinical Trials of *Hypericum* Extracts in Depressed Patients—An Overview," *Pharmacopsychiatry* 30(Suppl):72-76, 1997.

Vorbach, E.U. "Efficacy and Tolerability of St. John's Wort Extract LI 160 Versus Imipramine in Patients with Severe Depressive Episodes According to ICD-10," *Pharmacopsychiatry* 30(Suppl):81-85, 1997.

STONE ROOT

HEAL-ALL, HORSE BALM, HORSEWEED, KNOB ROOT, KNOBWEED, KNOT ROOT, OX BALM, RICHLEAF, RICHWEED

Taxonomic class
Lamiaceae

Common trade names
Tincture Collinson

Common forms
Available as tincture of the root.

Source
Stone root is derived from the rhizome and root of *Collinsonia canadensis.* The plant is native to North America, growing wild from Mas-

---

sachusetts and Vermont west to Wisconsin and south to Florida and Arkansas.

Chemical components
The rhizome and roots of the *C. canadensis* contain saponins, tannins, mucilage, and resins.

Actions
The active chemical compounds of the plant show antifungal, astringent, and diuretic properties. Antifungal activity has been demonstrated in vitro using an alcoholic extract of the powdered roots. Tannins produce the characteristic astringent effect. The active ingredient responsible for the diuretic action is unknown. In the treatment of burns, the proteins of exposed tissue are precipitated. An antiseptic, protective coat forms and allows for regeneration of new tissue underneath (Tyler et al., 1988).

Reported uses
Stone root is used as a diuretic in several OTC preparations that claim to treat edema, hypertension, and menstrual distress. The herb has also been reported as useful in treating headaches and indigestion.

Its main use is claimed to be for the treatment of diarrhea, hemorrhoids, and varicose veins. These claims are based on the herb's astringent properties. There is no scientific evidence for any of these therapeutic claims.

Dosage
For diuretic action and for treating bladder stones, 15 to 60 gtt of the tincture P.O. t.i.d.

Adverse reactions
CV: increased blood pressure (with long-term use).

Interactions
Antihypertensives: May have an additive hypotensive effect. Monitor the patient's blood pressure.

Contraindications and precautions
Stone root is contraindicated in pregnant or breast-feeding patients; effects are unknown. Use cautiously in patients with hypertension.

Special considerations
• Monitor liver function test results; prolonged use of stone root may lead to hepatotoxicity.
• Urge the patient to seek appropriate medical advice before self-medicating for high blood pressure or edema.
• Instruct the patient to notify the prescriber and pharmacist of any herbal or dietary supplement he is taking when filling a new prescription.

Points of interest
• An FDA advisory review panel on menstrual drug products found little scientific evidence to support the use of stone root.

Commentary
The major therapeutic claims for the use of stone root include its astringent and diuretic activities. None of the therapeutic claims has been substantiated in the scientific literature in either animal or human models; therefore, this herb cannot be recommended.

References
Tyler, V.E., et al. *Pharmacognosy,* 9th ed. Philadelphia: Lea & Febiger, 1988.

SUNDEW

COMMON SUNDEW, DEW PLANT, GREAT SUNDEW, RED ROT, ROUND-LEAVED SUNDEW

Taxonomic class
Droseraceae

Common trade names
None known.

Common forms
Available as a fluid or solid dried extract and tincture.

Source
Drosera rotundifolia is a carnivorous plant named for the sticky, dewlike substance produced on its leaves and used to trap insects. The entire flowering plant and leaves, excluding the roots, are the components most medicinally used.

Chemical components
The sundew plant, *D. rotundifolia,* contains droserone, flavonoids, tannins, glycosides, vitamin C, pigments, traces of essential oils, and organic acids. The exudate from the leaves contain proteolytic enzymes and plumbagin (Bienenfeld et al., 1966).

Actions
Although sundew is claimed to have antispasmodic, demulcent, and expectorant activities, no supporting evidence is available. Some in vitro activity against staphylococci and pneumococci has been noted (Vinkenborg et al., 1969).

Reported uses
Traditionally, sundew has been used to treat such respiratory conditions as bronchitis, asthmatic coughs, tuberculosis, and whooping cough. It has also been used to treat stomach ulcers. No human studies support therapeutic use for any condition.

Bold italic type indicates that reaction may be life-threatening.

Dosage
The average daily dose is 3 g of herb.
Infusion: 1 tsp of dried herb mixed with 1 cup of boiling water; steep for 15 minutes and take P.O. t.i.d.
Tincture: 1 to 2 ml P.O. t.i.d.

Adverse reactions
GU: brownish orange urine discoloration.

Interactions
Disulfiram: Disulfiram reaction can occur if herbal product contains alcohol. Do not use together.

Contraindications and precautions
Sundew is contraindicated in patients with tuberculosis or hypotension.

Special considerations
• Advise the patient and laboratory staff that the patient's urine may be discolored.
• Caution the patient who is taking disulfiram against using an herbal product that contains alcohol.
• Urge the patient with suspected tuberculosis to seek standard medical treatment. Persistent cough should be evaluated by the primary health care provider.

Commentary
Data supporting any therapeutic use of sundew in humans are lacking. Potential use in respiratory conditions needs thorough clinical studies in humans.

References
Bienenfeld, W., et al. "Flavonoids from *Drosera rotundifolia* L.," *Arch Pharm Ber Dtsch Pharm Ges* 229:598-602, 1966.
Vinkenborg, J., et al. "The Presence of Hydroplumbagin Glucoside in *Drosera rotundifolia* L.," *Pharm Weekly* 104:45-49, 1969.

SWEET CICELY

BRITISH MYRRH, COW CHERVIL, ROMAN PLANT, SHEPHERD'S NEEDLE, SMOOTH CICELY, SWEET BRACKEN, SWEET CHERVIL, SWEET-FERN, SWEET-HUMLOCK

Taxonomic class
Apiaceae

Common trade names
None known.

Common forms
Available as an extract and an ointment.

Source
The whole plant (roots, leaves, seeds) of the *Myrrhis odorata* is used for medicinal and culinary purposes.

Chemical components
None known.

Actions
Sweet cicely's main effect is to act as a GI stimulant. It is also claimed to have an antiseptic effect when used topically (Bunney, 1984).

Reported uses
Sweet cicely is claimed to be useful as an antiflatulent, a diuretic, an expectorant, and a GI stimulant. Topical application of sweet cicely is thought to be useful for treating gout pain, ulcers, and small, external bite wounds (Heinerman, 1996). Scientifically based studies supporting these claims are lacking in the medical literature. The plant is being studied for use as an artificial sweetener in diabetic foods.

Dosage
No consensus exists.

Adverse reactions
None reported.

Interactions
Diuretics: May increase diuretic effect. Avoid administration with sweet cicely.

Contraindications and precautions
High doses of sweet cicely are contraindicated in pregnant or breast-feeding patients. Use cautiously in patients with peptic ulcer disease or ulcerative colitis.

Special considerations
• Urge the patient not to self-treat symptoms of GI illness before seeking appropriate medical evaluation because this may delay diagnosis of a serious medical condition.
• Caution the patient taking diuretics against using sweet cicely because of additive effects.
• Monitor serum electrolyte levels in patients taking this herb.
• Instruct the patient to notify the prescriber and pharmacist of any herbal or dietary supplement he is taking when filling a new prescription.

Points of interest
• The root from the *Osmorrhiza longistylis,* also known as American sweet cicely, is claimed to have similar medicinal properties. It is used to make a tea for treating abdominal cramps, flatulence, heartburn, and indigestion and for improving appetite.

Commentary
The entire sweet cicely plant is edible and considered safe for consumption. Thus, its use in medicine is probably harmless in moderate amounts. The medicinal claims have yet to be scientifically proven. Little information is available surrounding the use of this herb. Identification of active ingredients, standardized formulations, and clinical trials are warranted to support claims.

References
Bunney, S., ed. *The Illustrated Book of Herbs. Their Medicinal and Culinary Uses.* London: Octopus Books Ltd., 1984.
Heinerman, J. *Heinerman's Encyclopedia of Healing Herbs and Spices.* Englewood Cliffs, N.J.: Prentice-Hall, 1996.

SWEET FLAG

BEE WORT, CALAMUS, RAT ROOT, SWEET MYRTLE, SWEET ROOT, SWEET SEDGE

Taxonomic class
Araceae

Common trade names
None known.

Common forms
Available as liquid extract, dried powder, and tincture. Not commonly available in the United States.

Source
The dried rhizome and roots of *Acorus calamus* are used. Sweet flag is believed to have originated in India but now grows in most parts of the world in wet soil or shallow water.

Chemical components
The active ingredients are the bicyclic sesquiterpines alpha- and beta-asarone.

Actions
Asarone has been shown to be carcinogenic (Hasheninejad and Caldwell, 1994). Sweet flag is claimed to have analgesic, anticholinergic, euphoric, hypotensive, psychoactive (hallucinogenic), sedative (beta-asarone), stimulatory (alpha-asarone), and laxative activities. Asarone has some anticoagulant effect and nematodocidal activity in animals (Sugimoto et al., 1995); it is metabolically converted to TMA-2, a potent hallucinogen.

Reported uses
Native Americans of the Cree tribe chewed the root for its euphoric, hallucinogenic, and stimulant effects. They also used the drug as an analgesic and an antidiabetic agent. In Ayurvedic medicine, it is used

mostly for digestive disorders. Western herbalists recommend sweet flag as an antispasmodic for GI disturbances. Clinical data supporting any claim in humans are lacking.

Dosage
Dried rhizome: 1 to 3 g P.O. t.i.d.
Liquid extract: 1 to 3 ml P.O. t.i.d.
Tincture: 2 to 4 ml P.O. t.i.d.

Adverse reactions
CNS: confusion, disorientation, hallucinations.
GI: nausea, vomiting.
Other: mutagenic effects.

Interactions
Disulfiram: Disulfiram reaction can occur if herbal product contains alcohol. Avoid use together.
Psychoactive, sedative, or stimulating drugs: May increase effects of these drugs. Use cautiously with sweet flag.
Sedatives, other CNS depressants: Antagonistic effects. Do not use together.

Contraindications and precautions
Sweet flag is contraindicated in pregnant patients and in those with psychiatric disorders. Use cautiously in patients at risk for hepatotoxicity.

Special considerations
• Monitor the patient for adverse CNS reactions.
• Monitor for misuse or abuse of sweet flag.
• Caution the patient to avoid hazardous activities until the herb's CNS effects are known.
• At least one case of toxicity has been related to sweet flag ingestion (Vargas et al., 1998).
• Instruct women to report planned or suspected pregnancy.
• Caution the patient taking disulfiram against using an herbal product that contains alcohol.

Points of interest
• Hepatocarcinogenicity associated with the asarones has been observed in animals (Hasheninejad and Caldwell, 1994).
• Sweet flag abuse by people seeking the herb's psychoactive effects has been reported.
• The oil is used by the Cree for anointing in religious ceremonies.

Commentary
Sweet flag has been used for 2,000 years worldwide for several conditions and in religious ceremonies for its psychoactive properties. Its use as a food additive or supplement is banned in the United States because of its mutagenic potential.

Bold italic type indicates that reaction may be life-threatening.

References

Hasheninejad, G., and Caldwell, J. "Genotoxicity of the Alkylbenzenes Alpha- and Beta-Asarone, Myristin and Elmicin as Determined by the UDS Assay in Cultured Rat Hepatocytes," *Food Chem Toxicol* 32:223-31, 1994.

Sugimoto, N., et al. "Mobility Inhibition and Nematocidal Activity of Asarone and Related Phenylpropanoids on Second-stage Larvae of *Toxocara canis*," *Biol Pharm Bull* 18:605-9, 1995.

Vargas, C.P., et al. "Getting to the Root *(Acorus calamus)* of the Problem," *J Toxicol Clin Toxicol* 36(3):259-60, 1998.

SWEET VIOLET

ENGLISH VIOLET, FLOR DE PROSEPINA, VIOLA, *VIOLA SUAVIS*, VIOLETA, *VIOLETA CHEIROSA*, *VIOLETA COMUN*

Taxonomic class
Violaceae

Common trade names
None known.

Common forms
Available as dried and fresh flowers and leaves.

Source
Active compounds have been derived from the roots, seeds, flowers, and leaves of *Viola odorata.*

Chemical components
Chemical compounds isolated from the seeds, roots, leaves, and flowers of *V. odorata* include saponin, myrosin, violamin, viola-quercetin, gaultherin, an emetine-like alkaloid (viola-emetin), 2-nitropropionic acid, and odoratine (alkaloid). Methylsalicyclic acid can be found after hydrolysis of gaultherin. More than 100 volatile oils have been isolated from the leaves.

Actions
Leaf extracts of *V. odorata* were found to be comparable with aspirin in reducing pyrexia in animals; a significant reduction in temperature was noted (Khattak et al., 1985).

Reported uses
V. odorata has been claimed to have several therapeutic uses. Decoctions and syrups made from the leaves and flowers have been used as a cough remedy and sedative and applied topically as an anti-inflammatory. The dried root has been used for treating constipation and as an emetic. Extracts of the leaves and flowers are also used in manufacturing perfumes.

Dosage

No consensus exists. Various concentrations of decoctions, extracts, and powders have been used, making standardized dosage identification difficult.

Adverse reactions

GI: cathartic effects.

Interactions

Laxatives: Additive effect. Monitor the patient.

Contraindications and precautions

Sweet violet is contraindicated in pregnant or breast-feeding patients; effects are unknown.

Special considerations

• Inform the patient that insufficient data exist for therapeutic use of sweet violet.
• Advise the patient to consult a health care provider before using herbal preparations because a treatment that has been clinically researched and proved effective may be available.
• Monitor the patient taking this herb for excessive vomiting and diarrhea.
• Instruct the patient who is pregnant or breast-feeding to avoid using sweet violet.

Points of interest

• *Viola tricolor*, also known as wild pansy, is a related species used for treating several skin conditions, including eczema.

Commentary

Few data are available concerning the pharmacologic and therapeutic effects of *V. odorata*. Studies in animals have shown that leaf extracts have antipyretic action comparable to aspirin. The therapeutic usefulness of *V. odorata* cannot be established.

References

Khattak, S.G., et al. "Antipyretic Studies on Some Indigenous Pakistani Medicinal Plants," *J Ethnopharmacol* 14:45-51, 1985.

Bold italic type indicates that reaction may be life-threatening.

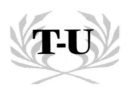

T-U

TANGERINE PEEL

CHEN PI ("AGED PEEL"), CHU SHA CHU, *CITRUS RETICULATA*, *CITRUS RETICULATA* BLANCO, KAN, MANDARINE, MANDARIN ORANGE PEEL, PERICARPIUM CITRI RETICULATAE, TRAN BI

Taxonomic class
Rutaceae

Common trade names
None reported.

Common forms
The two forms of tangerine peel are aged tangerine peel and green (young) tangerine peel. It is available as a peel and in pill form.

Source
After tangerines ripen, the skins are collected and dried.

Chemical components
Tangerine peel contains dietary fibers and bioflavonoids (naringin and hesperidin). Tangerine seeds contain three limonoids: limonin, nomilin, and obacunone.

Actions
Information regarding the mechanism of action of tangerine peel is limited. Naringin acts as an antimicrobial and hesperidin acts as a blood pressure depressant. Both bioflavonoids have been pharmacologically evaluated as potential anticancer agents and anti-inflammatories and are thought to be associated with preventing hyperlipidemia (Bok et al., 1999).

Reported uses
Tangerine peel has been used to treat anorexia, bloating, diarrhea, flatulence, hyperlipidemia, indigestion, muscle pain, nausea, and vomiting. It can also be used as a diuretic, an expectorant, and a sedative.

Dosage
None reported.

Adverse reactions
None reported.

Interactions
None reported.

Contraindications and precautions

Some sources suggest that tangerine peel may be contraindicated in patients who have a dry cough or red tongue or in those who are spitting up blood. The red tongue could be a sign of inflammation or infection, which would be aggravated and cause pain in tangerine peel is taken.

Special considerations

• Advise the patient to consult a health care provider before using herbal preparations because a treatment that has been clinically researched and proved effective may be available.
• Instruct the patient to report new adverse reactions if using tangerine peel.
• Although no known chemical interactions have been reported in clinical studies, consideration must be given to the pharmacologic properties of the herbal product and the potential for exacerbation of the intended therapeutic effect of conventional drugs.

Points of interest

• Tangerine peel essential oil is popular in aromatherapy.
• A red or orange peel is favored by some herbalists.

Commentary

Because of the lack of human clinical data, the use of tangerine peel is not recommended. One study in rats appears to show a connection between tangerine peel extracts and the prevention of hyperlipidemia, but further clinical trials are needed to confirm its safety and efficacy.

References

Bok, S.H., et al: "Plasma and Hepatic Cholesterol and Hepatic Activities of 3-Hydroxy-3-methyl-glutaryl-CoA Reductase and Aacyl CoA; Cholesterol Transferase Are Lower in Rats Fed Citrus Peel Extract or a Mixture of Citrus Bioflavonoids," *J Nutr* 129(6):1182-85, 1999.

TANSY

BITTER BUTTONS, GOLDEN BUTTONS, YELLOW BUTTONS

Taxonomic class

Asteraceae

Common trade names

Tansy Extract, Tansy Herb Liquid, Tansy Herb LQ, Tansy Oil

Common forms

Available as an essential oil, fluidextract, and tea.

Source

Active components are derived from the dried leaves and flowering tops of *Tanacetum vulgare*. It should not be confused with other plants referred to as tansy, including the tansy ragwort (*Senecio jacobaea*).

Chemical components
A range of tansy strains exist that yield extracts of varying chemical composition, which is determined more by the genetic makeup of the plant than by environmental factors. Fresh tansy contains 0.12% to 0.18% volatile oil. Some strains yield an oil composed almost entirely of a toxic terpene, thujone, with several minor sesquiterpene and flavone components; others yield an oil that is nearly thujone-free. Besides thujone, these oils contain artemisia ketone, chysantheyl acetate, beta-caryophyllene, germacrene-D, borneol, camphor, isopinocamphone, isothujone, piperitone, gamma-terpinene, umbellulone, and other unidentified terpenes.

Actions
Tansy oil has shown in vitro activity against gram-positive bacteria but not gram-negative bacteria. Toxic effects are probably attributable to thujone. The plants or extracts may cause contact dermatitis, possibly because of the sesquiterone lactones, arbusculin-A, or tanacetin components (Guin and Skidmore, 1987; Paulsen et al., 1993).

Reported uses
In ancient Greece, tansy was believed to impart immortality and was, therefore, used for embalming. It has been used as an anthelmintic, an anti-inflammatory, an antispasmodic, a menstrual stimulant, and a tonic and to treat bruises, diarrhea, fever, headaches, sore throat, and swelling. The Micmac and Malecite Indians used tansy to prevent pregnancy (largely as an abortifacient) and as a diuretic (Chandler et al., 1982). Tansy leaves have been used to prepare a tea and as a food flavoring.

Dosage
No consensus exists. Because these plants vary considerably from one genetic "race" to another, it is impossible to predict the thujone content and the strength or toxicity of a given tansy preparation.

Adverse reactions
CNS: personality changes.
EENT: allergic rhinitis, sneezing.
GU: renal damage (with long-term use).
Skin: contact dermatitis.

Interactions
None reported.

Contraindications and precautions
Tansy is contraindicated in pregnant patients because of its potential abortifacient effects and in patients who are hypersensitive to tansy or its components.

Special considerations
- Inform the patient who wants to use tansy that the chemical composition of the oil cannot be predicted unless specifically analyzed; thus, the safety profile is not known.
- ▲ ALERT   Tansy contains essential oils (thujone, camphor, and cineole) that have epileptogenic potential. In particular, thujone, a relatively toxic compound, is probably responsible for the toxicity associated with tansy (Burkhard et al., 1999). As few as 10 drops of tansy oil has been reported to be fatal. Symptoms of tansy poisoning include rapid, weak pulse; seizures; severe gastritis; and violent muscle spasms. Patients with known seizure disorders should be counseled to avoid consumption of tansy or its component, thujone.
- Caution the patient taking tansy about the risk of allergic dermatitis and rhinitis.
- Instruct women to report planned or suspected pregnancy immediately.

Commentary
No clinical data support the use of tansy for any medical condition. The most frequent indication for tansy in folk medicine has been as an anthelmintic and insect repellent, but safer and more effective products are available for these purposes. Because of the herb's unpredictable toxicity and allergenic properties, it cannot be recommended for use.

References
Burkhard, P.R., et al. "Plant-Induced Seizures: Reappearance of an Old Problem," *J Neurol* 246:667-70, 1999.

Chandler, R.F., et al. "Herbal Remedies of the Maritime Indians: Sterols and Triterpenes of *Tanacetum vulgare* L. (Tansy)," *Lipids* 17:102-6, 1982.

Guin, J.D., and Skidmore, G. "Compositae Dermatitis in Childhood," *Arch Dermatol* 123:500-02, 1987.

Paulsen, E., et al. "Compositae Dermatitis in a Danish Dermatology Department in One Year," *Contact Dermatitis* 29:6-10, 1993.

Stingeni, L., et al. "T-lymphocyte Cytokine Profiles in Compositae Airborne Dermatitis," *Br J Dermatol* 141:689-93, 1999.

TEA TREE
AUSTRALIAN TEA TREE OIL, *MELALEUCA ALTERNIFOLIA*, MELALEUCA OIL, TEA TREE OIL

Taxonomic class
Myrtaceae

Common trade names
Jason Winter's Tea Tree Oil, Swanson Ultra Tea Tree Oil, Thursday Plantation Tea Tree Oil

---

Common forms
Available as creams, lotions, ointments, and soaps. It is also included in cosmetics, household products, and toiletries. Concentrations of melaleuca oil in these products range from less than 1% to 100%.

Source
Tea tree oil, or melaleuca oil, is an essential oil distilled from the leaves and branches of *Melaleuca alternifolia,* a member of the myrtle family that is native to coastal areas of Australia.

Chemical components
The steam distillation of the leaves yields about 2% oil. The colorless to pale yellow oil is composed of terpene hydrocarbons (pinene, terpinene, cymene), cineol, and various minor sesquiterpenes and related alcohols. Composition of the extract is varied; the oxygenated terpene, terpinen-4-ol, can constitute up to 60% of the total oil. Some oils contain high concentrations of 1,8-cineol, which is the main component of eucalyptus oil. Most commercially available tea tree oils contain little or no cineol. More than 100 compounds (all plant terpenenes) have been identified in melaleuca oil.

Actions
Terpinen-4-ol, a main component of tea tree oil, has significant antibacterial and antifungal activity in vitro; susceptible organisms include *Escherichia coli, Staphylococcus aureus, Proprionibacterium acnes, Pseudomonas aeruginosa, Streptococcus* species, and *Candida albicans.* Controversy exists as to the precise mechanism of action for the melaleuca. One report suggests that tea tree oil disrupts cell membrane permeability, promoting leakage of intracellular ions and proteins (Cox et al., 2000). Earlier data have suggested that the antiseptic effect of tea tree oil was related to its ability to activate WBCs (Budhiraja et al., 1999). Still other information suggests that organic matter and surfactants that accompany melaleuca oil were responsible for the antibacterial effect (Hammer et al., 1999). Tea tree oil may be effective against MRSA carriers that have previously been treated with topical mupirocin (Carson et al., 1995). There is in vitro evidence as well that tea tree oil has antimicrobial activity against vancomycin-resistant enterococci (VRE) (Nelson, 1997). Polymyxin B may enhance melaleuca's antibacterial effect against *P. aeruginosa* by enhancing permeability of the organism cell membrane to the tea tree oil components (Mann et al., 2000).

Cooling appears to be an effective modality for the therapy of burn wounds. An investigation in piglets was undertaken to determine the effect of melaleuca gel on artificially induced burn wounds (Jandera et al., 2000). Melaleuca gel, applied immediately or in a delayed manner, reduced intradermal temperature (cooling) and promoted more rapid healing as compared with untreated controls. Cold water compresses appeared to fare as well as melaleuca.

RESEARCH FINDINGS
Tea tree oil for oral candidiasis infections in AIDS

In vitro data suggest that melaleuca oil may be effective for certain fungal infections (Hammer et al., 1998; Concha et al., 1998). Subsequently, a small prospective, open-label study of patients at an AIDS clinic in Detroit identified a potential role for melaleuca oral solution in the treatment of oropharyngeal candidiasis (thrush; Jandourek et al., 1998). Thirteen patients who were refractive to oral fluconazole therapy (up to 14 days of fluconazole, 400 mg P.O. once daily, with minimum inhibitory concentrations no greater than 20 mcg/ml of fluconazole) were switched to melaleuca oral solution (15 ml P.O. four times a day; swish and expel) for 4 weeks. Weekly evaluations were conducted. At the end of 4 weeks, six patients had improved, two had been cured of their candidiasis; four were considered nonresponders, and one had worsened. The two cured patients had not relapsed as of a few weeks after the treatment had been discontinued. Despite their low success rate, the investigators considered melaleuca oral solution an effective alternative for AIDS patients with refractory oral candidiasis. These results are intriguing, but the clear lack of a control group, the nonblinded study design, and the study's small sample size make any conclusion preliminary.

Reported uses

Tea tree oil has long been used primarily as a local antiseptic. Australian aborigines used it for athlete's foot, burns, cuts, and insect bites, among other disorders. Some studies indicate that the oil is promising as a treatment for skin problems, including acne, chronic cystitis, eczema, furuncles, bacterial and fungal infections of the skin and oral mucosa, lice infestation, psoriasis, vaginal candidiasis, and wound infections (Nenoff et al., 1996).

Melaleuca oil has also been compared with tolnaftate and clotrimazole solution for various skin conditions with some effect. A cream comprising 2% butenafine and 5% melaleuca oil was studied in patients with onychomycosis (Syed et al., 1999). In this double-blind, randomized, placebo-controlled study, 60 patients with onychomycosis of at least 6 months' duration were followed for 16 weeks after initiation of therapy. The results were rather dramatic, with 80% of the treatment group cured as compared with none in the placebo group. After several additional weeks of follow-up, no improvements in either group were demonstrated but no relapses were seen. Butenafine itself has activity against several typical fungal pathogens.

Bold italic type indicates that reaction may be life-threatening.

Melaleuca oil has also been studied against 5% benzoyl peroxide for the treatment of acne vulgaris (Bassett et al., 1990). More research is needed to prove its use in this area.

Preliminary information suggests a role for melaleuca in the treatment of oral thrush infections. (See *Tea tree oil for oral candidiasis infections in AIDS.*)

Dosage
Tea tree oil is applied locally in concentrations ranging from 0.4% to 100%, depending on the type of product and the nature and location of the skin disorder.

Adverse reactions
CNS: CNS depression (ataxia, drowsiness).
EENT: stomatitis.
GI: diarrhea, GI mucosal irritation, vomiting.
Skin: dermatitis (in sensitive people).

Interactions
None reported.

Contraindications and precautions
Use tea tree oil cautiously in patients who are hypersensitive to the components of melaleuca oil or in those who are prone to contact dermatitis from plants. Some data point to the sesquiterpenoid fraction of the oil as the allergenic agent of melaleuca (Rubel et al., 1998). Avoid using tea tree oil in pregnant or breast-feeding patients; effects are unknown.

Special considerations
• Monitor for worsening of skin condition or infection.
• Inform the patient that melaleuca oil is ubiquitous in commercially available products and that concentration of the oil varies greatly.
• Because essential oils are more appealing to olfactory senses and exhibit more natural appeal than available topical drugs, melaleuca may be preferred for antiseptic use. Encourage the patient to consider conventional therapy until substantial testing is done with the oil.
• Caution the patient that the oil should not be ingested and should be kept out of the reach of young children. Even small amounts of oil taken internally may produce CNS depression. A 17-month-old child who ingested less than 10 ml of tea tree oil experienced ataxia and drowsiness but recovered fully (Jacobs et al., 1994).
• Advise women to avoid using tea tree oil during pregnancy or when breast-feeding.

Commentary
Interest in melaleuca oil has erupted with reports of favorable in vitro antimicrobial activity against multiple pathogens (gram-negative and gram-positive bacteria, MRSA, VRE, and some fungal pathogens), suggesting many potential therapeutic topical applications. Although an-

timicrobial activity has been well documented in vitro, human clinical trials evaluating melaleuca's efficacy and safety profile are still preliminary. Topical application as an antifungal appears promising, but it seems prudent not to ingest the essential oil of the plant until more is known.

References

Bassett, I.B., et al. "A Comparative Study of Tea-Tree Oil Versus Benzoylperoxide in the Treatment of Acne," *Med J Aust* 153:455-58, 1990.

Budhiraja, S.S., et al. "Bioogical Activity of *Melaleuca alternifolia* Oil Component, Terpinen-4-ol, in Human Myelocytic Cell Line HL-60," *J Manipulative Physiol Ther* 22(7):447-53, 1999.

Carson, C.F., et al. "Susceptibility of Methicillin-resistant *Staphylococcus aureus* to the Essential Oil of *Melaleuca alternifolia*," *J Antimicrob Chemother* 35:421-24, 1995.

Concha, J.M., et al. "Antifungal Activity of *Melaleuca alternifolia* Oil Against Various Pathogenic Organisms," *J Am Podiatr Med Assoc* 88(10):489-92, 1998.

Cox, S.D., et al. "The Mode of Antimicrobial Action of the Essential Oil of *Melaleuca alternifolia* (Tea Tree Oil)," *J Appl Microbiol* 88(1):170-75, 2000.

Hammer, K.A., et al. "Influence of Organic Matter, Cations and Surfactants on the Antimicrobial Activity of *Melaleuca alternifolia* (Tea Tree) Oil In Vitro," *J Appl Microbiol* 86(3):446-52, 1999.

Hammer, K.A., et al. "In Vitro Activity of Essential Oils, in Particular *Melaleuca alternifolia* Oil and Tea Tree Oil Products, Against *Candida* spp," *J Antimicrob Chemother* 42(5):591-95, 1998.

Jacobs, M.R., et al. "Melaleuca Oil Poisoning," *Clin Toxicol* 32(4):461-64, 1994.

Jandera, V., et al. "Cooling the Burn Wound: Evaluation of Different Modalities," *Burns* 26(3):265-70, 2000.

Jandourek, A., et al. "Efficacy of Melaleuca Oral Solution for the Treatment of Fluconazole Refractory Oral Candidiasis in AIDS Patients," *AIDS* 12(9):1033-37, 1998.

Mann, C.M., et al. "The Outer Membrane of *Pseudomonas aeruginosa* NCTC 6749 Contributes to Its Tolerance to the Essential Oil of *Melaleuca alternifolia*," *Lett Appl Microbiol* 30(4):294-47, 2000.

Nelson, R.R.S. "In-Vitro Activities of Five Plant Essential Oils Against Methicillin-Resistant *Staphylcoccus aureus* and Vancomycin-resistant *Enterococcus faecium*," *J Antimicrob Chemother* 40:305-6, 1997.

Nenoff, P., et al. "Antifungal Activity of the Essential Oil of *Melaleuca alternifolia* (Tea Tree Oil) Against Pathogenic Fungi In Vivo," *Skin Pharmacol* 9:388-94, 1996.

Rubel, D.M., et al. "Tea Tree Oil Allergy: What Is the Offending Agent? Report of Three Cases of Tea Tree Oil Allergy and Review of the Literature," *Australas J Dermatol* 39(4):244-47, 1998.

Syed, T.A., et al. "Treatment of Toenail Onychomycosis with 2% Butenafine and 5% *Melaleuca alternifolia* Oil in Cream," *Trop Med Int Health* 4(4):284-87, 1999.

THUJA

EASTERN WHITE CEDAR, FALSE WHITE CEDAR, HACKMATACK, TREE OF LIFE, YELLOW CEDAR

Taxonomic class
Cupressaceae

Bold italic type indicates that reaction may be life-threatening.

Common trade names
None known.

Common forms
Available as liquid extract and tincture.

Source
Active components are obtained from the needles and young twigs of *Thuja occidentalis*, an evergreen conifer that is native to eastern North America.

Chemical components
Thuja contains the volatile oil thujone, tannin, flavonoid glycoside, and a resin, thujin.

Actions
Thuja's actions appear related to its stimulating and blood-purifying volatile oil. Thuja has some mitogenic activity, inhibits HIV-1 antigens and HIV-1 specific reverse transcriptase, and is an inducer of a subset of T cells and various cytokines in vitro (Offergeld et al., 1992). It has also been shown to be an immunostimulant in a rat liver model (Vomel, 1985). Thujone oil can cause seizures in animals (Elsasser-Beile et al., 1996).

Reported uses
Therapeutic claims for thuja include its use as an antiseptic, an astringent, a diuretic, and an expectorant. Although thuja has become popular as a cancer treatment, all the supporting data are from in vitro (Offergeld et al., 1992) or anecdotal case reports and not from controlled human trials.

Dosage
No consensus exists.
Infusion: 1 tsp of dried herb added to 1 cup of boiling water, steeped for 10 to 15 minutes, and taken P.O. t.i.d.
Tincture: 1 to 2 ml P.O. t.i.d.

Adverse reactions
CNS: CNS stimulation, *seizures.*
GI: flatulence, indigestion, nausea, vomiting.
GU: uterine stimulation (may lead to *spontaneous abortion*).
Respiratory: *asthma* (Cartier et al., 1986).

Interactions
Anticonvulsants: Lowered seizure threshold. Adjust anticonvulsant dosage as needed.
Caffeine, other stimulants: Additive effect. Avoid administration with thuja.

Contraindications and precautions
Thuja is contraindicated during pregnancy because of the risk of spontaneous abortion. Internal use is contraindicated in patients with seizure disorders. Use cautiously in patients with gastritis or ulcers because of its GI stimulating effects.

Special considerations
• Monitor the patient for adverse reactions, such as excess stimulation.
• Urge women to report planned or suspected pregnancy.
• Caution the patient against using thuja because little evidence regarding its medicinal use exists.

Commentary
Insufficient data exist in humans to support a medicinal use of thuja. Further studies are needed to evaluate its effects in AIDS and cancer therapy. Safer alternatives are available for the traditional use of thuja as a diuretic and an expectorant.

References
Cartier, A., et al. "Occupational Asthma Caused by Eastern White Cedar (*Thuja occidentalis*) with Demonstration that Plicatic Acid Is Present in this Wood Dust and Is the Causal Agent," *J Allergy Clin Immunol* 77:639-45, 1986.

Elsasser-Beile, U., et al. "Cytokine Production in Leukocyte Cultures During Therapy with *Echinacea* Extract," *J Clin Lab Anal* 10:441-45, 1996.

Offergeld, R., et al. "Mitogenic Activity of High Molecular Polysaccharide Fractions Isolated from the *Cuppressaceae Thuja occidentalis* L. Enhanced Cytokine-Production by Thyapolysaccharide, G-Fraction (TPSg)," *Leukemia* 6(Suppl. 3):189S-91S, 1992.

Vomel, T. "Effect of a Plant Immunostimulant on Phagocytosis of Erythrocytes by the Reticulohistiocytary System of Isolated Perfused Rat Liver," *Arzneimittelforschung* 35:1437-39, 1985.

THYME

COMMON THYME, GARDEN THYME, RUBBED THYME, THYMI HERBA, TIMO

Taxonomic class
Lamiaceae

Common trade names
Multi-ingredient preparations: Autussan "T," Olbas, Pertussin, Pertussin N

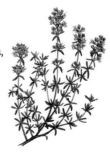

Common forms
Extract: 12% to 14%
Ointment: 1% to 2% thymol
    Also available as an essential oil.

Source
Active components are derived from the dried leaves and flowering tops of *Thymus vulgaris,* a member of the mint family; the plant is native to Spain and Italy and widely cultivated worldwide.

Chemical components
The composition of thyme essential or volatile oil is varied. Phenols, principally thymol, constitute 25% to 70% of the oils. Other components include carvacrol, camphene, sabinene, beta-pinene, 1,8-cineol, linalol, borneol, geraniol, geranyl acetate, sesquiterpine, and alcohol.

Actions
Thyme extract contains thymol and other phenols, which have antiseptic, antitussive, and expectorant properties. Thymol acts as an expectorant by directly irritating GI mucosa. Therefore, thymol is usually taken orally or applied topically.

Thyme exerts antifungal action, both topically and systemically. In vitro studies have also identified inhibitory effects on protozoa (Mikus et al., 2000) and certain bacteria (Dorman and Deans, 2000).

Thyme liquid extracts have shown spasmolytic action in animal models (van Den Broucke and Lemli, 1981) and antioxidant effects (thyme oil) in rats (Youdim and Deans, 1999).

Reported uses
Thyme products have been used most widely as food additives, flavoring agents, and condiments. Therapeutic claims include use as an anthelmintic, an antiflatulent, an antifungal, an antiseptic, an antispasmotic, an antitussive, an expectorant, a diaphoretic, and a digestive aid. It is commonly used as an antitussive in respiratory tract disorders. Its antiseptic properties are exploited in toothpastes, mouthwashes, and tooth fillings. Other anecdotal uses include treatment of dysmenorrhea, dyspepsia, headache, and hysteria.

Thyme has been tested against actinomycosis in humans (Myers, 1937). Its systemic action is apparently greatly diminished in the presence of protein.

Dosage
For itchy skin, 1% to 2% ointment applied topically as needed.
Cough syrup: 1 tsp P.O. every 2 hours as needed.
Essential oil: 5 to 10 gtt in some water P.O. b.i.d. or t.i.d.
Tea: 1.5 to 2 g of dried herb P.O. t.i.d.

Adverse reactions
CNS: dizziness, headache.
CV: *bradycardia.*
EENT: cheilitis, glossitis (with toothpaste).
GI: diarrhea, nausea, vomiting.
Musculoskeletal: muscle weakness.
Respiratory: slow respiratory rate.

Skin: dermatitis.
Other: systemic allergic reaction.

Interactions
None reported.

Contraindications and precautions
Thyme is contraindicated in patients with a history of gastritis and intestinal disorders and in those who are hypersensitive to various plants, such as grass. Internal use is contraindicated in patients with enterocolitis or cardiac insufficiency and during pregnancy.

Special considerations
• Inform the patient that there are few clinical data to support thyme's use for any medical condition.

◆ **ALERT** Systemic allergic reactions have occurred when thyme is used as a flavoring agent. Symptoms include dysphagia, dysphonia, edema, hypotension, nausea, pruritus and swelling of the lips and tongue, progressive upper respiratory difficulty, and vomiting. Treatment involves antihistamine, corticosteroid, and epinephrine administration and fluid therapy (Benito et al., 1996).

• Caution the patient with sensitive skin or known allergies to avoid thyme.

• Although no known chemical interactions have been reported in clinical studies, consideration must be given to the pharmacologic properties of the herbal product and the potential for exacerbation of the intended therapeutic effect of conventional drugs.

Points of interest
• The volatile oils of *T. vulgaris* have proved effective against certain agricultural insects and have been suggested as an abundant, inexpensive, safe, and environmentally friendly alternative to commonly used pesticides in Egypt.

Commentary
Thyme preparations have been used for centuries to treat several disease states. In light of the limited availability of clinical studies that assess the safety and efficacy of thyme, these products cannot be recommended for therapeutic purposes. The use of thymol as an antiseptic may be useful in dental products, but well-designed studies are needed.

References
Benito, M., et al. "Labiatae Allergy: Systemic Reactions Due to Ingestion of Oregano and Thyme," *Ann Allergy Asthma Immunol* 76:416-18, 1996.

Dorman, H.J., and Deans, S.G. "Antimicrobial Agents from Plants: Antibacterial Activity of Plant Volatile Oils," *J Appl Microbiol* 88(2):308-16, 2000.

Mikus, J., et al. "In Vitro Effect of Essential Oils and Isolated Mono- and Sesquiterpenes on *Leishmania major* and *Trypanosoma brucei*," *Planta Med* 66(4):366-68, 2000.

Myers, H.B. "Thymol Therapy in Actinomycosis," *JAMA* 108:1875, 1937.

Bold italic type indicates that reaction may be life-threatening.

van Den Broucke, C.O., and Lemli, J.A. "Pharmacological and Chemical Investigation of Thyme Liquid Extracts," *Planta Med* 41:129-35, 1981.

Youdim, K.A., and Deans, S.G. "Dietary Supplementation of Thyme Essential Oil During the Lifetime of the Rat: Its Effects on the Antioxidant Status in Liver, Kidney and Heart Tissues," *Mech Ageing Dev* 109(3):163-75, 1999.

TONKA BEAN

CUMARU, TONKA SEED, TONQUIN BEAN, TORQUIN BEAN

Taxonomic class
Lamiaceae

Common trade names
Tonka Bean

Common forms
Tonka bean is difficult to obtain commercially; availability is rare.

Source
Active components are extracted from the fruits and seeds of *Dipteryx odorata*, a tree that is native to South America, specifically Brazil and Venezuela. The tonka bean tree belongs to the legume family.

Chemical components
The primary chemical components of tonka bean are coumarin, dihydrocoumarin, and *o*-coumaric acid. Other components include melilotic acid, methyl melilotate, ethyl melilotate, 5-hydroxymethylfurfural, fat, and starch.

Actions
Coumarin is metabolized within the body to 7-hydroxycoumarin, which then undergoes glucuronidation in the intestines and liver; this extensive first-pass metabolism results in a low absolute bioavailability of coumarin. Both coumarin and 7-hydroxycoumarin have inhibited growth of selected types of malignant human cell lines in vitro. The glucuronide metabolite of 7-hydroxycoumarin appears to be inactive (Marshall et al., 1994).

Reported uses
Tonka bean is claimed to relieve abdominal cramps and nausea; the fruit is also thought to act as an aphrodisiac. It is known as a folk remedy for whooping cough as well. Coumarin has long been used as a flavoring agent in foods and a scent in pharmaceutical products. It has shown therapeutic benefit against lymphedema in clinical trials (Overik et al., 1995; Vettorello et al., 1996).

Dosage
The usual dose used is 60 mg of coumarin P.O. daily. (Some studies have based doses on the coumarin content of the product.)

Adverse reactions
CV: potential cardiac effects (with large doses).
Hepatic: *hepatotoxicity.*

Interactions
Anticoagulants: May cause excessive bleeding. Avoid administration with tonka bean.
Drugs that cause hepatotoxicity: Risk of additive toxicity. Avoid administration with tonka bean.

Contraindications and precautions
Tonka bean is contraindicated in patients with underlying hepatic dysfunction because of the potential for toxicity. Avoid its use in pregnant or breast-feeding patients; effects are unknown.

Special considerations
• Inform the patient that tonka bean is on the FDA's list of unsafe herbs.
• Advise the patient to consult a health care provider before using herbal preparations because a treatment that has been clinically researched and proved effective may be available.
• Monitor liver function test results.
• Advise women to avoid using tonka bean during pregnancy or when breast-feeding.

Points of interest
• Do not confuse this herb with the synthetic anticoagulant *bis*-hydroxycoumarin.
• Extracts of tonka bean have been used as a flavoring for castor oil preparations.

Commentary
Several tonka bean components, especially coumarin and 7-hydroxycoumarin, show promise as future therapeutic agents. Because efficacy and safety data are lacking, the herb cannot be recommended for any medicinal use.

References
Marshall, M.E., et al. "Growth-inhibitory Effects of Coumarin (1,2-Benzopyrone) and 7-Hydroxycoumarin on Human Malignant Cell Lines In Vitro," *J Cancer Res Clin Oncol* 120(Suppl):S3-S10, 1994.

Overvik, E., et al. "Activation and Effects of the Food-derived Heterocyclic Amines in Extrahepatic Tissues," *Princess Takamatsu Symp* 23:123-33, 1995.

Vettorello, S., et al. "Contribution of a Combination of Alpha and Beta Benzpyrones, Flavonoids and Natural Terpenes in the Treatment of Lymphedema of the Lower Limbs at the 2d Stage of Surgical Classification," *Minerva Cardioangiol* 44:447-55, 1996.

Bold italic type indicates that reaction may be life-threatening.

TORMENTIL ROOT

BISCUITS, BLOODROOT, EARTHBANK, ENGLISH SARSAPARILLA, EWE DAISY, FIVE-FINGERS, FLESH AND BLOOD, SEPTFOIL, SEVEN LEAVES, SHEPHERD'S KNAPPERTY, SHEPHERD'S KNOT, THORMANTLE

Taxonomic class
Rosaceae

Common trade names
None known.

Common forms
Available as powder, rootstock, and tincture.

Source
Active components are derived primarily from the rhizome and roots of *Potentilla tormentilla*, a perennial herb that belongs to the rose family and is native to Europe and Asia.

Chemical components
The rhizome contains mainly tannic acid, tormentol (a triterpine alcohol), a glycoside, tormentillin, starch, sugars, a bitter compound (chinovic acid), and essential oils (Stodola, 1984). Many other components have also been identified, such as adimericellagitannin, agrimoniin, gallic acid, ellagic acid, and catechol gallates.

Actions
Because it is rich in tannic acid, the herb is a strong astringent and has some tonic properties as well. Tormentil has also been reported to have antiallergic, antihypertensive, and antiviral effects. It has demonstrated antielastase, antioxidant, and immunostimulant properties as well (Bos et al., 1996).

Reported uses
The astringent properties of *P. tormentilla* are reportedly useful topical agents as compresses or ointments for burns, grazes, rashes, sunburn, and slow-healing wounds. The tincture is claimed to be valuable as a gargle for throat and mouth inflammations (Grieve, 1997). Internal use of *P. tormentilla* has been touted as a treatment for diarrhea (Carr et al., 1987). Clinical trials are lacking for these indications and for its antielastase and immunostimulant properties.

Dosage
For diarrhea, mix 1 oz each of powdered tormentil, powdered galangal, and powdered marshmallow root with 240 grains of powdered ginger and 1 pt of boiling water. Strain mixture, and take 5 to 10 ml (3 tsp) t.i.d. or q.i.d. Do not use for longer than 4 days.
Gargle: 2 oz of bruised root boiled in 50 oz of water until reduced by one-third. Strain the cooled liquid and use as gargle.

Powder: ¼ to ½ tsp of powder P.O. t.i.d.
Tea: 1 tbsp of rootstock mixed with 1 cup of water and steeped for 30 minutes. Strain and drink during the day in mouthful doses.
Tincture: 20 to 30 gtt P.O. b.i.d. or t.i.d.

Adverse reactions

With acute ingestion of more than 1 g of tannins
GI: abdominal pain, constipation, gastroenteritis, nausea, vomiting.
Hepatic: *hepatic necrosis.*

Interactions

Alkaloids, glycosides: May cause precipitation and reduced absorption of these drugs. Avoid internal administration with tormentil.
Disulfiram: Disulfiram reaction if tincture contains alcohol. Avoid administration with tormentil.
Iron and other minerals: Tormentil interferes with absorption of iron and other minerals when taken internally. Separate administration times.

Contraindications and precautions

Tormentil is contraindicated in patients with diverticulitis, diverticulosis, duodenal or gastric ulcers, reflux esophagitis, spastic colitis, or ulcerative colitis. Also avoid its use in pregnant or breast-feeding patients; effects are unknown.

Special considerations

• Advise the patient to consult a health care provider before using herbal preparations because a treatment that has been clinically researched and proved effective may be available.
• Monitor for adverse GI reactions.
• Advise women to avoid using tormentil during pregnancy or when breast-feeding.
• Caution the patient taking disulfiram not to use herbal products that contain alcohol.

Points of interest

• In ancient Athens, Hippocrates used tormentil to treat malaria.
• The 17th-century British herbalist Nicholas Culpeper recommended packing tormentil root into a painful tooth. In the days before the discovery of dental plaque, the herb was used to dry up the "flux of humors" thought to cause toothaches (Carr et al., 1987).

Commentary

No clinical data exist to support taking tormentil for any medical condition. Because little is known about its toxicologic properties, this herb is best avoided.

References

Bos, M.A., et al. "Procyanidins from Tormentil: Antioxidant Properties Towards Lipoeroxidation and Anti-Elastase Activity," *Biol Pharm Bull* 19:146-48, 1996.

Bold italic type indicates that reaction may be life-threatening.

Carr, A., et al. *Encyclopedia of Herbs*. Emmaus, Pa.: Rodale Press, 1987.

Grieve, M. *A Modern Herbal*. London: Tiger Books International, 1997.

Stodola, J. *The Illustrated Book of Herbs*. London: Octopus Books Ltd., 1984.

TRAGACANTH

ADRILEL, E413, GOMA ALATIRA, GUM DRAGON, GUM
TRAGACANTH, HOG GUM, SHAGAL EL KETIRA, SYRIAN
TRAGACANTH, TRAGACANTH TREE

Taxonomic class
Fabaceae

Common trade names
None known; usually sold as tragacanth or gum tragacanth.

Common forms
Available as a gel, gum, powder, tablets, and viscous solution.

Source
Tragacanth is obtained by drying the gummy substance that exudes from the cut tap root and branches of *Astracantha gummifer* or other *Astracantha* species, low thorny shrubs that belong to the legume family. The plants are native to the Middle East.

Chemical components
Tragacanth gum consists of two major fractions, tragacanthin and bassorin, with trace amounts of starch, a cellulose-like substance, amino acids, and amino acid derivatives. Tragacanthin is water-soluble and consists of an arabinogalactan and tragacanthic acid; bassorin is a complex of methoxylated acids that swells to form a gel or viscous solution that is insoluble in water. Tragacanth may also contain some karaya, India gum, or acacia, other natural gums used for similar purposes.

Actions
When added to water, tragacanth swells to form a viscous jelly that is mixed with other ingredients to create the desired consistency in the final product. This action is probably attributable to the bassorin content; high-quality gums contain less tragacanthin. The herb also exerts a mild laxative effect (Iwu, 1993).

Tragacanth appears to be a relatively innocuous substance. In one study, large doses (10 g) of tragacanth reduced intestinal transit time and increased fecal fat levels (Eastwood et al., 1984). Plasma biochemistry, hematologic indexes, urinalysis parameters, glucose tolerance, breath hydrogen, methane concentrations, and serum cholesterol, triglyceride, and phospholipid were not significantly changed. The quantity of tragacanth used in this study far exceeds the normal annual dietary intake. Other claims are that tragacanth stimulates phagocytosis, increases plasma cell counts of T lymphocytes, and acts against some experimental tumors (Iwu, 1993). Confirmatory data are lacking.

Tragacanth is not allergenic, mutagenic, or teratogenic. No adverse toxicologic effects have been observed in nonallergic people (Eastwood et al., 1984).

Reported uses
FDA guidelines state that tragacanth may be used in concentrations of 0.2% to 1.3% to thicken, emulsify, stabilize, or flavor foods (Eastwood et al., 1984). The concentration in medicinal products ranges from 4.8% to 6% in oral liquids and from 0.42 to 100 mg in tablets (Smolinske, 1992). Because of its action with water, tragacanth is used for preparing adhesives, emulsions, protective or lubricating barriers, and suspensions. It may be used in oral and topical products with glycerin to create emulsions and suspensions.

Tragacanth is more resistant to acid hydrolysis than other hydrocolloids and is preferred in the preparation of acidic compounds. It has also been used as a binder and stabilizer in preparing cosmetics and hand lotions, to stiffen cloth, as a glue in bookbinding, and in making candy and other products (Smolinske, 1992). The herb is used as well in denture adhesives and toothpastes and as a bulk-forming laxative (Baker and Helling, 1986; Curry, 1986). In African folk medicine, tragacanth is used as a mild laxative; the leaves are used to prepare a first aid lotion (Iwu, 1993).

Dosage
FDA dietary guidelines allow concentrations of 0.2% and 1.3% as a thickener, stabilizer, and flavoring agent in foods. Little consensus exists, but the usual recommended dose ranges from 0.42 to 100 mg in tablet form P.O. b.i.d. or t.i.d.

Adverse reactions
EENT: rhinitis, sneezing.
GI: abdominal pain.
Musculoskeletal: arthralgia.
Respiratory: *asthma,* dyspnea.
Skin: contact dermatitis (with topical jelly; Smolinske, 1992), pruritus, rash, urticaria.
Other: *angioedema,* fever, hypersensitivity reactions (Danoff et al., 1978; Smolinske, 1992).

Interactions
Fat, fat-soluble nutrients: May decrease absorption of these agents if taken in excess. Avoid excessive use.

Contraindications and precautions
Tragacanth is contraindicated in patients who are hypersensitive to natural gums used in food or pharmaceutical products. Avoid its use in pregnant or breast-feeding patients; effects are unknown.

Bold italic type indicates that reaction may be life-threatening.

Special considerations

⚑ ALERT The gum may contain microbial contaminants, such as coliform and Salmonella bacteria (Farley and Lund, 1976). Monitor the patient closely for signs of infection.

• Monitor for hypersensitivity reactions.

• Advise women to avoid using tragacanth during pregnancy or when breast-feeding.

Points of interest

• Tragacanth's use in foods, cosmetics, and pharmaceutical products has declined in favor of synthetic substances with similar physical properties.

• The FDA lists tragacanth as a generally safe food additive.

• Tragacanth gets its name from the Greek words *tragos* (goat) and *akantha* (horn), probably in reference to the curved or twisted appearance of the dried exudate.

Commentary

Because other natural and synthetic suspending and emulsifying agents are available, tragacanth is no longer widely used in U.S. pharmaceuticals, except in extemporaneous compounding and some commercial suspensions or tablets. The herb is regarded as safe for use in foods and other products, and no known reports exist of adverse reactions in non-allergic people. Although it may be used as a mild bulk-forming laxative, safer and more effective products are readily available.

References

Baker, K.A., and Helling, D.K. "Oral Health Products," in *Handbook of Nonprescription Drugs,* 8th ed. Washington, D.C.: American Pharmaceutical Association, 1986.

Curry, C.E. "Laxative Products," in *Handbook of Nonprescription Drugs,* 8th ed. Washington, D.C.: American Pharmaceutical Association, 1986.

Danoff, D., et al. "Big Mac Attack," *N Engl J Med* 298:1095-96, 1978.

Eastwood, M.A., et al. "The Effects of Dietary Gum Tragacanth in Man," *Toxicol Lett* 21:73-81, 1984.

Farley, C.A., and Lund, W. "Suspending Agents for Extemporaneous Dispensing: Evaluation of Alternatives to Tragacanth," *Pharmaceutical J* 216:562-66, 1976.

Iwu, M.M. *Handbook of African Medicinal Plants.* Boca Raton, Fla.: CRC Press, 1993.

Smolinske, S.C. *Handbook of Food, Drug, and Cosmetic Excipients.* Boca Raton, Fla.: CRC Press, 1992.

TRUE UNICORN ROOT

AGUE GRASS, AGUE-ROOT, ALOE-ROOT, COLIC-ROOT, CROW CORN, DEVIL'S BIT, STAR GRASS, UNICORN ROOT, WHITETUBE STARGRASS

Taxonomic class

Liliaceae

Common trade names
Aletris-Heel, True Unicorn Root

Common forms
Available as a liquid and tea.

Source
Active components are derived from the rhizomes and roots of *Aletris farinosa,* a perennial herb of the lily family that is native to the eastern United States.

Chemical components
True unicorn root contains steroidal saponins—primarily diosgenin and gentrogenin—and alkaloids, essential oil, resin, and starch.

Actions
Diosgenin has been reported to have estrogen-like activity; hence, its use as a tonic. Lydia Pinkham's Vegetable Compound, a famous patent medicine made of *A. farinosa,* pleurisy root (*Asclepias tuberosa*), other herbs, and alcohol, was claimed to cure various gynecologic conditions. The alkaloids contribute to its CNS depressant effects (Lewis, 1977).

Reported uses
True unicorn root was popular with Native Americans. *A. farinosa* has been used to treat amenorrhea, colic, diarrhea, dysmenorrhea, flatulence, rheumatism, and snake bites. Other claims include its use as an antispasmodic, a cathartic, a diuretic, a narcotic, and a sedative and to prevent habitual miscarriage (Duke, 1985; Horn and Weil, 1996).

Dosage
No consensus exists. Some references state the dose as being 0.3 to 0.6 g P.O. t.i.d.

Adverse reactions
CNS: loss of balance caused by CNS depressant effects, stupor.
GI: diarrhea, nausea, vomiting.

Interactions
CNS depressants, narcotics: May increase sedative effects. Avoid administration with true unicorn root.
H₂ blockers, sucralfate: True unicorn root may increase acid production in the stomach, creating an antagonistic effect. Separate administration times.
Oxytocin: May cause antagonized effects of this drug. Avoid concomitant use.

Contraindications and precautions
Avoid using true unicorn root in pregnant patients (because of estrogenic activity and oxytocin antagonism) or breast-feeding patients; effects are unknown. Use cautiously in patients with GI disorders.

Bold italic type indicates that reaction may be life-threatening.

Special considerations
● Inquire about the patient's need to use true unicorn root.
● Advise the patient to consult a health care provider before using herbal preparations because a treatment that has been clinically researched and proved effective may be available.
● Caution the patient not to perform activities that require alertness and coordination until the CNS effects of the herb are known.
● Advise women to avoid using true unicorn root during pregnancy or when breast-feeding.

Points of interest
● True unicorn root should not be confused with false unicorn root (*Helonias luteum* or *Chamaelirium luteum*). These herbs differ in chemical composition and claimed uses.

Commentary
True unicorn root has been used chiefly to treat gynecologic and GI conditions and rheumatism. Although little is known about the chemical components, even small doses of the herb are associated with adverse reactions. No clinical data support the use of this herb for any medical condition.

References
Duke, J.A., ed. *Handbook of Medicinal Herbs.* Boca Raton, Fla.: CRC Press, 1985.
Horn, V., and Weil, C., eds. *The Encyclopedia of Medicinal Plants.* New York: DK Publishing Inc., 1996.
Lewis, W.H. *Medical Botany: Plants Affecting Man's Health.* New York: John Wiley & Sons, 1977.

TURMERIC

CURCUMA, INDIAN SAFFRON, INDIAN VALERIAN, JIANG HUANG, RADIX, RED VALERIAN

Taxonomic class
Zingiberaceae

Common trade names
Turmeric Root

Common forms
Available as capsules (100 mg, 450 mg), curry spices, dry rhizome, extract, oil, tincture, and turmeric spices.

Source
Active components are derived from the rhizome of *Curcuma longa,* a member of the ginger family. Turmeric is grown and harvested commercially in many areas of India, China, Asia, Indonesia, and other tropical countries.

Chemical components

Turmeric contains an orange-yellow volatile oil, curcumin. Curcuminoid compounds include tumerone, atlantone, diaryl heptanoids, and zingiberone; these substances are considered the active component of the plant. Other compounds include sugars (glucose, fructose, arabinose), resins, proteins, vitamins, and minerals.

Actions

Turmeric compounds, especially curcumin, have been extensively studied. Curcumin appears to inhibit carcinogenesis at all steps of cancer formation; it promotes detoxification of carcinogens in vitro and in vivo (Stoner and Mukhtar, 1995). Antioxidant properties were noted in protein isolated from a liquid extract of turmeric (Selvam et al., 1995). Rats pretreated with curcumin had fewer and smaller tumors than controls when exposed to chemical carcinogens; this action was partially attributed to the antioxidant properties (Broadhurst, 1997; Hastak et al., 1997).

Curcumin shows promise in the treatment of cholelithiasis (Kiso et al., 1983). Intestinal cholesterol uptake was significantly reduced in rats given curcumin (Roa, 1970). In animal studies, curcumin has demonstrated a natural cytochrome P-450 modulation by inhibiting the activity of CYP1A2 and glutathione S-transferase enzyme in animal hepatocytes (Oetari et al., 1996).

Curcuminoids inhibit leukotriene biosynthesis by way of the lipoxygenase pathways, which reduce prostaglandin formation. They also inhibit thromboxane B_4 without affecting prostacyclin synthesis (Lal et al., 1999; Grant et al., 2000). As a result, they are as effective as NSAIDs in the treatment of osteoarthritis, postoperative pain, and rheumatoid arthritis. They are thought to stimulate corticosteroid release, sensitize cortisol receptors, or increase the half-life of cortisol through alteration of hepatic degradation processes (Broadhurst, 1997).

Turmeric extract inhibited gastric secretion and protected gastroduodenal mucosa against ulcer formation induced by cysteamine, indomethacin, pyloric ligation, reserpine, and stress in rats. However, in high doses, it may be ulcerogenic (Rafatullah et al., 1990).

Curcumin has been used as an antiparasitic and antiseptic internally and externally; it has slowed the growth of most organisms associated with cholecystitis (Broadhurst, 1997). Curcumin has been found to interfere with the replication of viruses, including viral hepatitis and HIV. It has increased the CD4 count and inhibited the activity of enzymes that transport the virus into healthy cells (Broadhurst, 1997).

Reported uses

Turmeric has been used in cancer prevention and as a treatment adjunct. According to the American Institute for Cancer Research, curcumin helps to prevent breast, colon, esophageal, oral, skin, and stomach cancers. It is also used to treat atherosclerosis, cholelithiasis, GI bacterial overgrowth, GI diseases (flatulence, gastritis, ulcerations), hepatic disorders, inflammatory conditions (injuries, osteoarthritis, rheumatoid

---

Bold italic type indicates that reaction may be life-threatening.

arthritis), irritable bowel syndrome, parasitic infestation, and viral infections.

Traditional Chinese and Indian (Ayurvedic) philosophies of medicine involve the use of turmeric for bruises, chest pain, colic, flatulence, hematuria, hemorrhage, jaundice, menstrual problems, and toothache. Poultices of turmeric have been used to relieve local inflammation and pain.

Dosage
The recommended dosage of curcumin is 400 to 600 mg P.O. t.i.d. For turmeric, an equivalent dosage of 8 to 60 g P.O. t.i.d. is needed. Turmeric should be taken on an empty stomach.

Adverse reactions
GI: GI ulceration (with high doses or prolonged use).
Skin: contact dermatitis.

Interactions
Anticoagulants: May cause additive effects on platelets. Avoid administration with turmeric.
Immunosuppressants: Decreased immunosuppressive effect. Use cautiously, if at all, in combination.
NSAIDs: May inhibit platelet function and increase risk of bleeding. Avoid administration with turmeric.

Contraindications and precautions
Avoid using turmeric in pregnant or breast-feeding patients; effects are unknown. The American Herbal Products Association has classified turmeric as a menstrual stimulant; therefore, it can induce miscarriage. It is also contraindicated in patients with bleeding disorders and bile duct obstruction. Use cautiously in patients with a history of ulcers.

Special considerations
• Monitor coagulation studies if medicinal doses are being used.
• Urge the patient to report unusual bruising or bleeding.
• Advise women to avoid using turmeric during pregnancy or when breast-feeding.
• Caution the patient to keep turmeric preparations out of the reach of children and pets.

Points of interest
• The antioxidant activity of curcumin is comparable with standard antioxidants, such as vitamins C and E, butylated hydroxyanisole, and butylated hydroxytoluene. Curcumin strongly inhibits the peroxidation of fats, thus helping to retard food spoilage. Because of its bright yellow color, curcumin is commonly added to butter, margarine, cheese, curry power, mustard, and other food products.

Commentary
Turmeric has shown potential as an anti-inflammatory because it appears to be as effective as NSAIDs and cortisol and has a lower inci-

dence of the dangerous adverse reactions associated with these drugs. More clinical research is needed to prove safety and efficacy in humans before turmeric can be recommended for any medical condition.

References

Broadhurst, L. "Curcumin, a Powerful Bioprotectant Spice, or...Curry Cures!" Botanical Medicine Conference. Philadelphia: May 15, 1997.

Grant, K., et al. "Tumeric," *Am J Health-Syst Pharm* 57:1121-22, 2000.

Hastak, K., et al. "Effect of Turmeric Oil and Turmeric Oleoresin on Cytogenic Damage in Patients Suffering from Oral Submucous Fibrosis," *Cancer Lett* 116:265-69, 1997.

Kiso, Y., et al. "Antihepatotoxic Principles of *Curcuma longa* Rhizome," *Planta Med* 49:185-87, 1983.

Lal, B., et al. "Curcumin Successful Treats Chronic Anterior Uveitis," *Phytotherapy Res* 13:318-22, 1999.

Oetari, S., et al. "Effects of Curcumin on Cytochrome P-450 and Glutathione S-transferase Activity in Rat Liver," *Biochem Pharmacol* 51(1):39-45, 1996.

Rafatullah, S., et al. "Evaluation of Turmeric (*Curcuma longa*) for Gastric and Duodenal Antiulcer Activity in Rats," *J Ethnobotany* 29:25-34, 1990.

Roa, D.S. "Effect of Curcumin on Serum and Liver Cholesterol Levels in the Rat," *J Nutr* 100:1307-16, 1970.

Selvam, R., et al. "The Anti-oxidant Activity of Turmeric (*Curcuma longa*)," *J Ethnobotany* 47:59-67, 1995.

Stoner, G.D., and Mukhtar, H. "Polyphenols as Cancer Chemoprotective Agents," *J Cell Biochem* 22(Suppl):169-80, 1995.

Bold italic type indicates that reaction may be life-threatening.

V

VALERIAN

ALL-HEAL, AMANTILLA, BALDRIANWURZEL, GREAT WILD VALERIAN, HERBA BENEDICTA, KATZENWURZEL, PHU GERMANICUM, PHU PARVUM, *PINNIS DENTATIS*, SETEWALE CAPON'S TAIL, SETWALL, THERIACARIA, VALERIANA, *VALERIANA FOLIIS PINNATIS*, *VALERIANA RADIX*

Taxonomic class
Valerianaceae

Common trade names
Valerian Easy Step, Valerian
Extract, Valerian Nighttime,
Valerian Root, Valerian Root
Extract

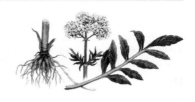

Multi-ingredient preparations: Alluna Sleep (combination of valerian root 500 mg, and hops 120 mg, extracts)

Common forms
Standardized capsules, tablets (0.8% valerenic acid): 180 mg, 200 mg, 250 mg, 400 mg, 410 mg, 450 mg, 493 mg, 500 mg, 520 mg, 530 mg, 550 mg
Standardized tinctures: 2% essential oil
   Also available as tinctures and teas that contain crude dried herb and in combination with other dietary supplements.

Source
Active components are derived from rhizomes and roots of *Valeriana officinalis,* a perennial herb that is native to Eurasia and naturalized worldwide.

Chemical components
Valerian contains volatile oils, iridoid triesters known as valepotriates, aliphatic acids, alkaloids, amino acids, aromatic acids, flavonoids, free fatty acids, phenolic acids, sugars, and salts.

Actions
In vitro studies found that aqueous extracts of valerian inhibit the uptake and stimulate the release of gamma-aminobutyric acid (GABA), which may increase the extracellular concentration of GABA in the synaptic cleft and thereby contribute to the herb's sedative effect. The increased GABA release is independent of sodium-potassium-adenosinetriphosphatase activity. One study found that at higher concentrations, valerian inhibited binding to GABA (Ortiz et al., 1999). Most researchers attribute the sedative effect more to the valepotriates and less to the sesquiterpene

components of the volatile oils; others think that it is attributed to the valepotriate decomposition products (baldrinal and homobaldrinal). Because of their epoxide structure, the valepotriates are cytotoxic in cell cultures. They are also highly unstable, decompose easily, and are not readily absorbed. Most preparations contain only small amounts.

The extract has weak anticonvulsant and antidepressant properties (Sakamoto et al., 1992). The herb also has antispasmodic effects on GI smooth muscle (Hazelhoff et al., 1982), produces coronary dilation, and has antiarrhythmic activity (Petkov, 1979).

Reported uses

Valerian is widely used in Europe, particularly in France and Germany, as an antispasmodic and a sedative. The German Commission E recommends valerian for restlessness and nervous disturbances of sleep (Schulz et al., 1998). Multiple studies have demonstrated improvement in sleep (Donath et al., 2000; Fussel et al., 2000). Valerian is also used as a daytime sedative for restlessness and tension. Data on its anticonvulsant and antidepressant effects are lacking.

Dosage

The composition and purity of valerian preparations vary greatly.
For sleep disorders, 400 to 900 mg of standardized valerian extract P.O. 30 minutes to 1 hour before bedtime.
Tea: 2 to 3 g (1 tsp) of crude dried herb P.O. several times daily.
Tincture: 3 to 5 ml (½ to 1 tsp) P.O. several times daily.

Adverse reactions

With overdose or long-term use:
CNS: excitability, headache, insomnia.
CV: cardiac dysfunction.
EENT: blurred vision.
GI: hepatotoxicity, nausea.
Other: hypersensitivity reactions.

Interactions

Alcohol, CNS depressants: Risk of additive effects. Avoid administration with valerian.
Disulfiram: Disulfiram reaction if herbal product contains alcohol. Avoid administration with valerian.

Contraindications and precautions

Valerian is contraindicated in patients who are hypersensitive to this herb. Because of the risk of hepatotoxicity, avoid its use in patients with hepatic dysfunction. Also avoid its use in pregnant or breast-feeding patients; effects are unknown.

Special considerations

◗ **ALERT** Caution the patient about the risk of hepatotoxicity from combination products that contain valerian (Shepard, 1993) and from overdosage averaging 2.5 g (Chan et al., 1995).

Bold italic type indicates that reaction may be life-threatening.

- Monitor liver function test results periodically in patients with preexisting hepatic disease or with prolonged use.
- Inform the patient that many extract products contain 40% to 60% alcohol and may not be appropriate for all patients.
- Caution the patient taking disulfiram not to take an herbal form that contains alcohol.
- Inform the patient about valerian's sedative effects, and advise him to avoid hazardous activities until the CNS effects are known.
- Advise women to avoid using valerian during pregnancy or when breast-feeding.
- Inform the patient that safety and efficacy data in children are lacking.

Commentary

Valerian appears to exert mild sedative-hypnotic effects; the extract improved the subjective-recalled quantity of sleep and decreased sleep latency without causing hangover effects. Most studies have been flawed methodologically: they were of short duration, used small sample sizes, and defined patient populations inadequately. Better planned and well-controlled studies are needed. A USP expert advisory panel has determined that evidence supporting the use of valerian for treating insomnia is insufficient.

References

Chan, T.Y.K., et al. "Poisoning Due to an Over-the-Counter Hypnotic, Sleep-Qik (Hyoscine, Cyprohepatadine, Valerian)," *Post Grad Med J* 71:227-28, 1995.

Donath F., et al. "Critical Evaluation of the Effect of Valerian Extract on Sleep Structure and Sleep Quality," *Pharmacopsychiatry* 33(2):47-53, 2000.

Fussel, A., et al. "Effect of a Fixed Valerian-Hop Extract Combination (Ze 91019) on Sleep Polygraphy in Patients with Nonorganic Insomnia: A Pilot Study," *Eur J Med Res* 5(9):385-90, 2000.

Hazelhoff, B., et al. "Antispasmodic Effects of *Valeriana* Compounds: An In-Vivo and In-Vitro Study on the Guinea Pig Ileum," *Arch Intern Pharmacodyn* 257:274-87, 1982.

Ortiz, J.G., et al. "Effects of *Valeriana officinalis* Extracts on [3H]Flunitrazepam Binding, Synaptosomal [3H]GABA Uptake, and Hippocampal [3H] GABA Release," *Neurochem Res* 24(11):1373-78, 1999.

Petkov, V. "Plants with Hypotensive Antiatheromatous and Coronarodilating Action," *Am J Chin Med* 7:197-236, 1979.

Sakamoto, T., et al. "Psychotropic Effects of Japanese Valerian Root Extract," *Chem Pharm Bull* 40:758-61, 1992.

Schulz, V., et al. *Rational Phytotherapy: A Physicians' Guide to Herbal Medicine,* 3rd ed. New York: Springer Publishing Co., 1998.

Shepard, C. "Sleep Disorders. Liver Damage Warning with Insomnia Remedy," *Br Med J* 306:1472, 1993.

VANADIUM
VANADATE, VANADYL, VANADYL SULFATE

Common trade names
None known.

Common forms
Available as capsules and powder and in beverages and other herbal formulas.

Source
Vanadium is a trace mineral that is found in the earth's crust and in rocks, some iron ores, and crude petroleum deposits. In nature, it is often found as crystals. It usually combines with other elements such as oxygen, sodium, sulfur, and chloride.

Chemical components
Vanadium is found combined with other elements and particles in soil and in low levels in plants.

Actions
Vanadium is an antioxidant that may play a role in the mineralization of bones and teeth. Animal studies have also suggested that vanadium may improve insulin action or mimic insulin in rats (Uthus et al., 1990). These studies also imply that vanadium may inhibit cholesterol synthesis. The amount of vanadium needed to mimic insulin was high, to the point of toxicity, causing poor appetite and growth, diarrhea, and death in many of the animals.

Reported uses
Therapeutic claims for vanadium include its use as a muscle, strength, or performance enhancer and as a supplement to improve glucose metabolism and to treat and prevent diabetes and high cholesterol levels. These claims have not been supported by human trials and are based on animal trials in which high doses were used that produced toxic symptoms. Deficiency symptoms have not yet been identified in humans (French et al., 1993), and even the most nutritionally inadequate diet has been shown to contain sufficient quantities to prevent deficiency (Harland et al., 1994).

Dosage
No RDA has been established. Estimated requirements for adults are 1 to 3 mcg/day P.O. with dietary intake usually 10 to 60 mcg. Available dosage forms supply a wide range of dosage strengths (1-100 mg).

Adverse reactions
CNS: confusion.
EENT: eye inflammation, green tongue.
GI: anorexia, diarrhea.

Bold italic type indicates that reaction may be life-threatening.

Hematologic: anemia.
Respiratory: cough, pleurisy, wheezing.
Musculoskeletal: growth retardation.
Other: *death.*

Interactions
Chromium and vanadium: May interfere with each other's absorption. Separate administration times.
Smoking: Decreased vanadium absorption. Avoid smoking when taking this herb.

Contraindications and precautions
Vanadium is contraindicated in pregnant patients; birth defects were reported in animal studies.

Special considerations
• Caution the patient against using vanadium because little evidence regarding its medicinal use exists.
• Advise the patient to consult a health care provider before using herbal preparations because a treatment that has been clinically researched and proved effective may be available.
• Monitor for adverse reactions in patients who are taking more than 10 mcg/day.
• Advise the female patient to report planned or suspected pregnancy.

Commentary
Insufficient data exist in humans to support any medicinal use of vanadium. Animal studies have produced some insulin-like effects but at doses that are known to be toxic. The danger of toxicity warrants that this supplement not be recommended.

References
French, R., et al. "Role of Vanadium in Nutrition: Metabolism, Essentiality, and Dietary Considerations," *Life Sci* 52:339-46, 1993.

Harland, B.F., et al. "Is Vanadium of Human Nutritional Importance Yet?" *J Am Diet Assoc* 94:891-94, 1994.

Uthus, E., et al. "Effect of Vanadium, Iodine, and Their Interactions on Growth, Blood Variables, Liver Trace Elements, and Thyroid Status Indicies in Rats," *Mag Tr El* 9:219-26, 1990.

VERVAIN

Aмerican vervain, blue vervain, enchanter's herb,
European vervain, herba veneris, herbe sacrée,
herb of grace, holy herb, pigeon's grass, purvain,
simpler's joy, traveler's joy, wild hyssop

Taxonomic class
Verbenaceae

Common trade names
Blue Vervain, Blue Vervain Herb

Common forms
Available in capsules (360 mg), dried leaves, liquid, and
tea.

Source
Active components are obtained from the leaves and
flowering heads of European vervain, *Verbena officinalis,* a
member of the vervain or verbena family. Originally native to the
Mediterranean, the herb is now cultivated widely throughout Europe,
Asia, and North America. A related species, the American vervain, *V.
hastata,* is native to the central and eastern United States and also used
medicinally.

Chemical components
Vervain contains tannin, flavonoids (mainly luteolin 7-diglucuronide),
glycosides (verbenalin, hastatoside, verbenin), volatile oils (geraniol,
limonene, verbenone), and vitamin K. The leaves contain adenosine
and beta-carotene. The roots and stems contain stachyose.

Actions
In large doses, the glycoside verbenin has been thought to stimulate
milk excretion in low doses and inhibit sympathetic nerve endings on
the heart, blood vessels, intestines, and salivary glands. Two studies
failed to show antidiarrheal, antigonadotropic, or antithyrotropic activity (Almeida et al., 1995; Auf'Mkolk et al., 1984).

Various extracts of aerial parts of *V. officinalis* demonstrated anti-
inflammatory activity (Deepak and Handa, 2000).

Reported uses
Traditionally, vervain has been claimed to be useful in anemia, bronchitis, colds, cramps, dysuria, eczema, edema, fever, hemorrhoids, insomnia, kidney stones, malaria, neuralgia, ocular disease, pertussis, pleurisy,
rheumatism, tumors, tympany, ulcers, and uterine disorders. It has also
been used as an analgesic, an anthelmintic, an antispasmodic, an aphrodisiac, an astringent, a diaphoretic, a diuretic, an emetic, and an expectorant. Clinical data are lacking.

Bold italic type indicates that reaction may be life-threatening.

One study of vervain for use against kidney stones concluded that more effective pharmacologic therapies are available (Grases et al., 1994).

Dosage
As a purgative and for bowel pain, a decoction of 2 oz to 1 qt of water P.O. daily has been used (Almeida et al., 1995).
As a sedative, 360 mg (1 capsule) P.O. at bedtime.

Adverse reactions
CNS: CNS paralysis, ***clonic and tetanic seizures*** (with large doses), stupor.
Other: contact dermatitis.

Interactions
Anticoagulants: The vitamin K found in vervain may reduce anticoagulant effect. Monitor INR and consider adjusting dose, if necessary.
Iron supplements: Herbal teas that contain vervain may significantly impair iron absorption (Hurrell et al., 1999). Do not use together.

Contraindications and precautions
Use vervain cautiously in patients with multiple allergies or in those with asthma or other respiratory disorders. Also use it cautiously in patients with a history of seizure disorders; in large doses, vervain is capable of inducing seizures.

Special considerations
• Inform the patient with seizure disorder that vervain may exacerbate seizure activity if taken in excessive amounts.
• Inform the patient that no clinical data support the use of vervain for any medical condition.
• Caution the patient taking anticoagulants that even though vervain has been known in folk medicine to slow blood coagulation, it still may diminish the effectiveness of warfarin. Additional monitoring and dosage adjustments may be necessary.

Points of interest
• The FDA has classified vervain as an herb of undefined safety.

Commentary
Although vervain has had many traditional uses, there is little, if any, clinical information to support its use for any medical condition. Therefore, it cannot be recommended for use. Patients who take iron supplements or warfarin should be informed of the potential for interactions with their drug therapy.

References
Almeida, C.E., et al. "Analysis of Antidiarrheic Effects of Plants Used in Popular Medicine," *Revista De Saude Publica* 29:428-33, 1995.
Auf'Mkolk, M., et al. "Inhibition by Certain Plant Extracts of the Binding and

Adenylate Cyclase Stimulatory Effect of Bovine Thyrotropin in Human Thyroid Membranes," *Endocrinology* 115:527-34, 1984.

Deepak, M., and Handa, S.S. "Antiinflammatory Activity and Chemical Composition of Extracts of *Verbena officinalis*," *Phytother Res* 14(6):463-65, 2000.

Grases, F., et al. "Urolithiasis and Phytotherapy," *Int Urol Nephrol* 26:507-11, 1994.

Hurrell, R.F., et al. "Inhibition of Non-haem Iron Absorption in Man by Polyphenolic-containing Beverages," *Br J Nutr* 81(4):289-95, 1999.

VINPOCETINE

CEZAYIRMENEKSESI, ETHYL APOVINCAMINATE, ETHYL APOVINCAMINOATE, LESSER PERIWINKLE, MYRTLE VINCAPERVINC, PERIWINKLE, VINCA MINOR

Taxonomic class
Apocynaceae

Common trade names
Cavinton, Eusenium, Intelectol, Remedial, VinpocetineRx, VinRx

Common forms
Available as capsules and tablets (5 mg, 10 mg) and as an injection.

Source
Vinpocetine is derived from vincamine, an alkaloid from the extract of the periwinkle plant, *Vinca minor*. It is a semisynthetic ethyl ester of apovincamine. *V. minor* is indigenous to northern Spain and parts of central and southern Europe. The medicinal parts of the plant include the dried leaves and the flowering plant.

Chemical components
V. minor contains indole alkaloids (vincamine, vincin, apovincamine, vincadifformin) and flavonoids.

Actions
The actual mechanism of action of vinpocetine is not fully understood. Potentially, it is a vasodilator and enhancer of cerebral metabolism. It is thought to have a stimulating effect on memory and increases metabolic activity in the brain by increasing blood flow. There are also claims that vinpocetine inhibits platelet aggregation and increases the release of serotonin and norepinephrine. Vinpocetine may have direct or indirect cholinergic activity, increase the turnover of brain catecholamine levels, and enhance norepinephrine effects on cortical cAMP levels (Nicholson, 1990; Groo et al., 1987). Vinpocetine may also block sodium ion channels (Molnar and Erdo, 1995).

Reported uses
A study of eight patients with renal failure who were undergoing hemodialysis reported that vinpocetine, 15 mg P.O. daily, treated intractable tumoral calcinosis after 6 to 12 months of therapy (Ueyoshi and Ota, 1992).

Bold italic type indicates that reaction may be life-threatening.

In Europe, vinpocetine is commonly administered to patients with cerebrovascular disorders. It is claimed to be useful for memory and cognitive function enhancement and to increase brain function. Vinpocetine has been evaluated but not shown to be effective in improving symptoms of Alzheimer's disease (Thal et al., 1989). Another study evaluated the use of vinpocetine in Alzheimer's disease patients (Leon et al., 1989). This study determined the safety of vinpocetine but suggested that vinpocetine did not decrease the rate of disease progression. Vinpocetine, 30 mg P.O. daily, did demonstrate clinical improvement in patients with vascular or degenerative cerebral dysfunction (Manconi et al., 1986; Nicholson, 1990). Another report reviewed the use of vinpocetine in acute ischemic stroke and determined that evidence to recommend vinpocetine to these patients was insufficient (Bereczki and Fekete, 1999). Vinpocetine has been claimed to treat aphasia, unstable blood pressure, poor coordination, depression, dizziness, headache, impaired hearing and vision, insomnia, irritability, mood instability, motor disorders, nervousness, ophthalmic diseases, acute stroke, and vertigo.

Dosage
For Alzheimer's dementia, up to 20 mg P.O. t.i.d.
For vascular or degenerative cerebral insufficiency, 5 to 10 mg P.O. t.i.d.
For mild to moderate organic psychosyndrome, 10 to 20 mg P.O. t.i.d.

Adverse reactions
CNS: dizziness, pressure headache, restlessness, sleep disturbances.
CV: slight reduction in blood pressure, rapid or irregular heartbeat.
GI: abdominal pain, bloating, nausea.
Metabolic: decreased blood glucose levels.
Other: facial flushing.

Interactions
Glyburide: May alter glyburide concentrations; unlikely to have clinical significance.
Oxazepam: May alter oxazepam pharmacokinetics; unlikely to have clinical significance.
Warfarin: May alter PT; unlikely to have clinical significance. Regular monitoring of INR is advised; minor adjustments in warfarin dosing may be necessary (Hitzenberger et al., 1990).

Contraindications and precautions
Vinpocetine is contraindicated in patients who are hypersensitive to this herb. Avoid its use in pregnant or breast-feeding patients. Use vinpocetine cautiously in patients with a history of allergic phenomena during treatment with other vinca alkaloids, in those with hepatic disease, and in those with nonorganic psychoses.

Special considerations
• Patients with nonorganic psychoses or other mental illnesses should be evaluated before initiating therapy.

- Elderly patients may require higher doses of vinpocetine because they have significantly higher plasma clearance and a larger volume of distribution of vinpocetine.
- Monitor the patient for improvement of neurologic parameters, dementia symptoms, and daily functioning.
- Monitor the patient with seizure disorder closely.
- Routine blood chemistry, blood pressure, and pulse rate monitoring should be performed during long-term therapy with vinpocetine.
- Advise the patient to take vinpocetine tablets or capsules with meals and fluids and not to chew them.

Points of interest

- In Italy, the flower of *V. minor* is called "The Flower of Death" because it was used in ancient custom to make garlands placed on dead children. Ironically, in Germany, it is called the "Flower of Immortality." In France, the flower is considered a symbol of friendship.

Commentary

Although there have been studies in both animals and humans, there is contradictory information for use in the treatment of Alzheimer's disease, dementia, and ischemic stroke. Additional studies are needed to evaluate the efficacy and safety of vinpocetine.

References

Bereczki, D., and Fekete, I. "A Systematic Review of Vinpocetine Therapy in Acute Ischaemic Stroke," *Eur J Clin Pharmacol* 55:349-52, 1999.

Groo, D., et al. "Effects of Vinpocetine in Scopolamine-induced Learning and Memory Impairments," *Drug Develop Res* 11:29-36, 1987.

Gruenwald, J., et al., eds. *PDR for Herbal Medicines*. Montvale, N.J.: Medical Economics Company, 1998.

Hitzenberger, G., et al. "Influence of Vinpocetine of Warfarin-induced Inhibition of Coagulation," *Int J Clin Pharmacol Ther Toxicol* 28:8:323-28, 1990.

Leon, J., et al. "The Safety and Lack of Efficacy of Vinpocetine in Alzheimer's Disease," *J Am Geriatr Soc* 37:6:515-20, 1989.

Manconi, E., et al. "A Double-blind Clinical Trial of Vinpocetine in the Treatment of Cerebral Insufficiency of Vascular and Degenerative Origin," *Curr Ther Res* 40:702-9, 1986.

Molnar, P., and Erdo, S.L. "Vinpocetine Is as Potent as Phenytoin to Block Voltage-gated Na^+ Channels in Rat Cortical Neurons," *Eur J Pharmacol* 273:303-6, 1995.

Nicholson, C.D. "Pharmacology of Nootropics and Metabolically Active Compounds in Relation to Their Use in Dementia," *Psychopharmacology* 101:147-59, 1990.

Thal, L.J., et al. "The Safety and Lack of Efficacy of Vinpocetine in Alzheimer's Disease," *J Am Geriatr Soc* 36:515-20, 1989.

Ueyoshi, A., and Ota, K. "Clinical Appraisal of Vinpocetine for the Removal of Intractable Tumoral Calcinosis in Hemodialysis Patients with Renal Failure," *J Int Med Res* 20:435-43, 1992.

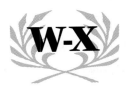

W-X

WAHOO

ARROWWOOD, BITTER ASH, BLEEDING HEART, BURNING
BUSH, BURSTING HEART, FISH-WOOD, INDIAN
ARROWWOOD, PIGWOOD, PRICKWOOD, SKEWERWOOD,
SPINDLE TREE, STRAWBERRY BUSH, STRAWBERRY TREE

Taxonomic class
Celastraceae

Common trade names
Multi-ingredient preparations: GB Tablets,
Indigestion Mixture, Jecopeptol, Ludoxin, Stago,
Stomachiagil

Common forms
Available as extracts, dried powders, syrups, tablets,
teas, and tinctures,

Source
Active components are obtained from the dried bark of the root and,
sometimes, the stem of *Euonymus atropupureus*, a shrub or tree that is
native to the central eastern United States and Canada.

Chemical components
Wahoo bark and extracts contain euonymol, euonysterol, atropurol, at-
ropurpurin, asparagine, homoeuonysterol, phytosterol, galactitol, tri-
acetin, citrullol, dulcitol, and various tartaric acids.

Actions
The herb is said to promote biliary function and intestinal secretions by
acting as a direct bile stimulant. It also acts as a mild laxative and increases capillary circulation (Grieve, 1997). Other *Euonymus* species appear to have attracted more attention from investigators than wahoo.
The bark of *E. sieboldianus* yields euonymoside, a cytotoxic cardenolide
glycoside that may prove to be active against human lung and ovary
carcinomas (Baek et al., 1994).

Reported uses
Wahoo is claimed to be useful as an antipyretic, a cathartic, a digestive
aid, a diuretic, an emetic, an expectorant, a liver stimulant, a menstrual
stimulant, and a tonic. An oil or powder form of wahoo has been used
to kill head lice.

Dosage

Dried root: 1 oz added to 1 pt of water, simmered slowly; 1 cup taken b.i.d. or t.i.d.
Euonymin extract: 1 to 4 grains P.O. t.i.d. as needed.

Adverse reactions

CNS: chills, ***seizures***, syncope, weakness.
GI: diarrhea, vomiting.

Interactions

None reported.

Contraindications and precautions

Avoid using wahoo in pregnant or breast-feeding patients; effects are unknown.

Special considerations

• Advise the patient that no clinical data support the use of wahoo for any medical condition.
• Discourage the patient from consuming wahoo because of its potential toxicity.
• Advise the patient to consult a health care provider before using herbal preparations because a treatment that has been clinically researched and proved effective may be available.
• Advise women to avoid using wahoo during pregnancy or when breast-feeding.

Commentary

Wahoo has been used to treat several conditions. Because clinical data are lacking and the ingestion of large quantities of wahoo may be hazardous, this herb cannot be recommended for any indication.

References

Baek, N.I., et al. "Euonymoside: A New Cytotoxic Cardenolide Glycoside from the Bark of *Euonymus sieboldianus*," *Planta Med* 60:26-29, 1994.
Grieve, M. *A Modern Herbal.* London: Tiger Books International, 1997.

WALNUT

ENGLISH WALNUT, EUROPEAN WALNUT, JUGLONE, JUPITER'S NUTS, PERSIAN WALNUT, WALNUT HULL, WALNUT LEAF

Taxonomic class

Juglandaceae

Common trade names

None known.

Common forms
Available as a decoction, an extract, and a tincture and used externally as a bath additive and a compress.

Source
The leaves of the deciduous tree *(Juglans regia)*, the bark, the hull of the nut, and the nut itself have been used for various preparations.

Chemical components
The leaves contain about 10% tannins of the ellagitannin type; naphthalene derivatives, especially the monoglucosides of juglone (=5-hydroxy-1,4-naphtholquinone) and hydrojuglone; more than 3% flavonoids (such as quercetin, quercitrin, hyperoside, and kaempferol derivatives); 0.8% to 1% ascorbic acid, plant acids, including gallic, caffeic, and neochlorogenic acids; and 0.001% to 0.03% volatile oil, mainly germacrene D. The main active components are the tannins and juglone.

Actions
J. regia is mainly used externally as an astringent, based on its tannin content (10%). Juglone and the essential oils may have in vitro antifungal activity (Ahmad et al., 1973) and, possibly, antitumorigenic effects in mice. The actual nut has been studied as a substitute (replacing 20% to 35% of monounsaturated fat foods) in cholesterol-lowering diets with success in further reducing total cholesterol and LDL levels in human subjects (Sabate et al., 1993; Zambron et al., 2000).

Reported uses
Walnut preparations have been used externally for acne, eczema, eyelid inflammation, excessive perspiration of the hands and feet, pyodermia, tuberculosis, and various skin ulcers. It has been used internally for catarrhs of the GI tract and as an anthelmintic and a blood-purifying agent.

Dosage
Dosing is highly dependent on various factors. Because no standard production exists, dosage ranges must be viewed as relative guidelines.
External: 3 to 6 g/day; 100 g per full bath.
Extracts: 2 to 3 g P.O. once to several times a day.
Tincture: 1 to 3 ml P.O. once to several times a day.

Adverse reactions
Hepatic: *hepatotoxicity* (caused by tannin content).
Other: carcinogenic effects (potential with long-term use of *J. regia* as an external preparation).

Interactions
None reported.

Contraindications and precautions
Excessive oral ingestion and topical application of walnuts should be avoided in pregnant or breast-feeding patients.

Special considerations
- Caution the patient who is at risk for heptatotoxicity about ingesting considerable quantities of walnut because the tannin content may increase the risk of hepatic injury.
- Advise the patient who is looking for a natural agent to reduce serum cholesterol levels to pursue more stringently studied and proven alternatives.
- Inform the patient that walnut preparations that contain juglone compounds can discolor the skin or mucous membranes yellowish brown.
- Caution the patient that daily topical application of walnut preparations may increase the risk of tongue cancer and leukoplakia of the lips.

Commentary
Little, if any, evidence exists other than in vitro studies to support most of the claims for the use of walnut. Larger human trials are needed to demonstrate its effectiveness in hypercholesterolemic men and women. More research is needed before definitive recommendations can be put forward.

References
Ahmad, S., et al. "Fungistatic Action of *Juglans*," *Antimicrob Agents Chemother* 3(3):436-38, 1973.

Sabate, J., et al. "Effects of Walnuts on Serum Lipid Levels and Blood Pressure in Normal Men," *N Engl J Med* 328(9):603-7, 1993.

Zambron, D., et al. "Substituting Walnuts for Monounsaturated Fat Improves the Serum Lipid Profile of Hyperchloesterolemic Men and Women," *Ann Intern Med* 132(7):538-46, 2000.

WATERCRESS

GARDEN CRESS, SCURVY GRASS, WASSERKRESSE

Taxonomic class
Brassicaceae

Common trade names
None known.

Common forms
Available as juice from the leaves, the whole plant, and tea.

Source
All plant parts of *Nasturtium officinale* are used for medicinal purposes. A low-growing aquatic that belongs to the mustard family, the plant is native to Europe. It is naturalized in the United States and should not be confused with the garden nasturtium or Indian cress (*Tropaeolum majus*), a popular annual flower that belongs to a different plant family.

Chemical components

Watercress contains gluconasturtiin, the glucosinolate precursor of phenethyl isothiocyanate, benzyl glucosinolate, benzyl isothiocyanate (BITC), vitamins A and C, iron, phosphates, and oils.

Actions

The body converts gluconasturtiin to phenethyl isothiocyanate (PEITC). PEITC is also released when the fresh plant is chewed. The N-acetylcysteine metabolite of PEITC is detectable in human urine (Chung et al., 1992, 1997). PEITC and synthetic isothiocyanates acted as inhibitors of the tobacco-specific carcinogen nitrosamine 4-(methylnitrosamino)-1-(3-pyridyl)-1-butanone (NNK) in animal models. PEITC is thought to inhibit the metabolic activation NNK and inhibit lung tumorigenesis (Hecht, 1995). In animals, BITC has demonstrated some ability to inhibit lung tumor formation induced by NNK. Doses of 200 mg/kg in rats did not reduce tumor mass and caused toxic effects (Pintao et al., 1995).

Other in vitro studies suggest that the chemical components of watercress inhibit histamine release (Goda et al., 1999).

Reported uses

The plant is a popular salad green. It has been used as an anti-inflammatory and antimicrobial, and the juice of the leaves has been used to treat acne, eczema, rashes, and topical infections.

Dosage

A dose of 2 oz of fluidextract (juice) P.O. t.i.d. was used in a human clinical study (Hecht et al., 1995).

Adverse reactions

None reported.

Interactions

Acetaminophen: May inhibit acetaminophen's oxidative metabolism (Chen et al., 1996). Avoid administration with watercress.

Contraindications and precautions

Avoid using watercress in pregnant or breast-feeding patients; effects are not clearly documented in humans.

Special considerations

● Several cases of fascioliasis of the liver (parasitic fluke infection) have been reported after ingesting wild watercress (Rivera et al., 1984).
● Advise women to avoid using watercress during pregnancy or when breast-feeding.
● Instruct the patient to carefully wash the fresh herb before use if collecting from the wild to reduce the risk of ingesting waterborne parasites or pathogens.
● Inform the patient using other drugs to use watercress cautiously because interactions with watercress are largely unknown.

• Inform the patient that more safety and efficacy data for watercress are needed.

Points of interest
• Because it contains vitamin C, watercress was once used to prevent scurvy. The use of watercress in salads has been popular for centuries.

Commentary
Although research has shown watercress compounds to be promising anticancer agents, further research is needed. The role of PEITC as a protective agent in human cancers remains to be established. Watercress has no apparent activity against existing tumors. The fact that few reports of toxicity exist despite the consumption of watercress over a long period indicates that this herb is safe. Recommendations for consumption await additional safety research.

References
Chen, L., et al. "Decrease of Plasma and Urinary Oxidative Metabolites of Acetaminophen After Consumption of Watercress by Human Volunteers," *Clin Pharmacol Ther* 60:651-60, 1996.

Chung, F.L., et al. "Quantification of Human Uptake of the Anticarcinogen Phenethyl Isothiocyanate After a Watercress Meal," *Cancer Epidemiol Biomarkers Prev* 1:383-88, 1992.

Chung, F.L., et al. "Chemopreventative Potential of Thiol Conjugates of Isothiocyanates for Lung Cancer and a Urinary Biomarker of Dietary Isothiocyanates," *J Cell Biochem Suppl* 27:76-85, 1997.

Goda, Y., et al. "Constituents in Watercress: Inhibitors of Histamine Release from RBL-2H3 Cells by Antigen Stimulation," *Biol Pharm Bull* 22(12):1319-26, 1999.

Hecht, S.S. "Chemoprevention of Cancer by Isothiocyanates, Modifiers of Carcinogen Metabolism," *J Nutr* 129(3):768S-74S, 1999.

Hecht, S.S., et al. "Effects of Watercress Consumption on Metabolism of a Tobacco-specific Lung Carcinogen in Smokers," *Cancer Epidemiol Biomarkers Prev* 4:877-84, 1995.

Pintao, A.M., et al. "In Vitro and In Vivo Antitumor Activity of Benzyl Isothiocyanate: A Natural Product from *Tropaeolum majus*," *Planta Med* 61:233-36, 1995.

Rivera, J.V., et al. "Radionuclide Imaging of the Liver in Human Fascioliasis," *Clin Nucl Med* 9:450-53, 1984.

WILD CHERRY

BLACK CHOKE, CHOKE CHERRY, RUM CHERRY

Taxonomic class
Rosaceae

Common trade names
Celestial Seasonings Tea, Wild Cherry Bark, Wild Cherry Bark Compound

Common forms
Available as liquid extract (1 oz, 2 oz) and teas.

Source
Active components are derived from the dried bark of *Prunus virginiana* and *Prunus serotina,* which are found in the woods and fields throughout northern United States. The fruit is edible, but the seeds should be discarded.

Chemical components
The bark, seeds, and leaves of wild cherry trees contain amygdalin, a cyanogenic glycoside. Beta-glucosidase, present in the human GI tract, converts amygdalin to hydrogen cyanide (HCN). Wild cherry also contains emulsin, b-methylaesculetin, phytosterol, L-mandelic acid, oleic acid, *p*-coumaric acid, trimethyl gallic acid, ipuranol, dextrose, sugar, tannin, starch, and calcium oxalate (Ellenhorn, 1997).

Actions
Wild cherry has been touted to possess analgesic, antitussive, astringent, and sedative properties.

Reported uses
Wild cherry has been used to treat colds, coughs, and other respiratory problems as well as certain cancers and diarrhea.

Dosage
Liquid extract: 1 to 2 g in 1 cup of boiling water P.O. t.i.d.

Adverse reactions
The following reactions result from cyanide poisoning:
CNS: *coma,* headache, stupor, tremor.
GI: GI ulceration, nausea, vomiting.
Musculoskeletal: muscle spasms and weakness.
Respiratory: respiratory failure.
Other: *death.*

Interactions
None reported.

Contraindications and precautions
Wild cherry is contraindicated in pregnant or breast-feeding patients because of the presence of cyanogenic glycosides and their possible teratogenic effect.

Special considerations
🔺 **ALERT** Because all plant parts contain HCN, wild cherry is considered toxic. Death has occurred in children who ate seeds, drank tea made from the plant, or chewed on the leaves. Ingestion of the leaves by livestock has also resulted in death. Wilted leaves contain more HCN than do dried leaves.
🔺 **ALERT** Symptoms of HCN poisoning include difficulty breathing, coma leading to death, muscle twitching and spasms, stupor, and vocal paralysis. In mild cases, symptoms include headache, irregular heartbeat, muscle weakness, nausea, and vomiting (Ellenhorn, 1997).

- Inform the patient that consumption of wild cherry extracts can be dangerous and may cause death from cyanide poisoning.
- Urge the patient to keep wild cherry plant parts out of the reach of children.
- Inform the patient that data supporting any therapeutic use of the extracts are inadequate.

Points of interest

- Congenital malformations caused by cyanogenic glycosides in a related species, black cherry (*P. serotina*), have been reported in animals (Selby et al., 1971).
- The lethal adult dose of HCN is 50 mg. Lethal doses for cyanogenic plants cannot be predicted because of variations in content, extraction methods, and metabolism (Ellenhorn, 1997).
- Application of some chemical herbicides have been shown to reduce the hydrocyanic acid content in wild cherry (Williams and James, 1983).

Commentary

Although wild cherry has been used for various conditions, wild cherry bark, seeds, and leaves are potentially toxic. Clinical data substantiating the use of wild cherry extracts for any medical condition are insufficient.

References

Ellenhorn, M.J., ed. *Ellenhorn's Medical Toxicology: Diagnosis and Treatment of Human Poisoning.* Baltimore: Williams & Wilkins, 1997.

Selby, L.A., et al. "Outbreak of Swine Malformations Associated with the Wild Black Cherry, *Prunus serotina,*" *Arch Environ Health* 22:496-501, 1971.

Williams, M.C., and James, L.F. "Effects of Herbicides on the Concentration of Poisonous Compounds in Plants: A Review," *Am J Vet Res* 44:2420-22, 1983.

WILD GINGER

CANADA SNAKEROOT, COLIC ROOT, FALSE COLTSFOOT, INDIAN GINGER, VERMONT SNAKEROOT

Taxonomic class

Aristolochiaceae

Common trade names

None known.

Common forms

Available as capsules and the whole root.

Source

Active components are derived from the dried rhizome and roots of *Asarum canadense,* a low-growing perennial herb that is native to the northern and central United States and southern Canada.

Chemical components
Wild ginger contains 2.5% volatile oil, which comprises such terpenoids as methyl eugenol, borneol, linalool, geraniol, and pinene. Other compounds include a pungent resin, starch, gum, a fragrant principle called asarol, and traces of a fixed oil.

Actions
Volatile oil components linalool, geraniol, and eugenol have demonstrated antibacterial and antifungal activity (Pattnaik et al., 1997). Geraniol inhibited pancreatic tumor growth in animals receiving wild ginger as part of their diet (Burke et al., 1997).

Reported uses
Wild ginger reportedly has been used as an antiflatulent, an aromatic stimulant, and a tonic and for treating angina and arrhythmias. Methyl eugenol is a rapid-acting anodyne used in dentistry.

Dosage
No consensus exists.

Adverse reactions
EENT: burning sensation in mouth, cheilitis, stomatitis.
Skin: contact dermatitis.

Interactions
Hepatically eliminated drugs: Conflicting reports exist on the effects of certain terpenoids (citral, linool) on hepatic metabolism. Some reports indicate that they may induce the hepatic oxidative pathway (Roffey et al., 1990). Effects on specific isoenzymes and on particular drugs are unknown, but these terpenoids could potentially lower levels of other hepatically eliminated drugs. Monitor the patient closely.

Contraindications and precautions
Avoid using wild ginger in pregnant or breast-feeding patients; effects are unknown. Use cautiously, if at all, in patients with a history of allergic contact dermatitis, especially to any of the volatile oils or terpenoid compounds.

Special considerations
• Inform the patient that no clinical data support the use of wild ginger for any medical condition.
• Advise the patient to consult a health care provider before using herbal preparations because a treatment that has been clinically researched and proved effective may be available.
• Instruct the patient with a history of allergic contact dermatitis to avoid using wild ginger.
• Advise women to avoid using wild ginger during pregnancy or when breast-feeding.

Commentary

Preliminary data appear to warrant further study of components of wild ginger as antimicrobial and potential anticancer agents. Insufficient evidence exists to support any therapeutic application at this time.

References

Burke, Y.D., et al. "Inhibition of Pancreatic Cancer Growth by the Dietary Isoprenoids Farnesol and Geraniol," *Lipids* 32:151-56, 1997.

Pattnaik, S., et al. "Antibacterial and Antifungal Activity of Aromatic Constituents of Essential Oils," *Microbios* 89:39-46, 1997.

Roffey, S.J., et al. "Hepatic Peroxisomal and Microsomal Enzyme Induction by Citral and Linalool in Rats," *Food Chem Toxicol* 28:403-8, 1990.

WILD INDIGO

FALSE INDIGO, HORSE-FLY WEED, INDIGO WEED, *PODALYRIA TINCTORIA*, RATTLEBUSH, RATTLESNAKE WEED, *SOPHORA*, YELLOW INDIGO

Taxonomic class

Fabaceae

Common trade names

Wild Indigo, Wild Indigo Root

Common forms

Available as a tincture (1 oz).

Source

Active components are derived from the leaves and dried roots of *Baptisia tinctoria,* a perennial herb that belongs to the legume family and is native to central and eastern United States and Canada.

Chemical components

Wild indigo contains glycoproteins that comprise arabinose, arabinogalactans, and alkaloids (baptitoxine, baptisine, baptisin, and quinolizindine). The root of the plant contains gum, albumen, starch, a yellowish resin, and a crystalline substance.

Actions

Wild indigo is claimed to act as an antiseptic, an astringent, and an emetic. Immunomodulating properties are attributed to the plant's arabinogalactan components and other glycoproteins (Beuscher et al., 1989; Beuscher and Kopanski, 1985; Egert and Beuscher, 1992). When used in combination with other plant extracts, a stronger phagocytic stimulant activity than in echinacea extract alone was noted in mice (Wagner and Jurcic, 1991).

Reported uses
Wild indigo has been claimed to be useful as an antimicrobial and a laxative. Evidence surrounding therapeutic effects is sparse and poorly documented.

Dosage
Tincture: 10 to 20 gtt P.O. t.i.d.

Adverse reactions
GI: vomiting (with high doses).

Interactions
None reported.

Contraindications and precautions
Wild indigo is contraindicated in patients who are hypersensitive to this or related plant species. Avoid its use in pregnant or breast-feeding patients; effects are unknown.

Special considerations
● Inform the patient that there is little information about wild indigo's therapeutic benefit or risk.
● Caution the patient that although there are no reports of toxic ingestion in humans, the alkaloids have toxic potential.
● Advise the patient with allergies to wild indigo or related plant species not to use this herb.
● Advise women to avoid using wild indigo during pregnancy or when breast-feeding.

Commentary
Despite the folkloric use of wild indigo as an antiseptic, safety and efficacy data in humans are lacking. Immunomodulating properties of wild indigo are based on in vitro experiments but appear promising and warrant additional investigation.

References
Beuscher, N., and Kopanski, L. "Stimulation of Immunity by the Contents of *Baptisia tinctoria*," *Planta Med* Oct(5):381-84, 1985.

Beuscher, N., et al. "Immunologically Active Glycoproteins of *Baptisia tinctoria*," *Planta Med* 55:358-63, 1989.

Egert, D., and Beuscher, N. "Studies on Antigen Specificity of Immunoreactive Arabinogalactan Proteins Extracted from *Baptisia tinctoria* and *Echinacea purpurea*," *Planta Med* 58:163-65, 1992.

Wagner, H., and Jurcic, K. "Immunologic Studies of Plant Combination Preparations. In-Vitro And In-Vivo Studies on the Stimulation of Phagocytosis," *Arzneimittelforschung* 41:1072-76, 1991.

WILD LETTUCE

BITTER LETTUCE, GERMAN LACTUCARIUM, LETTUCE OPIUM

Taxonomic class
Asteraceae

Common trade names
Lactucarium, Lettuce Hash, Lettucine, Lopium

Common forms
Available as dried juice (sap) from stems, dried leaves, lettuce leaf cigarettes, liquid (1 oz, 2 oz), and tincture.

Source
The dried leaves of *Lactuca virosa* are rolled (with tobacco or other additives) into a cigarette and smoked. The stem juice may be taken directly from the plant for various purposes. The plant should not be confused with the garden lettuce, *L. sativa*.

Chemical components
The plant contains flavonoids (apigenin, luteolin), terpenoids (lactucin, lactupicrin, germanicol), lactucone (lactucerin), coumarins (aesculin, cichoriin), various acids (citric, malic, cichoric, and oxalic), mannitol, proteins, resins, and carbohydrates. The milky white latex sap contains lactucin and lactucopicrin. The leaves contain polycyclic aromatic hydrocarbons and two isoenzymes of carbonate dehydratase (Wickstrom et al., 1986).

Actions
Lactucin and lactucopicrin are claimed to produce CNS depression and sedative effects. A study in rabbits concluded that wild lettuce has no hypoglycemic activity (Roman-Ramos et al., 1995). Another study showed that the latex of *L. sativa* had mild antifungal activity against *Candida albicans* (Giordani et al., 1991).

Reported uses
Smoking lettuce leaf cigarettes has been used to produce an alleged euphoric effect (Huang et al., 1982). The sap of the plant has been used to induce sleep and treat coughs.

Dosage
Dried leaves (tea): 0.5 to 3 g P.O. t.i.d.
Lactucarium (dried latex extract): 0.3 to 1 g P.O. t.i.d.
Liquid extract (1:1 in 25% alcohol): 0.5 to 30 ml P.O. t.i.d.
Tincture: 2 to 4 ml P.O. t.i.d.

Adverse reactions
Skin: contact dermatitis.
Other: allergic reactions (Krook, 1977).

Bold italic type indicates that reaction may be life-threatening.

Interactions
None reported.

Contraindications and precautions
Avoid using wild lettuce in pregnant or breast-feeding patients; effects
are unknown. It is also contraindicated in patients who are hypersensitive to any member of the lettuce family.

Special considerations
• Inform the patient that no clinical data support the use of wild lettuce
for any medical condition.
⚠ ALERT Crude I.V. preparations of wild lettuce have been used recreationally by drug abusers. One case report describes three subjects who
became very ill (abdominal and back pain, chills, fever, flank pain,
headache, mild hepatic dysfunction, leukocytosis, and neck stiffness) after an I.V. dose of wild lettuce and valerian extract (Mullins and Horowitz, 1998).
⚠ ALERT Caution the patient that smoking large quantities of wild lettuce can be toxic. Overdose may be characterized by coma, shallow
breathing, and stupor; death may occur (Huang et al., 1982).
• Caution the patient about the risk of hallucinogenic effects from
smoking wild lettuce leaves.
• Advise women to avoid using wild lettuce during pregnancy or when
breast-feeding.

Points of interest
• Ancient Egyptians used wild lettuce for its supposed ability to induce
sleep.
• During the 1970s, wild lettuce was smoked in the United States as an
alternative hallucinogen.
• Some sources state that trace amounts of morphine exist in some *Lactuca* species, but there is not enough to exert any clinical pharmacologic
effect (Huang et al., 1982).

Commentary
Claims of hallucinogenic effects from smoking wild lettuce leaves are
unsubstantiated. Because little is known about potential toxicity from
using this herb, its use is not recommended.

References
Giordani, R., et al. "Glycosidic Activities of *Candida albicans* After Action of Vegetable Latex Saps (Natural Antifungals) and Isoconazole (Synthetic Antifungal)," *Mycoses* 34:67-73, 1991.
Huang, Z.J., et al. "Studies on Herbal Remedies. Part I: Analysis of Herbal Smoking Preparations Alleged to Contain Lettuce (*Lactuca sativa* L.) and Other Natural Products," *J Pharm Sci* 71:270-71, 1982.
Krook, G. "Occupational Dermatitis from *Lactuca sativa* (Lettuce) and *Cichorium* (Endive): Simultaneous Occurrence of Immediate and Delayed Allergy as a Cause of Contact Dermatitis," *Contact Dermatitis* 3:27-36, 1977.

Mullins, M,E,, and Horowitz, B.Z. "The Case of the Salad Shooters: Intravenous Injection of Wild Lettuce Extract," *Vet Human Toxicol* 40(5):290-91, 1998.

Roman-Ramos, R., et al. "Anti-hyperglycemic Effect of Some Edible Plants," *J Ethnopharmacol* 48:25-32, 1995.

Wickstrom, K., et al. "Polycyclic Aromatic Compounds (PAC) in Leaf Lettuce," *Z Lebensum Unters Forsch* 183:182-85, 1986.

WILD YAM

COLIC ROOT, MEXICAN WILD YAM, RHEUMATISM ROOT

Taxonomic class
Dioscoreaceae

Common trade names
Mexican Wild Yam, Natrol Wild Yam, Wild Yam Extract, Wild Yam Root

Common forms
Available as a cream, liquid extract, powder, tincture, tea, and topical oil.

Source
Wild yam, *Dioscorea villosa* L., grows wild in the damp woodlands of North and Central America. A deciduous perennial vine that often climbs to 20', it is characterized by heart-shaped leaves and tiny green flowers.

Chemical components
Wild yam contains steroidal saponins, diosgenin, dioscenin, DHEA, phytosterols (beta-sitosterol), alkaloids, and tannins. It is most noted for its component DHEA. (See earlier monograph on DHEA for a complete discussion of this agent.)

Actions
Wild yam was historically the sole source of raw materials for manufacturing contraceptive hormones, cortisone, and anabolic hormones. Wild yam contains large amounts of dioscin, which has anti-inflammatory activity.

DHEA, a constituent of wild yam, is a steroid hormone produced in the adrenal gland in humans; it is the most abundant adrenocorticoid hormone in the body. DHEA is believed to be useful in several conditions, including AIDS, Alzheimer's disease, cancer, CV disease, hypercholesterolemia, multiple sclerosis, obesity, psychological disorders, and systemic lupus erythematosus (SLE).

In a double-blind study, patients with SLE who were given DHEA for 3 months showed marked improvement compared with placebo (Morales et al., 1994). Wild yam itself has not been proven to promote anabolic effects in humans.

Reported uses
Wild yam is claimed to be useful in treating abdominal cramps, adrenal exhaustion, spasmodic asthma, biliary stones, diverticulosis, dysentery,

---

Bold italic type indicates that reaction may be life-threatening.

gallstones, intermittent claudication, menopausal symptoms, muscle cramps, ovarian and uterine pain, inflammatory rheumatism, and rheumatoid arthritis and as an antispasmodic and a diaphoretic.

Dosage

The average dose is 2 to 4 g or its fluid equivalent P.O. t.i.d.

As a food supplement, DHEA dosage should not exceed 50 mg/day; medical approval is required for higher doses. DHEA doses over 25 mg/day should be avoided in women because of reports of irreversible voice changes and hirsutism.

Liquid extract: 2 to 4 ml in water P.O. t.i.d., or 5 to 30 gtt P.O. t.i.d.

Tincture (1:5 in 45% alcohol): 2 to 10 ml in water P.O. t.i.d.

Oil: external use only.

Tea: ½ tsp to 1 cup of boiling water, steep 15 minutes; ½ to 1 cup P.O. t.i.d.

Powder: 0.5 to 2 g P.O. t.i.d.

Adverse reactions

CNS: headache.

GU: menstrual irregularities, potential for stimulating growth of prostate cancer.

Skin: acne, hair loss, hirsutism, oily skin.

Interactions

None reported for wild yam itself, but a few interactions may be relevant for the DHEA component in wild yam. The following list comes from reports of drugs and their potential effect on endogenous DHEA or DHEA-S serum levels. The absolute effect on serum DHEA or DHEA-S levels may or may not be similar when exogenous DHEA is ingested in combination with the interacting drug.

Alprazolam: May increase serum levels of endogenous DHEA. DHEA-S levels are not changed. Evaluate need for combination therapy.

Calcium channel blockers: Increased serum levels of endogenous DHEA and DHEA-S l in obese, hypertensive men. Monitor the patient.

Carbamazepine: Decreased serum levels of endogenous DHEA-S. Monitor the patient.

Dexamethasone: Decreased endogenous levels of DHEA-S. Monitor the patient.

Insulin (exogenous): Decreased serum DHEA and DHEA-S levels in men. Monitor the patient.

Insulin-sensitizing drugs (metformin, other oral hypoglycemics): May increase serum DHEA and DHEA-S levels. Monitor the patient.

Although not specifically documented, DHEA may interact with other exogenous androgen or estrogen hormone therapies. Monitor the patient if used together.

Contraindications and precautions

Avoid using wild yam in pregnant patients because of the possibility of fetal masculinization. Use cautiously in patients with hepatic disease because of hepatic damage with high doses in animal models. Also avoid its use in patients with a family history of hormone-induced cancer, including breast, ovarian, prostate, and uterine cancer.

Special considerations
• Advise the patient to acquire DHEA, or any other natural product, only from the most reliable sources to ensure quality, purity, and strength.
• Advise women to avoid using wild yam during pregnancy.
• Inform women that irreversible voice changes and hirsutism may occur if more than 25 mg of DHEA is taken daily.

Commentary
The majority of interest surrounding wild yam is in regard to its naturally occurring neurosteroid hormone, DHEA. DHEA in wild yam is touted to be useful for several conditions, but data are lacking about the proper dose and long-term effects. Many claims for DHEA use are based on in vitro and animal studies. Larger and more comprehensive trials are needed to determine a role for DHEA, the primary focus of investigators of wild yam.

References
Morales, A.J., et al. "Effects of Replacement Dose Dihydroepiandrosterone in Men and Women of Advancing Age," *J Clin Endocrinol Metab* 78:1360-67, 1994.

WILLOW

BLACK WILLOW, WHITE WILLOW

Taxonomic class
Salicaceae

Common trade names
Multi-ingredient preparations: Aller g Formula 25, White Willow Bark, Willowprin

Common forms
Available as cut bark, capsules (375 mg, 400 mg), and liquid extract (1 oz, 2 oz).

Source
Active components are derived from the bark of various willows, such as the white willow *(Salix alba)* and the black willow *(S. nigra)*. White willow is native to Europe and naturalized in the United States; black willow is native to North America.

Chemical components
Willow bark contains phenolic glycosides (salicin, salicortin, salireposide, and picein), esters of salicylic acid and salicyl alcohol, tannins, catechins, and flavonoids. Concentrations of the salicylate-like agent salicin range from 0.5% to 10% in the bark, depending on the species.

Bold italic type indicates that reaction may be life-threatening.

Actions
The salicylate-like compounds exert analgesic, anti-inflammatory, antipyretic, and uricosuric effects. Tannins exert astringent effects. Flowers of a Russian species (*S. daphnoides)* have yielded thromboplastin-like agents that trigger procoagulant effects in animals.

Reported uses
In ancient Egypt, extracts of willow bark were commonly used to treat inflammatory conditions. Willow is claimed to be an effective analgesic and antipyretic and thought to be useful in treating rheumatism, other systemic inflammatory diseases, and influenza.

A double-blind study was undertaken to evaluate the efficacy and safety of willow bark extract in patients with back pain. More than 200 patients with exacerbations of low back pain were randomized to one of three groups: a high-dose (240 mg of salicin) group or a low-dose (120 mg of salicin) group of willow bark extract or placebo (Chrubasik et al., 2000). Treatment was continued for 4 weeks, and subjects were allowed rescue pain relief with therapeutic doses of tramadol. The primary outcome measurement was the incidence of patients who were pain-free for at least 5 days out of the 4th week (last) of the study without the use of rescue medication. Subjects were determined to be pain-free by an interview conducted over the telephone. Information obtained with respect to the subject's use of rescue doses and adverse reactions was also obtained in this manner. At study conclusion, 5% of placebo recipients were considered responsive to treatment; 21% of the low-dose–salicin group and 39% of the high-dose–salicin group were also determined to be responsive to therapy. Although the number was not quantified, significantly more patients in the placebo group required rescue tramadol doses than those in either the high- or low-dose treatment group for each week of therapy. The investigators concluded that willow bark extract was an effective and safe analgesic therapy for acute low back pain exacerbations.

Dosage
The average daily dose of salicin is 60 to 120 mg P.O. In some cases, doses as high as 240 mg of salicin daily have been used.
Dried bark: 1 to 3 g as a decoction (cold tea) P.O. t.i.d.
Liquid extract (1:1 in 25% alcohol): 1 to 3 ml P.O. t.i.d.

Adverse reactions
GI: *GI bleeding.*
GU: renal damage.
Hematologic: increased bleeding time.
Hepatic: hepatic dysfunction.
Respiratory: allergic rhinitis from aerosolized willow pollen, *asthma.*
Skin: contact dermatitis, local irritation.
Other: allergic reactions, *anaphylaxis, salicylate toxicity* (confusion, diarrhea, dizziness, lethargy, metabolic acidosis, nausea, tinnitus, vomiting).

Interactions
Anticoagulants: Increases risk of bleeding. Avoid administration with willow.

Antihypertensives: May reduce effectiveness of these drugs. Avoid administration with willow.

Diuretics: Increases risk for salicylate toxicity; may reduce effectiveness of these drugs. Avoid administration with willow.

NSAIDs: May increase risk of GI ulceration and bleeding. Avoid administration with willow.

Contraindications and precautions
Willow is contraindicated in patients with salicylate hypersensitivity. Avoid its use in pregnant or breast-feeding patients; effects are unknown. Use cautiously in patients with allergic rhinitis, asthma, or history of plant allergy and in those who are prone to systemic thromboembolism, such as those with history of venous thromboembolic disease or thromboembolic stroke, previous MI, poor ejection fraction, or atrial fibrillation. Also use cautiously in patients with renal insufficiency, history of GI bleeding, and peptic ulcers and in those with bleeding tendencies.

Special considerations
• Urge the patient with a history of allergy or asthma to avoid using willow products.

• Advise the patient taking anticoagulants to avoid using willow because of the risk of increased bleeding.

• Inform the patient that insufficient evidence exists to confirm a therapeutic application for willow. Commercial products containing salicylic acid are readily available. Advise the patient to use standardized products.

Points of interest
• Autopsy reports of the great composer Ludwig von Beethoven suggest a probable link between his chronic use of powdered willow bark and the development of renal papillary necrosis (Schwarz, 1993).

• In a Norwegian study, cadmium was found to accumulate in some bird species that fed on willow seeds and insects (Hogstad, 1996).

Commentary
Willow has a long history of anecdotal use as an analgesic and anti-inflammatory. Despite the use of some subjective outcome measurements, published clinical trial data appear to support its potential application as an analgesic. Because salicylate-like compounds naturally occur in varying strengths in the plant, only standardized salicylate products can be typically recommended.

References
Chrubasik, S., et al. "Treatment of Low Back Pain Exacerbations with Willow Bark Extract: A Randomized, Double-blind Study," *Am J Med* 109:9-14, 2000.

Bold italic type indicates that reaction may be life-threatening.

Hogstad, O. "Accumulation of Cadmium, Copper, and Zinc in the Liver of Some Passerine Species Wintering in Central Norway," *Sci Total Environ* 183:187-94, 1996.

Schwarz, A. "Beethoven's Renal Disease Based on His Autopsy: A Case of Papillary Necrosis," *Am J Kidney Dis* 21:643-52, 1993.

WINTERGREEN

BOXBERRY, CANADA TEA, CHECKERBERRY, DEERBERRY, GAULTHERIA OIL, MOUNTAIN TEA, OIL OF WINTERGREEN, PARTRIDGE BERRY, TEABERRY

Taxonomic class
Ericaceae

Common trade names
Aura Cacia Essential Oil of Wintergreen, Koong Yick Hung Fa Oil (KY-HFO), Wintergreen Altoids, Wintergreen Sucrets

Common forms
Available as creams, liniments, lotions, lozenges, oil, ointments, and teas.

Source
The active component is obtained from the leaves and bark of *Gaultheria procumbens*, a low-growing herb that is native to parts of Canada and the eastern United States.

Chemical components
Wintergreen contains less than 1% of wintergreen oil. This oil is about 98% methyl salicylate. No drug product should contain more than 5% methyl salicylate. Other compounds include gaultherin and carbohydrates (D-glucose, D-xylose).

Actions
Methyl salicylate produces counterirritant and skin-reddening effects. Analgesia may result from the masking of pain caused by counterirritation or the analgesic properties of the salicylate itself. Antiflatulent effects occur when taken internally (not recommended).

Reported uses
Wintergreen has been used to treat inflamed and swollen muscles, ligaments, and joints. It is also claimed to provide relief for neurologic pain from sciatica and trigeminal neuralgia.

Dosage
Apply 10% to 30% wintergreen oil or methyl salicylate product to the skin, not to exceed t.i.d. or q.i.d.

Adverse reactions
With oral use:
CNS: lethargy.

GI: indigestion, vomiting.
Respiratory: hyperpnea.

With topical application:
Other: *salicylate poisoning.*

Interactions

Anticoagulants: May increase INR and produce subsequent bleeding when combined with use of topical wintergreen oil (Chow et al., 1989; Yip et al., 1990). Discourage concomitant use.

Contraindications and precautions

Wintergreen is contraindicated for internal use in patients with gastroesophageal reflux disease. Avoid its use in pregnant or breast-feeding patients; effects are unknown. Use cautiously in patients receiving anticoagulants.

Special considerations

• Instruct the patient who is sensitive to aspirin to avoid wintergreen.
• Advise the patient taking oral anticoagulants to reduce the use of wintergreen.
• Instruct the patient not to use topical wintergreen agents with heating devices or warmed towels to avoid skin irritation.
◆**ALERT** Methyl salicylate is highly soluble in lipids and may cause salicylate poisoning from overgenerous topical application. Heat and physical activity increase its absorption through the skin. Symptoms of salicylate poisoning include acid-base disturbances, bleeding, CNS toxicity, coagulopathy, endocrine abnormalities, fluid and electrolyte disturbances, hepatitis, pulmonary edema, rhabdomyolysis, nausea, tinnitus, and vomiting. Cases of fatal poisonings have been reported with oil of wintergreen (Hofman et al., 1998; Chan, 1996).
• Advise the patient to avoid using the oil topically after strenuous exercise and in hot humid weather to avoid toxic effects.
• Urge the patient to keep wintergreen (methyl salicylate) products out of the reach of children. (See *Wintergreen toxicity.*)
• Advise women to avoid using wintergreen products during pregnancy or when breast-feeding.

Points of interest

• Oil from sweet birch (*Betula lenta*) is also rich in methyl salicylate.
• An old folk remedy for children who developed "bad chests" during the winter months involved their wearing a paper "jacket" made from a large brown paper bag with holes cut in it for the head and arms that was coated with camphor and wintergreen oil (Watson, 1992).
• Most commercial products that contain methyl salicylate use the synthetic compound.

Bold italic type indicates that reaction may be life-threatening.

RESEARCH FINDINGS
Wintergreen toxicity

Because products containing wintergreen oil have a tantalizing, candylike aroma, young children are at risk for ingesting potentially lethal quantities. Its aroma, together with unprotected packaging and lack of knowledge about its potential hazards, makes wintergreen dangerous. As little as 4 ml has caused extreme illness and death.

In one report, a 21-month-old infant ingested wintergreen oil, which was labeled as a flavoring or candy. Although the child's parents witnessed only one swallow, the salicylate concentration was 81 mg/dl 6 hours after ingestion. The infant experienced repeated hyperpnea, lethargy, and vomiting. Emergency treatment consisted of I.V. bicarbonate and fluids and supportive care; recovery was uneventful (Howrie and Moriarty, 1985).

The toxic hazard can be minimized by restricting bottle size and methyl salicylate concentration; mandating FDA regulation of labeling with clear, concise descriptions of ingredients and adverse effects; and providing warnings about the risks if the herb is misused. Also, child-resistant containers should be used for all liquid products that contain more than 5% wintergreen by weight.

Commentary
Because there are few efficacy data for wintergreen in any medicinal capacity, endorsements for its therapeutic application cannot be substantiated. Wintergreen oil should not be taken internally, and topical application, although seemingly benign, is not without risk if misused, especially in children.

References
Chan, T.Y. "Potential Dangers from Topical Preparations Containing Methyl Salicylate," *Hum Exp Toxicol* 15:747-50, 1996.

Chow, W.H., et al. "Potentiation of Warfarin Anticoagulation by Topical Methyl Salicylate Ointment," *J Soc Med* 82:501-2, 1989.

Hofman, M., et al. "Oil of Wintergreen Overdose," *Ann Emerg Med* 31(6):793-94, 1998.

Howrie, D.L., and Moriarty, R. "Candy Flavoring as a Source of Salicylate Poisoning," *Pediatrics* 75:869-71, 1985.

Watson, R. "Senna-Pod and Wintergreen," *Nursing Times* 88:64, 1992.

Yip, A.S.B., et al. "Adverse Effects of Topical Methyl Salicylate Ointment on Warfarin Anticoagulation: An Unrecognized Potential," *Postgrad Med J* 66:367-69, 1990.

WITCH HAZEL

HAMAMELIS, SNAPPING HAZEL, SPOTTED ALDER, TOBACCO WOOD, WINTER BLOOM

Taxonomic class
Hamamelidaceae

Common trade names
Witch Doctor, Witch Hazel Cream, Witch Hazel Liquid, Witch Hazel Lotion, Witch Hazel Pads, Witch Hazel Soap, Witch Stik

Common forms
Available as dried bark, cream, dried leaves, liquid extract, lotion, medicated pads, soap, and witch hazel water (milder form of extract).

Source
The active components are derived from the leaves and bark of *Hamamelis virginiana,* a shrub that is native to North America. Witch hazel is prepared by distilling twigs of the plant and adding alcohol to the distillate. Commercial sources originate in western Virginia, North Carolina, and Tennessee. Witch hazel water distillate is prepared from wintergreen twigs and contains 13% to 15% alcohol in water with a trace of volatile oil.

Chemical components
Witch hazel contains tannins, flavonoids (kaempferol, quercetin, and others), traces of volatile oil (eugenol, safrole, sesquiterpenes), a bitter principle, calcium oxalate, fixed oil, resin, wax, saponins, and gallic acid.

Actions
Witch hazel is reported to exert astringent, antihemorrhagic, and anti-inflammatory effects. Some studies have shown that witch hazel distillate reduces swelling and inflammation of skin after exposure to ultraviolet B radiation (Hughes-Formella et al., 1998; Masaki et al., 1995); another study failed to show this effect (Duwieija et al., 1994). Other components from witch hazel bark have demonstrated antimutagenic properties (Dauer et al., 1998).

Reported uses
Witch hazel has long been used to relieve anal and vaginal itching and irritation, hemorrhoids, and postepisiotomy or posthemorrhoidectomy discomfort. It is also claimed to be useful for treating bruises, local swelling, and varicose veins. Witch hazel has been used as a gargle to decrease inflammation of mucous membranes of the mouth, gums, and throat.

Dosage
Dried leaves: 2 g as a tea t.i.d. or a gargle.
Liquid extract (1:1 in 45% alcohol): 2 to 4 ml P.O. t.i.d.
Witch hazel water: apply topically t.i.d. or q.i.d.

Bold italic type indicates that reaction may be life-threatening.

Adverse reactions
GI: constipation (more than 1,000 mg), nausea, vomiting.
Hepatic: *hepatotoxicity* (tannin component), increased risk of liver cancer (controversial; related to safrole component [Dauer et al., 1998]).
Skin: contact dermatitis.

Interactions
None reported.

Contraindications and precautions
Avoid using witch hazel in pregnant or breast-feeding women; effects are unknown.

Special considerations
• Caution the patient not to ingest witch hazel.
• Advise the patient to consult a primary health care provider if his condition worsens or does not improve after a few days of topical use of witch hazel.
• Caution the patient to keep witch hazel out of the reach of children.

Commentary
Witch hazel products are known to be effective astringents and produce hemostatic effects. Although they are apparently safe for external use, they are not for internal use.

References
Dauer, A., et al. "Proanthocyanidins from the Bark of *Hamamelis virginiana* Exhibit Antimutagenic Properties Against Nitroaromatic Compounds," *Planta Med* 64:324-27, 1998.
Duwieja, M., et al. "Anti-inflammatory Activity of *Polygonum bistorta, Guaiacum officinale* and *Hamamelis virginiana* in Rats," *J Pharm Pharmacol* 46:286-90, 1994.
Hughes-Formella, B.J., et al. "Anti-inflammatory Effects of Hamamelis Lotion in a UV-B Erythema Test," *Dermatology* 196:316-22, 1998.
Masaki, H., et al. "Protective Activity of Hamameli Tannin on Cell Damage of Murine Skin Fibroblasts Induced by UVB Irradiation," *J Dermatol Sci* 10:25-34, 1995.

WORMWOOD

ABSINTHE, ABSINTHIUM, GREEN GINGER

Taxonomic class
Asteraceae

Common trade names
None known.

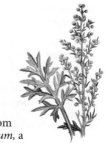

Common forms
Available as an essential oil and dried leaves.

Source
Active components of wormwood are extracted from the leaves and flowering tops of *Artemisia absinthium,* a

shrubby perennial herb that is native to Europe, northern Africa, and western Asia.

Chemical components
Extracts of *A. absinthium* contain the glucosides absinthin and anabsinthin, lactones (including santonin), and other compounds. The plant contains a sweet-smelling volatile oil consisting of terpenes, primarily thujone, with smaller amounts of phellandrene, pinene, and azulene.

Actions
Santonin has shown analgesic, anti-inflammatory, and antipyretic activity in mice (al-Harbi et al., 1994). Thujone exerts narcotic-like analgesic effects (Rice and Wilson, 1976); it is believed to be responsible for causing the symptoms associated with absinthism. This syndrome is marked by digestive disorders, hallucinations, insomnia, loss of intellect, paralysis, paresthesia, psychosis, seizures, tremor, and, possibly, brain damage.

Crude extracts of *A. absinthium* have also demonstrated preventive and curative effects on acetaminophen hepatotoxicity in mice (Gilani and Janbaz, 1995).

Reported uses
Common therapeutic claims for wormwood include its use as an anthelmintic, an antipyretic, and a sedative. Lay publications promote wormwood as an insect repellent. These sources encourage the planting of wormwood hedges or use of powders and infusions around gardens and other areas where insects may be a problem (Sherif et al., 1987).

Dosage
No consensus exists.

Adverse reactions
CNS: absinthism, *seizures.*
GU: *renal failure* (Weisbord et al., 1997).
EENT: xanthopsia (Arnold and Loftus, 1991).
Metabolic: *anion gap acidosis* (Weisbord et al., 1997).
Musculoskeletal: *rhabdomyolysis* (Weisbord et al., 1997).
Skin: allergic reactions (with topical use in sensitized people).
Other: porphyria (Bonkovsky et al., 1992) .

Interactions
None reported.

Contraindications and precautions
Avoid using wormwood in pregnant or breast-feeding patients; effects are unknown. Internal and long-term use is contraindicated.

Special considerations
• Advise the patient to consult a health care provider before using herbal preparations because a treatment that has been clinically researched and proved effective may be available.

Bold italic type indicates that reaction may be life-threatening.

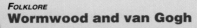

FOLKLORE
Wormwood and van Gogh

Wormwood extract was the main ingredient in absinthe, a toxic emerald green liqueur that was popular until its ban early in the 20th century. Vincent van Gogh was believed to be addicted to absinthe and craved other substances that contain terpenes, such as paints. It is now believed that the predominance of yellow in his paintings and the hallucinations he experienced were related to his consumption of absinthe and other thujone-related compounds (Arnold and Loftus, 1991; Bonkovsky et al., 1992).

• Inform the patient that wormwood should not be taken internally.
ALERT Absinthism may result from chronic intake of wormwood compounds. (See *Wormwood and van Gogh.*) Monitor the patient who uses wormwood for symptoms of absinthism.

Points of interest
• Wormwood, derived from *A. absinthium*, should not be confused with other substances termed wormwood. Sweet wormwood, or Chinese wormwood, derived from *A. annua,* has been used in China for almost 2,000 years for fever, and the active component, artemisinin, has received much attention as an antimalarial (van Agtmael et al., 1999; van Geldre et al., 1997).
• A thujone-free extract of wormwood is used as a flavoring agent for alcoholic beverages, such as vermouth.

Commentary
Wormwood shows some promise as an anthelmintic, an antipyretic, an anti-inflammatory, and a hepatoprotective agent, but more animal and human clinical data are needed. Because wormwood extract has been associated with potentially serious CNS toxicity, it cannot be recommended for internal use.

References
al-Harbi, M.M., et al. "Studies on the Antiinflammatory, Antipyretic and Analgesic Activities of Santonin," *Jpn J Pharmacol* 64:135-39, 1994.

Arnold, W.N., and Loftus, L.S. "Xanthopsia and van Gogh's Yellow Palette," *Eye* 5:503-10, 1991.

Bonkovsky, H.L., et al. "Porphyrogenic Properties of the Terpenes Camphor, Pinene, and Thujone (with a Note on Historic Implications for Absinthe and the Illness of Vincent van Gogh)," *Biochem Pharmacol* 43:2359-68, 1992.

Gilani, A.H., and Janbaz, K.H. "Preventative and Curative Effects of *Artemisia absinthium* on Acetaminophen and CCl4-induced Hepatotoxicity," *Gen Pharmacol* 26:309-15, 1995.

Rice, K.C., and Wilson, R.S. "(-)-3-Isothujone, a Small Nonnitrogenous Molecule with Antinociceptive Activity in Mice," *J Med Chem* 19:1054-57, 1976.

Sherif, A., et al. "Drugs, Insecticides and Other Agents from *Artemisia*," *Med Hypotheses* 23:187-93, 1987.

van Agtmael, M.A., et al. "Artemisinin Drugs in the Treatment of Malaria: From Medicinal Herb to Registered Medication," *Trends Pharmacol Sci* 20(5):199-205, 1999.

van Geldre, E., et al. "State of the Art Production of the Antimalarial Compound Artemisinin in Plants," *Plant Mol Biol* 33:199-209, 1997.

Weisbord, S.D., et al. "Poison on Line: Acute Renal Failure Caused by Oil of Wormwood Purchased Through the Internet," *N Engl J Med* 337:825-27, 1997.

WOUNDWORT

ALL-HEAL, CLOWN'S WOUNDWORT, DOWNEY WOUNDWORT, HEDGE WOUNDWORT, MARSH STACHYS, MARSH WOUNDWORT, OPOPANEWORT, PANAY, RUSTICUM VULNA HERBA

Taxonomic class
Lamiaceae

Common trade names
None known.

Common forms
Available in ointment, tea, and tincture forms and prepared as a poultice.

Source
Active components are derived from the leaves and stems of *Stachys palustris* (marsh woundwort) and *S. sylvatica* (hedge woundwort), members of the mint family.

Chemical components
Woundwort contains various flavonoids (including palustrin), stachydrine, and iridoids.

Actions
Mechanisms of action are not well described for this herb. Investigations have focused on other *S.* species. *S. sieboldii* may contain a promising agent (acteoside) for preventing glomerulonephritis (Hayashi et al., 1996*)*. Flavonoids isolated from *S. candida* and *S. chrysantha* have been reported to inhibit prostaglandin E_2 and leukotriene C4 in murine macrophages and thromboxane B_2 production in human platelets (Skaltsa et al., 2000). The essential oils of these two species have also been evaluated for antibacterial activity (Skaltsa et al., 1999).

Reported uses
Both varieties of woundwort have been used externally to stop bleeding and promote healing of wounds. The herb has also been used as an antiseptic, an astringent, and a disinfectant. Internally, woundwort is

---

Bold italic type indicates that reaction may be life-threatening.

claimed to be useful as an antispasmodic, to ease abdominal cramps and joint pain, and to treat diarrhea, dysentery, fever, menstrual disorders, and vertigo.

Dosage
For abdominal cramps or diarrhea, 1 to 2 ml of tincture P.O. t.i.d.
Tea: 1 tsp of dried herb steeped in 1 cup of boiling water for 10 to 15 minutes; drink tea t.i.d.
Poultice: apply bruised leaves to wound.
Ointment: incorporate dried leaves into an ointment base and apply topically.

Adverse reactions
None reported.

Interactions
None reported.

Contraindications and precautions
Avoid using woundwort in pregnant or breast-feeding patients; effects are unknown.

Special considerations
• Inform the patient that no clinical data support the use of woundwort for any medical condition.
• Advise women to avoid using woundwort during pregnancy or when breast-feeding.
• Inform the patient that several plant species are referred to by the common name woundwort, including *Achillea millefolium, Anthyllis vulneraria, Prunella vulgaris, Solidago canadensis, Solidago virgaurea,* and *Stachys officinalis.*

Commentary
Although woundwort has traditionally been used to promote wound healing and been taken internally for other complaints, there is no scientific evidence to support these uses. This herb cannot be recommended for use until safety and efficacy data become available.

References
Hayashi, K., et al. "Acteoside, a Component of *Stachys sieboldii* MIQ, May Be a Promising Antinephritic Agent (3): Effect of Acteoside on Expression of Intercellular Adhesion Molecule-1 in Experimental Nephritic Glomeruli in Rats and Cultured Endothelial Cells," *Jpn J Pharmacol* 70:157-68, 1996.

Skaltsa, H., et al. "Inhibition of Prostaglandin E_2 and Leukotriene C4 in Mouse Peritoneal Macrophages and Thromboxane B_2 Production in Human Platelets by Flavonoids from *Stachys chrysantha* and *Stachys candida*," *Biol Pharm Bull* 23:47-53, 2000. Abstract.

Skaltsa, H.D., et al. "Composition and Antibacterial Activity of the Essential Oils of *Stachys candida* and *S. chrysantha* from Southern Greece," *Planta Med* 65:255-56, 1999. Abstract.

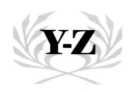

Y-Z

YARROW

Taxonomic class
Asteraceae

Common trade names
Diacure, Lasadoron, Rheumatic Pain Remedy, Yarrow Flowers

Common forms
Capsules: 320 mg, 340 mg
Liquid extract: 1 oz, 2 oz
   Also available as cut herb, essential oil, powder, and tincture.

Source
The drug is extracted from the dried leaves and flowering tops of *Achillea millefolium*, a plant that is native to Europe and Asia and naturalized in North America. The plant is a member of the daisy family.

Chemical components
Yarrow contains tannins, amino acids, fatty acids, sesquiterpene lactones, and peroxides.

Actions
Yarrow is claimed to have anti-inflammatory and antispasmodic actions. It is also believed to have astringent, diaphoretic, GI stimulatory, and vasodilatory effects. Some sesquiterpenoid compounds isolated from the herb have been reported to display activity against mouse P-388 leukemia cells in vivo (Tozyo et al., 1994).
   Other studies in mice have demonstrated an antispermatogenic effect from daily administration of a yarrow extract (Montari et al., 1998).

Reported uses
Yarrow has been used as an emergency styptic applied externally to heal wounds and as an external wash for eczema. Taken internally, the herb is thought to reduce phlegm and other symptoms associated with respiratory tract infections; it has also been used in disorders of the digestive, female reproductive, and urinary systems.

Dosage

Dried herb: 2 to 4 g as a tea P.O. t.i.d.
Liquid extract (1:1 in 25% alcohol): 2 to 4 ml P.O. t.i.d.
Tincture (1:5 in 45% alcohol): 2 to 4 ml P.O. t.i.d.

Adverse reactions

GU: uterine stimulant (with increased doses).
Skin: allergic contact dermatitis (in up to 50% of patients [Hausen et al., 1991; Rucker et al., 1991]), photosensitivity (conflicting reports).

Interactions

Anticoagulants: May increase anticoagulant effect. Use cautiously with yarrow.
Antihypertensives: May increase hypotensive effect. Monitor the patient.
CNS depressants: May increase sedative effect. Use cautiously with yarrow.
Disulfiram: May cause a disulfiram reaction if the herbal product contains alcohol. Avoid administration with yarrow.

Contraindications and precautions

Yarrow is contraindicated in patients who are hypersensitive to yarrow or other members of the Asteraceae family. Avoid its use in pregnant or breast-feeding patients; effects are unknown. Use cautiously in men because of a potential inhibitory effect on spermatogenesis that has been documented in animal studies.

Special considerations

• Monitor for adverse CNS effects.
• Monitor blood pressure of the patient who is also taking an antihypertensive.
• Caution the patient taking disulfiram to avoid using an herbal product that contains alcohol.
• Advise women to avoid using yarrow during pregnancy or when breast-feeding.
• Caution the patient to avoid hazardous activities until yarrow's CNS effects are known.
• Advise the patient with skin allergies to avoid handling the plant.
• Instruct the patient to discontinue using yarrow if bleeding, rash, or unusual signs or symptoms occur.

Points of interest

• Yarrow obtained its scientific name, *Achillea*, from the warrior Achilles of Homeric legend. At the battle of Troy, a Greek god appeared and showed Achilles how to stop bleeding by applying yarrow leaves.

Commentary

Although yarrow has many folk uses, there are no clinical studies for any disease state in humans. Therefore, it should be used cautiously in view of its apparent tendency to cause contact dermatitis.

Bold italic type indicates that reaction may be life-threatening.

References

Hausen, B.M., et al. "Alpha-Peroxyachifolid and Other New Sensitizing Sesqui-terpene Lactones from Yarrow (Achillea millefolium L., Compositae)," *Contact Dermatitis* 24:274-80, 1991.

Montari, T., et al. "Antispermatogenic Effect of *Achillea millefolium* L. in Mice," *Contraception* 58(5):309-13, 1998.

Rucker, G., et al. "Peroxides As Plant Constituents. Part 8. Guaianolide-Peroxides from Yarrow, *Achillea millefolium* L., a Soluble Component Causing Yarrow Dermatitis," *Arch Pharm* 324:979-81, 1991.

Tozyo, T., et al. "Novel Antitumor Sesquiterpenoids in *Achillea millefolium*," *Chem Pharm Bull (Tokyo)* 42:1096-1100, 1994.

YERBA MATÉ

ARMINO, BARTHOLOMEW'S TEA, BOCA JUNIORS, CAMPECHE, EL AGRICULTOR, ELACY, FLOR DE LIS, GAUCHO, HERVEA, ILEX, JAGUAR, JESUIT'S BRAZIL, JESUIT'S TEA, LA HOJA, LA MULATA, LA TRANQUERA, LONJAZO, MADRUGADA, MATÉ, MATÉ BULK LOOSE TEA, *MATE FOLIUM*, MATE LEAF, NOBLEZA GAUCHA, ORO VERDE, PARAGUAY TEA, PAYADITO, ROSAMONTE, SAFIRA, *ST. BARTHOLOMEW'S TEA*, *THE DE PARAGUAY*, UNION, YERBA-DE-MATÉ, YI-YI, ZERBONI

Taxonomic class
Aquifoliaceae

Common trade names
None known.

Common forms
Available as leaves, liquid extract, and tea.

Source
Yerba maté is a drink made from the dried leaves of *Ilex paraguariensis* of the holly family, an evergreen tree that is native to Paraguay, Argentina, and Brazil.

Chemical components
The leaves of yerba maté contain tannin, methylxanthines (including caffeine, theobromine, and theophylline), resin, and crude fiber. Other compounds include the antitumorigenic compound ursolic acid, sterols (related to cholesterol and ergosterol), fats, carotene, vitamins A and B, riboflavin, ascorbic acid, and nicotinic acid. Pyrrolizidine alkaloids have also been detected (McGee et al., 1976).

Actions
The pharmacologic properties of caffeine, theophylline, and theobromine have been evaluated in humans and are well documented. Unlike caffeine and theophylline, theobromine has no stimulant effects on the

---

RESEARCH FINDINGS
Yerba maté drinking and increased cancer risk

Consumption of large quantities of yerba maté has been associated with increased risk of esophageal and bladder cancers. One case-control study showed an association between yerba maté drinking and mouth, laryngeal, and pharyngeal cancers.

The unadjusted relative risk for all upper digestive tract cancers was 2.1. After controlling for tobacco smoking, alcohol use, and coffee or tea drinking, the relative risk was 1.6. Most of the excess risk for yerba maté drinkers was for oral and pharyngeal cancers (Pintos et al., 1994).

In another case-control study, yerba maté was linked to increased risk of bladder cancer. After adjustment for age, social class, and tobacco smoking, a sevenfold increase in risk of bladder cancer was seen among the heavy tea drinkers (De Stefani et al., 1991).

CNS. Theobromine also has a weaker diuretic effect and is a less powerful stimulant of smooth muscle than theophylline. Large doses of theobromine may result in nausea and vomiting.

Reported uses
Aside from its popularity as a tea drink in South America, yerba maté has been claimed to be used as an analgesic, an antidepressant, an antirheumatic, a cathartic, a CNS stimulant, and a diuretic. It has been promoted for the management of diabetes and GI, heart, and nervous disorders. In Germany, yerba maté is used to manage physical and mental fatigue because of its purported analeptic properties. In China, yerba maté is reportedly given parenterally for its hypotensive effect and used as an appetite suppressant.

Dosage
Liquid extract (1:1 in 25% alcohol): 2 to 4 ml P.O. t.i.d.
Tea: 2 to 4 g of dried leaf in pot of boiling water P.O. t.i.d.

Adverse reactions
CNS: irritability, nervousness, withdrawal headache.
CV: palpitations.
GI: nausea, vomiting.
Hepatic: *hepatotoxicity.*
Musculoskeletal: muscle twitching.
Other: flushing; increased cancer risk with prolonged consumption of yerba maté. (See *Yerba maté drinking and increased cancer risk*).

Interactions
Benzodiazepines, other CNS depressants: May counteract effects of these drugs. Avoid administration with yerba maté.
Caffeine, other CNS stimulants (including tobacco): Additive effects. Monitor the patient.
Clozapine: May inhibit metabolism and increased toxicity of clozapine. Avoid administration with yerba maté.
Disulfiram: May cause disulfiram reaction if herbal product contains alcohol. Avoid administration with yerba maté.
Diuretics: May cause an additive effect of these drugs. Do not use together.
Hepatic microsomal enzyme inhibitors (cimetidine, ciprofloxacin, verapamil): May decrease clearance of yerba maté methylxanthines, causing toxicity. Use together cautiously.
Lithium: May increase lithium excretion. Monitor the patient.
MAO inhibitors: Risk of hypertensive reactions. Avoid administration with yerba maté.

Contraindications and precautions
Yerba maté is contraindicated in patients with hypertension and anxiety. Avoid its use in pregnant or breast-feeding patients; effects are unknown. It is also contraindicated in children, who may be especially susceptible to its toxic effects.

Special considerations
• Inform the patient that heavy consumption of yerba maté may increase the risk of bladder cancer, upper digestive tract cancers, hepatic disease, and renal cell cancer.
• Monitor liver function test results, and observe for signs and symptoms of methylxanthine toxicity.
• Caution the patient taking disulfiram to avoid using an herbal form that contains alcohol.
• Advise the patient to avoid caffeine and other CNS stimulants while using this herb.
• Advise the patient to report unusual signs or symptoms.

Points of interest
• Yerba maté is a popular beverage, much like coffee or tea, in parts of South America (primarily Brazil, Paraguay, and Argentina).
• Yerba maté was originally served in a small gourd (maté) and sipped through a filter straw to prevent ingestion of plant material. Sometimes burnt sugar, lemon juice, or milk is added to the drink.

Commentary
Yerba maté is a popular beverage, but little evidence exists to support its medicinal uses. Risks appear to outweigh any potential benefits. The herb contains methylxanthines and potentially hepatotoxic compounds that could have detrimental effects in patients with chronic medical

---

Bold italic type indicates that reaction may be life-threatening.

conditions. Chronic consumption of yerba maté has been linked to an increased risk of certain cancers.

References

De Stefani, E., et al. "Black Tobacco, Maté, and Bladder Cancer. A Case-Control Study from Uruguay," *Cancer* 67:536-40, 1991.

De Stefani, E., et al. "Meat Intake, 'Mate' Drinking and Renal Cell Cancer in Uruguay: A Case-Control Study," *Br J Cancer* 78:1239-43, 1998.

McGee, I., et al. "A Case of Veno-Occlusive Disease of the Liver in Britain Associated with Herbal Tea Consumption," *J Clin Pathol* 29:788-94, 1976.

Pintos, J., et al. "Maté, Coffee, and Tea Consumption and Risk of Cancers of the Upper Aerodigestive Tract in Southern Brazil," *Epidemiology* 5:583-90, 1994.

YERBA SANTA

BEAR'S WEED, CONSUMPTIVE'S WEED, *ERIODICTYON*, GUM BUSH, GUM PLANT, HIERBA SANTA, HOLY HERB, HOLY WEED, MOUNTAIN BALM, SACRED HERB, TARWEED

Taxonomic class
Hydrophyllaceae

Common trade names
Multi-ingredient preparations: EarSol-HC, Feminease, Fen-Tastic, Herbal Gold Cigarrettes, Lung-Mend, Magic Cigarettes, MouthKote, Nature's Sunshine SN-X, Nettle-Reishi Virtue, Oragesic, Pretz-D, Pretz Irrigation, Pretz Spray, Respirtone, Respitonic, Tot Tonic, #493 VRM3 Micro Pathogens, Yerba Manza-Eyebright Virute, Yerba Prima, Yerba Santa-Echinacea Virtue, Yerba Santa Resin-Rich Leaf

Common forms
Available as a liniment, liquid extract (1:5), powder, syrup, and tea.

Source
Active components are derived from the leaves and roots of *Eriodictyon californicum* (syn. *E. glutinosum* Benth. and *Wigandia californicum* Hook. & Arn.), an evergreen shrub that belongs to the waterleaf family and is native to the mountains of California, Oregon, and northern Mexico.

Chemical components
The plant contains various acids (cerotinic, formic, and butyric), a resin (pentacontane, xanthoeriodictyol, priodonal, and chrysoeriodictyol), phenols (eriodictyol, homoeriodictyol, chrysocriol, zanthoeridol, and eridonel), chrysoeriol, cirsimaritin, glycerides of fatty acids, a phytosterol, eriodictyonine, tannins, a volatile oil, sugar, fixed oil, and a gum.

Actions
Physiologic mechanisms of action are poorly described. It is reported that yerba santa exerts expectorant and mildly diuretic effects. Two fla-

vonoid isolates from the plant, cirsimaritin and chrysoeriol, show some promise as anticancer agents (Liu et al., 1992).

Reported uses

Native Americans used yerba santa externally for bruises and inflammation, and they smoked or chewed the leaves for asthma. The herb has also been used to treat bronchial conditions, the common cold, cough, fever, hay fever, hemorrhoids, excessive mucus production, rheumatic pain, sore throat, and tuberculosis. The mashed leaves have been prepared as a poultice to treat insect bites, sores, sprains, and wounds.

Dosage

No consensus exists, but some sources suggest that a tea made from the leaves may be used for asthma, colds, coughs, and tuberculosis. Powdered leaves are used as a stimulating expectorant. A liniment formulation of the leaves is applied topically to reduce fever. Fresh leaves are applied as poultices for bruises, and younger leaves are applied to relieve rheumatism.

Adverse reactions

None reported.

Interactions

Iron, other minerals: Yerba santa reportedly interferes with the absorption of iron and other minerals when taken internally. Separate administration times.

Contraindications and precautions

Avoid using yerba santa in pregnant or breast-feeding patients; effects are unknown.

Special considerations

• Advise the patient not to chew yerba santa leaves because they leave a gummy residue on the teeth.
• Inform the patient that no clinical data support the use of yerba santa for any medical condition.
• Advise the patient not to depend on yerba santa alone to treat such conditions as asthma and tuberculosis.

Points of interest

• Spanish colonists named this plant yerba santa (holy weed) after learning of its medicinal uses from the American Indians. Yerba santa is available in several OTC herbal preparations and as a pharmaceutical flavoring to mask the flavor of bitter drugs. The liquid extract is also used in foods and beverages.

Commentary

Information regarding the safety and efficacy of yerba santa is scant. No clinical trials or published case reports are available for evaluation. As a result, its use cannot be recommended.

Bold italic type indicates that reaction may be life-threatening.

References
Liu, Y.L., et al. "Isolation of Potential Cancer Chemopreventative Agents from *Erio-dictyon californicum*," *J Nat Prod* 55:357-63, 1992.

YEW

AMERICAN YEW, CALIFORNIA YEW, CHINWOOD, GLOBE-BERRY, GROUND HEMLOCK, OREGON YEW, WESTERN YEW

Taxonomic class
Taxaceae

Common trade names
Vital Yew, Yew Antiviral Tea, Yew Tea

Common forms
Available as an extract (concentrated tincture), capsules (with olives), and salve.

Source
Active components are derived from the bough tips and bark of the Pacific or Western yew (*Taxus brevifolia*), which is native to the north-western United States and British Columbia.

Chemical components
Several alkaloids are found in yew plants. The most notable include tax-ine (a mixture of alkaloids), taxol (or paclitaxel, a diterpenoid taxane), taxicatin, milossine, and ephedrine. Other compounds include lignans, tannins, and resin.

Actions
Paclitaxel inhibits cell division by interfering with microtubule forma-tion. Microtubules are necessary for proper division of cellular genetic information (O'Leary et al., 1998).

Reported uses
Herbal extracts of yew were used by Native Americans for arthritis, fever, and rheumatism. The plant's toxicity is well recognized; all parts of the plant are poisonous except the succulent red outer covering of the seeds (Howard and DeWolf, 1974).

Paclitaxel is FDA-labeled for metastatic ovarian cancer after failure of first-line chemotherapy. Numerous studies have documented its effica-cy in metastatic ovarian and breast cancer (O'Leary et al., 1998).

Paclitaxel has been identified in lesser quantities in other yew species, such as the American yew and *T. cuspidata*, the Japanese yew. The Eng-lish yew contains a similar compound called docetaxel, which is also known as taxotere.

Dosage
Consumption of this herb can be hazardous; it should be used only un-der the supervision of a qualified health care provider.

Salve: apply as needed.
Tea: 1 cup P.O. daily.
Tincture: 10 to 60 gtt P.O. b.i.d. to q.i.d.

Adverse reactions

The following reactions have been reported with paclitaxel; some or all may also appear with ingestion of large amounts of yew products.
CNS: peripheral neuropathy.
CV: *arrhythmias,* hypercholesterolemia, hypotension.
GI: elevated liver function test results, nausea, vomiting.
Hematologic: anemia, *leukopenia, neutropenia, thrombocytopenia.*
Musculoskeletal: arthralgia, myalgia.
Skin: alopecia, rash.
Other: hypersensitivity reaction.

Interactions

Chemotherapeutic agents: May increase myelosuppressive effects. Do not use together unless the benefits outweigh possible harmful effects.
Ketoconazole: Inhibited paclitaxel metabolism. Avoid administration with yew products.

Contraindications and precautions

Avoid using yew products in pregnant or breast-feeding patients; effects are unknown.

Special considerations

- Monitor liver function test results.
- Although paclitaxel (and its derivative, docetaxel) are highly effective anticancer drugs, consumption of yew products (as entire plant or whole plant extracts) has not been studied for the treatment of cancer. These agents are also toxic. Thus, advise patients with cancer to avoid using nonpharmaceutical yew products for treatment.
- Some patients have attempted to abuse yew plants to intentionally harm themselves (Stebbing et al., 1995).

Points of interest

- Paclitaxel was formerly referred to as taxol. Subsequently, Bristol-Myers Squibb named their brand of paclitaxel Taxol after approval by the FDA for chemotherapy-refractive metastatic ovarian cancer.
- Other chemical components of yew species are being studied for their chemotherapeutic potential (Huxtable 1995; O'Leary et al., 1998; von Hoff, 1997).

Commentary

There are no clinical data to support the use of this herb (as derived from raw plant parts) for any medical condition. Paclitaxel and other components of yew are effective chemotherapeutic agents that can be used only under medical supervision.

Bold italic type indicates that reaction may be life-threatening.

References

Howard, R.A., and DeWolf, G. "Poisonous Plants," *Arnoldia* 34:41-96, 1974.

Huxtable, R.J. "Regional Sources of Natural Products: *Taxomyces andreanae*," *Proc West Pharmacol Soc* 38:1-4, 1995.

O'Leary, J., et al. "Taxanes in Adjuvant and Neoadjuvant Therapies for Breast Cancer," *Oncology* 12:23-27, 1998.

Stebbing, J., et al. "Deliberate Self-harm Using Yew Leaves (*Taxus baccata*)," *Br J Clin Pract* 49:101, 1995.

Von Hoff, D.D. "The Taxoids: Same Roots, Different Drugs," *Semin Oncol* 24(S13):3-10, 1997.

YOHIMBE

APHRODIEN, *CORYNANTHE YOHIMBE*, CORYNINE, JOHIMBE, *PAUSINYSTALIA YOHIMBE*, QUEBRACHINE, YOHIMBEHE, YOHIMBENE, YOHIMBIME, YOHIMBINE

Taxonomic class
Rubiaceae

Common trade names
Multi-ingredient preparations: Aphrodyne, Dayto Himbin, Potensan, Vikonon Combination, X-action with Yohimbe, Yobinol, Yocon, Yohimbe Max, Yohimbe Royale, Yohimbine HCl, Yohimex

Common forms
Available as extract and tablets (3 mg, 5.4 mg).

Source
Active components are derived from the bark of *Pausinystalia yohimbe*, a West African tree that is native to Congo, Cameroon, and Gabon. The main agent, yohimbine, is also found in the roots of *Rauwolfia serpentina*.

Chemical components
Yohimbe bark contains a mixture of about 6% alkaloids, of which yohimbine is most important. Chemically, yohimbine possesses some structural similarity to reserpine and lysergic acid.

Actions
The alkaloid yohimbine is relatively selective for alpha$_2$-adrenoceptors. In high concentrations, yohimbine may also interact with alpha$_1$-adrenoceptors, serotonin, and dopamine receptors. Yohimbine is also an MAO inhibitor that acts centrally and peripherally. CNS effects include excitation, irritability, and tremor; CV effects are elevated blood pressure and increased heart rate. It also produces antidiuresis because of the release of antidiuretic hormone in the CNS. Peripherally, yohimbine affects autonomic nervous system activity by reducing adrenergic activity and increasing cholinergic activity.

Reported uses

Yohimbe has long been used in Africa as an aphrodisiac; it has also been used as a hallucinogenic (Siegel, 1976). Yohimbine has been used for orthostatic hypotension and clonidine overdose (Roberge et al., 1996), but it has been most heavily studied for possible use in treating vasculogenic male impotence. The mechanism of action is believed to be improved cavernous arterial blood flow and corporeal smooth-muscle relaxation. Clinical trials have produced contradictory results.

One study demonstrated a positive benefit from yohimbine in men, some of whom were diabetic (Morales et al., 1982). Two other studies found no improvement. No significant benefit was found when yohimbine was compared with placebo in patients with organic erectile dysfunction (Teloken et al., 1998). A randomized, crossover study of patients treated with yohimbine and isoxsuprine in combination or pentoxifylline alone found neither regimen effective against mixed vasculogenic erectile dysfunction (Knoll et al., 1996).

Dosage

For male impotence, 5.4 mg P.O. t.i.d. based on clinical studies. If adverse effects occur, reduce to 2.7 mg P.O. t.i.d. and gradually increase to 5.4 mg. Dosage of 20 to 30 mg/day may increase heart rate and blood pressure. One trial used a single daily dose of 100 mg.

For orthostatic hypotension, 12.5 mg/day P.O. More research is needed on the use and dosage of yohimbe for orthostatic hypotension (Roberge et al., 1996).

Adverse reactions

CNS: anxiety, dizziness, headache, manic reactions, nervousness, irritability, tremor.
CV: hypertension, tachycardia.
GI: anorexia, diarrhea, nausea.
GU: dysuria, genital pain, ***acute renal failure.***
Skin: flushing.

Interactions

OTC stimulants: Additive effects. Decrease dose or avoid administration with yohimbe.
Selective serotonin reuptake inhibitors, venlafaxine: Increased stimulation. Do not use together.
Tricyclic antidepressants: Increased serum levels of these drugs. Reduce dose of these agents with concomitant use.
Tyramine-containing foods (cheese, wine, liver): May cause high blood pressure. Avoid administration with yohimbe.

Contraindications and precautions

Yohimbe is contraindicated in patients with psychiatric disorders, renal or hepatic disease, hypersensitivity to yohimbe, or a history of gastric or duodenal ulcer. It is also contraindicated in children and in pregnant or breast-feeding patients. Use cautiously in patients with hypertension.

Bold italic type indicates that reaction may be life-threatening.

Special considerations

ALERT Manic reactions occurred when an average daily dose of 12.5 mg of yohimbe was given to psychiatric patients who were experiencing orthostatic hypotension from psychotropic drugs (Price et al., 1984).

- Yohimbe is usually not used by women.
- Monitor for adverse CNS and cardiac effects.
- Inform the patient that the effects of using yohimbe for longer than 10 weeks are unknown.
- Advise the patient to avoid caffeine.

Points of interest

- Yohimbe has no FDA-sanctioned use in humans.
- Yohimbe has been on the USDA's unsafe herb list since March 1977.

Commentary

Yohimbe has been used primarily as an aphrodisiac and for treating male erectile dysfunction. Clinical trials have produced contradictory results. The most convincing data suggest a role in male organic impotence associated with diabetes. To date, no studies have compared yohimbe with other available treatments for male impotence. Until further studies define the precise role of yohimbe in this disorder, the drug cannot be recommended.

References

Knoll, L.D., et al. "A Randomized Crossover Study Using Yohimbine and Isoxsuprine versus Pentoxifylline in the Management of Vasculogenic Impotence," *J Urol* 155:144-46, 1996.

Morales, A., et al. "Nonhormonal Pharmacological Treatment of Organic Impotence," *J Urol* 128:45-47, 1982.

Price, H.L., et al. "Three Cases of Mania Symptoms Following Yohimbine Administration," *Am J Psychiatry* 141:1267-68, 1984.

Roberge, R.J., et al. "Yohimbine as an Antidote for Clonidine Overdose," *Am J Emerg Med* 14(7):678-80, 1996.

Siegel, R.K. "Herbal Intoxication: Psychoactive Effects from Herbal Cigarettes, Tea, and Capsules," *JAMA* 236:473-76, 1976.

Teloken, C., et al. "Therapeutic Effects of High Dose Yohimbine Hydrochloride on Organic Erectile Dysfunction," *J Urol* 159:124, 1998.

APPENDICES
&
INDEX

Therapeutic monitoring guidelines

As with traditional medicines, many alternative agents require close monitoring to detect adverse reactions. This table lists tests that should be monitored for selected alternative agents.

	Complete blood count	Liver function tests	Renal function & electrolytes	Coagulation studies	Blood glucose
alfalfa				x	x
aloe			x		
American cranesbill		x			
androstenedione		x			
angelica				x	
basil					x
bayberry		x			
bearberry			x		
bee pollen					x
betony		x			
bistort		x			
bitter melon					x
black catechu					x
black haw				x	
blackroot		x			
blue cohosh					x
bogbean				x	
boneset		x			
borage		x			
buchu		x			
cascara			x		
castor bean			x		
cat's claw				x	
celandine		x			
chaparral		x			
chondroitin	x			x	

	Complete blood count	Liver function tests	Renal function & electrolytes	Coagulation studies	Blood glucose
comfrey		x			
condurango		x			
couch grass			x		
cowslip		x			
creatine			x		
cucumber			x		
damiana		x			
dandelion					x
dill			x		
dock, yellow			x		
dong quai				x	
fenugreek				x	x
garlic	x				
ginger				x	
ginkgo				x	
ginseng					x
glucomannan					x
goldenseal	x				
gossypol	x	x	x		
gotu kola					x
guggul				x	
hesperidin				x	
horehound					x
horse chestnut		x		x	
Iceland moss		x			
Irish moss				x	
jaborandi tree		x			
jambul					x
kava	x				
kelp				x	

(continued)

	Complete blood count	Liver function tests	Renal function & electrolytes	Coagulation studies	Blood glucose
kelpware			x	x	x
khat		x			
khella		x			
lady's mantle		x			
licorice			x		
lovage			x		
lungwort				x	
male fern		x			
mayapple	x	x	x		
meadowsweet				x	
milk thistle		x			
mistletoe			x		
motherwort				x	
myrrh					x
myrtle		x			x
oaks		x			
oleander			x		
olive leaf					x
parsley		x		x	
pau d'arco				x	
pennyroyal oil		x	x		
pomegranate		x			
poplar		x		x	
prickly ash				x	
pumpkin			x		
ragwort		x			
red clover				x	
rhatany		x			
rosemary			x		

	Complete blood count	Liver function tests	Renal function & electrolytes	Coagulation studies	Blood glucose
royal jelly					X
sarsaparilla			X		
sassafras		X			
savory	X	X			
scented geranium		X	X		
schisandra		X			
sea holly			X		
shark cartilage		X			
skullcap		X			
soapwort		X	X		
sorrel		X	X		
squaw vine		X			
stevia			X		X
stone root		X			
tansy			X		
tonka bean		X		X	
tormentil		X			
turmeric				X	
valerian		X			
walnut		X			
willow		X	X	X	
wintergreen				X	
witch hazel		X			
wormwood			X		
yarrow				X	
yerba maté		X			
yew		X			
yohimbe			X		

Potentially unsafe plants

The following table identifies some of the more popular plant species that may possess chemical components harmful to mammalian tissue. Not all plants cited here have been documented to be life-threatening, but they have usually appeared several times on other notable poisonous plant lists and possess the potential to be extremely harmful. Much of the toxicologic symptom information is obtained from studying the effects of accidental ingestion of the plant by previously healthy livestock.

Botanical name	Common names	Potential harmful effects
Aconitum spp.	Monkshood, aconite, wolfsbane	Arrhythmias, cardiotoxicity, hypotension, neurotoxicity
Acorus calamus	Sweet flag	Dermatitis, bloody diarrhea, nephrotoxicity
Actaea spp.	Baneberry, doll's eyes	Abdominal pain, diarrhea, oral mucosal irritation, salivation, vomiting
Aesculus spp.	Buckeye, horse chestnut	Bleeding
Amanita phalloides	Death cap mushroom	Death, hepatotoxicity
Angelica archangelica	Dong quai	Carcinogenicity, bleeding diasthesis, phototoxicity, uterine stimulation
Apocynum spp.	Bitterroot, dogbane	Arrhythmias (cardiac glycosides), cardiac stimulation, cardiotoxicity
Areca catechu	Betel palm	Teratogenicity
Aristolochia fangchi	None	Carcinogenicity, renal failure
Arnica montana	Arnica	Collapse, violent gastroenteritis, muscle weakness, nervous disorders
Artemisia absinthium	Wormwood	Absinthism, hallucinations, mental disorders, renal failure, rhabdomyolysis, seizures
Asclepias spp.	Milkweed	Cardiotoxicity
Astragalus spp.	Locoweed	Heart failure, hepatotoxicity (Swainsonine), neurotoxicity
Atropa belladonna	Belladonna, deadly nightshade	Anticholinergic poisoning
Barbarea vulgaris	Wintercress	Renal damage in animals
Borago officinalis	Borage	Veno-occlusive hepatotoxicity (pyrrolizidine alkaloids)

Botanical name	Common names	Potential harmful effects
Caltha palustris	Cowslip, marsh marigold	Death of livestock (accidental ingestion)
Catha edulis	Khat	Cirrhosis, hypertension, hyperthermia, mutagenicity, myocardial infarction, optic atrophy, oral cancer, stroke, teratogenicity
Cheiranthus cheiri	Wallflower	Bradycardia, cardiotoxicity, heart failure
Chelidonium majus	Celandine	CNS depression, death, diarrhea, headache, skin irritation
Chenopodium ambrosioides	Wormseed	Dizziness, nausea, paralysis, seizures
Cicuta spp.	Cowbane, water hemlock	Multiple organ dysfunction syndrome, paralysis, seizures
Claviceps spp.	Ergot	Hallucinations, hypertension, tissue ischemia, St. Anthony's fire
Colchicum autumnale	Autumn crocus	GI toxicity, neurotoxicity, renal failure, vomiting
Conicum maculatum	Poison hemlock	Birth defects, crooked calf disease
Convallaria majalis	Lily-of-the-valley	Cardiotoxicity
Cytisus scoparius	Broom	Arrhythmias, diarrhea, nausea, shock, tachycardia, uterine contractions, vertigo
Datura spp.	Jimson weed, devil's trumpet, thorn-apple	Anticholinergic toxicity
Digitalis purpurea	Foxglove	Arrhythmias, cardiotoxicity
Ephedra spp.	Ma huang, Mormon tea, squaw tea	Angina, hypertension, myocardial infarction, myopathy, neuropathy, psychosis, stroke, tachycardia
Equisetum arvense	Horsetail	Diarrhea, neurotoxicity progressing to muscle weakness
Euonymous spp.	Spindle tree, wahoo root bark	Cardiotoxicity, death, diarrhea, hallucinations, seizures, vomiting
Eupatorium rugosum	White snakeroot	CNS stimulation, tremor (animals)

(continued)

Botanical name	Common names	Potential harmful effects
Euphorbia spp.	Leafy spurge, poinsettia, snow-on-the-mountain	Dermatitis, diarrhea, GI irritation
Exagonium purga	Jalap root	Dramatic purgative catharsis
Gelsemium sempervirens	Jessamine, yellow jessamine	Death, paralysis
Glycyrrhiza lepidota	Wild licorice	Hypernatremia, hypertension, hypotension, muscle weakness
Gossypium hirsutum	Cotton	Heart failure (high doses), hypokalemia, male sterility
Griffonia sylvestre	Griffonia	Eosinophilia-myalgia syndrome (contaminants)
Heliotropium europaeum	Heliotrope	Veno-occlusive hepatotoxicity (pyrrolizidine alkaloids)
Hydrastis canadensis	Golden seal	Hyperreflexia, hypertension, respiratory failure, seizures
Hyoscyamus niger	Henbane	Anticholinergic toxicity
Hypericum perforatum	St John's wort	Phototoxicity
Ilex paraguariensis	Paraguay tea	CNS stimulation, esophageal cancer, hepatotoxicity
Ipomoea purpurea	Morning glory	Hallucinations, psychosis
Laburnum anagyroides	Golden chain, laburnum	Abdominal pain, CNS depression, confusion, death (cytisine component), dizziness, hyperthermia, vomiting
Larrea tridentata	Chaparral, creosote bush	Hepatotoxicity (may be irreversible)
Lobelia spp.	Cardinal flower, great lobelia, Indian tobacco	Coma, death, defecation, emesis, GI upset, hepatotoxicity, hypotension, lacrimation, respiratory depression, salivation, tachycardia, urination
Lotus corniculatus	Bird's foot trefoil	Cyanide poisoning: coma, death, paralysis, seizures
Mandragora officinarum	Mandrake	Anticholinergic toxicity, hallucinations
Medicago sativa	Alfalfa, lucerne	Listeriosis (contaminant), pancytopenia, systemic lupus erythematosus

Botanical name	Common names	Potential harmful effects
Melilotus spp.	White sweetclover, yellow sweetclover	Bleeding
Menispermum canadense	Moonseed	Purging, tachycardia, severe vomiting
Mentha pulegium	Pennyroyal	Multiple organ dysfunction syndrome, neurotoxicity
Narcissus pseudonarcissus	Daffodil	Coma, CNS depression, death, miosis, salivation, vomiting
Nerium oleander	Oleander	Cardiotoxicity
Papaver spp.	Opium poppy	CNS and respiratory depression
Pausinystalia yohimbe	Yohimbe	Renal failure, seizures
Phoradendron flavescens	American mistletoe	Hypertension, hypertensive crisis
Physostigma venenosum	Calabar bean	Cholinergic toxicity
Phytolacca americana	Pokeweed	Coma, gastroenteritis, hypotension, mitogenesis, seizures
Podophyllum peltatum	Mandrake (not *Mandragora* spp.), May apple	Severe GI irritation, multiple organ dysfunction syndrome, nausea, vomiting
Polygonum mutliflorum	Fo-Ti	Hepatotoxicity
Prunus spp.	Black, choke, pin, wild cherries	Dyspnea, seizures, vertigo
Quercus spp.	Oak tree	Gastroenteritis, hepatotoxicity (tannins), renal failure
Ranunculus spp.	Buttercup, crowfoot	Diarrhea, GI and oral irritation, salivation
Ricinus communis	Castor bean	Abdominal distention, dehydration, GI toxicity, shock
Robina pseudoacacia	Black locust	Bradycardia, dizziness, nausea, vomiting
Rumex spp.	Curly-leafed dock sorrel, dock	Calcium and oxalate deposits in kidneys, hypocalcemia, muscle weakness

(continued)

Botanical name	Common names	Potential harmful effects
Ruta graveolens	Rue	Hepatotoxicity
Salix spp.	Willow bark	GI toxicity, adverse effects in pregnancy, salicylate intoxication (CNS disturbances, confusion, nausea, vision changes, vomiting)
Sambucus canadensis	Elderberry	Cyanide poisoning (seeds)
Sanguinaria canadensis	Bloodroot	Tissue destruction on contact
Senecio spp.	Groundsels, life root, ragwort, senecio	Veno-occlusive hepatotoxicity (pyrrolizidine alkaloids)
Solanum spp.	Black nightshade, common bittersweet, horse nettle	Cardiotoxicity
Sophora flavenscens	None	Seizures
Spigelia marilandica	Indian pink	Death (large ingestions)
Stillingia sylvatica	Queen's delight	GI toxicity, mutagenicity
Strychnos nux vomica	Strychnine tree	CNS stimulation leading to cardiac arrest and seizures
Symphytum spp.	Comfrey, prickly comfrey, Russian comfrey	Veno-occlusive hepatotoxicity (pyrrolizidine alkaloids)
Symplocarpus foetidus	Eastern skunk cabbage	Dysphagia, mouth irritation
Tabebuia heptaphylla	Pau d'arco	Death, hepatotoxicity
Teucrium chamaedrys	Germander	Hepatotoxicity
Toxicodendron spp.	Poison ivy, poison oak, poison sumac	Severe skin irritation
Tussilago farfara	Colt's foot	Veno-occlusive hepatotoxicity (pyrrolizidine alkaloids)
Veratrum californicum	Corn lily, false hellebore	Hypotension, teratogenicity (animals)
Vicia spp.	Common vetch, hairy vetch, purple vetch	Cyanide toxicity (seeds), diarrhea, granulomatous disorders, seizures

Botanical name	Common names	Potential harmful effects
Vinca spp.	Periwinkle	Cytotoxicity, hepatic failure, neurologic damage, renal failure
Wisteria spp.	Wisteria	Abdominal pain, dehydration, diarrhea, nausea, vomiting
Xanthium strumarium	Cocklebur	Abdominal pain, hepatotoxicity, seizures, vomiting
Zigadenus spp.	Death camas	Coma, death, hypotension, muscle weakness, salivation, seizures, vomiting

Alternative medicines to avoid in pregnancy

Certain alternative medicines may pose a risk to pregnant women and fetuses. This table lists common and botanical names of proven or suspected uterine stimulants and teratogens.

Common name	Botanical name
aloe	*Aloe vera*
arnica	*Arnica montana*
barberry, common	*Berberis vulgaris*
betel palm	*Areca catechu*
bethroot	*Trillium erectum*
betony	*Stachys officinalis*
bitter melon	*Momordica charantia*
black cohosh	*Cimicifuga racemosa*
bloodroot	*Sanguinaria canadensis*
blue cohosh	*Caulophyllum thalictrioides*
borage	*Borago officinalis*
broom	*Cytisus scoparius*
buchu	*Agathosma betulina*
burdock	*Arctium lappa*
butterbur	*Petasites hybridus*
capsicum	*Capsicum annum*
carline thistle	*Carlina vulgaris*
catnip	*Nepeta cataria*
celandine	*Chelidonium majus*
celery	*Apium graveolens*
chamomile	*Chamaemelum nobile*
chaparral	*Larrea tridentata*
chicory	*Chicorium intybus*
coltsfoot	*Tussilago farfara*
comfrey	*Symphytum officinale*
cumin	*Cumina Cyminum*
damiana	*Turnera diffusa var aphrodisiaca*
devil's claw	*Harpagophytum procumbens*

Common name	Botanical name
ephedra	Ephedra sinica
fenugreek	Trigonella foenum-graecum
feverfew	Chrysanthemum or Fanacetum parthenium
flax	Linum usitatissimum
garlic	Allium sativum
ginger	Zingiber officinale
goldenrod	Solidago virgauria
goldenseal	Hydrastis canadensis
gotu kola	Centella asiatica, Hydrocotyle asiatica
guggul	Commiphora mukul
hawthorn	Crataegus monogyma, C. oxyacantha, C. laevigata
hops	Humulus lupulus
horehound, black	Marrubium vulgare
horehound, white	Ballota nigra
hyssop	Hyssopus officinalis
jaborandi tree	Pilocarpus jaborandi
Jamaican dogwood	Piscidia piscipula
juniper	Juniperus communis
kelp	Laminara digata, L. japonica
khat	Catha edulis
lady's mantle	Alchemilla mollis
licorice	Glycyrrhiza glabra
madder	Rubia tinctorium
magnolia	Magnolia lilifora
male fern	Dryopteris filix-mas
marjoram	Origanum majorana
mayapple	Podophyllum peltatum, other Podophyllum spp.
meadowsweet	Filipendula ulmaria
milk thistle	Silybum marianum

(continued)

Common name	Botanical name
mistletoe	*Viscum alba, Phoradendron serotinum*
motherwort	*Leonurus cardiaca*
mugwort	*Artemisia vulgaris*
mustard	*Brassica nigra*
myrrh	*Commiphora molmol*, other *Commiphora spp.*
nettle	*Urtica dioica*
notoginseng root	*Panax notoginseng*
nutmeg	*Myristica fragrans*
papaya	*Carica papaya*
pareira	*Chondrodendron tomentosum*
parsley	*Petroselinum crispum*, other *Petroselinium spp.*
passion flower	*Passiflora incarnata*, other *Passiflora spp.*
peach	*Prunus persica*
pennyroyal	*Hedeoma pulegioides, Mentha pulegium* (mint)
pepper, black	*Piper nigrum*
pill-bearing spurge	*Euphoria hirta*
pineapple	*Ananas comosus*
plantains	*Plantago major, P. lanceolata, P. media, P. psyllium*
pokeweed	*Phytolacca americana*
poplars	*Populus spp.*
prickly ash	*Zanthoxylum americanum*
pulsatilla	*Pulsatilla vulgaris*
Queen Anne's lace	*Daucus carota*
ragwort	*Packera aurea, Senecio aureus*
raspberry	*Rubus idaeus*
rauwolfia	*Rauvolfia serpentina*
red clover	*Trifolium pratense*
rosemary	*Rosmarinus officinalis*
rue	*Ruta graveolens*
saffron	*Crocus sativus*

Common name	Botanical name
sage	*Salvia officinalis*
St. John's wort	*Hypericum perforatum*
sassafras	*Sassafras albidum*
senega	*Polygala senega*
senna	*Cassia senna, C. acutifolia*
shepherd's purse	*Capsella bursa-pastoris*
skullcap	*Scutellaria laterifolia*
skunk cabbage	*Symplocarpus foetidus*
slippery elm	*Ulmus rubra*
southernwood	*Artemisia abrotanum*
squaw vine	*Mitchella repens*
squill	*Urginea maritima*
tansy	*Tanacetum vulgare*
thuja	*Thuja occidentalis*
turmeric	*Curcuma longa*
vervain	*Verbena officinalis*
watercress	*Tropaeolum majus*
wild cherry	*Prunus virginiana, P. serotina*
wild ginger	*Asarum canadense*
wild yam	*Dioscorea villosa*
willow	*Salix nigra*, other *Salix spp.*
wormwood	*Artemisia absinthum*
yarrow	*Achillea millefolium*

Plant families

This list identifies plants and their related species. Plants of the same species often have similar chemical characteristics, suggesting similar pharmacology and similar allergic and adverse effects.

Apiaceae (formerly Umbelliferae)
Angelica
Anise
Caraway
Celery
Coriander
Cumin
Dill
Dong quai
Fennel
Gotu kola
Khella
Lovage
Parsley
Queen Anne's lace
Sea holly
Sweet cicely
Apocynaceae
Ibogaine
Oleander
Rauwolfia
Aquifoliaceae
Yerba maté
Araceae
Glucomannan
Skunk cabbage
Sweet flag
Araliaceae
Ginseng
Ginseng, Siberian
Arecaceae
Betel palm
Saw palmetto
Aristolochiaceae
Wild ginger
Asclepiadaceae
Condurango

Asteraceae (formerly Compositae)
Arnica
Blessed thistle
Boneset
Burdock
Butterbur
Carline thistle
Chamomile
Chicory
Colt's foot
Daisy
Dandelion
Echinacea
Elecampane
Feverfew
Goldenrod
Lutein
Marigold
Milk thistle
Mugwort
Ragwort
Safflower
Santonica
Southernwood
Tansy
Wild lettuce
Wormwood
Yarrow
Berberidaceae
Barberry
Blue cohosh
Mayapple
Oregon grape
Betulaceae
Birch
Bignoniaceae
Pau d'arco
Boraginaceae
Borage
Comfrey
Lungwort

Brassicaceae (formerly Cruciferae)
Horseradish
Mustard
Shepherd's purse
Watercress
Bromeliaceae
Pineapple
Burseraceae
Boswellia
Guggul
Myrrh
Cactaceae
Night-blooming cereus
Peyote
Campanulaceae
Lobelia
Cannabaceae
Hops
Caprifoliaceae
Black haw
Elderberry
Caricaceae
Papaya
Caryophyllaceae
Chickweed
Soapwort
Celastraceae
Khat
Wahoo
Clusiaceae
Garcinia
Cucurbitaceae
Bitter melon
Cucumber
Cycladol
Pumpkin
Cupressaceae
Juniper
Thuja

Dioscoreaceae
  Wild yam
Droseraceae
  Sundew
Dryopteridaceae
  Male fern
Ephedraceae
  Ephedra
Equisetaceae
  Horsetail
Ericaceae
  Bearberry
  Bilberry
  Cranberry
  Pipsissewa
  Wintergreen
Euphorbiaceae
  Castor bean
  Pill-bearing spurge
Fabaceae (formerly Leguminosae)
  Alfalfa
  Astragalus
  Balsam of Peru
  Black catechu
  Broom
  Cabbage
  Fenugreek
  Goat's rue
  Gum arabic
  Indigo
  Jamaica dogwood
  Kudzu
  Licorice
  Red clover
  Senna
  Tonka Bean
  Tragacanth
  Wild indigo
Fagaceae
  Oaks
Flacourtiaceae
  Chaulmoogra
Fucaceae
  Kelpware
Fumariaceae
  Fumitory

Gentianaceae
  Bogbean
  Centaury
  Gentian
Geraniaceae
  American cranesbill
  Scented geranium
Gigartinaceae
  Irish moss
Ginkgoaceae
  Ginkgo
Gramineae
  Barley
Hamamelidaceae
  Witch hazel
Hippocastanaceae
  Horse chestnut
Hydrophyllaceae
  Yerba santa
Hypericaceae
  St. John's wort
Iridaceae
  Blue flag
  Saffron
Krameriaceae
  Rhatany
Lamiaceae (formerly Labiatae)
  Basil
  Betony
  Bugleweed
  Catnip
  Chaste tree
  Clary
  Ground ivy
  Horehound
  Hyssop
  Lavender
  Lemon balm
  Marjoram
  Mint
  Motherwort
  Oregano
  Pennyroyal
  Rosemary
  Sage

  Self-heal
  Skullcap
  Stoneroot
  Thyme
  Woundwort
Laminariaceae
  Kelp
Lauraceae
  Bay
  Cinnamon
  Sassafras
Liliaceae s.l.
  Aloe (Asphodelaceae)
  Bethroot
  Butcher's broom
  Daffodil (Amaryllidaceae)
  False unicorn root
  Galanthamine (Amaryllidaceae)
  Garlic (Alliaceae)
  Hellebore American lily-of-the-valley
  Squill (Hyacinthaceae)
  True unicorn root (Melanthiaceae)
Linaceae
  Flax
Malvaceae
  Gossypol
  Mallow
  Marshmallow
Menispermaceae
  Calumba
  Pareira
Monimiaceae
  Boldo
Moraceae
  Fig
Myricaceae
  Bayberry
Myristicaceae
  Nutmeg

(continued)

Myrtaceae
  Allspice
  Cloves
  Eucalyptus
  Jambul
  Myrtle
  Tea tree
Oleaceae
  Ash
Onagraceae
  Primrose, evening
Orchidaceae
  Lady's slipper, yellow
Oscillatoriaceae
  Spirulina
Papaveraceae
  Bloodroot
  Celandine
  Red poppy
Parmeliaceae
  Iceland moss
Passifloraceae
  Passion flower
Pedaliaceae
  Devil's claw
Phytolaccaceae
  Pokeweed
Pinaceae
  Pinebark
Piperaceae
  Kava
  Pepper, black
Poaceae (formerly Gramineae)
  Couch grass
  Oats
Polygalaceae
  Senega
Polygonaceae
  Bistort
  Chinese rhubarb
  Dock, yellow
  Plantains
  Sorrel
Primulaceae
  Cowslip

Pulmonaceae
  Lungmoss
Punicaceae
  Pomegranate
Ranunculaceae
  Aconite
  Black cohosh
  Golden seal
  Hellebore, black
  Pulsatilla
Rhamnaceae
  Buckthorn
  Cascara sagrada
Rosaceae
  Agrimony
  Avens
  Hawthorn
  Lady's mantle
  Meadowsweet
  Parsley piert
  Peach
  Quince
  Raspberry
  Rose hips
  Tormentil
  Wild cherry
Rubiaceae
  Coffee
  Madder
  Squaw vine
  Yohimbè
Rutaceae
  Bitter orange
  Buchu
  Grapefruit seed extract
  Jaborandi tree
  Prickly ash
  Rue
Salicaceae
  Poplar
  Willow
Sapindaceae
  Guarana
Schisandraceae
  Schisandra

Scrophulariaceae
  Blackroot
  Eyebright
  Figwort
  Mullein
Simmondsiaceae
  Jojoba
Smilacaceae
  Sarsaparilla
Solanaceae
  Capsicum
  Corkwood
  Jimson weed
Sterculiaceae
  Chocolate
  Cola tree
  Karaya gum
Styracaceae
  Benzoin
Taxaceae
  Yew
Theaceae
  Green tea
Turneraceae
  Damiana
Ulmaceae
  Slippery elm
Urticaceae
  Nettle
Valerianaceae
  Valerian
Verbenaceae
  Vervain
Violaceae
  Pansy
  Sweet violet
Viscaceae
  Mistletoe
Vitaceae
  Grapeseed
Zingiberaceae
  Cardamom
  Galangal
  Ginger
  Tumeric
Zygophyllaceae
  Chaparral

Alternative medicine resource list

Health care providers can obtain more information on herbs and the status of complementary and alternative medicine in general by consulting the related resources listed below. Specific Internet addresses may change without notice.

Alternative Health News Online
Alternative Health News, Inc.
Publisher, Frank Grazian
www.altmedicine.com

Alternative Medicine Foundation, Inc.
5411 West Cedar Lane
Suite 205-A
Bethesda, MD 20814
Tel: (301) 581-0116
Fax: (301) 581-0119
www.amfoundation.org

American Botanical Council
P.O. Box 144345
Austin, TX 78714-4345
Tel: (512) 926-4900
Fax: (512) 926-2345
www.herbalgram.org

American Foundation of Traditional Chinese Medicine
505 Beech Street
San Francisco, CA 94133

The American Preventative Medical Association
9912 Georgetown Pike
Suite D-2
P.O. Box 458
Great Falls, VA 22066
Tel: (800) 230-APMA
Fax: (703) 759-6711
www.healthy.net/pan/pa/Natural Therapies/apma

APRALERT
College of Pharmacy
The University of Illinois at Chicago
Contact: Mary Lou Quinn
Tel: (312) 996-2246
Fax: (312) 996-7107
www.pmmp.uic.edu

The Australasian College of Herbal Studies
USA Office
P.O. Box 57
530 First Street
Lake Oswego, OR 97034
Tel: (503) 635-6652 or
   (800) 48-STUDY
Fax: (503) 636-0706
www.achs@herbed.com

Botanical Society of America
Office of Publications
1735 Neil Avenue
Columbus, OH 43210-1293
Tel: (614) 292-3519
Fax: (614) 247-6444
www.botany.org

Centers for Disease Control and Prevention
Public Health Service
U.S. Department of Health and Human Services
1600 Clifton Road NE
Atlanta, GA 30333
Tel: (404) 639-3311
www.cdc.gov

Herb Research Foundation
1007 Pearl Street
Suite 200
Boulder, CO 80302
Tel: (303) 449-2265
Fax: (303) 449-7849
www.herbs.org

The Herb Society of America
9019 Kirtland Chardon Road
Kirtland, OH 44904
Tel: (440) 256-0514
Fax: (440) 256-0541
www.herbsociety.org

Integrative Medicine
  Communications
1029 Chestnut Street
Newton, MA 02464
Tel: (617) 641-2300
Fax: (617) 641-2301
www.onemedicine.com

The Lloyd Library and Museum
917 Plum Street
Cincinnati, OH 45202
Tel: (513) 721-3707
Fax: (513) 721-6575
www.libraries.uc.edu/lloyd/index.htm

National Center for Complementary
  and Alternative Medicine
  (NCCAM) Clearinghouse
P.O. Box 8218
Silver Spring, MD 20907-8218
Tel: (888) 644-6226
Fax: (301) 495-4957
www.nccam.nih.gov

Natural Medicine Online
825 Challenger Drive
Green Bay, WI 54311
Tel: (920) 469-1313
Fax: (920) 469-1313

Office of Dietary Supplements
National Institutes of Health
Building 31, Room 1B25
31 Center Drive, MSC 2086
Bethesda, MD 20892-2086
Tel: (301) 435-2920

U.S. Food and Drug Administration
Public Health Service
Department of Health and Human
  Services
5600 Fishers Lane
Rockville, MD 20857
Tel: (888) 463-6332
www.fda.gov

U.S. National Library of Medicine
National Institutes of Health
8600 Rockville Pike
Bethesda, MD 20894
Tel: (888) 346-3656
www.nlm.nih.gov

Alternative medicine information sheet

Patient _____ **Date** _____

Health care provider _____ **Phone** _____

Dear Patient,

When taking an alternative medicine, keep in mind the following general tips.

- Be sure to tell your health care provider about *all* the medicines you take, including herbs and vitamins.
- Make sure your health care provider is aware of your medical history, including allergies.
- Women of childbearing age should consider using appropriate contraception because little is known about the effects of alternative medicines on a fetus.
- Purchase your alternative medicine from a reputable source, such as a pharmacy.
- Read labels carefully when purchasing alternative medicines. Check that the term "standardized" is on the label. Standardized means that the dose of medicine in each tablet or capsule in that package is the same. Also check that the label states specific percentages, amounts, and strengths of active ingredients.
- When taking alternative medicines, follow the prescription exactly. Taking too much of an herb or taking it inappropriately may diminish its effectiveness and increase the risk of dangerous side effects.
- Never ignore symptoms you may be experiencing.
- Never use alternative medicines to delay seeking more appropriate therapy.
- Be aware that alternative medicines are not necessarily a substitute for traditional, proven medical therapy.
- Contact your health care provider if you experience side effects of this alternative medicine or if you have other health concerns that would normally require medical attention.

(continued)

Professional's Handbook of Complementary & Alternative Medicines, Second Edition.
© Springhouse Corporation, 2001.

• Call your health care provider if you experience abdominal cramping; abnormal bleeding or bruising; changes in heart rate or rhythm; changes in vision; dizziness or fainting; hair loss; hallucinations, inability to concentrate, or other mental changes; hives, itching, rash, or other allergic symptoms; loss of appetite; or dramatic weight loss.

• Never allow other people to take your medicine. Store these alternative medicines out of the reach of children and pets.

• If you have questions about the alternative medicine you're taking, seek advice from a qualified health care provider. If your health care provider isn't knowledge-able about alternative medicines, ask for a referral to someone experienced in the use of these agents.

About this alternative medicine

This agent is called _____

You are taking this agent to _____

The recommended dosage is _____

Special instructions for how to take or store this agent include _____

_____

_____

Side effects of this agent include _____

_____

_____

_____

Other instructions _____

_____

_____

_____

_____

Index ✿

F

K

L

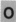
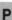

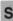

X

Y